Human Nutrition

ELEVENTH EDITION

Edited by

Catherine A. Geissler BDS MS PHD RNutr

*Professor of Human Nutrition, Department of Nutrition and Dietetics,
King's College London, London, UK, and Director, Higher Education Academy,
Health Sciences and Practice, UK*

Hilary J. Powers BSC PHD RNutr

*Professor in Nutritional Biochemistry and Head of Human Nutrition Unit,
University of Sheffield, Sheffield, UK*

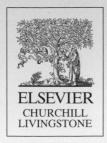

ELSEVIER
CHURCHILL
LIVINGSTONE

EDINBURGH LONDON NEW YORK OXFORD PHILADELPHIA ST LOUIS SYDNEY TORONTO 2005

ELSEVIER
CHURCHILL LIVINGSTONE

© E. & S. Livingstone 1959, 1963, 1966, 1969
© Longman Group Ltd 1972, 1975, 1979, 1986
© Longman Group UK Ltd 1993
© Harcourt Publishers Limited 2000
© 2005, Elsevier Limited. All rights reserved.

First edition 1959
Second edition 1963
Third edition 1966
Fourth edition 1969
Fifth edition 1972
Sixth edition 1975
Seventh edition 1979
Eighth edition 1986
Ninth edition 1993
Tenth edition 2000
Eleventh edition 2005

ISBN 0 443 07356 2

British Library Cataloguing in Publication Data
A catalogue record for this book is available from the British Library

Library of Congress Cataloging in Publication Data
A catalog record for this book is available from the Library of Congress

Dewey no.	Subject headings		
613. 2	*nutrition diet therapy*		
Location FHSW	Abstract *May 2006*		
3 Week / 1 Week / LUO / Reference	Order details *PO 23833 C*	*40·05*	

Note
Knowledge and best practice in this field are constantly changing. As new research and experience broaden our knowledge, changes in practice, treatment and drug therapy may become necessary or appropriate. Readers are advised to check the most current information provided (i) on procedures featured or (ii) by the manufacturer of each product to be administered, to verify the recommended dose or formula, the method and duration of administration, and contraindications. It is the responsibility of the practitioner, relying on their own experience and knowledge of the patient, to make diagnoses, to determine dosages and the best treatment for each individual patient, and to take all appropriate safety precautions. To the fullest extent of the law, neither the publisher nor the editors and contributors assume any liability for any injury and/or damage.

The Publisher

Working together to grow libraries in developing countries

www.elsevier.com | www.bookaid.org | www.sabre.org

ELSEVIER   BOOK AID International   Sabre Foundation

ELSEVIER   your source for books, journals and multimedia in the health sciences

www.elsevierhealth.com

The Publisher's policy is to use paper manufactured from sustainable forests

Printed in China

Contents

Contents

Part 6 PUBLIC HEALTH NUTRITION

Section editors and contributors

Section editors

Lawrence Haddad PhD (Stanford California)
Director, Institute of Development Studies at the University of Sussex, Brighton, UK

David A. Bender BSc PhD RNutr
Senior Lecturer in Biochemistry, Department of Biochemistry and Molecular Biology, University College London, London, UK

Catherine A. Geissler BDS MS PhD RNutr
Professor of Human Nutrition, Department of Nutrition and Dietetics, King's College London, London, UK and Director, Higher Education Academy, Health Sciences and Practice, UK

Patricia Judd MSc PhD RD
Professor of Nutrition and Dietetics, Lancashire School of Health and Postgraduate Medicine, University of Central Lancashire, Preston, UK

Hilary Powers BSc PhD
Professor in Nutritional Biochemistry and Head of Human Nutrition Unit, University of Sheffield, Sheffield, UK

Contributors

Nils-Georg Asp MD PhD
Professor of Applied Nutrition, Department of Food Technology, Engineering and Nutrition, Lund University, Lund, Sweden

Arne Astrup MD PhD
Director and Professor, Research Department of Human Nutrition, Royal Veterinary and Agricultural University, Copenhagen, Denmark

Margo E. Barker BAgr(Hons) MSc PhD
Lecturer, Human Nutrition Unit, Division of Clinical Sciences (North), University of Sheffield, Northern General Hospital, Sheffield, UK

Christopher J. Bates MA DPhil(Oxon)
Formerly Head of Micronutrient Status Research, MRC Human Nutrition Research, Elsie Widdowson Laboratory, Cambridge, UK

David A. Bender BSc PhD RNutr
Senior Lecturer in Biochemistry, Department of Biochemistry and Molecular Biology, University College London, London, UK

Aubrey Blumsohn MBBCh PhD MRCPath
Senior Lecturer, Bone Metabolism Group, Division of Clinical Sciences (North), University of Sheffield, Sheffield, UK

Eric Brunner PhD
Senior Lecturer in Epidemiology, Department of Epidemiology and Public Health, University College London, London, UK

B. Capaldo MD
Department of Clinical and Experimental Medicine, Federico II University, Naples, Italy

V. A. Chudleigh BA(Hons) PGDip SRD
Research Dietitian, Gastroenterology Research, Addenbrooke's Hospital, Cambridge, UK

Marc J. Cohen PhD
Research Fellow, Food Consumption and Nutrition Division, International Food Policy Research Institute (IFPRI), Washington DC, USA

Maureen B. Duggan MD MSc(HumanNutrition) FRCP FRCPCH DCH DTM&H
Visiting Lecturer, Human Nutrition Unit, University of Sheffield, Sheffield; formerly Senior Lecturer in Paediatrics, University of Sheffield, and Professor of Paediatrics, Mbarara University, Uganda

Abdul Dulloo PhD
*Lecturer and Researcher, Department of Medicine,
Division of Physiology, University of Fribourg,
Switzerland*

Christopher G. Fairburn DM FRCPsych FMedSci
*Wellcome Principal Research Fellow and Professor of
Psychiatry, Department of Psychiatry, University of
Oxford, Oxford, UK*

The late **Anne Ferguson** PhD FRCP
*Formerly at the Institute of Child Health, University
College London, London, UK*

Robert Fraser MBChB MD(Sheffield) FRCOG DCH
*Reader in Obstetrics and Gynaecology, University of
Sheffield, Sheffield, UK*

Salah Gariballa MD FRCP
*Clinical Senior Lecturer, Sheffield Institute for Nutritional
Studies on Ageing, University of Sheffield, Sheffield, UK*

John Garrow MD PhD FRCPE FRCP(Lond)
*Emeritus Professor of Human Nutrition, St Bartholomew's
Hospital Medical School, London, UK*

Catherine A. Geissler BDS MS PhD RNutr
*Professor of Human Nutrition, Department of Nutrition
and Dietetics, King's College London, London, UK and
Director, Higher Education Academy, Health Sciences
and Practice, UK*

Barbara E. Golden BSc MBBCh BAD MD FRCPI
FRCPCH DCH RNutr
*Clinical Senior Lecturer and Honorary Consultant in
International Child Health, Department of Child
Health, University of Aberdeen Medical School,
Aberdeen, UK*

Michael H. Gordon MA DPhil MIFST
*Senior Lecturer, Hugh Sinclair Unit of Human
Nutrition, School of Food Biosciences, University of
Reading, Reading, UK*

George Grimble BSc PhD
*Group Leader for Nutrition, Dietetics, Food and
Consumer Sciences, Department of Health & Human
Sciences, London Metropolitan University, London, UK*

Lawrence Haddad PhD (Stanford, California)
*Director, Institute of Development Studies at the
University of Sussex, Brighton, UK*

Andrew J. Hill PhD CPsychol
*Senior Lecturer in Behavioural Sciences, Academic Unit
of Psychiatry and Behavioural Sciences, School of
Medicine, University of Leeds, Leeds, UK*

J. O. Hunter MA MD FRCP FACG
*Consultant Physician, Addenbrooke's Hospital,
Cambridge; Visiting Professor of Medicine, University
of Cranfield, Shrivenham, Swindon, UK*

Ross Hunter BSc MD
*Department of Nutrition and Dietetics, King's College
London, London, UK*

John M. Kearney BScAgr PhD Dip(Epidemiology &
Biostatistics)
*Lecturer in Epidemiology/Nutrition, Department of
Biological Sciences, Dublin Institute of Technology,
Dublin, Ireland*

Timothy J. Key BVM&S MSc DPhil
*Professor of Epidemiology and Deputy Director,
Cancer Epidemiology Unit, University of Oxford,
Radcliffe Infirmary, Oxford, UK*

Jim I. Mann CNZM DM PhD FRACP FRSNZ
*Professor in Human Nutrition and Medicine,
Department of Human Nutrition, University of Otago,
Dunedin, New Zealand*

D. Joe Millward DSc PhD RPHN
*Professor of Human Nutrition, University of Surrey,
Guildford, Surrey, UK*

Anne Marie Minihane BSc PhD
*Lecturer in Human Nutrition, School of Food
Biosciences, University of Reading, Reading, UK*

Jane B. Morgan MSc PhD SRD RPHNutr
*Reader in Childhood Nutrition, School of Biomedical
and Molecular Sciences, University of Surrey,
Guildford, Surrey, UK*

Annhild Mosdøl MSc PhD
*Research Fellow, Department of General Practice and
Community Medicine, University of Oslo, Oslo, Norway*

Paula Moynihan BSc PhD SRD RPHNutr
*Senior Lecturer in Nutrition, School of Dental Sciences,
University of Newcastle, Newcastle upon Tyne, UK*

Michael Nelson BSc MSc PhD
*Reader in Public Health Nutrition, Department of
Nutrition and Dietetics, King's College London,
London, UK*

Timothy J. Peters DSc PhD FRCP FRCPE FRCPath
*Department of Clinical Biochemistry, King's College
London, London, UK (retired)*

Elizabeth M. E. Poskitt MB BChir FRCP FRCPCH
*Senior Lecturer, Public Health Nutrition Group, London
School of Hygiene and Tropical Medicine, London, UK*

Hilary J. Powers BSc PhD
Professor in Nutritional Biochemistry and Head of Human Nutrition Unit, University of Sheffield, Sheffield, UK

Victor Preedy DSc PhD FIBiol FRCPath
Professor, Department of Nutrition and Dietetics, King's College London, London, UK

Gabrielle Riccardi MD
Professor of Endocrinology – Metabolic Diseases, Chief of the Diabetes Unit, Federico II University, Naples, Italy

A. A. Rivellese MD
Department of Clinical and Experimental Medicine, Federico II University, Naples, Italy

Tom A. B. Sanders BSc PhD DSc RPHNutr
Professor of Nutrition and Dietetics, Head of the Research Division of Nutritional Sciences, King's College London, London, UK

W. H. M. Saris PhD MD
Professor of Human Nutrition, Department of Human Biology, Maastricht University, Maastricht, The Netherlands

Yves Schutz PhD
Institute of Physiology, Faculty of Medicine, University of Lausanne, Switzerland

Paul Sharp BSc PhD
Senior Lecturer in Nutritional Sciences, School of Health and Life Sciences, King's College London, London, UK

Alan J. Sinclair MSc MD FRCP(Edin) FRCP(Lond)
Professor of Medicine and Consultant Physician, Walsgrave Hospital and Centre for Health Services Studies, University of Warwick, Coventry, UK

Stephan Strobel MD PhD FRCP FRCPCH
Professor of Paediatrics and Clinical Immunology and Director of Clinical Education, Peninsula Postgraduate Health Institute, Peninsula Medical School, Plymouth, UK

Jane Thomas SRD BSc MMedSci
Senior Lecturer in Nutrition, Department of Nutrition and Dietetics, King's College London, London, UK

David I. Thurnham BSc PhD
Howard Professor of Human Nutrition, Northern Ireland Centre for Food and Health, School of Biomedical Sciences, University of Ulster, Coleraine, Northern Ireland

A. M. Tomkins MBBS FRCP FRCPCH FFPHM FMedSci
Professor and Director of Centre for International Child Health, Institute of Child Health, University College London, London, UK

Paul Trayhurn DSc FRSE
Professor of Nutritional Biology and Director, Neuroendocrine & Obesity Biology Unit, Liverpool Centre for Nutritional Genomics, School of Clinical Sciences, University of Liverpool, Liverpool, UK

Stanley J. Ulijaszek BSc MSc MA PhD
Professor of Human Ecology, Institute of Social and Cultural Anthropology, University of Oxford, Oxford, UK

L. J. C. van Loon PhD
Medical Physiologist, Department of Movement Sciences, Maastricht University, Maastricht, The Netherlands

Christine M. Williams BSc PhD
Professor of Human Nutrition, School of Food Biosciences, University of Reading, Reading, UK

I. Stuart Wood BSc(Hons) PhD
Lecturer, Neuroendocrine & Obesity Biology Unit, Liverpool Centre for Nutritional Genomics, School of Clinical Sciences, University of Liverpool, Liverpool, UK

Parveen Yaqoob MA DPhil
Reader in Cellular and Molecular Nutrition, School of Food Biosciences, University of Reading, Reading, UK

Preface

This edition of *Human Nutrition* has a long pedigree, being the 11th edition of the textbook previously called *Human Nutrition and Dietetics*, which has been the leading British textbook in the field for almost half a century. The 9th and 10th editions were edited by John Garrow and Philip James, together with Ann Ralph in the latter edition. John Garrow was Professor of Human Nutrition at St Bartholomew's Hospital Medical School in London, and Professor Philip James was Director of the Rowett Research Institute in Aberdeen, also the work base of Ann Ralph.

The forerunner of the first edition was *A Textbook of Dietetics*, published in 1940 and written by Professor Stanley Davidson and Dr Ian Anderson, both of the Edinburgh University Medical School, with a preface by Lord Boyd Orr, the first Director of the Rowett Research Institute, a distinguished adviser on government food policy during World War II and subsequently Director-General of the newly formed United Nations Food and Agricultural Organization. The textbook was further developed in collaboration with Dr Reg Passmore, also at the Medical School in Edinburgh, into the first edition of *Human Nutrition and Dietetics*, which was published in 1959. Sir Stanley Davidson died in 1981 but Reg Passmore continued to ply his excellent editorial skills with the assistance of other colleagues in Edinburgh up to the 8th edition, which was published in 1986. This continuity contributed greatly to the long-term success of the textbook.

Garrow and James took over the editing of the 9th edition, published in 1993, retaining the essential format of the 8th edition but bringing in experts to contribute chapters in the many specialist areas of nutrition. There was also a change in the balance of content, so that clinical nutrition no longer focused on deficiency diseases, but considered in more depth the clinical implications of overconsumption. The developments in food processing meant that nutrient content of foods had altered and the 'health food' industry was offering nutrients singly or in combination, leading to new risks of excessive intakes of certain nutrients and to a blurring of the boundaries between nutrition and toxicology. The 9th and 10th editions also explored the economic, political and cultural pressures that influence a nation's diet and which tend to distort the sound advice that should be offered to the public.

Significant advances in scientific knowledge over the past decade, and changes in the social and technological context of these changes, have been the stimulus to this, the 11th edition in terms of both content and form. Many of the basic principles of previous editions remain strong tenets of the current edition, such as providing the important scientific principles of nutrition and its social and economic context, to allow students to distinguish between fact and fiction in advertising and the popular press. However, as the scientific base of nutrition has grown and the core knowledge base essential to the student of nutrition has become larger, it has become unrealistic to offer all aspects of nutrition in a single text. For this reason the textbook concentrates on the principles and context of human nutrition, leaving the application to dietetics to be dealt with by existing excellent textbooks of dietetics.

Over the last decade a revolution has occurred in electronic information sources. Much of higher education is computer based and the internet has completely altered the availability of information worldwide. Hence a major change in this edition is the provision of a CD-ROM to support the textbook. The CD-ROM offers a valuable additional resource to allow students to explore certain topics in more detail, through expanded text for many chapters as well as more comprehensive reference lists, including website addresses.

Foremost in scientific advances relevant to nutrition is the completion of the human genome project, which underpins developments in nutritional genomics and the study of gene–nutrient interactions. Progress in this field will eventually lead to improved targeting of nutritional interventions and advice, based on the genetic inheritance of the individual. Lifestyle changes that have occurred in the context of nutrition include further developments in work patterns and food technology, engendering a plethora of new food products with a huge range of ready prepared foods, fast food outlets, and a reduction in cooking skills in the younger generations. An epidemic of obesity and related diseases such as diabetes has emerged to such an extent that it has reached the political agenda in most of the 'developed' or 'industrialised' countries. At the same time many of the 'developing' countries are going through the so-called 'nutrition transition' in which food patterns are shifting from mainly vegetable sources to increasing animal content, with related nutritional changes, reduced activity with mechanisation, and shifts in disease patterns from deficiency diseases towards the 'diseases of affluence' – CHD, diabetes, cancer, etc. While pockets of poverty remain in the affluent countries, internal conflict in many poorer countries, including the growing population of refugees, fuels the existence of severe acute malnutrition and chronic malnutrition.

The new format, incorporating a CD-ROM, has allowed us to offer the essential information about nutrition in its broadest sense in one textbook. The chapters have been kept short to distil what the specialist authors consider to be the most important aspects of the topic, whilst further reading, diagrams, case studies, and additional references are given for most chapters on the accompanying CD-ROM. Each chapter has been written by a recognised authority or authorities on the topic, and the universality of the importance of nutrition is reflected in the ten countries represented.

The structure of the book has been altered to reflect the revised content and is now divided into six parts. Part 1 starts with food, and explores the various patterns of food consumption and reasons for food availability and choice. It also outlines the chemical structure of food and nutrients. Part 2 concerns the physiology and biochemistry of digestion, body composition and metabolism of the macronutrients and energy. Part 3 describes the function of micronutrients, vitamins and minerals that have special importance in human nutrition, and explores their interactions with each other and with environmental and pharmacological substances. Part 4 considers the dietary requirements of particular age groups and groups with specific preferences and activities. Part 5 deals with the main nutrition-related diseases and Part 6 with public health nutrition, including the epidemiological and individual assessment methods, the factors affecting food supply and the development of food and nutrition policies and interventions worldwide.

Human Nutrition is intended as an authoritative, comprehensive textbook on nutrition for both undergraduate and graduate students of nutrition and other health sciences, and a concise source of information for all working in the field of nutrition.

The editors would like to thank the section editors for their excellent support and the fifty authors for contributing their expertise to this new edition and for their patience with frequent requests concerning deadlines, content and format.

CAG

HJP

London and Sheffield, 2005

Part 1

Food and nutrients

Edited by Lawrence Haddad

1

Food and nutrient patterns

John Kearney, Jane Thomas and Lawrence Haddad

Objectives

By the end of this chapter you should be able to:

- identify the main sources of nutrients in Western diets
- understand the social, psychological, geographic and economic factors determining food choices and diet patterns
- appreciate the similarities and variability in food and nutrient patterns in different population groups and countries
- be aware of changing trends over time including novel foods.

1.1 INTRODUCTION

This chapter examines food and nutrient patterns in the context of the major foods and food products in the Western diet and their nutritional importance. Taking the UK as an example of a country with a typical Western diet, it considers the main food groups and identifies the main sources of nutrients in the Western diet. It also outlines the main contributors to the nutrient and non-nutrient content of the UK diet. Another important aspect of this chapter is the exploration of the variations in dietary patterns in terms of the causes of variation such as availability (geographic, trade, demand) as well as economics, food beliefs and cultural differences. Examples of variations in dietary patterns in population subgroups such as vegetarians, and those defined by religion and region (national and international) are also outlined. This should enable the reader to appreciate the similarities and variability in different population groups and to clarify the social, psychological and geographical factors influencing food intake patterns. The variability in the consumption of foods, nutrients and non-nutrients, in terms of time (secular trends) and place (geographical differences – between developing and developed countries as well as between different developed countries), is described. This highlights the ability of different diets (foods consumed) to provide optimal nutrient intake. The wide diversity in the quantities of foods consumed between different countries and the changes with nutritional transition will serve to illustrate this.

In summary, in this chapter the major food groups in the diet are examined in terms of their nutrient and non-nutrient contribution, their variability between countries and between subgroups in the population, as well as changing trends in food intake patterns (including novel foods) over time.

1.2 MAJOR FOOD GROUPS IN THE WESTERN DIET

Western diets are composed of several food groups collectively providing the nutritional needs of the body. The particular food groups in the Western diet that provide all the nutrients and non-nutrients for optimum health include: cereals and cereal products (e.g. bread); vegetables and fruit; roots and tubers; milk and other dairy products; meats, fish, eggs and other sources of protein; fats and oils. A typical pattern of the Western diet may be illustrated in terms of the food intake patterns for British adults (Table 1.1). How these patterns vary between countries (i.e. geographically) is discussed below in Section 1.3, while changes over time are discussed in Section 1.4. The non-nutrients discussed in this chapter are those believed to have a potentially beneficial effect on human health. They include both dietary fibre and phytoprotectants such as flavonoids and phytoestrogens. Other non-nutrients in foods such as contaminants, allergens and food additives do not have specific health benefits and are not discussed here (see Sections 2.3, 2.5, 2.6 in Ch. 2).

Nutritional importance of food groups in the Western diet

For a fuller version of this section see Section CD 1.2. For main food sources of macronutrients, vitamins, minerals and dietary fibre in UK adults see Tables CD 1–4.

Table 1.1 **Food intakes in grams/day among British adults (n = 2197)**

Food group	Foods	g/day
Cereal	White bread	64
	Wholemeal bread	28
	Other bread	13
	Pasta and rice	34
	High fibre breakfast cereals	15
	Other cereals	5
	Potatoes (not fried)	68
	All starchy foods	**227**
Dairy	Whole milk	162
	Reduced fat milk	62
	Cheese and dairy desserts	28
	All dairy products	**253**
Meat, fish etc.	Meat and poultry	165
	Eggs	25
	Fish and shellfish	30
	Nuts and pulses	18
	All meats and alternatives	**238**
Vegetables and fruit	Vegetables	143
	Fresh fruit	59
	Canned fruit and other fruit	77
	All vegetables and fruit	**279**

Data from DNSBA, Gregory et al (1990).

Cereals and cereal products

Cereals represent the most important plant foods in the human diet for their contribution to energy and carbohydrate intake and many micronutrients. They are all seeds from domesticated members of the grass family. Their contribution to energy intake varies markedly between developing and developed countries. In developing countries such as those in Africa and parts of Asia, cereals contribute as much as 70% of energy intakes. By contrast in developed countries, such as the UK, they provide approximately 30% of the energy intake. In the UK, cereals also provide about 10% of fat, 25% of protein and 50% of available carbohydrates. They also make a significant contribution to dietary fibre as non-starch polysaccharides (NSP). The major cereals in the human diet are wheat and rice followed by maize, barley, oats and rye.

Cereals are the staple foods in almost all populations. Carbohydrates form the major part of the cereal grain and consequently these are often referred to as carbohydrate foods.

Vegetables and fruit

These include a wide range of plant families and consist of any edible portion of the plant including roots, leaves, stems, buds, flowers and fruits. The leaves, stems, buds, flowers and some fruits (tomatoes, cucumbers, marrows and pumpkins) are commonly classified as vegetables while the fruits that are sweet are classified as fruits. Root crops are usually classified separately for human consumption rather than botanically. Vegetables and fruits are primarily seen as sources of vitamins and are important contributors to the intake of dietary fibre. Fruits tend to be high in potassium and low in sodium. Although quite low in B vitamins (with the exception of folates, for which leafy vegetables are rich sources), they are the most important source of vitamin C. Also, fruits and vegetables are important sources of such non-nutrients as the phytoprotectants, carotenoids and anthocyanins (flavonoids in berries).

Roots and tubers

Roots and tubers are the underground organs of many plants and could be included in the vegetable and fruit group. However, due to differences in their nutrient composition and the important role they play in the Western diet (especially the potato) they are being discussed separately.

Root crops: Most roots have a high water content and tend to be rich in carbohydrates as free sugars (with small amounts of starch in mature organs). They are generally low in dietary fibre, protein and micronutrients.

Tubers: Tubers are not true roots but rather underground stems that store large quantities of carbohydrate, usually starch. The potato is a stem tuber native to the Andes and was brought into Europe in the seventeenth century. The nutrient composition of the potato varies according to variety but all contain large amounts of starch (Table 1.2). They also contain significant amounts of vitamin C and their high levels of consumption make them an important source of this vitamin.

Meat and meat products

Meat has comprised an important part of the human diet for a large part of our history and still is the centrepiece of most meals in developed countries. In many developing countries, non-animal-based sources of protein such as legumes are still dominant. In the USA and the UK the most important meat sources are pigs, sheep and cattle. In other regions such as India, the Middle East and Africa, goats and camels are the main meats consumed. Other meat sources include wild animals such as rabbits and venison and poultry (chicken, ducks, turkey and

Table 1.2 **Contribution to energy and selected nutrient intakes from potatoes, all other vegetables and total fruits**

	Potatoes	Other vegetables	Total fruits
Energy (MJ)	6.8	3.1	4.0
Protein (g)	4.2	4.9	1.9
Carbohydrate (g)	10.2	4.2	6.8
Dietary fibre (g)	14.7	23.3	11.2
Iron (mg)	6.2	9.2	3.0
Carotenes (μg)	0	79.0	2.8
Vitamin C (mg)	13.8	19.0	44.8
Folates (μg)	13.8	18.3	6.3

Data from Ministry of Agriculture, Fisheries and Food (1994) The Dietary and Nutritional Survey of British Adults – Further Analysis. HMSO, London.

geese). In the UK poultry (chicken) has now become the most popular meat source. Apart from the muscle, other parts of the animal collectively described as offal are also consumed. The liver, kidneys, brain and pancreas (sweetbreads) are the most commonly consumed organs. Meat products such as sausages, pork pies etc. count for almost half of total meat consumption. Conventionally viewed as protein foods, meats as a whole are a major source of protein of high biological value. In developed countries such as the UK, where meat consumption is relatively high, it provides the main source of protein. Meats are also an important source of fat in the diet.

Fish
While fish catches worldwide are on the increase according to the Food and Agriculture Organization (FAO), fish stocks are being depleted due to over-fishing. The main fish consumed are white fish, oily fish and sea-food invertebrates. Fish are an important source of good quality protein and are low in fat (except for the oily fish which provide a very good source of long-chain polyunsaturated fatty acids (PUFA)). Fish are also a major source of iodine which has been accumulated from their environment. Also, they may be an important source of calcium (in fish with fine bones) and vitamin D.

Eggs
The most widely consumed eggs in the UK are hens' eggs. The proteins found in eggs contain the amino acids essential for the chick embryos' complete development. Because of this it was considered the 'reference protein' for biological evaluation of other protein sources in terms of their amino acid patterns.

Lipids found in eggs are rich in phospholipids and cholesterol. The fatty acid profile shows a high proportion of polyunsaturated fatty acids to saturated fatty acids (high P:S ratio).

Milk (and other dairy products)
Cows provide the bulk of all milk consumed in the UK, with goat and sheep making only a minor contribution to overall milk consumption. Milk is an excellent source of many nutrients. The major protein in milk is casein, comprising up to 80% of the protein in cow's milk. Other proteins include lactalbumin, and immunoglobulins that are responsible for the transfer of maternal immunity of the young animal for a short period following birth. Milk from ruminant animals, such as the cow, contains a large proportion of short chain fatty acids produced from the fermentation of carbohydrates in the rumen. Milk and its products are excellent sources of many inorganic nutrients especially calcium and certain vitamins (both fat-soluble and water-soluble). Other dairy products include:

- cheese, which contains, in a concentrated form, many of milk's nutrients; and
- yoghurt, which is produced from the culturing of a mixture of milk and cream products with the lactic acid-producing bacteria *Lactobacillus bulgaricus* and *Streptococcus thermophilus* and other bacterial cultures (e.g. *Lactobacillus acidophilus, Bifidobacteria*).

The contribution of dairy products to the UK diet (and to that of many other northern European countries) is very important. They can be an important source of calcium and riboflavin, especially in children and adolescents.

Fats and oils
These are distinguished by their physical characteristics, with fats being solid at room temperature (due to a high relative concentration of saturated fatty acids) while oils are liquid and usually of plant origin, either from the flesh of the fruit (olive oil) or from the seed (sunflower and linseed). They have a higher concentration of unsaturated fatty acids. Lipids that are isolated from animal products tend to be solid fats (e.g. butter, lard and suet). In recent years there has been increased consumption of margarine made from highly unsaturated fats such as sunflower due to the beneficial effects on serum cholesterol. Margarines are required by legislation in many countries, including the UK, to be fortified with vitamins A and D so that they are nutritionally equivalent to butter.

Food sources of nutrients and health-related non-nutrients

The importance of specific foods as sources of macro- and micronutrients for particular populations depends not only on the level of the nutrient in the food or food product (and its availability to the body), but also on the extent to which the food is consumed (the quantity and the proportion of the population that consumes that food). The way the food is consumed (raw, cooked or processed) will also influence its nutritional importance. Thus, it is important to distinguish between the nutritional importance of various foods generally and 'the main contributors' from food sources to nutrient intakes of a particular population. Such information is obtained from individual dietary surveys including diet histories or food records (see Ch. 31). One such survey was the Diet and Nutrition Survey of British Adults commissioned by the former Ministry of Agriculture, Fisheries and Food (now FSA and DEFRA) and the Department of Health. The main food sources of carbohydrates in the UK are cereal products and potatoes. Biscuits, cakes and snacks also make a sizeable contribution. Important contributors to protein and fat intakes are meat, fish and eggs as well as dairy products, while vegetables and fruit make important contributions to a considerable number of the micronutrients (vitamins and minerals), dietary fibre and other non-nutrients (the phytoprotectants).

Dietary fibre

Fibre (total fibre) in the diet has a new definition based upon dietary fibre (indigestible carbohydrate and lignin which are intrinsic and intact in plants) and functional fibre (isolated non-digestible carbohydrates that have beneficial physiological effects) (see Ch. 6). Previous definitions were based upon methods of analysis. The main contributors to fibre in the diet of British adults are cereal products and potatoes.

Phytoprotectants

Epidemiological studies indicate that a diet rich in fruits and vegetables has health benefits particularly related to protection against certain chronic diseases such as cancer. Experimental studies are being conducted to help establish causality and to elicit mechanisms for these observations, and this currently focuses on the antioxidant potential of certain nutrients and non-nutrients. The term 'phyto' originates from a Greek word meaning plant. Also known as phytochemicals and bioactive compounds, they are derived from foods of plant origin and, while not regarded as nutrients, they may be beneficial to health (e.g. reduce risk of certain cancers and cardiovascular disease, and of age-related blindness). Fruits, vegetables, grains, legumes, nuts and teas are rich sources of phytonutrients. Phytoprotectants are extremely varied in their chemical composition, the plants in which they are found and their putative beneficial effects. There are tens of thousands of phytonutrients in plants that have not yet been tested. The best way to benefit from these phytonutrients is to increase consumption of plant foods. Indeed, variety in colour appears to be important. (A more detailed description of phytoprotectants and their effects is given in Ch. 13.) Some of the common classes of phytonutrients include: flavonoids (polyphenols) including isoflavones (phytoestrogens), inositol phosphates (phytates), lignans (phytoestrogens), isothiocyanates, indoles, phenols and sulphides and thiols.

Polyphenols: Polyphenolic compounds are natural components of a wide variety of plants; they are also known as secondary plant metabolites. Much of the total antioxidant activity of fruits and vegetables is related to their phenolic content. Research suggests that many flavonoids are more potent antioxidants than vitamins C and E. Chlorogenic acid and caffeic acid are important phenolic compounds in our diet. The interest in these compounds is increasing because phenolic compounds have antioxidant activity in vitro. It has recently been shown that chlorogenic acid and caffeic acid are absorbed in humans, which increases the possibility that they might affect health. Food sources rich in polyphenols include onion, apple, tea, red wine, red grapes, grape juice, strawberries, raspberries, blueberries, cranberries, and certain nuts. The average polyphenol/flavonoid intake in the USA has not been determined with precision, as there is presently no US national food database for these compounds. (USDA scientists and their colleagues are in the process of developing a database for foods rich in polyphenols.) It has been estimated that in the Dutch diet a subset of flavonoids (flavonols and flavones) provides 23 mg per day. Polyphenols can be classified as non-flavonoids and flavonoids.

The flavonoids quercetin and catechins are the most extensively studied polyphenols relative to absorption and metabolism. The flavonol quercetin belongs to the group of flavonoids, one of the large groups of secondary plant metabolites occurring widely throughout the plant kingdom. Experimental studies in animals suggest that dietary quercetin, at relatively high doses, could inhibit the initiation and development of tumours in humans. These results are supported by in vitro studies showing that quercetin inhibits the growth of isolated human tumour cell lines. Furthermore, quercetin, the most commonly consumed flavonoid, is reported to exhibit antioxidant activity. A relationship has been reported between quercetin intake and reduced risk of cancer and coronary heart disease in a Finnish population. Further studies on epidemiology, mechanisms and interventions are needed before firm conclusions on the health protective effects of quercetin can be drawn. Examples of other beneficial effects from phytoprotectants include lycopene, in tomatoes, which may decrease risk of developing prostate cancer, and lutein, found in dark green leafy vegetables, which is believed to reduce age-related blindness. Table 1.3 summarises some types of flavonoid and non-flavonoid polyphenols.

Contribution of macronutrients to energy needs

Energy is required by the body to do its work, in particular to maintain basal metabolic rate and also for physical activity and for thermogenesis (see Ch. 5). The energy needs of the body are served by the contribution of the three macronutrients: carbohydrate, fat and protein. Alcohol is the other energy source. Carbohydrate and fat are the primary fuel sources and for this purpose they can be largely used interchangeably. To a large extent the body can synthesise de novo the carbohydrates and lipids it needs, with the exception of the requirement for small amounts of carbohydrate and n-6 and n-3 fatty acids. Thus a mixture of the macronutrients is required as a source of fuel to meet the energy requirements of the body. Defining the optimal mix of energy sources to optimise health and promote

Table 1.3 Examples of sources of non-flavonoid and flavonoid polyphenols

	Sources
Non-flavonoids	
Ellagic acid	Strawberries, blueberries, raspberries
Coumarins	Citrus fruits, some herbs
Flavonoids	
Anthocyanins	Berry fruits
Catechins	Tea, wine
Flavanones	Citrus fruits
Flavones	Fruits and vegetables
Flavonols	Fruits, vegetables, tea, wine
Isoflavones	Soya beans

longevity is not easy. There are no clinical trials that compare various macronutrient combinations with longevity in humans.

Patterns of consumption of the macronutrients have changed radically from those of our ancient ancestors, where the relative contribution to energy of these macronutrients has been estimated as 34% protein, 45% carbohydrate and 21% fat, contrasting to that of a typical current Western diet of 12% protein, 46% carbohydrate and 42% fat. A contrast also exists in the energy contribution of these macronutrients between developing countries, having a much higher contribution from carbohydrates relative to fat, and developed countries where fat constitutes well over a third of energy intake. The acceptable (i.e. healthy) macronutrient distribution ranges (AMDR) are 10–15% of energy for protein, 25–30% of energy for fat and 45–65% of energy for carbohydrate. The recommendations (dietary reference values – DRV) for total fat are 33% of total energy or 35% of food energy. Considerable debate exists on the importance of total fat (quantity versus the qualitative composition of the fat) in relation to cardiovascular disease and certain cancers (see Ch. 7).

1.3 VARIATIONS IN DIETARY PATTERNS

Examples of variations in diet

For further details see Section CD 1.3(a).

Developing versus developed countries

Diets in the developing world are very different from those in the rich countries, although there is

some evidence of convergence between the two. The diets of the former tend to be characterised by lower total calorie intake, more calories from cereals and roots and tubers, less diversity in terms of food groups consumed, fewer animal source foods (and less fat), less processed food and less food away from home. Many of these differences are explained

Table 1.4 **Mean energy intake and macronutrient energy intakes in 13 EU member states**

Country	Energy (MJ/day)	% Energy Carbohydrate	Protein	Fat
Northern Europe				
Belgium	13.2	38.7	14.3	41.8
Denmark	10.2	43.5	14.5	37.0
Finland	9.0	47.7	16.1	33.8
France	8.6	38.2	17.4	38.9
Germany	9.6	39.2	15.1	40.7
Ireland	9.4	47.8	14.8	35.2
Netherlands	9.7	43.6	15.4	37.5
Sweden	8.8	46.0	15.0	36.5
UK	8.6	42.3	14.7	38.4
Southern Europe				
Greece	7.6	44.0	14.2	40.3
Italy	8.7	47.5	16.9	32.6
Portugal	9.7	49.1	18.0	28.5
Spain	8.9	40.2	19.6	38.0

Source: British Journal of Nutrition (1999) Food-based dietary guidelines – a staged approach. Volume 81, Supplement Number 2.

by socioeconomic factors, but there is considerable variation in consumption patterns even accounting for such factors (as an example, see Section CD 33.4(b) on South Korea's attempts to promote a 'traditional' diet).

Europe and the USA

For further details see also Section CD 1.3(b).

Differences in European diets can be examined from two main sources: a questionnaire based survey carried out by the World Health Organization (WHO) Regional Office for Europe; and food supply data published by the Food and Agriculture Organization of the United Nations (FAO). Table 1.4 shows the total energy and macronutrient energy intakes in 13 EU member countries. For the comparative consumption of selected foods by men in selected European countries see Table CD 1.5.

Both the WHO dietary intake and the FAO food available for consumption data show that fruit and vegetable intake is higher in southern European countries than it is in northern, western, central and eastern European countries. Indeed, large variations were found with up to a five-fold variation in mean vegetable intakes from 100 g/day in Norway and Iceland to 370–500 g/day in Greece. Such a marked north–south variation in vegetable intakes is not as clear for fruit intakes, although wide inter-country variations do exist. For example, both sets of data

indicate that people in Spain eat twice as much fruit and vegetables as people in the UK and three times as much as people in Kazakhstan (see Table CD 1.6). Whereas the intakes of polyunsaturated fatty acids (PUFA) are generally similar for countries in the north and south of Europe, the intakes of monounsaturated (MUFA) and saturated fatty acids (SFA) differ markedly. The intakes of SFA as % energy are higher in northern European countries, ranging from 14 to 18% energy compared with 9 to 13% in southern European countries, while intakes of monounsaturated fatty acids (MUFA) as % energy are higher in southern European countries (12 to 20%) compared with 11 to 15% in northern European countries. This difference in MUFA intake may be directly attributed to the higher consumption of olive oil in the southern countries of Europe. For % energy from fats and fatty acid categories in selected European countries see Tables CD 1.7 and 1.8.

One specific diet survey, the SENECA (Survey in Europe on Nutrition and the Elderly project), examined cross-cultural variations in intakes of food groups among elderly Europeans (Schroll et al 1997) in four European countries (Denmark, the Netherlands, Switzerland and Spain). The dietary pattern followed a typical Western diet, with all participants from all four countries consuming milk, grain products and vegetables and virtually all consuming meat and fruit. Fewer participants consumed fish, eggs and sugar. While variation was found between these food groups, the main variation seen between countries was in the types of foods comprising the food groups and with which meals the foods are consumed.

Variation within the UK

The UK National Expenditure and Food Survey (ONS 2002) enables comparison of different patterns according to socioeconomic group and region (see Tables CD 1.9 and CD 1.10). There is considerable variation between regions with the lowest and highest levels of consumption of particular foods. For example, the highest consumption of fruit is in London and the lowest in Scotland whereas the highest consumption of meat products, bread confectionery and sugar and preserves is in Wales and the lowest in London. The low levels of vegetable and fruit consumption recorded in Scotland are the result of a number of historical and economic factors, and this observation is clearly linked to the current high levels of cardiovascular disease.

A number of important variations are also evident in relation to income. Non-pensioner households in which the head of household received less than £180 per week consumed less than the all-household average amounts of fresh fruits and fresh vegetables (excluding potatoes) and less skimmed milk, cheese, fish, fruit juices, breakfast cereals, alcoholic drinks and confectionery. However, they consumed more liquid whole milk, eggs, fats and oils, sugar and preserves, fresh potatoes, frozen and canned vegetables, bread and beverages than the average for all households.

For further details about economic and regional variation in food consumption in the UK see Section CD 1.3(c).

Factors in dietary variations

So far in this chapter we have considered foods and the nutritional contribution of food groups. But of course in practice, people do not eat 'food groups' any more than they eat 'nutrients'. They choose foods to eat which usually contain ingredients from a number of the groups, for example pizza, apple pie, beef stew. Food groups are useful tools for nutritionists, especially in relation to public nutrition policy, but they are not entirely satisfactory in picturing the way in which people eat. The way that people think about foods and group them together when making choices about what to eat may be very different from the nutritionists' view of food groups.

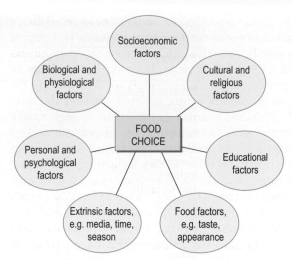

Figure 1.1 The main factors determining dietary variation.

Of all the animal and plant species that could be safely consumed, humans choose from a relatively narrow range of species. Those which may be considered a delicacy by some groups are rejected as inedible by others. Individuals' food choice at any given time will be influenced not only by what they consider to constitute 'food' and whether it is available (either physically accessible or affordable) but also by what is appropriate according to a variety of sociocultural factors, ideas, beliefs and attitudes as well as psychological factors and their level of hunger or satiety.

This section describes the main factors in dietary variation for developed and developing countries (Fig. 1.1).

Biological and physiological factors

Human physiology places few restrictions on food choice. Clearly the quantity of food consumed is limited to some extent by the capacity of the gastrointestinal tract, which results in the necessity to feed regularly, at least once a day and preferably more often. The quality of the diet is also limited, for example, by the fact that humans are monogastric, which renders plants with very high fibre contents impossible to digest.

Although factors such as age, gender, pregnancy, lactation and activity patterns all affect nutritional requirements, humans are unable to perceive their specific needs and act in response. No convincing evidence has been produced by studies that have attempted to demonstrate 'gustatory sensibility' (the innate ability of an individual to select foods that meet variations in nutritional status with regard to specific nutrients). However, studies with infants fed solely on milk have shown an innate ability to regulate energy intake in early life by adjusting the quantity of milk consumed in response to the level of dilution in order to maintain energy intake (Fomon et al 1969). This ability appears to decline when the diet becomes more varied, and is easily overridden by other factors influencing the timing of eating and the amount and types of food consumed in later life. Nonetheless the familiar experience of a decrease in pleasantness in association with increasing consumption of a particular food serves to limit the amount of that food which is eaten (Rolls 1986). This innate mechanism (sensory specific satiety) serves to ensure that humans eat a varied diet and are therefore more likely to meet their requirements for all nutrients. While this may have served humans well from a survival point of view in earlier times, it is potentially more problematic when surrounded by a huge variety of different, highly palatable, food items.

Humans experience general and non-specific feelings of hunger or satiety as a result of complex physiological processes which are not fully understood but involve an integrated set of feedback mechanisms.

In recent years there has been growing interest in the possible identification of gene-related determinants of nutritional behaviour. It has been proposed that these might be modulated through sensory sensitivity to specific chemical substances and reflected in taste preferences. However, it appears that while biology determines humans' nutritional needs, it does not substantially affect food choices. For further information on hunger and satiety see Section CD 1.3(d).

Economic factors

Access to food is a primary determinant of food choice and dietary variation. The availability of food will be influenced by (a) geography, season and factors such as food preservation and distribution systems which affect physical availability and (b) the ability of the individual to acquire what is available. These two elements are closely interlinked and the relative importance of either will depend on the situation.

In remote rural areas, with poorly developed food markets, decisions about what to produce have

an important effect on what is consumed, both at the village and at household levels. In these cases, decisions about production and consumption cannot be treated as entirely separate. Where markets are stronger, physical access to foods becomes less important and economic constraints assume a greater role. About 20% of the world's 6 billion population participate in the cash economy and about 90% of the world's food consumption occurs where it is produced. In towns and cities people depend almost entirely on purchased foods, while in rural populations people consume around 60% of the food they produce (McMichael 2001).

In situations where food must be purchased, there are two key aspects in the relationship between income and food consumption patterns. The first relates to the overall level of expenditure on food, the second to the types of food consumed. As income levels increase, families will spend more on food, although as a proportion of overall expenditures food is likely to decline in importance (called Engels' law). This may occur within a fairly narrow range in an industrialised country, such as the UK, where expenditure may range from 15% to 29% of reported expenditure between high income and low income households. However, in developing countries the differences may be far more dramatic. While the most affluent group may be spending a similar proportion on food to their counterparts in Western countries, around 15%, studies have indicated that in the lowest income groups, food may account for 70–80% of household expenditure.

One important outcome of this is the increased vulnerability of low income groups to changes in the price of foodstuffs and other necessities. This may be particularly important to the urban poor in less industrialised countries. If a diet which requires a high level of expenditure is barely adequate nutritionally, then any increase in price which leads to the purchase of reduced quantities of food may have serious nutritional consequences. Income may also be very unreliable. People are likely to be casually employed, or receive small amounts of cash intermittently as a result of different activities, and there is usually only enough money to buy small quantities of food at a time. Low income families have few opportunities to accumulate savings. As a result it is not possible to take advantage of the economies which are possible through bulk purchase. The urban poor may also be disadvantaged in the range and quality of foodstuffs available to them as well as the price they pay for food.

The cost of utilities – fuel, water, clothing, transport, rent – also affect food choices. The budgets of low income households leave very little room for manoeuvre and often food is the most flexible element of expenditure. If the price of cooking fuel increases, disposable income goes down and food purchases are affected. This may result in a change in the types of food purchased and a reduction in the amount of food eaten. Some or all of the family members may go without meals. It is commonly a priority to maintain the diet of the 'breadwinner', while women and children are particularly adversely affected by any shortfall.

The second area where income has a marked influence on food intake is in relation to the type of foods eaten. It is an internationally observed phenomenon that as income levels rise, people diversify away from a reliance on cereals and roots/tubers and begin to purchase more animal source foods, fruits and vegetables. In the UK more affluent households eat more fruit and vegetables, polyunsaturated margarine, low fat products and carcass meat. In contrast, low income families eat less fruit and more of the cheaper 'meat products', meat pies and sausages. The use of high fat foods such as these contributes to the observation that in a European context, energy-dense diets tend to cost less (Darmon et al 2004). Prices of one food can affect the consumption of other foods. If two foods are complements (i.e. they are eaten in combination), a price increase in one, will, in the short run, lead to a lower demand for it and a lower demand for its complement. For two foods that are substitutes (e.g. one type of cereal for another), if the price of one increases, people will switch to the substitute, increasing the demand for it. These food prices can be dramatically affected by food policies that subsidise the consumption and production of certain foods, typically not based on nutritional goals (see Ch. 33).

Food prices are not the only prices that affect food consumption and diets. Financial needs and the availability of paid employment may cause men and women to work outside the home. As a result, less food will be prepared at home and more food will be consumed away from home. This has an effect on the types of food which are eaten. Only certain foods are 'portable' and suitable for advance preparation and consumption elsewhere, especially in the absence of refrigeration. Food choices become increasingly influenced by the types of food produced by others and available at times and in places convenient to the work schedule. The tendency to consume food away from home increases in urban areas, associated with a greater concentration of food vendors and restaurants.

Cultural and religious factors

The human is basically an omnivore who has to learn what to eat, and what is learned is strongly influenced by culture and religion. This includes learning what is acceptable or not acceptable as food and appropriate foods for different occasions and different types of people according to age, gender and social status. Rules about the preparation of food and how it is eaten may also be culturally determined. Food has many important social uses and although the food items associated with these uses may vary from society to society and change over time, these 'non-nutritional' functions persist.

Communication

An invitation to share food or drink, in a range of different settings, is widely used to initiate and maintain personal relationships. The actual foods and drinks that are consumed will vary according to the nature of those relationships and are hence imbued with layers of social meaning. What may be considered appropriate when the setting is a casual encounter between old friends will probably be very different from what might be served on a more formal occasion with people who are less well known and whom the host might want to impress. Food can be used as a means of demonstrating status and prestige. Arrangements for feeding guests at a wedding celebration may well be designed to reflect the status of the bride's father rather than being a response to the perceived hunger and nutritional needs of the guests. In addition to cementing relationships through hospitality and demonstrating social status, food is widely used to reward, punish or influence the behaviour of others. This may range from the use of sweets by parents to reward children for good behaviour to, in the wider world, the giving/withholding of food aid to particular countries, depending on whether the politics of the regime in power are acceptable to the donor government.

Identity

As part of the socialisation process, children grow up learning the conventions of their social, gender and age group concerning appropriate food choices and the manner in which such foods should be prepared and consumed. In some parts of the world, notably northern India and Pakistan, such conventions may have a marked impact on the diets of women and children, particularly girls, as a result of restrictions on the amount and types of foods which are considered suitable. More generally, the selection of foods that are deemed as inappropriate for a particular situation may have social consequences. The saying 'Tell me what you eat, and I will tell you who you are' is attributed to Brillat-Savarin and encapsulates this phenomenon. People's choice of food identifies them in various aspects of social background and may demonstrate whether they do or do not 'fit in' with another social group. The existence of clearly defined 'food rules' may play an important role in reinforcing 'in-group' identity. This may assume considerable importance in the context of religion, where such rules operate to set those with particular beliefs apart from others who do not share their beliefs.

Ethics and religion

Food may play a very special role in the 'living out' of an individual's beliefs. Since food is ultimately incorporated into the body, food choices become part of who we are in a very real sense and as food must be eaten every day it serves as a constant reminder of what we believe. In recent years vegetarianism and veganism have become increasingly popular in the UK (see Ch. 17) and for many people this choice has been based on ethical concerns about the exploitation of farm animals. In contrast to ethical considerations, which operate primarily on an individual level, religious food rules serve not only to enhance the spiritual life of the individual but also to enhance allegiance to a community of believers.

An individual may use the restriction of food choice or fasting as a means to enhance personal spiritual growth through the rejection of worldliness, or use foods in rituals associated with communication with God/supernatural forces. Following specified food rules can also be used to express separateness from non-believers and enhance feelings of identity and belongingness with co-religionists. The 2001 UK census showed a culturally diverse population. While the eating habits of the majority, white Christian population are relatively unaffected by their religious affiliation, nearly 3% of the population are Muslim (1 591 000) whose religion requires the following of particular food rules as is the case for the next largest groups, Hindus (559 000), Sikhs (336 000) and Jews (267 000).

Some dietary restrictions are based on direct injunctions from the holy texts of the religions concerned, while others have their origins in the commemoration of particular events in religious history. For example, the prohibition against pork in Judaism is firmly based on Leviticus 11:4, whereas the eating of matzahs by Jewish people at Passover commemorates the deliverance from Egypt, when their ancestors had no time to allow the bread to rise.

Such rules may affect different aspects of food choice. This includes the items which are considered acceptable as food. For example, those that are acceptable to Muslims are described as 'halal' and those that are forbidden, such as pork and alcohol, as 'haram'. Certain foods may be proscribed on particular days – Roman Catholics should not eat meat on Fridays during Lent. The time of day at which food is eaten may also be restricted – Buddhist monks should not eat after midday. Rules may include the preparation of food. Ritual slaughter is important in rendering meat acceptable to both Muslims (halal) and Jews (kosher). In addition, meat and dairy products must be kept separate and no food prepared on the Sabbath in Jewish households. Fasting is important to the followers of many religions and may take different forms, varying in length and the extent of restriction. In the case of the Ramadan fast for Muslims, no food or drink should be taken between sunrise and sunset for one month. In the Greek Orthodox Church it is expected that during the 40 days of Lent, which precede Easter, the faithful will abstain from all animal foods. In contrast, Hindus may 'fast' once or twice a week throughout the year, restricting themselves to 'pure' foods.

To prevent and treat illness

Later chapters of this book will examine in detail the scientific basis for our understanding of nutritional requirements and how dietary intake can affect health. However, popular beliefs about the links between diet, health and disease are shaped by their cultural context and consequently vary in different parts of the world. Not only do ideas vary geographically, but they also change over time. The history of medicine (using the term broadly) is not characterised by a linear succession in which old systems of thought are exchanged wholesale for new ones. We can see this clearly in relation to diet. Despite an enormous growth in the understanding of physiology and the origins of disease, popular advice in the early nineteenth century in England was still

The appeal of different textures may also vary throughout life. A crisp and crunchy apple may be much more attractive to a teenager than to an elderly person who has lost all their teeth. Furthermore, the role of texture in food acceptance is highly product dependent. In the case of meat, celery and mashed potato, for example, perception of texture makes a major contribution to the overall acceptability of the food. Socially and culturally learned expectations also play an important part in evaluating texture.

Awareness of the sensory attributes of food which appeal to consumers is clearly of major importance to food manufacturers. Insights into how the senses interact in the experience of eating can also have implications for product formulation; for example, consumers of a fruit drink with a deeper colour will report a stronger fruit taste. Foods are also made tastier through the use of fats, sugars and salts, all items that in modest excess can lead to health problems such as diabetes, hypertension and some forms of heart disease and cancer.

Extrinsic factors

Huge amounts of money are spent each year marketing foods in rich and middle income countries. In the UK the top ten food and drink companies spent over £130 million on advertising in 2000. Advertising is a very powerful influence on food choice, especially for highly processed and packaged foods. Some groups of the population may be much more susceptible to this influence and there has been particular concern about the impact on children. In experimental situations, young children clearly have high levels of recall of advertisements and are more likely to request advertised products. The extent to which this results in increased consumption will depend on the relationship with the parent or food provider and the extent to which that person is resistant to 'pester power'. Once children are older and have more money to spend they are clearly in a position to make their own purchases. Advertising also contributes to the creation of social norms – projecting images about what 'people do' and offering images of people who the audience might want to identify with. This has been the focus of extensive debate in relation to the contribution that media images make to the development of eating disorders, particularly anorexia nervosa, in young girls.

The types of foods that are advertised are often high in fat and simple sugars and the emphasis on the promotion of these types of foods in contrast to the low level of marketing of fruit and vegetables is also considered to have a distorting effect on food habits. In less affluent countries it is also the nature of the foods which are promoted (expensive and nutrient-poor) and the distortion that consumption of these may cause to already overstretched food budgets that raises ethical questions, when western food companies are involved.

Seasonality

In parts of the world where food markets are not well integrated, local physical availability is a key determinant of food consumption. In rich countries, there are fewer and fewer seasonal food items as foods are sourced from all corners of the globe.

1.4 CHANGING DIETARY PATTERNS

Changing dietary patterns – migration

The large-scale rural–urban and international migration seen around the world in the second half of the twentieth century has been accompanied by major changes in eating habits as people have adapted to the demands of their new environments. As people move from the countryside to the city they are forced to enter into a cash economy, while at the same time often having few employment-related skills. Lack of cash may severely limit access to food and food choice. Income generation may also often involve several jobs spread over long working hours. This has particular implications for women in relation to food preparation and child care. Facilities for cooking are often limited and living conditions poor.

Access to familiar foods, economic factors and food preparation facilities may also contribute to changes in the eating habits of international migrants. But the eating habits of the host community will also have an impact, depending on the extent to which the migrants are exposed to these and the strength of individual factors which may affect their resistance to change (Table 1.5). The dietary changes that are made first usually involve the adoption of foods that are convenient, affordable

Table 1.5 Factors associated with changes in international migrants' eating habits

1. Food availability:
   - physical
   - economic
   - time and cooking facilities

2. Exposure:
   - length of stay
   - social contacts
   - education and language skills
   - mass media

3. Individual:
   - age
   - religious beliefs
   - beliefs about diet and health

and do not clash with religious or cultural beliefs. The adoption of ready-to-eat breakfast cereals and the decline in cooking traditional foods at breakfast has been widely observed in migrants to the USA and UK. Breakfast is also a meal with less social significance, whereas traditional dishes and foods are more often retained at evening meals when family members gather to eat. The presence of children in a family can accelerate the incorporation of non-traditional foods and eating patterns and the gradual development of eating patterns that incorporate elements of both the traditional and new food environments.

For further details see Section CD 1.4(a).

Changing patterns – supply and demand

In response to changing lifestyle and popular demand (initially among more affluent, more industrialised Western countries and subsequently the growing middle classes in developing countries) global food supply systems have been transformed, through changes in agriculture, food technology and transport in the past fifty years.

These trends are linked to two major developments in relation to patterns of diet and health on a global basis. The first of these is the demographic transition – the shift from high fertility and high mortality to low fertility and low mortality which has been associated with increased industrialisation. The second is the epidemiological transition, the shift from a pattern of high levels of infectious diseases associated with unreliable food supply, malnutrition and poor environmental sanitation to a

high prevalence of chronic degenerative diseases associated with urban-industrial lifestyles. These two changes underpin the so-called 'nutrition transition' (Popkin 2002).

At one time, nutrition-related non-communicable diseases (NR-NCDs) were referred to as 'diseases of affluence', more commonly found in industrialised Western countries than the developing world. However, it has long been recognised that this name was misleading in higher income countries, where these diseases were in fact more common in lower income groups, associated with lifestyle and dietary differences. It has also become apparent that NR-NCDs are emerging increasingly among lower and middle income groups in less affluent countries. This shift from a high prevalence of undernutrition to a situation where NR-NCDs predominate is referred to as the 'nutrition transition'.

The dietary changes associated with the nutrition transition are outlined below and commented on in relation to global trends in the following sections of this chapter.

Against a background of urbanisation, economic growth, technological changes for work, leisure and food processing, mass media growth, the changes in dietary and activity patterns can be summarised in three stages:

1. Receding famine pattern characterised by: diet – starchy, low variety, low fat, high fibre; labour intensive work/leisure
2. Degenerative disease pattern characterised by: increased fat, sugar, processed foods; shift in technology of work and leisure
3. Behavioural change pattern characterised by: reduced fat, increased fruit and vegetables, carbohydrate, fibre; increased activity (Popkin 2002).

Although lifestyle and other factors clearly lie behind these changes in eating habits (Fig. 1.2) there are other aspects of the 'globalisation' process that need to be recognised as having a powerful part to play in shaping food choice. Throughout history foods have 'migrated' and been incorporated into the diets of people thousands of miles away – the tomato and potato, originally from America, transformed the cuisines of Europe. These dietary changes have sometimes had huge social consequences, as in the case of sugar and the slave trade or the development of the Irish dependence on the potato and subsequent impact of the potato famine. What is different about the changes in the past 50 years is

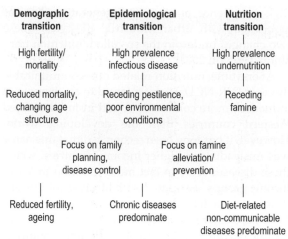

Figure 1.2 The demographic, epidemiological and nutrition transitions. (Modified from Popkin 2002, with permission.)

Table 1.6 Supply of vegetables per capita, by region, 1979 and 2000 (kg per capita per year)		
Region	**1979**	**2000**
World	66.1	101.9
Developed countries	107.4	112.8
Developing countries	51.1	98.8
Africa	45.4	52.1
North and Central America	88.7	98.3
South America	43.2	47.8
Asia	56.6	116.2
Europe	110.9	112.5
Oceania	71.8	98.7

the pace and scale of change. This is in part due to the application of marketing techniques to mould changes in taste. Most cuisines have traditionally included 'fast foods' but the spread of the hamburger has been achieved through systematic and sophisticated marketing strategies. For a case study on the hamburger in Hong Kong see Section CD 1.4(b). The current phase of globalisation is also marked by concentration at regional, national and international levels. This applies throughout the food chain including production, processing and retailing. Decisions in all these areas affect the choices that people can exercise about what they actually eat. A relatively small number of companies dominate the world food markets, affecting every aspect of the route from farm to consumer. Supermarkets place contracts with distant suppliers to enable previously seasonal foods to be available all year round. The UK's food manufacturing sector is also highly concentrated. In 1995, three companies (Unilever, Cadbury Schweppes and Associated British Foods) dominated UK food manufacturing, and half the world's top 100 food sector companies are US-owned. Estimates suggest that the global food industry will come to be dominated by up to 200 groups who account for approximately two-thirds of sales. In the classical market economy, many suppliers compete for the attention of the consumer, responding to what the consumer wants. It has been suggested that in the evolving hypermarket economy, sophisticated systems of contracts and specifications and tight managerial control enable the retailer rather than the primary food producer or consumer to control the entire supply chain.

Selection of foods which are *acceptable* to an individual increasingly takes place in a context where *availability* is substantially influenced by the food industry and food retailers.

Examples of variation in diets over time

For more detailed information see Section CD 1.4(c).

Worldwide

On a worldwide basis the consumption of meat, milk, and eggs varies widely among countries, reflecting differences in food production resources, production systems, income, and cultural factors. Per capita consumption is much higher in developed countries but the current rapid increase in many developing countries is projected to continue. Total meat consumption in developing countries is projected to more than double by the year 2020, while, in developed countries, it is projected to increase no more and, in some cases, less than population growth. Because most of the world's population is in developing countries, which are experiencing the most rapid growth rates, global demand for meat is projected to increase by more than 60% of current consumption by 2020. Thus, diets in developing countries are changing with rising incomes. The share of staples, such as cereals, roots and tubers, is declining, while that of meat, dairy products and oil crops is rising. Between 1964–1966 and 1997–1999, per capita meat consumption in developing countries rose by 150% and that of milk and dairy products by 60% (see Ch. 32).

Table 1.6 outlines world trends in the supply of vegetables and indicates the regional and temporal variations in the per capita availability of vegetables

Table 1.7 **Trends in the dietary supply of fat**

Region	Supply of fat (g per capita per day)				% increase from
	1967–69	1977–79	1987–89	1997–99	1978–79 to 1997–99
North Africa	44	58	65	64	10
Sub-Saharan Africa	41	43	41	45	5
North America	117	125	138	143	14
Latin America and the Caribbean	54	65	73	79	22
China	24	27	48	79	193
East and Southeast Asia	28	32	44	52	63
South Asia	29	32	39	45	41
European Community	117	128	143	148	16
Eastern Europe	90	111	116	104	−6
Near East	51	62	73	70	13
Oceania	102	102	113	113	11
World	53	57	67	73	28

Note: Sub-Saharan Africa excludes South Africa.
Source: SCN 2004 The Firth Report on the World Nutrition Situation. UN Standing Committee on Nutrition, Geneva.

per year over the past few decades. In 2000, the global annual average per capita vegetable supply was 102 kg, with the highest level in Asia (116 kg), and the lowest levels in South America (48 kg) and Africa (52 kg).

Diets in developing countries are changing rapidly, as incomes grow, populations urbanise and age, and food choice options change. The latter occurs due to transformations in food technology (such as global positioning systems and other information and communications technology) and food distribution systems (such as a reduction in the numbers of wholesalers and retailers and longer food chain linkages). The transition in diets is happening most rapidly in China (see Ch. 33 and Table 1.7, and in middle income, urbanising countries such as Brazil, Mexico, Indonesia and Nigeria. The diet transition is causing a relative shift in the causes of disease away from those related to undernutrition only, towards those related to both under- and over-nutrition – the nutrition transition.

Europe

As trade and cultural links within the European Union (EU) have strengthened over time, the consumption patterns of the first 15 EU members (EU-15) have been converging. A new study from FAO's Global Perspectives Studies Group, based on Food Balance Sheets (FBS), shows that the diets of the UK and Sweden were much more similar to the USA in the 1960s, but are now more similar to the EU average. Similarly Mediterranean diets have moved more towards the EU mainstream although variations persist. There has been little convergence of diets between the EU average and the USA; they are still relatively distinct, with the latter consuming much higher levels of added sugars.

Examples of temporal changes in a southern European country may be seen in Italy. In the early 1960s the diet consumed in the rural population of southern Italy was based mainly on cereals, fresh vegetables and olive oil. It was low in animal fat, protein and cholesterol and high in fibre. Since then, there has been a progressive move towards a higher nutrient density with fat intake increasing from 28% energy at that time to 36% in the 1980s. For trends in cereals consumption in selected European countries between 1972 and 1997, see Figure CD 1.1.

The UK

Consistent survey-based estimates of diets are available only for the rich countries. In the UK, the National Food Survey (NFS) reveals 50-year trends in food intakes from 1940 to 1990 (MAFF 1991).

World War II and its aftermath had a significant effect on the UK diet. During the war years and in the early post-war years dietary habits were shaped by the prevailing scarcity and restriction of many foods at that time. While many foods such as fruits and meat were restricted others such as foods rich in starch including potatoes and wholemeal brown bread (known as national bread) were increased.

From 1954, consumers were able to return to their pre-war diets, higher in butter, sugar, fresh meat and white bread. It was not until the 1980s that the brown and wholemeal breads considered as healthier foods become more popular again. The 50-year trend shows a marked decline in total bread consumption. While brown bread declined sharply it was only partly replaced by white bread.

Recent changes in the pattern of milk products in the UK are reflected in a lower proportion of the population consuming full fat milk and more consuming semi-skimmed and skimmed milk. This may have resulted from dietary guidelines recommending a reduction in total fat and more specifically saturated fat intake (see Section CD 33.4(a)). Thus, there is now a substantial demand for low fat and skimmed milk. In addition, butter has been partly replaced by margarines and low fat spreads. These changes are most evident from the early 1980s when lower fat products became readily available. The decreasing consumption has also been accompanied by an increase in vegetable oils.

The main temporal changes in meat consumption between 1940 and 1990 were the rise in consumption of beef, lamb and pork in the early 1950s and the subsequent decline in lamb consumption. This has been accompanied by a huge rise in the consumption of chicken, which was rarely consumed 50 years ago in the UK and has now become the most common form of dietary protein. Overall, fish consumption trends show little change from a low intake level. Taken together fruit and vegetable consumption has not changed appreciably in the last 50 years in the UK. Vegetables have declined slightly but this has been offset by the increase in fruit consumption. There has been a decline in intakes of brassica vegetables including cabbage, cauliflower and Brussels sprouts as well as the traditional root vegetables. On the other hand, there has been an increase in salad vegetables and frozen vegetables. The consumption of frozen vegetables has increased by a factor of 6 since 1965, of which frozen peas are the single largest contributor accounting for 25% of all frozen vegetables consumed. The sizeable increase in the consumption of the fruit group since the 1970s may be attributed to fruit juice (now accounting for 75% of fruit products) as well as the increasing year-round availability of fresh fruit. Apples are the most commonly consumed fruit followed by bananas and oranges. The changes in consumption of specific fruit and vegetables between 1975 and 1995 may be seen in Figure CD 1.2.

Novel foods

'Novel foods' are foods or food ingredients that do not have a significant history of consumption in the European Union before 1997 (see also Section CD 1.4(d)). A novel food may be defined as: (1) a substance, including a microorganism, that does not have a history of safe use as a food; (2) a food that has been manufactured, prepared, preserved or packaged by a process that (i) has not been previously applied to that food, and (ii) causes the food to undergo a major change; (3) a food that is derived from a plant, animal or microorganism that has been genetically modified such that (i) the plant, animal or microorganism exhibits characteristics that were not previously observed in that plant, animal or microorganism, (ii) the plant, animal or microorganism no longer exhibits characteristics that were previously observed in that plant, animal or microorganism, or (iii) one or more characteristics of the plant, animal or microorganism no longer fall within the anticipated range for that plant, animal or microorganism.

Most of these products are crop plants (e.g. corn, canola (rape), potatoes and soya bean) that have been genetically modified to improve agronomic characteristics such as crop yield, hardiness and uniformity, insect and virus resistance, and herbicide tolerance. Tomatoes that express delayed ripening characteristics have also been assessed and approved. A few of the products have been modified to intentionally change the composition, e.g. canola oil with increased levels of lauric acid. In the UK, the Food Standards Agency has a research programme on the safety of novel foods, with specific emphasis on GM foods. However, other novel foods, including 'functional foods', also fall within the scope of this programme.

Genetically modified foods

Genetically modified foods (GM foods) have ingredients in them that have been modified by a technique called gene technology (see Ch. 32 for further details). This technology allows food producers to alter certain characteristics of a food crop by introducing genetic material and proteins from another source. An example of this is a corn plant with a gene that makes it resistant to insect attack. With this technology it is possible to speed up the breeding of new and 'improved' crop varieties and to introduce completely new genetic information, for example from bacteria or animals into plants. Currently, only genetically modified soya beans and maize have been approved within the EU market. However, several others have been notified to the Commission as being substantially equivalent to traditional varieties according to the 1997 *Novel Food Directive*. In the USA more than 50 new recombinant-DNA (r-DNA) derived foods have been evaluated successfully by the Food and Drug Administration. The USA is the market leader in the total area occupied by genetically modified crops at 68%, while in Europe the figure is close to zero. For almost a decade genetically modified foods such as corn, soya beans, canola and tomatoes have been part of the American diet. This is not the case in Europe. It may well be that recent food safety issues such as the BSE outbreak in Europe and the way they were dealt with (or more importantly perceived to be inadequately dealt with) and the decided lack of trust in government sources with respect to information on food safety have resulted in the slower adoption of GM foods in Europe. (See also Section CD 1.4(e).)

Functional foods

Consuming a nutritionally balanced diet was formerly considered as eating an adequate diet to avoid deficiency. But among developed countries, consuming a nutritionally balanced diet has come to mean consuming an optimal diet for promoting health as well as reducing the risk of diet-related chronic diseases. Optimal nutrition focuses on optimising the quality of the diet in terms of its quantity of nutrients and non-nutrients that favour the maintenance of health. This is where functional foods may have an important role to play since they are considered to have a specific role in relation to disease or the promotion of health. Indeed, a functional food is one claiming to have additional benefits other than nutritional value, for example a margarine that contains a cholesterol-lowering ingredient.

A functional food may be a natural food in which one of the components has been naturally enhanced through special growing conditions, a food to which a component has been added to provide benefits, a food from which a component has been removed so that the food has less adverse health effects (e.g. the reduction of saturated fatty acids), a food in which the nature of one or more components has been chemically modified to improve health (e.g. the hydrolysed protein in infant formulas to reduce the likelihood of allergenicity) or a food in which the bioavailability of one or more components has been increased to provide greater absorption of a beneficial component. A recent and comprehensive review of the role of functional foods in health is published in a recent supplement to the British Journal of Nutrition, including their possible future role (Westrate et al 2002). (See also Section CD 1.4(f).)

⊃ Key points

⊃ The typical Western diet is characterised by a diet relatively high in fat and low in carbohydrates when compared to the typical diet of most developing countries.

⊃ While nutrient intakes and even broad food groups may not differ dramatically between developed countries (for example in Europe) the foods that contribute to these nutrient intakes do differ markedly. Despite some recent convergence within the EU, there is no single 'Western diet', or even European diet. The European diet differs considerably in the foods that compose it. Factors in dietary variations include those that are: physiological, such as age, gender, pregnancy, lactation, activity; economic; cultural and religious; psychological; beliefs and perceptions, such as risk, benefit; educational; related to food characteristics such as taste, appearance, texture; and extrinsic, such as advertising.

⊃ Diets in developing countries are changing rapidly, driven by urbanisation, food distribution and retail technology, increased trade, income growth and food price policies. Rather than transition from undernutrition through health to overnutrition, many countries are moving to a situation of a double burden of malnutrition. This double burden is characterised by many people in a given population not getting enough food in terms of quality and quantity coexisting with many who are in danger of chronic disease due to excess calorie, fat, sugar or salt consumption.

⊃ While nutrient intakes have remained remarkably consistent in the last 50 years (in the UK) there have been certain notable changes in food consumption patterns, e.g. the partial replacement of butter by low fat spreads and vegetable-based margarines, the partial replacement of full fat milk by low fat and skimmed milk, an increase in fruit juice consumption, a decrease in certain vegetables (e.g. swedes, turnips and Brussels sprouts), which have been replaced by salad vegetables and mushrooms. This changing pattern in food intakes is also evident in other countries.

⊃ The most important sources of dietary fibre in the British diet are cereal products and vegetables (including potatoes) and fruits.

⊃ Novel foods, including genetically modified and functional foods, are increasing in the Western diet with increasing emphasis on an optimal diet for promoting health as well as reducing the risk of diet-related chronic diseases. The rigorous safety evaluations that these foods must undergo should increase their consumer acceptance.

References and further reading

References

Birch L L, Zimmerman S, Hind H 1980 The effect of social-affective context on pre-school children's food preferences. Child Development 51:856–861

Cardello A 1996 The role of human senses in food acceptance. In: Meiselman H L, MacFie H J H (eds) Food choice, acceptance and consumption. Blackie Academic & Professional, London, pp 1–82

Darmon N, Briend A, Drewnowski A 2004 Energy-dense diets are associated with lower diet costs: a community study of French adults. Public Health Nutrition 7(1):21–27

Fomon S J, Filer L J, Thomas L N et al 1969 Relationship between formula concentration and rate of growth in normal children. Journal of Nutrition 198:241–243

Gregory J, Foster K, Tyler H, Wiseman M (Ministry of Agriculture, Fisheries and Food) 1990 The dietary and nutritional survey of British adults. HMSO, London

Ministry of Agriculture, Fisheries and Food 1991 Fifty years of the National Food Survey, 1940–1990 (ed. J M Slater). HMSO, London

McMichael P 2001 The impact of globalisation, free trade and technology on food and nutrition in the new millennium. Proceedings of the Nutrition Society 60:215–220

Office for National Statistics 2002 Expenditure and Food Survey 2001–2002. The Stationery Office, London

Popkin B M (Special Editor) 2002 The Bellagio Conference on the Nutrition Transition and its implications for health in the developing world. Public Heath Nutrition (Special Issue) 5(1A):1–280

Rolls B J 1986 Sensory-specific satiety. Nutrition Reviews 44:93–101

Schroll K, Moreiras-Varela O, Schlettwein-Gsell D et al 1997 Cross-cultural variations and changes in food-group intake among elderly women in Europe: results from the survey in Europe on nutrition and the elderly a concerted action: (SENECA). American Journal of Clinical Nutrition 65(suppl):1282S–1289S

Weststrate J A, van Poppel G, Verschuren P M 2002 Functional foods, trends and future. British Journal of Nutrition 88(suppl 2):S233–S235

Further reading

Fieldhouse P 1995 Food and nutrition: customs and culture. Chapman & Hall, London

Gibney M J 1999 Nutrition, physical activity and health status in Europe: an overview. Public Health Nutrition (Special Issue) 2(3A):329–334

Lang T 1999 Diet, health and globalisation: five key questions. Proceedings of the Nutrition Society 58:335–343

Meiselman H L, Macfie H J H (eds) 1996 Food choice, acceptance and consumption. Blackie Academic and Professional, London

Paul A A, Southgate D A T 1978 McCance and Widdowson's The composition of foods, 4th edn. HMSO, London

Roberfroid M B 2000 Defining functional foods. In: Gibson G, Williams C (eds) Functional foods. Woodhead Publishing, Cambridge, UK

Vaughan J G, Geissler C A 1997 The new Oxford book of food plants. Oxford University Press, Oxford

CD-ROM contents

Expanded material

Section CD 1.2 Nutritional importance of major foods and food products in the Western diet

Section CD 1.3(a) Examples of variations in diets

Section CD 1.3(b) Europe and the USA

Section CD 1.3(c) Economic and regional variation in food consumption in the UK

Section CD 1.3(d) Hunger, and satiety – the satiety cascade

Section CD 1.4(a) Migration and eating habits – minority ethnic groups in the UK

Section CD 1.4(b) The hamburger in Hong Kong

Section CD 1.4(c) Examples of variation in diets over time

Section CD 1.4(d) Novel foods

Section CD 1.4(e) Genetically modified foods

Section CD 1.4(f) Functional foods

Tables

Table CD 1.1 Food groups making important contributions to macronutrient intakes by UK adults

Table CD 1.2 Food groups making important contributions to vitamin intakes by UK adults

Table CD 1.3 Food groups making important contributions to mineral intakes by UK adults

Table CD 1.4 The main food sources of dietary fibre among UK adults

Table CD 1.5 Daily consumption of selected foods among men in selected European countries (grouped by consumption of total fat)

Table CD 1.6 Fruit and vegetable consumption in adults in selected European countries (by latest available year)

Table CD 1.7 Percentage of total energy from fat in adults in selected European countries (latest available year)

Table CD 1.8 Per cent energy from fatty acid categories in selected EU member countries

Table CD 1.9 Food consumption (Highest and Lowest) according to region in the UK 1998–2000

Table CD 1.10 Consumption of selected foods by income group of head of household, in the UK 2000

Figures

Figure CD 1.1 Trends in % total energy from cereals in selected European countries, 1972–1997

Figure CD 1.2 Consumption of fruit and vegetables in the UK between 1975 and 1995

Additional references related to CD-ROM material

Further reading

Further reading from the book

Useful websites

2

Food and nutrient structure

Michael H. Gordon

Objectives

By the end of this chapter you should be able to:

- describe the main structures of the macronutrients
- characterise the effects of food processing on nutrient content
- describe the main types of natural toxins, pollutants and pathogenic agents
- identify the classes and functions of phytoprotectants.

2.1 INTRODUCTION

Humans have found that a wide range of plant varieties, animals, and some microbial sources can be consumed as food. Originally, food raw materials were selected on the basis of materials that could be consumed without harmful effects, and it was subsequently found that processing of foods by heat could improve the texture, and in some cases inactivate harmful components within the food. As understanding of the composition of foods has developed, it has become convenient to classify food components into macronutrients, which are present as bulk components of foods, and micronutrients, which are present at lower levels. Energy is mainly derived from the macronutrients, which comprise carbohydrates, fat, proteins and alcohol, but both macronutrients and micronutrients provide dietary components that are essential for normal physiological processes. This chapter informs readers about the chemical structures, properties and functions of a wide range of food components including nutrients and toxic substances. The effects of processing and storage on these components are discussed.

2.2 CHEMICAL CHARACTERISTICS OF MACRONUTRIENTS

Carbohydrates

Carbohydrates are mainly important as a source of energy (16 kJ/g or 3.8 kcal/g) in the human diet, being converted to glycogen or fat as energy stores. Carbohydrates include simple sugars, such as glucose, fructose and sucrose, plus polymers of sugars, which are termed polysaccharides, of which starch is the most important dietary component. Other polysaccharides include glycogen and cellulose. Many properties of sugars and polysaccharides are very different, but the molecular formula of all carbohydrates approximates to $(CH_2O)_n$, and the presence of carbon and water in this structure is why the class gained its name. Carbohydrates are synthesised in plants from carbon dioxide and water during photosynthesis.

Sugars

Monosaccharides are the building blocks for oligosaccharides and polysaccharides. Monosaccharides and some oligosaccharides occur as sweet components in foods, with glucose and fructose being the most common monosaccharides, and lactose and sucrose being examples of oligosaccharides that are sweet and are classed as sugars. Oligosaccharides contain from 2 to 10 monosaccharide units linked together. The sweetness found in the monosaccharides disappears in the higher molecular weight oligosaccharides. Polysaccharides have very different properties from sugars, since they are non-sweet and their solubility in water is normally very low. They are commonly of significance as thickeners or gelling agents in foods.

Glucose occurs in fruits and vegetables, but it is also formed by the hydrolysis of oligosaccharides and polysaccharides during digestion in the small intestine.

Fructose occurs together with glucose in fruits and vegetables and in some sweet foods such as honey. Hydrolysis of sucrose in the small intestine is also a source of fructose.

The chemical structures of monosaccharides comprise chains of between four and six carbon atoms with multiple hydroxyl substituents. Each monosaccharide contains a carbonyl group along the chain, and this may either be at the end of the chain, in which case it corresponds to an aldehyde, e.g. glucose, or it may be away from the end of the chain, in which case it corresponds to a ketone group as in fructose. The chemical structures can be represented in several ways. The Fischer projection formula is often used to show sugar structures. Figures 2.1 and 2.2 show the orientation of the hydrogen atoms and hydroxyl groups relative to carbon atoms (which are not drawn but which are present at each point where four bonds meet). The ends of the carbon skeleton are behind the plane of the paper with the substituents above the plane of the paper (Fig. 2.1).

In solution, monosaccharides exist as the open chain form shown in Figure 2.1 in equilibrium with ring forms (Fig. 2.2), which develop when one of the hydroxyl groups forms an intramolecular bond with the carbonyl carbon atom. Since six-membered rings are most stable, glucose exists in solution as an equilibrium between the open chain form (2%) and the six-membered ring forms termed glucopyranose (98%). When the open chain form of a sugar closes to form a ring, the hydroxyl group at carbon-1 may either be in an axial position in the chair structure as in α-glucopyranose or in an equatorial position as in β-glucopyranose. These isomers are termed anomers.

Monosaccharide units may be linked together by an acetal or glycosidic link which is formed when the carbonyl group of one monosaccharide unit links to a hydroxyl group on a second monosaccharide unit. Molecules comprising a small number of monosaccharide units are termed oligosaccharides, with sucrose, maltose and lactose being common disaccharides, comprising two monosaccharide units. Raffinose and stachyose are examples of tri- and tetrasaccharides that occur in foods.

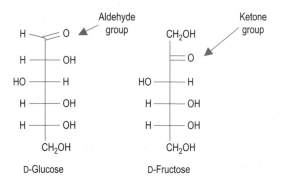

D-Glucose   D-Fructose

Figure 2.1   Common sugar structures.

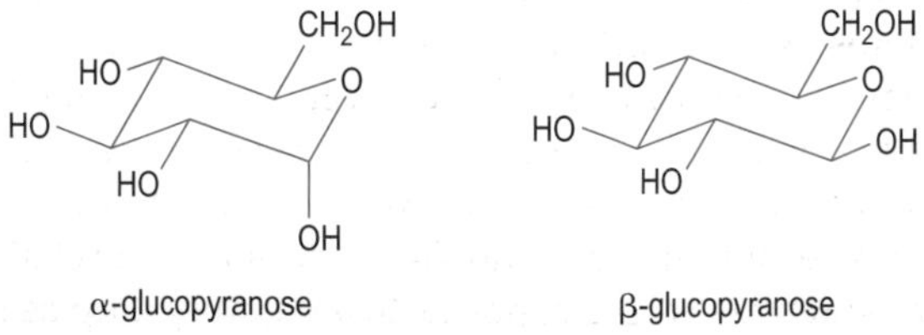

α-glucopyranose   β-glucopyranose

Figure 2.2   The ring forms of glucose and fructose.

Sucrose is well known as the most common sugar used in domestic kitchens and added to processed foods. It is refined on an industrial scale from sugar cane and sugar beet. Hydrolysis of sucrose during digestion provides glucose and fructose.

Lactose is present in cow's milk at about 4.7% of the milk, which corresponds to nearly 40% of the dry matter in milk. Its concentration in human milk is even higher at about 6.8% of the milk or nearly 60% of the dry matter in the milk. Hydrolysis of lactose forms galactose and glucose.

Polysaccharides

Polysaccharides contain large numbers of monosaccharide units linked together. Polysaccharides include starch, glycogen and cellulose, which are all polymers of glucose. They vary in whether the monosaccharide units are linked by α- or β-linkages, and whether they are linear or branched. These structural features are important since many enzymes including those of significance for digestion of the polysaccharides are selective in terms of which type of linkage are cleaved in the presence of the enzyme.

Starch, which is an important polysaccharide in plant foods including potatoes and bread, is a mixture of two polymers, amylose and amylopectin. Amylose contains glucose units linked by α-linkages between carbon-1 and carbon-4 of successive monosaccharide units, and these linkages cause the molecule to be linear. Amylopectin contains some α-1 → 6 linkages as well as α-1 → 4 linkages, and the α-1 → 6 linkages cause the polysaccharide to be branched. Starches from different plants differ in properties due to variations in the ratio of amylose to amylopectin present.

Glycogen is the form in which animals store carbohydrates, and this is similar to amylopectin in having both α-1 → 4 and α-1 → 6 linkages between glucose molecules, although there are rather more α-1 → 6-linkages than in amylopectin.

Cellulose is a polymer of glucose with β-1 → 4 linkages between the glucose units. As a consequence of this structure, cellulose is non-digestible because humans lack enzymes which are capable of hydrolysing polymers of glucose linked by β-glycosidic bonds. In contrast, starch is split by amylases, which are secreted by the salivary glands and by the small intestine, so that starch is initially hydrolysed to disaccharides which can be hydrolysed to monosaccharides for absorption.

Pectins are important polysaccharides for the food industry. They occur in fruits and vegetables including apples and carrots, but they are important for their gelling properties in acid foods with a high sugar content such as jam. Pectins are polymers mainly comprising α-1 → 4 linked galacturonic acid with some other sugars. The degree of esterification of the polysaccharide has a major effect on the gelling properties.

Fats

Fats are components of foods that are extractable with organic solvents such as hexane or diethyl ether, but are insoluble in water. Dietary fats are converted to energy (37 kJ/g or 8.8 kcal/g), but they are also sources of essential fatty acids. Dietary fatty acids or metabolites are incorporated into phospholipids in cell membranes to provide the membrane structure. Essential fatty acids are converted into prostaglandins and other biologically active compounds described as eicosanoids, which control biochemical reactions within cells.

Fats comprise several classes of chemical compounds, which are termed lipids. The bulk of the fats in food (often >95% of the fat) are triacylglycerols, which are often referred to by the more traditional name of triglycerides. These molecules consist of three fatty acid residues esterified to a glycerol backbone (see Fig. CD 2.1). The properties of triacylglycerols depend on the structures of the constituent fatty acid residues. The structure of fatty acids consists of a chain of carbon atoms with the required number of hydrogen atoms attached and a carboxylic acid residue at one end of the chain. The most common fatty acids have a chain of 16 or 18 carbon atoms, but fatty acids with between 4 and 22 carbon atoms occur in food lipids. Fatty acids with even numbers of carbon atoms occur almost exclusively because of the biosynthetic pathway by which they are formed in plants and animals. Fatty acids may be classified according to the number of carbon–carbon double bonds as saturated with 0, monounsaturated with 1, and polyunsaturated with 2–6 (Fig. 2.3; Fig. CD 2.2).

In polyunsaturated fatty acids, each of the carbon–carbon double bonds is separated from the next double bond by a methylene (CH_2) group. This allows a convenient short-hand nomenclature to be used for fatty acid structures with the number of carbon atoms in the fatty acid chain followed by a colon, the number of double bonds and then the position of the double bond nearest the methyl end of the fatty acid chain. The number of carbons (x) from the methyl end of the molecule is indicated by n-x. Hence linoleic acid may be represented as 18:2 (n-6). An alternative nomenclature is to denote the position of the double bond by ω, so that linoleic acid is denoted as 18:2 ω6.

The most common fatty acids in food lipids are oleic acid (18:1 n-9), palmitic acid (16:0), stearic acid (18:0), linoleic acid (18:2 n-6) and α-linolenic acid (18:3 n-3). The nutritionally important polyunsaturated fatty acids eicosapentaenoic acid (EPA) (20:5 n-3) and docosahexaenoic acid (DHA) (22:6 n-3) are present in fish oil. Linoleic and linolenic acids are important dietary components because humans lack the enzymes required to introduce double bonds into fatty acids at the n-6 or n-3 positions, but metabolism of linoleic and linolenic acids allows the biosynthesis of metabolites including arachidonic acid (20:4 n-6) and eicosapentaenoic acid (20:5 n-3) by desaturation and chain elongation. Although longer chain metabolites may be formed from 18:3 n-3, the consumption of EPA and DHA (22:6 n-3), which occur in fish oils, has been found to be beneficial in reducing inflammation and risk factors for coronary heart disease including plasma triacylglycerol levels.

Structure	Class
$CH_3-(CH_2)_4-CH=CH-CH_2-CH=CH-(CH_2)_7\ COOH$	Polyunsaturated (Linoleic acid, 18:2 n-6)
$CH_3-(CH_2)_7-CH=CH-(CH_2)_7\ COOH$	Monounsaturated (Oleic acid, 18:1 n-9)
$CH_3-(CH_2)_{16}\ COOH$	Saturated (Stearic acid, 18:0)

Figure 2.3   Fatty acid structures.

The substituents at carbon–carbon double bonds of fatty acids may be on the same side of the bond (*cis*) or on the opposite side of the double bond (*trans*), as shown in Figure 2.4. The configuration of the double bonds in natural plant lipids is exclusively *cis*, although small amounts of *trans*-unsaturated fatty acids are found in animal fats, such as milk fat, due to formation by hydrogenation of polyunsaturated fatty acids in the rumen of the animal. *Trans* fatty acids are also sometimes found in processed foods because fats containing these fatty acids can be prepared from liquid oils by an industrial process known as hydrogenation and these fats have the correct melting properties for use in foods such as margarine. However, because of concern about the health effects of excessive levels of intake of *trans* fatty acids, manufacturers in western Europe normally use other methods of preparing fats that do not form *trans* fatty acids. Low levels of *trans* fatty acids are consumed in foods containing animal products such as butter, or are present at very low levels in vegetable oils as a consequence of the heating that the oil is subjected to during refining. Although *cis* and *trans* unsaturated fatty acids are similar in chemical structure (Fig. 2.4), the different stereochemistry has important consequences. Polyunsaturated fatty acids containing one or more *trans* double bonds cannot act as essential fatty acids. Excessive dietary intake of *trans* unsaturated fatty acids may lead to increased risk of cardiovascular disease.

Besides triacylglycerols, phospholipids are the second major lipid class in foods.

Phospholipids are important structural components in biological membranes, and consequently are present in plants and animals consumed as food. The main phospholipids are phosphatidylcholine, phosphatidylethanolamine, phosphatidylserine, phosphatidylinositol and phosphatidic acid. These are acylglycerol derivatives with fatty acids at positions 1 and 2 of the glycerol molecule, with a phosphoric acid derivative at carbon-3 (see Fig. CD 2.3). Phospholipids are added to many foods as they act as emulsifiers, helping to stabilise emulsions such as mayonnaise.

Sterols occur as minor lipid components in biological membranes. Animal tissues contain almost exclusively cholesterol (see Fig. CD 2.4), whereas plant tissues contain a mixture of sterols, termed phytosterols, with β-sitosterol being a major component. Other phytosterols include campesterol and stigmasterol. Sterols are extracted with edible oils and fats from plant tissues, and they commonly occur at <1% concentration in edible oils such as sunflower oil. Their solubility in oils is limited but much higher levels of sterols have been incorporated into some functional foods by esterification of the sterols with fatty acids to form steryl esters. A functional food may be defined as a food having health-promoting benefits and/or disease-preventing properties over and above its usual nutritional value. In the case of foods containing steryl esters, the effect is to reduce blood serum cholesterol levels.

Other lipids occur as minor components in foods. These include glycolipids, sphingolipids, mono- and diacylglycerols and fat-soluble vitamins.

Proteins

Proteins are nitrogen-containing macromolecules that occur in major amounts in foods. Dietary proteins provide energy (17 kJ/g or 4.06 kcal/g) but they are also sources of amino acids that are essential for the synthesis of a wide variety of proteins with important functions including carriers of vitamins, oxygen, and carbon dioxide plus enzymes and structural proteins (Table 2.1). Proteins comprise polymers of amino acids with molecular weights varying from about 5000 up to several million. Twenty amino acids occur in most proteins (Fig. 2.5) but additional amino acids, namely hydroxyproline and hydroxylysine, occur in some animal proteins such as gelatine (see Fig. CD 2.5). In proteins, the amino acids are linked together by peptide linkages, which are formed when the carboxylic acid group of one amino acid condenses with the amine group of a second amino acid with the elimination of water.

Most amino acids have the chemical structure $H_2N-C(R)H -COOH$, with variation in chemical structure arising from the nature of the substituent R, which may correspond to an aromatic or aliphatic residue or to a hydrogen atom in the case of glycine. In the case of proline, the amino acid contains a

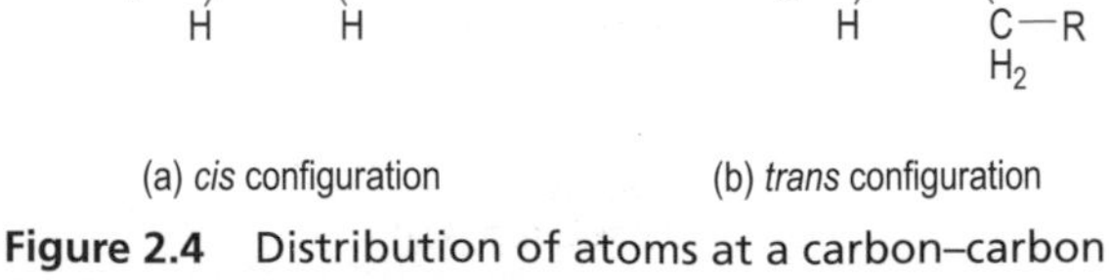

(a) *cis* configuration   (b) *trans* configuration

Figure 2.4 Distribution of atoms at a carbon–carbon double bond: (a) *cis* and (b) *trans* configuration.

Amino acid	Abbreviation	Side chain (R)
Alanine	Ala	CH_3-
Arginine	Arg	$\begin{array}{c} H_2N \\ \quad \diagdown \\ \qquad N-C-C-C- \\ HN \diagup \quad \underset{H}{|} \quad \underset{H_2}{|} \quad \underset{H_2}{|} \quad \underset{H_2}{|} \end{array}$
Aspartic acid	Asp	$HOOC-CH_2-$
Cysteine	Cys	$HSCH_2-$
Glutamic acid	Glu	$HOOC-CH_2-CH_2-$
Glycine	Gly	$H-$
Histidine	His	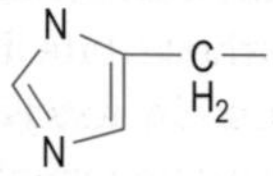 imidazole ring with $-\underset{H_2}{C}-$
Isoleucine	Ile	$CH_3-CH_2-\underset{\underset{CH_3}{|}}{CH}-$
Leucine	Leu	$\begin{array}{c} H_3C \\ \quad \diagdown \\ \qquad \underset{H_2}{C}- \\ H_3C \diagup \end{array}$
Lysine	Lys	$H_3\overset{+}{N}-\underset{H_2}{C}-\underset{H_2}{C}-\underset{H_2}{C}-\underset{H_2}{C}-$
Methionine	Met	$H_3C-S-\underset{H_2}{C}-\underset{H_2}{C}$
Phenylalanine	Phe	benzene ring $-CH_2-$
Serine	Ser	$HOCH_2-$
Threonine	Thr	$\begin{array}{c} H_3C-\underset{\underset{OH}{|}}{}- \end{array}$
Tryptophan	Trp	indole ring with $-\underset{H_2}{C}-$
Tyrosine	Tyr	$HO-$ phenyl ring $-CH_2-$
Valine	Val	$\begin{array}{c} H_3C \\ \quad \diagdown \\ \quad \diagup \\ H_3C \end{array}$
Proline	Pro	Formula: 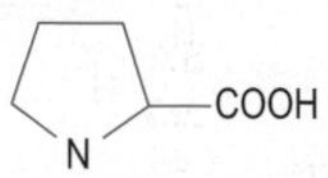 pyrrolidine ring $-COOH$

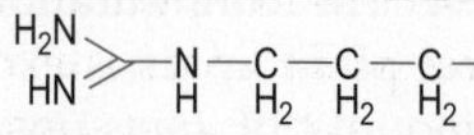

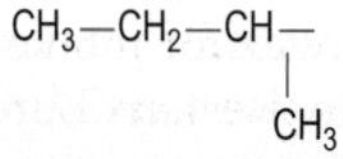

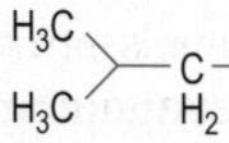

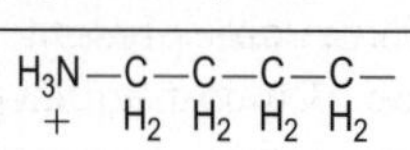

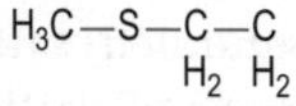

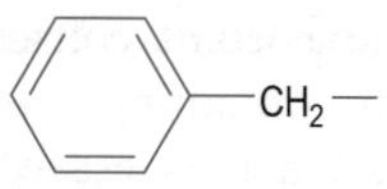

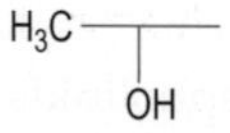

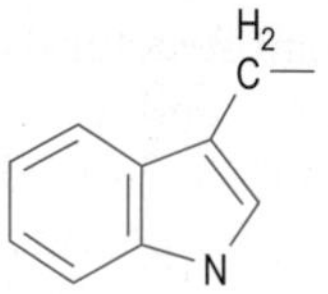

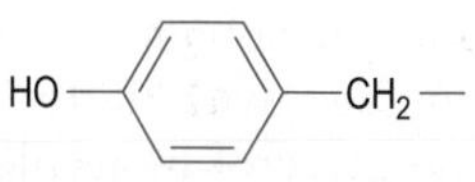

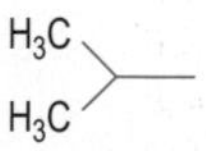

Figure 2.5 Amino acid structures.

secondary amine group in a ring instead of a primary amine group. The common amino acids comprise alanine, arginine, asparagine, aspartic acid, cysteine, glutamine, glutamic acid, glycine, histidine, isoleucine, leucine, lysine, methionine, phenylalanine, proline, serine, threonine, tryptophan, tyrosine and valine. These amino acids provide the common polypeptide backbone of proteins, with the identity of the amino acids determining the substituents along the polypeptide chain of the protein. The amino acid sequence of a protein is described as the primary structure of the protein.

Plants can synthesise all the amino acids they need from inorganic nutrients, but animals cannot synthesise the amine group. Animals must consume plants in order to introduce amino acids for protein synthesis, but they are able to synthesise some amino acids by transamination in which an amine group is shifted from one amino acid to another. Transaminases act with pyridoxal phosphate as a coenzyme to catalyse this reaction. However, isoleucine, leucine, lysine, methionine, phenylalanine, threonine, tryptophan and valine cannot be synthesised in this way and these amino acids are described as essential amino acids, because they can only be introduced into the body by eating foods that contain these amino

acids. The adult human body can maintain nitrogen equilibrium on a mixture of these amino acids as the sole source of nitrogen. If one or more of the essential amino acids is omitted from the diet, an adult would go into negative nitrogen balance. In the case of infants, histidine is also needed for growth.

The secondary structure of a protein is the conformation that the protein adopts along the long axis. The native protein adopts a certain conformation, which is energetically favourable. The precise conformation of a protein depends on the polarity, hydrophobicity and steric hindrance of the side-chains of the amino acids in the protein. The α-helix is a conformation that is adopted by many proteins. It has 3.6 amino acid residues per turn with a separation of 0.54 nm between successive coils of the helix (Fig. 2.6). The α-helix is stabilised by hydrogen-bonding between the backbone carbonyl of one residue and the backbone NH of the fourth residue along the chain.

The β-pleated sheet is another common secondary protein structure (Fig. 2.7). The sheet is formed from several individual β-strands, which are at a distance from each other along the primary protein sequence. The individual strands are aligned next to each other in such a way that the peptide carbonyl oxygens hydrogen-bond with neighbouring NH

Table 2.1 **Amino acid composition of selected proteins (%)**						
Amino acid	**Bovine serum albumin**	**Casein**	**Gelatin**	**Whole egg**	**Pork**	**Beef**
Alanine	6.3	3.1	11.0	5.4	15.3	20.0
Arginine	5.9	3.3	8.8	6.1	–	–
Aspartic acid	10.9	7.6	6.7	10.7	5.0	0.5
Cystine (0.5)	6.0	0.3	0.0	1.8	–	–
Glutamic acid	16.5	24.5	11.4	12.0	7.1	8.2
Glycine	1.8	1.9	27.5	3.0	10.0	4.2
Histidine	4.0	3.8	0.8	2.4	9.3	7.3
Hydroxyproline	0.0	0.0	14.1	0.0	–	–
Isoleucine	2.6	5.6	1.7	5.6	3.8	3.6
Leucine	12.3	9.2	3.3	8.3	9.8	6.8
Lysine	12.8	8.9	4.5	6.3	15.6	11.0
Methionine	0.8	1.8	0.9	3.2	2.5	3.6
Phenylalanine	6.6	5.3	2.2	5.1	1.9	2.4
Proline	4.8	13.5	16.4	3.8	2.3	–
Serine	4.2	5.3	4.2	7.9	10.8	13.4
Threonine	5.8	4.4	2.2	5.1	1.8	2.0
Tryptophan	–	–	–	1.8	–	–
Tyrosine	5.1	5.7	0.3	4.0	2.0	3.3
Valine	5.9	6.8	2.6	7.6	1.1	5.3
1-methylhistidine	–	–	–	–	1.8	8.5

Data from Deman J M (1999) Principles of food chemistry, 3rd edn; Aspen, Gaithersburg, MD; and Francis F J (2000) Encyclopedia of food science and technology, 2nd edn, John Wiley & Sons Inc., New York.

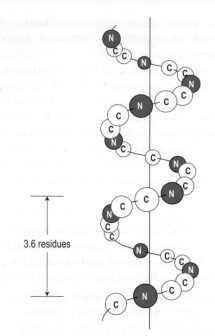

Figure 2.6   The α-helix structure.

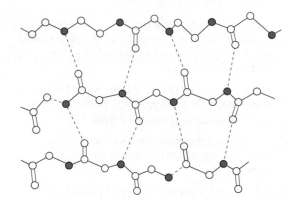

Figure 2.7   The β-pleated sheet structure.

groups. The atoms of the α-carbons alternate above and below the plane of the main chain of the polypeptide.

The tertiary structure of a protein is established when the chains are folded over into compact structures stabilised by hydrogen bonds, disulphide bridges and van der Waals forces. The quaternary structure of proteins is the non-covalent association of subunits of proteins due to hydrogen bonds and van der Waals forces. The full protein structure (see Figs CD 2.6, 2.7) is thus characterised by the amino acid sequence, the conformation along the *y* axis, the folding and the association of subunits.

Denaturation of proteins is the loss of structure that commonly occurs on heating proteins in solution.

It can also be caused by salts, pH, surface effects or freezing. No covalent bonds are broken, but the change in properties can be very large. Minor degrees of denaturation may be reversible when the denaturing agent is removed but if denaturation has proceeded further it is commonly irreversible. Enzymes lose activity on denaturation, and the texture of foods may change due to a reduction in protein solubility on denaturation. Thus, the change in eggs on boiling, or the toughening of fish on frozen storage are examples of changes in food texture due to denaturation.

Alcohol

Alcohol, which is more fully described as ethanol, C_2H_5OH, is formed by the fermentation of sugars during manufacture of beer, wines and spirits. Beer, wines, fortified wines and spirits contain ethanol at concentrations of about 30, 100, 150 and 300 g/l. Ethanol is fully miscible with water and fat. It is absorbed rapidly and metabolised in the liver to yield energy (29.7 kJ/g or 7.1 kcal/g). Many organic molecules are more soluble in aqueous ethanol solutions than in water and the presence of alcohol in a beverage may increase the bioavailability of minor components such as flavonoids from red wine.

Summary of relationship between structure and function

Fats provide a major contribution to the sensory quality of food, and they are also the richest energy source in foods. They are present at high levels in some foods such as butter and margarine, where the fat content is about 80%. Liquid oils provide foods with an oily texture, but semi-solid fats are important in foods such as chocolate, where the melting of the fat as it warms in the mouth is an important contributor to the sensory quality of the product. Fats are important in foods as carriers of the fat-soluble vitamins A, D, E and K, and they are also important as carriers of oil-soluble flavour compounds. Some liquid oils such as sunflower oil are rich in the essential polyunsaturated fatty acid linoleic acid (18:2 n-6), and some liquid oils also contain α-linolenic acid (18:3 n-3). Fish oils are the main source of the fatty acids eicosapentaenoic acid (20:5 n-3) and docosahexaenoic acid (22:6 n-3), which are considered as beneficial dietary components.

Proteins may be soluble or insoluble in water. If they are soluble they may be important as enzymes and they may contribute to a viscous texture in liquid foods, but when they are insoluble they are normally more important in determining the texture of foods such as meat. Proteins are sources of the essential amino acids isoleucine, leucine, lysine, methionine, phenylalanine, threonine, tryptophan and valine.

Carbohydrates vary in properties from low molecular weight components that contribute sweetness through to high molecular polysaccharides such as starch that may be important for food texture. If the carbohydrates are not hydrolysed in the small intestine, they are normally important as dietary fibre. Table 2.2 provides the typical values for protein, fat and carbohydrate content of selected foods.

Table 2.2 **Typical values for protein, fat and carbohydrate content of selected foods (% of wet weight)**

Food	Protein	Fat	Carbohydrate
Apple	0.4	0.1	11.8
Runner beans: raw	1.6	0.4	3.2
Runner beans: boiled	1.2	0.5	2.3
Beef	22.5	4.3	0.0
White bread	7.9	1.6	46.1
Hard cheese	24.9	34.5	0.1
Roast chicken	27.3	7.5	0
Baked cod	21.4	1.2	Trace
Sweetcorn	4.2	2.3	19.6
Egg	9.0	Trace	Trace
Haddock, steamed	20.9	0.6	0
Whole milk	3.3	3.9	4.5
Peas	5,8	0.7	13.8
Pork	21.8	4.0	0.0
Potatoes, new boiled	1.5	0.3	17.8
Rice: white, raw	7.3	3.6	85.8
Rice: cooked	2.6	1.3	30.9
Sardines, canned, drained	21.5	9.6	0
White wheat flour	9.4	1.3	77.7

From: Food Standards Agency (2002) McCance and Widdowson's The composition of foods. Sixth Summary Edition. Royal Society of Chemistry, Cambridge. Data from the Composition of Foods 6th Summary Edition Crown copyright material is reproduced with the permission of the Controller of HMSO and Queen's Printer for Scotland.

⊃ Key points

⊃ Carbohydrates include sugars and polysaccharides. They are important as an energy source or as dietary fibre.

⊃ Sugars are mainly monosaccharides (e.g. glucose) or disaccharides (e.g. sucrose).

⊃ Polysaccharides include thickeners (e.g. starch), gelling agents (e.g. pectin) and dietary fibre (e.g. cellulose).

⊃ Fats are mainly triacylglycerols. They are a source of the essential fatty acids linoleic acid and linolenic acid, which are utilised for eicosanoid synthesis.

⊃ Fish oils contain EPA and DHA, which have beneficial effects in reducing inflammation and risk of cardiovascular disease.

⊃ Proteins are macromolecules comprising chains of amino acids linked by a peptide bond.

⊃ The essential amino acids are isoleucine, leucine, lysine, methionine, phenylalanine, threonine, tryptophan and valine.

2.3 EFFECTS OF FOOD PROCESSING AND STORAGE

Types of food processing

Foods are processed either to improve their palatability or to extend their lifetime before deterioration reduces sensory or microbial quality to a level where they can no longer be consumed. The methods vary in the temperatures used and in the contact with water or oil as heat transfer media. Other variables that affect the rate of destruction of nutrients are the presence of oxygen, light and the pH of the aqueous phase.

Cooking processes such as roasting animals on a fire or boiling in a pot have been used for thousands of years. Preservation processes such as salting or drying in air have also been applied for hundreds of years. Modern industrial processes have been developed to maintain or improve flavour, texture, and nutritional or other quality aspects. Preservation techniques have been improved so as to improve the shelf life of products, whilst maintaining optimal quality.

Baking involves cooking cakes, pastry, potatoes or fruit in a dry oven at temperatures in the range 170–230°C. The surface of the food reaches the oven temperature, but in most foods, e.g. potatoes or fruit, the high water content limits the internal temperature to 100°C or less. Some loss of nutrients, e.g. vitamin C, may occur from the surface layer, but the bulk of the nutrients are retained. The loss of thiamin has been widely studied. In the mildly acid environment of many fermented products including bread, most thiamin is retained but if the pH rises above 6, most of the vitamin can be lost. Some of the amino acid lysine can be destroyed by baking due to the browning reactions between proteins and carbohydrates that contribute to the brown colour and aroma of baked products. Average losses of lysine during bread-making were reported to be about 15%.

Frying involves cooking in oil at temperatures in the range 160–200°C. Oil gives better heat transfer than air, so cooking times tend to be shorter than for baking. Losses of nutrients especially vitamin C may occur, but the food absorbs some oil which in the case of vegetable oils contains vitamin E. Plant foods rich in water such as potatoes tend to absorb more fat than meat does, because the fat is sucked into channels near the surface as the water is lost by evaporation. In potatoes, 80% of the ascorbic acid was converted to dehydroascorbic acid (DHA) during frying for 5 minutes at 180°C, with no residual ascorbic acid being detectable (Davey et al 2000). However, DHA is readily reduced by glutathione in cells, and this change should not reduce the bioavailability of ascorbic acid from fried foods. Longer frying periods can cause irreversible losses of ascorbic acid due to oxidation. Frying of meat causes losses of thiamin and riboflavin, with reductions of up to 72% and 55% respectively during the frying of chicken (Al-Khalifa & Dawood 1993).

Boiling involves cooking in water at about 100°C. It is commonly applied to vegetables and starch-rich foods such as rice or potatoes. Plant cell walls soften, and starch-rich foods absorb water and swell. Water-soluble vitamins such as vitamin C, thiamin, riboflavin and minerals leach out of the food and losses increase with the amount of added water and also if the food is over-cooked. Mashing of boiled potatoes increases losses of vitamin C by oxidation due to the increased exposure to oxygen. Immersing small amounts of vegetables into rapidly boiling water minimises loss of vitamin C by rapid denaturation of enzymes that catalyse oxidation of ascorbic acid. Losses of vitamin C during the boiling of spinach were 60%, compared to 46% through steaming and 58% through pressure cooking (Rumm-Kreuter & Demmel 1990). Braising of chicken led to losses of up to 52% thiamin and 37% riboflavin (Al-Khalifa & Dawood 1993).

Canning is a traditional food preservation technique. The times and temperatures applied in canning must be sufficient to ensure that all pathogens are inactivated or destroyed. The most heat-resistant pathogen normally found in canned food is *Clostridium botulinum*. Heating for 2.5 minutes at 121°C is sufficient to destroy *C. botulinum* spores. For foods with a pH of less than 4.5, a less severe heat treatment may be applied because *C. botulinum* spores are less heat stable and will not grow under these conditions. The amount of oxygen available in the headspace of canned food is small and this limits losses of vitamin C by oxidation. Losses of well over 50% vitamin C are typical for canned vegetables, but losses are much less for most fruits due to the stabilising effects of low pH. About 60% of the vitamin C content of green peas remains after the canning process, but about half of the remaining vitamin C is lost when the product is reheated before serving (Ang & Livingstone 1974).

Pasteurisation is a mild heat treatment applied to foods to reduce the number of spoilage organisms present and kill the pathogenic organisms, but it does not render the food sterile. Although commonly associated with milk, it is applied to a wide variety of foods. The process involves a temperature–time combination sufficient to kill enough organisms to achieve reduction to an acceptable number, but without unacceptable changes in the flavour or nutrients of the food. For heat treating milk, either a high temperature/short time process, which involves a temperature of 71.7°C for 15 seconds, or a low temperature holding process, which involves holding the milk at 62.8°C for 30 minutes, is applied. The milk must then be cooled rapidly to below 10°C. These conditions are sufficient to destroy tuberculosis organisms and other more sensitive pathogenic organisms in the milk. For liquid egg, the pasteurisation conditions require heating at 64.4°C for 2.5 minutes prior to cooling to below 3.3°C.

Fermentation is defined as the action of microorganisms or enzymes on food raw materials to cause biochemical changes. Fermentation is widely used as a processing method for improving the nutritional quality, digestibility, safety or flavour of food. Fermentation is a relatively low-energy process that can improve product life and reduce the need for refrigeration. Foods such as beer, cheese, mushrooms, bread, yoghurt, soy sauce, peperoni, tempeh and many others are produced by fermentation. Lactic acid bacteria which convert carbohydrates to lactic acid, thereby lowering the pH, and which also produce flavour compounds, are important in many fermented foods including fermented milk, cheese, meat and cereal products.

Storage of foods may cause deterioration by aerial oxidation or by enzyme action, which can lead to losses of nutrients and textural changes. Microorganisms may multiply in some foods, e.g. milk and yoghurt, unless the storage temperature is kept below 6°C, but dry foods can be kept at higher temperatures because micoorganisms will not grow in foods with a water activity below 0.6. In intermediate water foods (jam, dried and salted meats and fish, cakes, dried figs etc.) where the water activity is 0.70–0.90, mould and yeast spores, or pathogenic bacteria, can survive and then they can grow if the moisture content accidentally rises. The effect of water on microbiological changes is often discussed with reference to the water activity, a_w, where a_w is the ratio of the vapour pressure of water in a food to the saturated vapour pressure of water at the same temperature.

Refrigeration slows down changes in stored foods. A temperature below 5°C is recommended to retard the growth of microorganisms but chemical or enzymatic changes can still occur slowly at these temperatures. Leafy vegetables, e.g. spinach, are very vulnerable to vitamin C loss during storage, but reducing the storage temperature from 20°C to 4°C significantly reduces losses (Favell 1998).

Freezing slows down all chemical and enzymatic changes, but these processes can progress slowly even at −20°C, which is about the temperature in domestic freezers. Blanching, which involves heating briefly in hot water or steam, is commonly applied to vegetables prior to freezing in industrial processes in order to inactivate enzymes such as lipoxygenase that catalyse biochemical deterioration during frozen storage. Vitamin C is mainly lost at the blanching stage both due to thermal degradation and due to leaching into the blanching medium. Losses of 10–40% vitamin C throughout the freezing process are typical, but the extent of losses depends on exposure to air during the process and the type of blanching process that is used. Losses are generally lower for steam blanching than for water blanching (Favell 1998).

Drying or dehydration is the removal of water, and is traditionally achieved by leaving commodities in the sun. The larger the surface area the faster the drying process but the application of vacuum and heat accelerates the drying process. Drying reduces the activity of enzymes and also inhibits the growth of microorganisms. Industrially, dehydration is applied more widely to potatoes than to fruit and vegetables, and losses of about 75% of the vitamin C can occur. Vitamin C is commonly added to dehydrated potatoes, because of the importance of potatoes as a dietary source of vitamin C.

Freeze-drying is a process where water is removed under vacuum by sublimation from the frozen state of a food. Freeze-dried foods can normally be rehydrated to dissolve rapidly in water or to recover the original texture more closely than foods dried at higher temperatures. Thus freeze-drying is commonly applied in the manufacture of instant coffee powder because the powder has good solubility in water.

Salting is an effective way of preserving foods, e.g. meat, because the water activity is reduced. Salting in combination with smoking and drying was the main preservation method for centuries prior to the twentieth century. Salt-preserved products such as ham and bacon are still important in our diet but canning, refrigeration and freezing have become more common preservation techniques.

Irradiation is a physical method of processing food using ionising radiation. The radiation generates free radicals, which can react with the DNA of living insects and microorganisms. For food irradiation, maximum irradiation doses of 10 kGy are used, although lower doses are often used. Irradiation is permitted in Europe for fruits, vegetables, cereals, fish, shellfish and poultry, but the main application is herbs and spices, where chemical treatment is often required if irradiation is not used. Low irradiation doses, <1 kGy, inhibit sprouting, sterilise insects and delay ripening. At 1–3 kGy, the numbers of some spoilage microorganisms are reduced, but viruses and spores of sporulating bacteria such as *Clostridium botulinum* are not affected by food irradiation. Thiamin is the most sensitive of the water-soluble vitamins. More than 50% of the thiamin in chicken can be lost by an irradiation dose of 10 kGy at 10°C. Vitamin E is also sensitive to irradiation, with significant losses of vitamin E in irradiated cereals. However, although foods containing vitamins E and A are susceptible to irradiation, the main food sources of these vitamins are not irradiated. Losses of nutrients by irradiation are often no greater than losses by thermal processing methods. Irradiation of selected foods, especially herbs and spices, is a very safe procedure and it would be much more widely-applied if consumer concern about the effects of radiation on human tissues was not carried over into prejudice against irradiated foods, where no radiation is retained by the food.

High pressure processing: When high pressures up to 1000 MPa (10^4 bar) are applied to packages of food that are submerged in a liquid, the pressure is distributed instantly and uniformly throughout the food. The high pressure causes destruction of micro-organisms and inactivation of some enzymes, although a combination of heating and high pressure is often applied. The process has the potential for providing products with improved flavour, good retention of nutrients, and changed texture compared to products that are processed by heat alone. Fruit juices processed by high pressure processing are now sold in Europe and other products processed by this technique including jams, fruit jellies, sauces, fruit yoghurts and salad dressings are on sale in Japan.

Additives (including preservatives, flavours, colours, sweeteners and processing aids)

The use of additives in food in the UK is strictly controlled by legislation passed by Parliament. The legislation aims to protect the health of the consumer and to prevent fraud. Additives are allowed for specific functions (antioxidant, colour etc.) and are restricted to those listed in the regulations. In some cases additives may be allowed for use in selected foods and at limited levels. Prior to being included in the regulations, the technical need for an additive is assessed by the Food Advisory Committee. If a technical need is demonstrated, the Committee on Toxicity of Chemicals in Food, Consumer Products and the Environment is consulted before the additive is included in the legislation.

Preservatives are substances added to foods to inhibit microbial spoilage. Common foods including meats, cheeses, baked goods, fruit juices and soft drinks are likely to include preservatives. Even if sterile foods are produced initially by thermal processing, infection with bacteria, fungi and yeasts can occur in these foods, which are often not consumed at one sitting, and preservatives are required to extend the shelf life of the products. Sorbic acid, benzoic acid, sulphites, thiabendazole, nitrites and biphenyl are amongst the substances approved for use as food preservatives (see Fig. CD 2.8). Some food preservatives including benzoates and sulphur dioxide have been identified as causing sensitising or allergic reactions including chronic urticaria and asthma in susceptible individuals. Nitrites and nitrates, which are used in cured meats and some cheeses, have caused some concern because secondary amines may react with nitrite derivatives to form N-nitroso compounds that are possibly carcinogenic. However, nitrites are formed naturally in saliva within the body and nitrates are ingested in vegetables and water, so it is considered that the possibility of N-nitrosated compounds being formed in treated foods is of little consequence compared with other sources of these compounds. Sulphur dioxide is not used in foods containing thiamin because it brings about the destruction of the vitamin in the food.

Flavours added to food may be natural components derived from raw materials such as spices by physical processes such as extraction or distillation. A range of essential oils, including clove oil and orange oil, are isolated by these processes and they are widely used for flavouring foods. Other flavour compounds are synthesised by controlled chemical synthesis, by transformations using living biological systems, by enzyme-catalysed synthesis or by the reaction flavour approach which mimics established food-cooking techniques. Synthetic flavour compounds include vanillin, menthol, methyl salicylate, benzaldehyde, maltol, ethyl maltol and cinnamaldehyde (see Fig. CD 2.9).

Colours: The classes of natural or nature-identical colourings used for food include carotenoids, chlorophyll, anthocyanins and betalaines. Besides these, some synthetic compounds are allowed for addition to food. Synthetic food colours can be classified as azo (e.g. sunset yellow FCF), azo-pyrazolone (e.g. tartrazine), triarylmethane (e.g. green S), xanthene (e.g. erythrosine), quinoline (e.g. quinoline yellow) or indigoid compounds (e.g. indigo carmine) (see Fig. CD 2.10). Most of the allowed synthetic food colours are water-soluble. Some food colours have been found to cause allergic responses in susceptible individuals. Most concern has been expressed about tartrazine. It has been estimated that about 100 000 people in the USA are sensitive to tartrazine. Symptoms of the allergic response include urticaria, swelling, often of the face and lips, runny nose and occasionally asthma.

Sweeteners: Consumers are very interested in low calorie food and beverage products. Since the sugars present are significant contributors to the calorific content of many foods, the food industry has developed a range of zero or low calorie sweeteners. Aspartame, saccharin, acesulfame K and cyclamates are high potency sweeteners (see Fig. CD 2.11). Aspartame is used widely in foods because it is the sweetener that most closely mimics the taste of sucrose. It consists of two amino acids, aspartic acid and phenylalanine, and it is 180 times sweeter than sucrose. Aspartame is quite stable in acid foods but it is less stable in the neutral pH range found in baked foods. People with phenylketonuria, a rare inherited disorder, must avoid foods containing aspartame because they do not metabolise phenylalanine effectively.

Saccharin is a very stable, highly water-soluble and cheap food additive, but although it is a high potency sweetener, some consumers are sensitive to its bitter and metallic off-tastes. Although concerns about the safety of saccharin were raised following a Canadian study in the 1970s in which bladder tumours were found in the second generation of rats fed saccharin, there is no evidence that saccharin has caused cancer in humans. Some studies have suggested that it was the sodium component of sodium saccharin that caused the bladder tumours in rats at the high level of consumption, and there is no evidence that similar effects occur in humans at realistic consumption levels. Acesulfame K is structurally related to saccharin and suffers from similar taste defects. Although it is not as stable as saccharin, it is used together with other sweeteners especially aspartame in foods such as diet cola drinks. Cyclamates are sodium or calcium salts of cyclamic acid. The taste is considered better than that of saccharin, but the concentration is limited to 400 mg/l in soft drinks, and the Food Standards Agency has recommended that young children should not consume more than three beakers of dilutable soft drinks to avoid exceeding the acceptable daily intake (ADI). Weak biological effects for the main metabolite of cyclamate, cyclohexylamine, have limited the ADI to 11.0 mg/kg.

Sucralose was developed as a non-nutritive sweetener in the 1970s. It is a trichlorinated derivative of sucrose with excellent flavour and stability. It is currently allowed in some countries in the EU under temporary national legislation but it is being proposed for full acceptance.

Sugar alcohols including sorbitol, mannitol and xylitol have comparable sweetness and about the same calorific content as sucrose but they are absorbed more slowly from the digestive tract and do not raise postprandial blood sugar and insulin levels; thus they are suitable for sweetening diabetic foods.

Processing aids are substances used to facilitate food processing by acting as chelating agents, enzymes, antifoaming agents, catalysts, solvents, lubricants or propellants. They are not consumed as food ingredients by themselves, and are used during food processing without the intention that they should be present in the final product. Residues of the processing aids may be present in the finished product and it is a legal requirement that they do not present any risk to human health. Chymosin, which was developed as a replacement for rennet, the milk clotting enzyme traditionally used in cheese manufacture, was classified as a processing aid.

Genetically modified organisms (GMOs) are plants, animals or microorganisms which have had DNA inserted into them by means other than the natural processes of combination of an egg and a sperm or natural bacterial conjugation (see Ch. 32). The use of GMOs in food has been the subject of intense debate in recent years. GMOs have a number of potential benefits including improved nutritional attributes, e.g. reduction of anti-nutritive and allergenic factors, and increase of the vitamin A content in rice to reduce blindness in South-east Asia. Tomato puree produced from GM tomatoes was widely accepted for several years in the UK but it is no longer available. Advantages claimed for the product included better flavour, consistency and lower price than the non-GM alternative. However, concerns about antibiotic resistance, transferring allergenic components between plant species, and environmental concerns about the risks of GM crops to the agricultural environment have prevented widespread acceptance of GM foods amongst consumers.

2.4 TOXIC COMPONENTS FORMED BY PROCESSING

The processing of foods is essential to inactivate microorganisms and to allow flavour and texture development. However, processing may lead to losses of nutrients, and it may also lead to the formation of toxic components under certain conditions. A wide range of chemical reactions occur at high temperatures such as those that occur during frying or grilling of food. The following compounds are examples of toxic products that may be formed. **3-Monochloropropane-1,3-diol (3-MCPD)** (see Fig. CD 2.12) is an example of a chemical that may form in foods by the reaction of chloride with lipids. It has been shown to be a carcinogen by laboratory animal studies. 3-MCPD can be formed as a result of industrial processing of foods such as hydrolysed vegetable protein or soy sauce but it may also form during domestic cooking of foods or it may transfer into foods from packaging material. The European Commission's Scientific Committee on Food (SCF) have proposed a tolerable daily intake of $2\,\mu g/kg$ body weight.

Acrylamide (2-propenamide) (see Fig. CD 2.13) is found in fried and baked goods at levels up to $3\,mg/kg$. Highest levels are found in crisps, crispbread, chips and fried potatoes. The WHO classifies acrylamide as a probable human carcinogen based on experiments on laboratory animals and effects on humans exposed to high levels through industrial exposure. However, there is a lack of scientific information about the nature and extent of uptake from foods, and it is not known whether there is a relationship between the consumption of acrylamide in foods and cancer in humans. The Maillard reaction between the amino acid asparagine, which occurs in potatoes and cereals, and glucose is thought to be an important route for the formation of acrylamide.

Polycyclic aromatic hydrocarbons (PAHs) are a group of about 250 related compounds that are present in wood smoke and are detected at low levels in charred meat and in foods exposed to smoke. PAHs are chemically very stable and they are widespread in the environment, since they do not degrade easily. Consequently, a variety of food products that are not smoked including vegetable oils and fish contain detectable levels of PAHs. Many PAHs are carcinogenic to animals, and carcinogenic effects have

been demonstrated in humans following occupational exposure to high levels of PAHs. Benzo(a)-pyrene (BaP), benz(a)anthracene (BaA) and dibenz(ah)anthracene (DBahA) are PAHs about which there is most concern as potential carcinogens. Research by the Food Standards Agency showed that the average dietary intake of BaP, BaA and DBahA in the UK was less than $3\,ng/kg$ body weight per day in 2000, and this was 2–5 times less than in 1979.

> ⟳ **Key points**
>
> ⟳ Foods are processed either to improve their palatability or to extend their shelf life, especially by the destruction of microorganisms.
>
> ⟳ Food processing operations applied to foods include baking, frying, boiling, canning, pasteurisation, irradiation, freeze-drying, drying and high pressure processing.
>
> ⟳ Losses of water-soluble vitamins may occur by leaching into processing water. Vitamins may also be lost by reaction with oxygen or by thermal degradation. Vitamin C and thiamin are particularly susceptible to degradation.
>
> ⟳ Frying or grilling of foods may lead to the formation of toxic components in some products.
>
> ⟳ Temperatures below 6°C prevent the growth of microorganisms.
>
> ⟳ Food additives include preservatives, processing aids, flavours, colours, sweeteners.

2.5 NATURAL FOOD TOXINS

Many natural substances are harmful to health when consumed in foods at a sufficient dose. For example, fat-soluble vitamins cause toxic effects when excessive amounts are consumed and these can be fatal at a high level of intake. However, toxins are substances that cause harmful effects when foods are consumed at levels comparable to those which may be eaten by consumers. These may be natural products that accumulate in foods during processing or storage or they may be introduced into plants or animals that are subsequently consumed as foods. Some toxins, e.g. polychlorinated biphenyls, are cumulative but other toxins, e.g. glycoalkaloids, are completely harmless when consumed repeatedly at sub-toxic doses. Food components may cause toxic effects within hours, days or weeks of consumption

of the food or they may have mutagenic or carcinogenic effects in which an inheritable change in the genetic information of a cell may lead to cancer or other disease states over a period of years. When there is evidence from animal experiments that food components are toxic, regulatory authorities normally allow the components to be present in foods when the maximum amount consumed is 100 times less than the minimum amount shown to have an adverse effect in animals with due allowance for the body weight of the animal. Close monitoring of foods by government agencies helps to prevent chemical toxins reaching levels at which harmful effects occur, and pathogenic bacteria are much more common causes of human disease than chemical toxins.

Natural plant toxins

Glycoalkaloids: Solanine is the main glycoalkaloid, which commonly occurs with other glycoalkaloids including chaconine at low levels in potatoes. However, high levels of solanine may be found in green potatoes, since conditions which lead to an increase in chlorophyll content also cause increases in solanine levels (see Fig. CD 2.14).

Glycoalkaloid levels of over 200 mg/kg fresh weight may lead to harmful effects. Solanine acts by inhibiting the enzyme cholinesterase, which catalyses hydrolysis of acetylcholine to acetate and choline. The action of this enzyme is essential for the repolarisation of neurons following transmission of a nerve impulse. Increased gastric pain followed by nausea, vomiting and respiration difficulties, which may cause death, have been reported in individuals following consumption of potatoes with high levels of glycoalkaloids. Cholinesterase activity recovers within a few hours following ingestion of low doses of glycoalkaloids, so there are no ill-effects of repeat ingestion of small doses.

Lathyrus: Lathyrism is a disease caused by consumption of vetch peas, chickpeas, or garbanzos, which have the systematic name *Lathyrus sativus*. The illness occurs in two forms, which are osteolathyrism and neurolathyrism. Osteolathyrism is characterised by skeletal deformities and weakness in aortic and connective tissue. The toxic constituent of *L. sativus*, which causes osteolathyrism, is β-L-glutamylaminopropionitrile, which inhibits cross-linking of collagen, thereby affecting the structure of connective tissue and bone. Osteolathyrism mainly occurs in animals, but the second form of lathyrism, neurolathyrism, affects humans, especially young men, following long-term consumption of the peas. Neurolathyrism involves damage to the central nervous system, which causes paralysis of the legs, with general weakness and muscle rigidity developing. The disease mainly occurs in some areas of India, where *L. sativus* grows despite its cultivation being banned. The toxic component is β-*N*-oxalyl-L-α,β-diaminopropionic acid (see Fig. CD 2.15).

Marine toxins

The neurotoxin tetrodotoxin (see Fig. CD 2.16) occurs in some organs of the puffer fish, which is a culinary delicacy in Japan. Great skill is required by the chef to separate the muscles and testes, which are free of the toxin, from the liver, ovaries, skin and intestines. Tetrodotoxin is fatal above a dose of 1.5–4.0 mg, whereas the concentration may exceed 30 mg/100 g in the liver and ovaries. The toxin blocks movement of sodium ions across the membranes of nerve fibres, inhibiting transmission of nerve impulses, which causes distressing symptoms that develop into total paralysis and respiratory failure causing death within 6–24 hours. There is no known antidote to the poison, and fatalities continue to occur regularly. Japanese regulatory authorities require chefs to be licensed for cooking the puffer fish, and this has helped to reduce the number of fatalities in recent years.

Paralytic shellfish poisoning is caused by consumption of shellfish such as clams or mussels that have fed on dinoflagellate algae, which reach high concentrations in red tides that develop in seawater. The algal bloom is common in coastal waters close to Europe, North America, Japan and South Africa. The algae, especially *Gonylaux* sp., produce a toxin, saxitoxin (see Fig. CD 2.17), that accumulates in the flesh of the shellfish. Most shellfish break down or excrete the toxin within 3 weeks after ingestion ceases, but some species of clams may retain the toxin for several months. Saxitoxin is considered to be fatal at a dose of about 4 mg, with symptoms including numbness of lips, hands and feet that develop into vomiting, coma and death. A dose of 1 mg causes mild intoxication.

Fungal toxins

Mycotoxins

Many species of fungi produce metabolites that are toxic. Mycotoxins are produced by filamentous fungi. Epidemics due to the consumption of rye that had been stored in damp conditions were common in the Middle Ages. The grain was contaminated by the fungus *Claviceps purpurea*, known as ergot, and ergot poisoning was manifested either as gangrenous or convulsive ergotism. Gangrenous ergotism caused severe pain, inflammation and blackening of limbs, and loss of toes and fingers. Convulsive ergotism caused numbness, blindness, paralysis and convulsions.

The main pharmacologically active compounds in ergot are a series of alkaloid derivatives of lysergic acid (see Fig. CD 2.18). The most important alkaloids are ergotamine, ergonovine and ergotoxin. Some of these alkaloids have found applications in medicine for treatment of migraine.

Greater care over the harvesting and storage of grain has reduced the occurrence of ergot in grain very considerably, but a restricted outbreak occurred in France as recently as 1951. However, concern over the presence of mycotoxins in mouldy food has developed since the 1960s, when it was found that metabolites produced by the fungus *Aspergillus flavus* (aflatoxins) were toxic to animals. Aflatoxins occur in mouldy grain, soya beans or nuts and are carcinogenic at very low levels of intake. Toxin-producing fungi usually produce only two or three aflatoxins under a given set of conditions, but fourteen chemically related toxins have been identified. Aflatoxins are a series of bisfuran polycyclic compounds, which vary in the structure of at least one ring or substituent.

Aflatoxin B_1 is one of the most potent chemical carcinogens known (see Fig. CD 2.19). A high incidence of liver cancer is induced in rats by feeding diets containing $15\,\mu g/kg$ aflatoxin B_1. There have been many reports of animals suffering from toxic effects following the consumption of mouldy feeds. In 1960, over $100\,000$ turkeys died in England with extensive necrosis of the liver after consuming mouldy feed. Cattle consuming feed contaminated by aflatoxins excrete milk containing aflatoxin M_1. Aflatoxins may also be transmitted to humans via animals in meat or eggs. When food has been contaminated with mycotoxins, the toxins remain in the food even after the mould has been removed or has died. Aflatoxins and many other mycotoxins are quite stable during normal food processing operations.

Most toxins from other fungi are much less potent than the aflatoxins. Some mushrooms are toxic but sometimes they can be rendered edible by cooking, and only a few species are lethal if consumed. *Amanita muscaria* is a fleshy fungus that grows widely in temperate areas of the world. It causes hallucinogenic effects, and has commonly been used as a narcotic or intoxicant. The compounds responsible for the toxic effects are a series of isoxazoles including muscimol.

Pollutants

Pesticides are used to control weeds or insects that would otherwise reduce crop production or cause post-harvest losses. Several hundred pesticides, which correspond to several chemical classes, are used in agriculture. These include chlorinated hydrocarbons, organophosphates, carbamates and pyrethroids, which are used as insecticides; triazine, phenoxy, quaternary ammonium, and benzoic acids used as herbicides; and chlorinated phenols and ethylene bisdithiocarbamates, which are used as fungicides (see Fig. CD 2.20). The use of pesticides has made a major contribution to food production and preservation. Pesticides are designed to kill or adversely affect living organisms, and consequently there is in principle a risk to health. There is a balance between the benefits of pesticide use and the risks arising from their use, which government seeks to control by identifying allowed pesticides and by monitoring foods for traces of these residues to ensure that the residues that occur are unlikely to pose a risk to health.

Many pesticides degrade rapidly in the environment, but pesticide residues may be present in the meat or milk of animals that have drunk water contaminated by pesticide residues. Plant products can also be contaminated by residues of herbicides and fungicides used to produce foods of good quality. Maximum residue levels of many pesticides in foods such as fruit, vegetables and other plant and animal products are specified in the legal regulations.

Antibiotics used to treat animals may remain as residues in meat. Up to 10.6% of meat samples tested in Mexico contained sulfonamides, but chloramphenicol was less prevalent (Vazquez-Moreno et al 2002). There is concern that this may lead to the development of antibiotic resistance in humans, although it is only one of the mechanisms for the development of antibiotic-resistant organisms in humans, and resistant *E. coli* was more prevalent in vegetarians than in meat eaters (Berends et al 2001). The development in animals of antibiotic resistance in pathogenic bacteria and in commensal bacteria, which constitute a reservoir of resistance genes that may be transferred to pathogenic bacteria, are probably more significant pathways for the transfer of antibiotic resistance from animals to humans (van den Bogaard & Stobberingh 2000).

Hormones are used in the rearing of animals in some countries because they act as active growth promoters. Increases in yield of veal or beef of up to 15% may be produced. Although a total ban exists on the use of hormones in raising cattle in the EU, a black market exists and there is evidence that between 35 and 55 illegal hormones are used in the EU. In the USA, six hormones are allowed to be used. The levels of hormone residues found in beef are below the Maximum Residue Limit set by the FAO/WHO Expert Committee of Food Additives. Other food commodities contribute hormones to the diet. Eggs contribute more to the dietary level of oestradiol than beef, whether the animal is legally treated with hormones or not (Stephany 2001). However, the significance of hormones from food on human development and health is still a subject of debate between experts (Andersson & Skakkebaek 1999).

Heavy metals have received attention as widespread environmental contaminants and as accidental food contaminants. They enter the environment as a consequence of industrial pollution and they enter the food chain in various ways. The two metals of main concern are mercury and cadmium.

Mercury toxicity came to public attention after a mass poisoning incident in the Minamata Bay area of Japan. Symptoms were first evident in 1956, and by the end of the outbreak over 20 000 people were affected. The cause of the incident was identified as the consumption of fish and seafood, which was contaminated by methyl mercury, which had been discharged into the bay in waste water from chemical plants. The mercury had become concentrated in the fish tissues, and it is clear that fish are the main dietary source of methyl mercury. The symptoms of mercury toxicity are various neurological disorders which appear as loss of sight, hearing and ataxia, an inability to coordinate movement. Organic mercury attacks the central nervous system causing irreversible damage, and it is more toxic than inorganic mercury salts. Clinical signs of poisoning were evident when methyl mercury was consumed at $4\,\mu g/kg$ body weight, and a safe level of methyl mercury ingestion is less than $200\,\mu g$ per week with total mercury intake less than $300\,\mu g$.

Cadmium is widely distributed in the environment and is readily absorbed when eaten. Most foods contain less than $50\,\mu g/kg$, and ingestion of cadmium should be kept below 400–$500\,\mu g$ per week. Long-term exposure to cadmium causes damage to the renal tubules, anaemia, liver dysfunction and testicular damage.

Polychlorinated and polybrominated biphenyls (PCBs and PBBs)

PCBs and PBBs (see Fig. CD 2.21) are mixtures of inert molecules, which have been used as electrical insulators and fire retardants. They are resistant to chemical and biological breakdown and as a consequence of their stability, they have become widespread environmental contaminants, which are a potential hazard to human health. PCBs are frequently found at $\mu g/kg$ levels in fish, poultry, milk and eggs. PCBs may cause skin conditions including acne and rashes on acute exposure, but there is concern about the possible effects of long-term exposure to PCBs on the immune and endocrine function

and on the nervous system and cancer risk. PBBs entered the food chain in Michigan, USA in 1973, when a fire retardant was accidentally mixed with cattle feed. Several dairy herds suffered illness, but the possibility of ill effects in the human population consuming meat and milk from these animals is still being studied.

Radioactive fallout

Radioactive isotopes, or radionuclides, are atoms that are unstable and emit energy as radiation when they decay to more stable atoms. Some radionuclides such as carbon-14, uranium-238 and radon-222 occur naturally in the environment due to the effects of cosmic radiation or due to their creation in prehistoric times. However, fallout from nuclear power stations and the use of radioactive materials in industry, medicine and research have led to increases in the levels of radionuclides in the environment. When living tissue is exposed to ionising radiation it will absorb some of the radiation's energy and may become damaged, with the development of cancer.

The accident at the Chernobyl nuclear station in the Ukraine in 1985 led to long-term increases in strontium-90 and caesium-137 across long distances. Meat and milk from animals in the UK were widely monitored following the accident. Sheep who grazed on hills in the path of the wind from the Ukraine accumulated significant levels of caesium-137 in their bodies. Even 13 years after the accident, the movement, sale and slaughter of sheep on over 400 farms in the UK was still restricted because of excessive levels of caesium-137 from this accident.

Pathogenic agents

Pathogenic agents are a very common cause of food poisoning. Organisms may be associated with endogenous animal infections transmissible to humans (zoonoses) by consumption of meat or fish. This group includes bacterial, viral, fungal, helminthic and protozoan species. The second group of organisms are species that are exogenous contaminants of food, which may cause infections in humans. This group includes common food poisoning organisms such as *Salmonella*, *Staphylococcus* and *Clostridium botulinum*.

Seafood poisoning

Bacterial decomposition of fish that is stored at unacceptably high temperatures or for excessive time is the main cause of seafood poisoning.

Seafood poisoning is often called scombroid poisoning because fish of the *Scombroidea* species including mackerel and tuna are widely consumed. However, fish from other species including sardines and herring may also cause outbreaks. Consumption of contaminated fish may cause symptoms to appear within about 2 hours of the fish being eaten. The main symptoms include pain, vomiting and diarrhoea. Seafood poisoning has been attributed to the formation of histamine by bacterial decomposition of the amino acid histidine in fish. However, pure histamine has low oral toxicity, and it appears that other components in the fish such as putrescine and cadaverine are important in allowing the toxicity of histamine to be manifested.

Food poisoning organisms

Salmonella is one of the most common intestinal infections in the UK. In recent years, there have been about 30 000 reported cases per year. The most common organism involved is *S. enteritidis* followed by *S. typhimurium* but the known number of strains of the bacterium is over 2300. Eggs are the most common vehicle for the transmission of salmonellosis. The common contamination of eggs is due to the fact that hens lay eggs through a passageway called the vent, which is an exit shared by their intestines, where *Salmonella* is commonly present. Other foods of animal origin including unpasteurised milk, poultry and cheese are also possible sources. The organism is readily inactivated by cooking, but cross-contamination of cooked food by uncooked food is a common pathway for contamination of food in domestic kitchens. Symptoms normally follow ingestion of contaminated food within 6–48 hours. *Salmonella* causes diarrhoea, often with fever and abdominal cramps. The onset may be sudden and there may be nausea and vomiting initially.

Campylobacters are the leading cause of bacterial diarrhoea in humans. Campylobacteriosis commonly affects babies and young children. The WHO estimates that 1% of the population of western Europe is infected by *Campylobacter* spp. each year. The illness is a gastrointestinal infection caused by *C. jejuni* or *C. coli*. Symptoms may show themselves as bloody diarrhoea, fever, nausea and abdominal cramps. The illness normally lasts 2–10 days but some symptoms may persist for several months. The disease is usually self-limiting, so antibiotic treatment is not normally required except in serious cases. Campylobacters occur widely in the intestinal tract of many animals, especially chickens and turkeys. During slaughtering and preparation of raw bird, a large number of birds may become contaminated, and therefore undercooked poultry meat and offal are a major source of infection. Raw milk and poorly treated water supplies are also causes of campylobacter infections.

Verocytotoxin-producing *Escherichia coli* is an uncommon but important pathogen because serious infections particularly in children may result. The illness was first recognised in the early 1980s. Infection may produce mild diarrhoea or a severe or fatal illness. Cattle are the main source of infection, with most cases being associated with the consumption of undercooked beef burgers and similar food or raw milk. The infective dose appears to be very low, probably less than 10 cells. A temperature of 70°C for 2 minutes is sufficient to destroy the organism in meat.

Listeria monocytogenes is a potentially dangerous foodborne pathogen. The bacterium occurs in cheese. Hard cheeses do not support the multiplication of the bacterium and numbers less than 20/g do not present a hazard to health in hard cheese. However, the bacterium can multiply in soft cheeses at refrigeration temperatures, and the occurrence of the bacterium in cheese should be minimised by the use of Hazard Analysis Critical Control Point (HACCP) systems throughout the whole food chain. *L. monocytogenes* causes very serious illness including meningitis and septicaemia. The mortality rate can be as high as 30%, with pregnant women, infants, the elderly and people who are immune suppressed being most vulnerable.

Clostridium welchii is a common source of food poisoning, normally from meat that has been cooked and then stored at insufficiently low temperatures. The organism is anaerobic and spores that survive cooking may develop vegetative forms that multiply in the gut and produce an enterotoxin. Symptoms, which include diarrhoea and abdominal pain, normally occur within 8 to 24 hours following consumption of the food.

Staphylococcus aureus is a potentially pathogenic organism that is carried by large numbers of the population. Foods may be contaminated by carriers, and ingestion of contaminated food may be followed within 2 to 4 hours by vomiting and diarrhoea, which may be severe and may lead to collapse due to dehydration.

Clostridium botulinum is an organism found in soils, which may contaminate canned meats and meat pastes. The organism forms heat-resistant spores, which may develop vegetative forms anaerobically if not inactivated by heat. The vegetative forms of the organism produce a toxin that is extremely potent at very low levels. Difficulty in swallowing may develop into paralysis and death. Cases of botulism are rare, since the food industry uses nitrites to prevent anaerobic growth in processed meats.

Viral infections

Viruses have no cellular structure and possess only one type of nucleic acid (either RNA or DNA) wrapped in a protein coat. Consequently, they cannot multiply in foods, but food handlers with dirty hands or dirty utensils may allow foods to become contaminated by viruses, which can subsequently multiply in the intestinal tract by using the host cells' mechanism for replication. Viral infections often have much longer incubation periods of up to several weeks compared to several hours for bacterial infections.

Hepatitis A is a member of the genus *Enterovirus*, which causes symptoms of anorexia, fever, malaise, nausea and vomiting followed after a few days by symptoms of liver damage. Exposure to the virus is limited in the developed world due to good public hygiene and sanitation. In Delhi in 1955–6, 36 000 cases occurred in a waterborne epidemic of infectious hepatitis after the main water supply had been contaminated with sewage due to flooding. However, smaller numbers of cases have been caused by infected foods such as shellfish or fruit or by infected food handlers.

Poliomyelitis is another enterovirus that can be transmitted by contaminated food such as milk. However, it is now virtually eradicated in developed countries. Norwalk-like viruses, which have not been fully characterised, may cause gastroenteritis with an incubation period of 15–50 hours followed by diarrhoea and vomiting.

Prions

A prion protein is a small protein molecule that occurs mainly in the brain cell membrane. It differs in conformation from most proteins since it occurs mainly in a beta-sheet flattened form, which is heat resistant and protease resistant. Prions are believed to be the infectious agent causing humans to develop new variant Creutzfeldt–Jakob disease (vCJD). Cases of this disease were first reported in the early 1990s. Although CJD had been known as a rare disease that occurred worldwide since the 1920s, vCJD affected younger people than the earlier form, and there were unusual clinical features. This disease is believed to have developed in humans following consumption of meat from cattle affected by BSE (bovine spongiform encephelopathy), which is a fatal brain disease that affected large numbers of cattle in the UK in the 1980s and 1990s. The disease in cattle was reduced after 1993 by the removal of meat and bonemeal from cattle feed concentrates and by the slaughter of large numbers of animals. vCJD presents itself as psychiatric disorders including anxiety, depression and withdrawal but it develops over a period of months into forgetfulness and memory disturbance. A cerebellar syndrome develops with gait and limb ataxia and eventually death. The annual number of deaths identified as being due to vCJD in the UK reached 28 in the year 2000, but small reductions in the annual number of deaths have been recorded since that year.

Helminths and nematodes

Helminths and nematodes are flatworms and roundworms, which develop as parasites in humans following consumption of contaminated water or food, especially meat or raw salads. Liver flukes, *Fasciola hepatica*, and tapeworms of the genus *Taenia* are the most common helminths. The liver fluke develops as a leaf-like animal in humans, sheep or cattle. It grows up to 2.5 cm long by 1 cm wide and establishes itself in the bile duct after entering and feeding on the liver. When mature the liver fluke produces eggs, which are excreted in the faeces. Symptoms include fever, tiredness and loss of appetite with pain and discomfort in the liver region of the abdomen.

Tapeworms include *Taenia solium*, which occurs in pork, and *T. saginata*, which is associated with beef. The mature tapeworm develops in the human intestine, and may cause severe symptoms in the young and in individuals weakened by other diseases. Effects may include nausea, abdominal pain, gut irritation, anaemia and a nervous disorder resembling epilepsy. If gut damage allows eggs to be released in the stomach, the resulting bladder worms may invade the central nervous system with fatal consequences.

Trichinella spiralis is a nematode (roundworm) that causes trichinosis in humans with symptoms of discomfort, fever and even death. Consumption of raw or poorly cooked infected pork products is the normal source of foodborne illness.

➲ Natural plant toxins, marine toxins, fungal toxins and pollutants may contaminate food, but they rarely occur in foods sold in western Europe at levels which are harmful to health.

➲ Growth of pathogenic organisms including bacteria, yeasts and moulds may cause food poisoning.

➲ Processing of foods, e.g. heat treatment under selected conditions, reduces the levels of many

pathogenic organisms, so that the foods may be consumed safely. Cross-contamination of cooked products by unprocessed products during domestic storage, or storage at higher temperatures or for longer times than recommended by manufacturers, are common explanations of food poisoning incidents.

➲ Under certain conditions, processing of foods may cause the formation of potentially toxic compounds, although effects in humans have rarely been demonstrated.

2.6 PHYTOPROTECTANTS

There is strong evidence that a diet rich in fruits and vegetables can reduce heart disease and probably some cancers in the human population. However, identification of the individual components of the diet which may confer this protection is still a matter of intense study. Plants and plant extracts have been used for centuries in the treatment of chronic ailments. Foods and herbs to which the highest anticancer activity has been assigned include garlic, soya beans, cabbage, ginger, liquorice and the umbelliferous vegetables (carrots, celery, parsley and parsnips). Onions, flax, citrus, turmeric, cruciferous vegetables (broccoli, Brussels sprouts, cabbage and cauliflower), solanaceous vegetables (tomatoes and peppers), brown rice and whole wheat possess moderate levels of anticancer activity (Steinmetz & Potter 1991). Research has identified an array of phytochemicals including organosulphur compounds, carotenoids, terpenes and polyphenols including flavonoids and phytoestrogens that have been shown to produce beneficial physiological effects.

Phytoprotectants may inhibit tumour development by scavenging chemical carcinogens to prevent them binding to electron-rich sources in the cell including DNA, RNA and proteins. They may also act by their effect on phase I enzymes involved in activation of environmental and chemical carcinogens or phase II enzymes involved in detoxification pathways.

Organosulphur compounds present in garlic represent some of the more efficient phase I and II enzyme modulators. Diallyl sulphide (DAS), diallyl disulphide (DADS), triallyl sulphide and diallyl polysulphides are lipid-soluble components in garlic, and S-allylcysteine (SAC) and S-allylmercaptocysteine (SAMC) are among the water-soluble components that are considered important. DAS

and DADS from garlic, and isothiocyanates, which occur in cabbage, broccoli and cauliflower, have been shown to inhibit chemically induced cancers in animals. Sulforaphane, an isothiocyanate found in broccoli, is a potent inducer of phase II enzymes.

Carotenoids (see Fig. CD 2.22) are a class of structurally related compounds, which are strongly coloured red or orange, and which are found in foods that are coloured red, orange or green including tomatoes, carrots and spinach. Carotenoids comprise molecules with hydrocarbon structures including α-, β-, and γ-carotene and lycopene as well as molecules with one or more polar substituents attached to the hydrocarbon backbone including astaxanthin, zeaxanthin, lutein and β-cryptoxanthin. Some of the most common carotenoids act as provitamin A, being converted to vitamin A by β-carotene-15, 15'-oxygenase in the intestinal mucosa. Provitamin A activity is restricted to carotenoids such as β-carotene in which at least half of the molecule shares the ring and chain structure of vitamin A. The role of carotenoids in cancer prevention is uncertain (see Section 11.1, under 'Vitamin A and carotene in cancer prevention').

Carotenoids also have antioxidant properties and may contribute to a reduced risk of coronary heart disease by protecting low density lipoproteins against oxidation. Lycopene does not have provitamin A activity but it has been the subject of much research because it may provide some protection against prostate cancer in men. Processed tomato products are a good source of lycopene.

Polyphenols (vegetable tannins) are classes of plant components, the structure of which includes more than one aromatic ring and several phenolic hydroxyl groups. They are water-soluble compounds having molecular weights between 500 and 3000, and have the ability to precipitate proteins. The theaflavins and thearubigins, which contribute the colour to black tea, are examples of polyphenols.

Flavonoids are phenolic compounds, which occur widely in plant tissues, mainly as glycosides. All flavonoids have a C_6-C_3-C_6 structure in which a six-carbon aromatic ring is linked by a three-carbon bridging unit to a second aromatic ring (see Fig. CD 2.23). The nature of the central C_3 unit defines the class of flavonoid. The classes include: the anthocyanins, which contribute the red, purple or black colours to fruits such as strawberries, plums and blackcurrants; the flavonols, which occur widely in vegetables including onions, broccoli and beans; flavanols, which occur in green tea; flavones, which often accompany flavonols; and proanthocyanidins, which occur in cocoa, cider and wine.

The position of the benzenoid substituent on the C-ring divides the flavonoid class into flavonoids (2-position) and isoflavonoids (3-position). Isoflavones in soya products are of current nutritional interest because of their oestrogenic structure (see Fig. CD 2.23). Other flavonoids are of interest because of their antioxidant properties.

Phytoestrogens

Phytoestrogens are any plant substance or metabolite that induces biological responses in vertebrates and can mimic or modulate the actions of endogenous oestrogens, usually by binding to oestrogen receptors (UK Food Standards Agency Committee on Toxicity 2002). Most of the work investigating the properties of phytoestrogens has been on isoflavones, with a little work on prenylated flavonoids, coumestrol or lignans. Phytoestrogens mimic or block the action of the human hormone oestrogen, although they are much less potent. They are of interest because they may have benefits for prevention of certain cancers, as well as heart disease and osteoporosis in postmenopausal women. However, there are possible links to fertility problems in animals, which raises concerns that similar effects could occur in humans, particularly babies fed soya-based infant formulas.

Isoflavones are present in several legumes but soya beans are the primary human dietary source. The three main isoflavones are genistein, daidzein and glycitein, which are mainly present as the glycosides genistin, daidzin and glycitin. Isoflavones also occur as malonyl or acetyl esters but these derivatives are commonly hydrolysed during the processing of soya products such as tofu (Song et al 1998).

Metabolites of isoflavones such as equol, a bioactive metabolite of daidzein, and glucuronide and sulphate conjugates are formed by metabolism in the intestine and the liver.

➲ Key points

➲ Phytoprotectants include organosulphur compounds, flavonoids, carotenoids and phytoestrogens.

➲ The antioxidant activity of phytoprotectants may be important in inhibiting cardiovascular disease or cancer.

➲ They may also act to inhibit cancer by their effect on phase I enzymes that are involved in activation of environmental and chemical carcinogens or phase II enzymes that are involved in detoxification pathways.

References and further reading

References

Al-Khalifa A S, Dawood A A 1993 Effects of cooking methods on thiamine and riboflavin contents of chicken meat. Food Chemistry 48(1):69–74

Andersson A M, Skakkebaek N E 1999 Exposure to exogenous estrogens in food: possible impact on human development and health. European Journal of Endocrinology 140:477–485

Ang C Y W, Livingstone G E 1974 Nutritive losses in the home storage and preparation of raw fruits and vegetables. In: White P L, Selvey N (eds) Nutritional qualities of fresh fruit and vegetables. Futura Publishing, Mount Kisco, p 121–132

Berends B R, van den Bogaard A E, Van Knapen F, Snijders J M A 2001 Human health hazards associated with the administration of antimicrobials to slaughter animals – part II. Veterinary Quarterly 23:10–21

Davey M W, Van Montague M, Inze D et al 2000. Plant L-ascorbic acid chemistry, metabolism, bioavailability and effects of processing. Journal of the Science of Food and Agriculture 80:825–860

Favell D J 1998 A comparison of the vitamin C content of fresh and frozen vegetables. Food Chemistry 62:59–64

Rumm-Kreuter D, Demmel I 1990 Comparison of vitamin losses in vegetables due to various cooking methods. Journal of Nutrition Science and Vitaminology 36:S7–S15

Song T, Barua K, Buseman G, Murphy P 1998 Soy isoflavone analysis. American Journal of Clinical Nutrition 68:1474S–9S

Steinmetz K A, Potter J D 1991 Vegetables, fruit and cancer I. Epidemiology. Cancer Causes and Control 2:325–357

Stephany R W 2001 Hormones in meat: different approaches in the EU and in the USA. APMIS 109(suppl 103):S357–S363

UK Food Standards Agency Committee on Toxicity 2002 Draft report of the COT Working Group on phyto-estrogens, October 2002. Online. Available: http://www.food.gov.uk/multimedia/pdfs/phytoestrogenreport.pdf

van den Bogaard A E, Stobberingh E E 2000 Epidemiology of resistance to antibiotics – links between animals and humans. International Journal of Antimicrobial Agents 14:327–335

Vazquez-Moreno L, Almada M D B, Rico L G et al 2002 Study of toxic residues in animal tissues destined for consumption. Revista Cientifica-Faculdad de Ciencias Veterinarias 12:186–192

Further reading

Ballantine B, Marrs T, Turner P 1995 General and applied toxicology. Macmillan, Basingstoke

Coultate T P 2002 Food: The chemistry of its components, 4th edn. RSC, London

Deshpande S S 2002 Handbook of food toxicology. Marcel Dekker, New York

Ryley J, Kajda P 1994 Vitamins in thermal processing. Food Chemistry 49:119–129

Shahidi F (ed) 1997 Antinutrients and phytochemicals in food. American Chemical Society, Washington

Shibamoto T, Bjeldanes L F 1993 Introduction to food toxicology. Academic Press, San Diego

CD-ROM contents

Figures

Figure CD 2.1 Typical triacylglycerol structure
Figure CD 2.2 Fatty acids
Figure CD 2.3 Phospholipid structure
Figure CD 2.4 Cholesterol
Figure CD 2.5 Amino acids
Figure CD 2.6 Protein structure – β-strands in concanavalin A
Figure CD 2.7 Protein structure – retinol binding protein
Figure CD 2.8 Common food preservatives
Figure CD 2.9 Flavour compounds
Figure CD 2.10 Food colours
Figure CD 2.11 Sweeteners
Figure CD 2.12 MCPD
Figure CD 2.13 Acrylamide
Figure CD 2.14 Glycoalkaloids
Figure CD 2.15 BAPN and ODAP
Figure CD 2.16 Tetrodotoxin
Figure CD 2.17 Saxitoxin
Figure CD 2.18 Lysergic acid and related compounds
Figure CD 2.19 Aflatoxin B_1
Figure CD 2.20 Pesticides
Figure CD 2.21 Polychlorinated biphenyls and polybrominated biphenyls
Figure CD 2.22 Common carotenoids
Figure CD 2.23 Flavonoids

Further reading

Further reading from the book

Useful websites

Part 2

Body composition and macronutrient metabolism

Edited by David A. Bender

3

The physiology of nutrient digestion and absorption

George Grimble

Table 3.1 Regional anatomy of the intestine and sites of nutrient absorption

Region	Functions performed	Mucosal surface	Nutrients digested	Nutrients absorbed	Major site of absorption	Electrolytes absorbed
Mouth	Grinding food to smaller particle size Moistening food (saliva) Initial digestion by lipase and alpha amylase Initiation of satiety mechanisms	Small folds	Small amount of protein Starch	Small amounts of glucose, peptides and amino acids	No	No
Stomach	Intestinal defence (e.g. acid secretion) Homogenising food to smaller particle size Moistening food (gastric secretions) Further enzyme digestion Gastric emptying meters delivery of nutrients to the small intestine Feedback of satiety messages	Rugae and pits	Protein, lipid	Insignificant amounts	No	No
Small intestine	Completion of digestion by pancreatic enzymes Absorption of digestion products of carbohydrate, protein and fat Absorption of water and electrolytes Absorption of minerals and micronutrients Feedback of satiety messages	Rugae, villi and microvilli	Protein, lipid, carbohydrate	Amino acids, peptides, fatty acids, glucose, fructose and galactose	Carbohydrate, fat protein, water, electrolytes	Sodium, potassium, calcium, magnesium, chloride, phosphate
Colon	Final salvage of water and electrolytes Mucin breakdown Conversion of bilirubin to urobilinogen Cholesterol catabolism Organic acid production ('acetate buffer')	Rugae and pits	Dietary fibre – digested by bacteria and fermented to short-chain fatty acids	Acetate, propionate and butyrate and dicarboxylic acids	Short-chain fatty acids, water, electrolytes	Magnesium and calcium in form of soaps with fatty acids

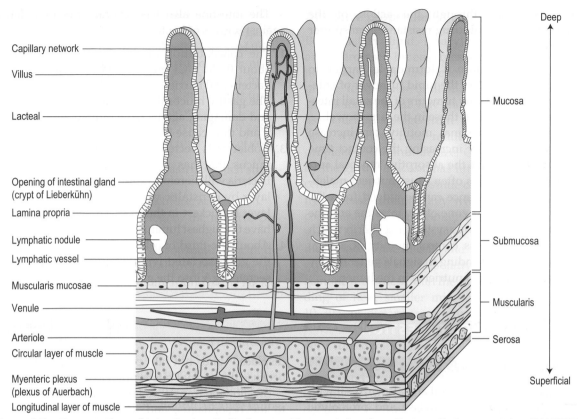

Deep

Capillary network

Villus

Lacteal

Mucosa

Opening of intestinal gland
(crypt of Lieberkühn)

Lamina propria

Lymphatic nodule

Lymphatic vessel

Submucosa

Muscularis mucosae

Venule

Muscularis

Arteriole

Serosa

Circular layer of muscle

Myenteric plexus
(plexus of Auerbach)

Superficial

Longitudinal layer of muscle

Figure 3.2 Cross-section of intestinal wall. (Redrawn with permission from Tortora G, Anagnostakos N P (1990) *Principles of anatomy and physiology* (Figure 24-18, p 760), Harper and Row, New York.)

The intestinal wall also has zoned anatomy (Fig. 3.2) the absorptive surface of which is amplified by three structures.

1. Folds or ridges (rugae) in the intestinal wall increase absorptive area.
2. Villi, finger-like projections 0.5–1.0 mm long covered with mucosal absorptive cells (enterocytes), further increase the absorptive capacity of mammals with higher continuous metabolic rates.
3. Enterocytes have further finger-like projections on their luminal surface, known as microvilli and these define the brush-border membrane.

These features increase the absorptive area of the human intestine to 200 m². Each villus is supplied by an arteriole and is drained by a venule and a lacteal. The venules drain into the hepatic portal vein and carry water-soluble nutrients, while the lacteals are part of the lymphatic system and carry the water-insoluble products of fat digestion and absorption.

Blood is supplied abundantly (500 ml/min) to the intestine by numerous small arteries that branch from the arch of mesenteric artery. This blood drains, via the portal vein, to the liver, which regulates the supply of nutrients to the periphery through the hepatic vein into the vena cava. Only one-quarter of this blood supplies the submucosa, muscularis and serosa; the remainder goes to the mucosal layer, which has very active metabolism (and needs a good oxygen supply) and where absorbed nutrients are quickly diluted out and removed to the portal vein, thus preventing any high osmotic loads developing. In some respects, the intestine behaves like a 'pre-liver' because it:

1. metabolises considerable amounts of dietary glucose and amino acids
2. completely degrades dietary arginine and nucleotides
3. detoxifies drugs and dietary toxins through the action of mucosal cytochrome P-450 enzymes and the UDP glucosyltransferases and sulphotransferases.

Pepsins are activated by acid and have an acid pH optimum but do not necessarily operate at acid pH. Meal-induced acid secretion is rapidly buffered by food so that the pH of the bulk-phase of the stomach lumen rises from pH 1.5 to pH 4.5 within 15 minutes of the end of a meal. Secreted zymogens are activated at the submucosal layer by gastric acid secretion whereas hydrolysis of bulk-phase dietary proteins, which have been acid denatured by contact with the mucosal surface, occurs at a relatively high luminal pH.

Control of the rate of gastric emptying

Gastric emptying matches not only the amount of food eaten during a meal, but also nutrients present in the food and the progress made in liquidising it within the stomach. Simple fluids like water will empty at a rate proportional to gastric volume, whereas nutrients will empty at a rate that depends on their energy density and potency in altering the duodenal brake.

Furthermore, fat that reaches the ileum exerts a profound inhibitory effect on gastric motility, known as the 'ileal brake'. After a meal, the two parts of the stomach show different motility responses:

- upper stomach (fundus, upper body) – slow, sustained contractions that generate pressure
- lower stomach (lower body, antrum) – powerful peristaltic contractions towards the pyloric sphincter.

These combined movements, together with hydrolysis of lipids and proteins, lead to liquidisation of food, which is released into the duodenum in spurts. The upper stomach acts as a 'pressure-pump'. In the lower stomach, solid food larger than 1–2 mm is recycled through the 'antral mill' until it has reached a size small enough to pass the pyloric sphincter.

Gastric emptying is controlled by neural or hormonal signals arising in response to nutrients in other parts of the gut (Rehfeld 1998). For example, the proximal and distal small bowel detect lipids and inhibit gastric motility; the effect is strongest with free fatty acids with a chain length > 10 carbon atoms. There seem to be four types of sensor.

1. Luminal lipid stimulates release of the regulatory peptide hormones cholecystokinin (CCK), neurotensin, peptide YY (PYY) and glucagon-like peptides (GLP) (see Fig. CD 3.6). CCK has local effects on motility.
2. CCK stimulates afferent nerve pathways in the intestine that inhibit gastric activity.
3. The products of lipid absorption, chylomicrons packaged for export to lymph (see 'Digestion and absorption of fat', below), are also sensed by an, as yet, unknown mechanism.
4. Short-chain fatty acids which reflux back into the ileum are sensed and signal the release of PYY, which inhibits gastric motility.

In this way, nutrient overload in the intestinal lumen is sensed and motility is inhibited so permitting more time before the remainder of the meal is released. Even at rest, the stomach is never quiescent since rhythmic waves of polarisation and depolarisation of gastric smooth muscle occur every 20 seconds, controlled by a pacemaker. Abnormalities in this pacemaker are associated with abnormal gastric emptying (e.g. 'dumping syndrome'). Slow emptying can be treated by prokinetic drugs and a new treatment for dumping is to give 1–2 grams of oleic acid before a meal to stimulate maximum inhibition of gastric motility by both the duodenal and ileal brakes.

Gastric emptying is also slowed by increased blood glucose concentration and is accelerated by insulin injection, which reduces blood glucose concentration. This is an example of a feedback mechanism that matches the amount of nutrient presented for absorption by the small intestine with the amount already absorbed. Another way in which gastric emptying is controlled is through inhibition of eating.

Gastric distension is a very powerful inhibitory signal that increases feelings of fullness and satisfaction (satiety) and hence counters the stimulatory afferent signals produced by eating tasty food. When the former signal predominates, eating is reduced and the stomach will, on balance, empty.

Digestive processes in the small intestine

Intestinal secretions and their control

Gastrin secreted by the stomach stimulates the secretion of enzymes by acinar cells in the pancreas. As the meal is released by the pylorus, acid-sensing cells in the duodenal mucosa release the hormone secretin, which stimulates water and bicarbonate secretion by pancreatic duct cells. This in turn flushes the pancreatic enzymes into the duodenum via the pancreatic duct. A second hormone, cholecystokinin, is also released and elicits two responses: (1) the acinar cells of the pancreas release large quantities of pancreatic enzymes as inactive zymogens; (2) the gallbladder contracts powerfully and squirts bile into the duodenum through the common bile duct.

Although digestion will increase luminal osmolality and mucosal water secretion, the absorption of digestion products reduces osmolality and the water will be reabsorbed. This is an impressive process; it is estimated that 7.5 litres of water are secreted and absorbed in this way, every day.

Digestive function of intestinal secretions

The pancreas secretes digestive enzymes in the form of inactive precursors (zymogens), and this may amount to up to 30% of the protein passing through the gastrointestinal tract with the meal. If these pancreatic enzymes were completely hydrolysed and the amino acids absorbed, a large amount of protein would need to be synthesised each day in order to digest 80–90 g of dietary protein. There is evidence that patients with an ileostomy (surgical fistula that drains ileal contents) do indeed excrete that amount of partially digested protein.

However, there is also evidence that pancreatic enzymes are absorbed intact and recycled in an enteropancreatic circulation that is analogous to the enterohepatic circulation of bile salts (Rothman et al 2002). Compelling arguments for this view are that pancreatic enzymes can be detected in the circulation and that the pancreas does not have the capacity to synthesise such a large amount of secretory enzymes each day. The mechanism of the proposed selective intestinal absorption of pancreatic enzymes is unknown.

Various pancreatic enzymes hydrolyse proteins (proteases), lipids (lipase, phospholipase), starch (amylase) and nucleic acids (ribonuclease, deoxyribonuclease) together with esterases and two specific proteases, gelatinase and elastase. These enzymes carry out luminal digestion of more highly polymerised substrates of >10 units (e.g. larger maltodextrins) whereas brush-border hydrolases favour shorter oligomers (e.g. maltose, maltotriose).

Proteases

The pancreatic proteases are either endopeptidases (trypsin, chymotrypsin and elastase) that cleave internal amino acid bonds or they are carboxypeptidases (A and B) that will sequentially cleave amino acids from the C-terminal of oligopeptides. The endopeptidases have specificities for bonds adjacent to dibasic amino acids (trypsin), hydrophobic amino acids (chymotrypsin) or small neutral amino acids (elastase). The combined actions of these enzymes will reduce dietary proteins to a mixture of free amino acids and peptides with a chain length of two to eight amino acids.

Like gastric pepsins, pancreatic proteases are secreted as inactive zymogens.

Enteropeptidase (sometimes known as enterokinase), a glycoprotein bound to the enterocyte brush-border, converts trypsinogen to trypsin by cleavage of a peptide sequence that blocks the active site of trypsinogen. Active trypsin which is released cannot catalyse further activation of trypsinogen, but does activate the zymogens of the other major proteases to yield chymotrypsin, elastase, carboxypeptidase A and carboxypeptidase B. The highest concentration of enteropeptidase is found in the duodenum and decreases distally; and its level of expression on the membrane depends on the luminal presence of pancreatic enzymes, amino acids or glucose.

Amylase

Both salivary and pancreatic α-amylases are most active at neutral pH and act as endoglucosidases that have an absolute specificity for α-1,4 glucose linkages with two adjacent α-1,4 linkages. Therefore, amylase will not cleave other glucose polymers such as β-glucans (oats), cellulose (plants) or dextran (dental plaque) or lactose or sucrose. The end-products of starch digestion are maltose, maltotriose and the α-1,6 branched limit dextrins.

No free glucose is released. Further digestion of the branched limit dextrins can only occur at the brush-border (catalysed by isomaltose or glucoamylase). The chain length of the linear, α-1,4-linked dextrins in the lumen after a starch meal depends on the extent to which α-amylase digestion has gone to completion, but is probably in the range 5–10 glucose units.

Lipases

There are three pancreatic lipases. Pancreatic triacylglycerol lipase (PL) is the most abundant and important in adult life; pancreatic lipase-related proteins 1 and 2 (PLRP-1, PLRP-2) are expressed pre- and perinatally but not in adulthood. PL has a preference for triacylglycerols rather than phospholipids. It is inhibited by bile salts but this inhibition is relieved by the colipase, another pancreatic protein, which binds to the C-terminal of the enzyme and helps it to bind to the lipid droplet surface. The N-terminal of the enzyme has a 'lid' sequence;

a highly mobile structure which, upon lipid binding, will swing aside to reveal the active site and thus allow lipid hydrolysis to occur. Fat digestion comprises the following steps:

1. Partial digestion and emulsification in the stomach.
2. Mixing of triacylglycerols, diacylglycerols, monoacylglycerols and fatty acids with detergent (bile salts), cholesterol and phospholipid to form mixed micelles that have a hydrophobic core and hydrophilic outer surface. Their small size and high surface area results in efficient hydrolysis.
3. Binding of colipase and lipase to the surface of these micelles leads to release of free fatty acids and retinol.
4. Osmotic pressures generated within the micelle by triacylglycerol hydrolysis causes budding of monoacylglycerol- and fatty-acid-rich micelles from the surface of these structures. These easily penetrate the unstirred water layer adjacent to the absorptive surface of the enterocyte.

Regulation of small intestinal motility

The pattern of intestinal motility depends critically on whether the subject is fasted, fed or postprandial. A typical peristaltic wave or migrating motor complex (MMC) will occur 4–6 hours after a meal and is a complex entity, comprising four phases that cycle continuously:

1. Phase I – inactivity (30–40 minutes)
2. Phase II – irregular pressure spike activity (30–40 minutes)
3. Phase III – intense repetitive high amplitude contractions (4–6 minutes)
4. Phase IV – irregular activity.

This cycle moves down the intestine at 4–6 cm/min before slowing in the terminal ileum and does not occur until 4–6 hours after a meal. Feeding initiates irregular activity throughout the small intestine, which resembles phase II of the MMC. It leads to greatly reduced rates of intestinal contraction and rate of movement, and this lengthens transit time in the bowel. The absorption of nutrients from the lumen of the small intestine is increased by the way in which the mucosa repeatedly dips into the chyme, minimising the diffusion barrier to absorption. At the same time, villous contractions help lymph and blood flow to carry away absorbed nutrients. These repetitive segmenting contractions are interspersed with erratic motile patterns that move chyme forwards rapidly by 10–30 cm before segmenting contractions recommence.

These responses are nutrient dependent. Lipid has particularly potent effects because it generates strong clustered contractions that enhance emulsification. In summary, fasting motility sweeps debris, shed cells and bacteria down the intestine whereas fed motility enhances digestion and absorption of nutrients. The transition between fasting and fed patterns is modulated by the presence of nutrients in the lumen. During a meal, a small portion of chyme (the head of the meal) will be rapidly swept down to the distal ileum, where the presence of digested fat evokes the ileal brake leading to a marked reduction in transit rate. In addition, the passage of food into the small bowel stimulates colonic segmental movement, known as the 'gastro-colonic reflex' (see Fig. CD 3.7A). This reflex is partially controlled by the cephalic phase of eating and leads to increased churning of colonic contents that increases absorption of nutrients, water and electrolytes from the colon and will eventually lead to defecation (see Fig. CD 3.7B). The short-chain fatty acids produced by bacterial fermentation in the colon not only stimulate water absorption, but if they reflux back through the ileocaecal valve into the ileum will simultaneously inhibit gastric emptying and stimulate peristalsis in the terminal ileum. The net effect is to sweep colonic bacteria from the distal small bowel.

Nasogastric tube-feeding is associated with diarrhoea. One cause is that the slow rate of nutrient infusion (4.2–6.3 kJ/minute) is insufficient to trigger a normal postprandial slowing of intestinal transit. It does, however, maintain colonic water secretion and hence provokes diarrhoea.

3.4 THE ABSORPTION AND SECRETION OF NUTRIENTS

Absorbed nutrients must cross four barriers to reach the bloodstream (Schultz 1998, Pacha 2000):

1. The mucus layer, a diffusion barrier which is rather thin in the small intestine.
2. The enterocyte apical membrane – a lipid bilayer, which requires transport proteins for water-soluble molecules
3. The enterocyte – a metabolic barrier which may metabolise the nutrient.

4. The basolateral membrane – a lipid bilayer which again requires transport proteins for water-soluble molecules.

In addition to transport proteins, absorption is enhanced by metabolic compartmentation or zonation within the enterocyte, which prevents excessive metabolism (e.g. only 10% of absorbed glucose).

The classification of transporters is shown in Figure CD 3.8 and the main intestinal transporters are listed in Table CD 3.1. Although different transporters carry very different substrates, they share many common structural features. They have regions of hydrophobic amino acids that can fold into helices which, when grouped together like the staves of a barrel, span the membrane and form a 'pore' through which substrates can be transported. Parts of the protein (bearing a sugar polymer) are outside the membrane and can act as a signalling receptor to allow other compounds to control the rate of transport of the main substrate. Alternatively, a transport protein may be linked to another regulatory protein that can chaperone the transporter into the membrane and thus modulate transport capacity. Transport may be either passive, allowing the transported nutrient to come to equilibrium across the membrane, or active, permitting a higher concentration to be achieved on one side of the membrane than the other.

Passive transporters

These comprise facilitated transporters and ion channels, which permit the transfer of a solute across the membrane in either direction. Transport therefore takes place down a concentration gradient (so-called 'downhill transport'). Net accumulation of the transported material in the cell can occur as a result of either onward metabolism to a compound that does not cross the membrane (e.g. vitamin B6 is accumulated intracellularly by phosphorylation to pyridoxal phosphate) or by binding to cytosolic proteins (e.g. ferritin, which binds iron).

Active transporters

These transport solutes against a concentration gradient, linked to either direct ATP utilisation (P-type transporters) or co-transport of an ion down its concentration gradient (symporters, which transport two solutes in parallel) (see Figs CD 3.8 and CD 3.9).

Direct utilisation of ATP involves phosphorylation of the transport protein, which permits it to transport one or more solute molecules in one direction only; solute transport causes dephosphorylation of the protein, so closing the pore.

Symporters commonly utilise a sodium ion gradient across the membrane, although some systems use a hydrogen ion gradient. The ionic gradient is generated by membrane ATPases that pump ions across the membrane. Intestinal absorption of glucose and some amino acids is by sodium-linked symporters.

Digestion and absorption of carbohydrates

The main dietary carbohydrates are starch, lactose and sucrose, as well as smaller amounts of glucose, sugar alcohols and fructose. Carbohydrates are only absorbed as monosaccharides, so starch assimilation proceeds in two phases.

Starch is hydrolysed by pancreatic amylase (and to some extent also by salivary amylase) to yield a mixture of glucose oligomers with a chain length in the range 5–10 glucose units. These are further hydrolysed by the brush-border glucosidases to glucose. In addition, some maltose and isomaltose are formed. Disaccharides are hydrolysed to their constituent monosaccharides by disaccharidases on the brush-border of the enterocytes: lactase, trehalase and a bifunctional enzyme, sucrase/isomaltase.

Glucose and galactose are taken up by the same active (sodium-linked) transporter (SGLT1) (see Fig. CD 3.10), while fructose, some other monosaccharides and sugar alcohols are carried by passive transporters. This means that only a proportion of fructose and sugar alcohols can be absorbed, and after a large dose much may remain in the lumen, leading to osmotic diarrhoea.

However, although SGLT1 has high affinity for glucose, it has a low transport capacity. There is a second glucose transporter, GLUT2, in the enterocyte that is only inserted into the membrane in response to glucose absorption via SGLT1. This process is controlled by insulin and dietary amino acids, mediated by protein kinase C activation. This leads to a great increase in transport capacity in response to dietary load.

Starch assimilation provides a good example of the distribution of digestive and absorptive function. It can be inferred that this occurs mainly in the duodenum, upper jejunum and proximal ileum because: (1) they have the highest mucosal expression of sucrase-isomaltase and the sodium glucose-linked transporter (SGLT1); (2) rapid appearance of blood glucose after a starch meal fits with this site of absorption; (3) removal of the distal small intestine hardly affects glucose assimilation. By contrast, most fat and fat-soluble vitamin assimilation occurs in the ileum, which has the highest transport capacity. Surgical removal of the ileum may therefore leave the patient at risk of essential fatty acid and fat-soluble vitamin deficiency.

Digestion and absorption of protein

The endopeptidases of gastric and pancreatic juice hydrolyse proteins to yield oligopeptides; aminopeptidases secreted by the intestinal mucosa and pancreatic carboxypeptidases then remove terminal amino acids sequentially from these oligopeptides, yielding free amino acids and di- and tripeptides. Early studies indicated the presence of amino acid transport systems with the following characteristics:

1. Stereospecific – L-amino acids are transported very much faster than D-amino acids.
2. Very specific so that only a small number of chemically related amino acids are transported by any one carrier system.
3. Duplicated – some amino acids are transported by more than one carrier system.

Some are sodium-linked, others are not. The main amino acid transports are shown in Table CD 3.1. The naming system is complex because it developed piecemeal: (1) system A (alanine) is a sodium symporter for small neutral aliphatic amino acids; (2) system ASC (i.e. alanine, serine and cysteine) is also a sodium-symporter; (3) system L (leucine) is not sodium-dependent and carries branched chain and aromatic amino acids; (4) system y+ is not sodium-dependent and carries dibasic amino acids; (5) system XAG is a sodium symporter and carries dicarboxylic (acidic) amino acids.

Di- and tripeptides are transported by separate systems from free amino acids. Patients with genetic defects of system ASC (cystinuria), which prevents intestinal absorption of arginine, lysine and cysteine, or system L (Hartnup disease), which prevents the absorption of aromatic and branched-chain amino acids, still absorb enough of the essential amino acids as small peptides to maintain nitrogen balance.

Di- and tripeptides are taken up into the enterocyte by peptide transporters (PEPT1 and PEPT2), hydrogen ion symporters that take advantage of the acid microclimate of the submucosal space. Unlike the amino acid transporters, PEPT1 and PEPT2 are:

1. Stereospecifically promiscuous – they will transport cyclic peptides, D-peptides, and *cis*-peptides.
2. Non-specific – they will transport most, if not all, of the theoretically possible 400 dipeptides and 8000 tripeptides, in addition to beta-lactam antibiotics (e.g. penicillin) and valacyclovir, an anti-herpes drug that has no peptide bond. The absorbed di- and tripeptides are hydrolysed by intracellular peptidases, and the resultant amino acids, together with those absorbed from the lumen as free amino acids, are transported into the villous microcirculation.

Some relatively large peptides (large enough to elicit antibody formation) enter the bloodstream intact, either by passing between cells or by uptake into mucosal cells. These are normally trapped by the gut-associated lymphoid tissue, but can enter the systemic circulation – this is the basis of food allergy (see Ch. 26).

Digestion and absorption of fat

The process of fat digestion is one of progressive emulsification of dietary lipids and hydrolysis of triacylglycerol to free fatty acids and monoacylglycerols. The final product of fat digestion is the mixed micelle, which buds smaller micelles (as a result of the osmotic action of the free fatty acids), which are transferred across the enterocyte membrane. Short-chain fatty acids enter the villus microcirculation, but most of the fatty acids are re-esterified to triacylglycerol in the mucosal cell, then are packaged into chylomicrons and secreted into the lacteals, and then into the lymphatic system (see Ch. 7).

Cholesterol and fat-soluble vitamins are absorbed dissolved in the hydrophobic core of the micelles. Much of the cholesterol destined for chylomicrons is esterified in the enterocyte, and competition between cholesterol and other sterols and stanols for the acyltransferase probably explains why these compounds reduce cholesterol absorption, and hence have a hypocholesterolaemic action.

Fatty acids can diffuse freely across the cell membrane. This occurs down a concentration gradient because of both intracellular binding to fatty acid binding proteins and esterification to triacylglycerol and also utilisation of fatty acids as a metabolic fuel inside the enterocyte. However, there is a strong body of experimental evidence to suggest that facilitated transport of fatty acids occurs. There is substrate selectivity of fatty acid uptake, and several membrane-bound proteins that can bind fatty acids have been identified (see Fig. CD 3.11A).

Within the enterocyte, fatty acids are transferred by intracellular fatty acid binding proteins (FABP) to the nascent lipid droplet where they are re-esterified to triacylglycerol. This lipid droplet enters the endoplasmic reticulum together with cholesterol, phospholipids, fat-soluble vitamins and apolipoproteins before moving to the Golgi apparatus where the chylomicron matures. Buds from the Golgi apparatus fuse with the enterocyte lateral membrane leading to exocytosis and the release of chylomicrons into the lymphatic system.

The rate-limiting step in this process is transfer of lipid from the endoplasmic reticulum to the Golgi apparatus, and triacylglycerol from excess dietary lipid may either be oxidised or temporarily stored within the endoplasmic reticulum. Components of chylomicrons (e.g. apoprotein A-IV) that enter the circulation can inhibit gastric emptying. This suggests that the intestinal motility is a key factor in controlling nutrient absorption because it is controlled by every stage of lipid digestion, absorption and repackaging.

The rate of movement of dietary fat into lymph depends on its fatty acid composition. Olive oil appears to be most rapidly absorbed, and cocoa butter and menhaden oil are most slowly absorbed. In malabsorption syndromes such as cystic fibrosis, medium chain triglycerides (MCT, chain length of 8–10 carbon atoms) are used because their shorter chain length and greater water solubility results in uptake into the portal circulation and hence a faster overall rate of macronutrient uptake.

The colonic microflora produce short-chain fatty acids (SCFAs), acetate, propionate and butyrate, by fermentation of resistant starch (see Ch. 6 and Fig. CD 3.11B) and non-starch polysaccharides. The presence of SCFAs in the colonic lumen is of interest because butyrate is a preferential fuel for the colonic mucosa, and promotes colonocyte differentiation. It may thus have a significant role in preventing colon cancer. Absorption of SCFAs can occur by diffusion across the colonocyte membrane, and they are also transported by a membrane transporter that co-transports Na^+ or K^+. Water uptake is stimulated by SCFA absorption and this is likely to be one of the major mechanisms for water and electrolyte salvage in the large intestine.

Absorption of vitamins

The fat-soluble vitamins A, D, E and K, and carotenoids (see Ch. 11) are absorbed dissolved in lipid micelles together with the products of fat digestion. Esters of vitamin A (retinyl esters) are hydrolysed in the duodenum by either pancreatic lipase or enterocyte brush-border phospholipase B. There is some evidence that there is a membrane transporter for retinol, then inside the cell, cellular retinol binding proteins (CRBP) bind retinol and channel it for resynthesis of retinyl esters by lecithin:retinol acyltransferase (LRAT) or acyl CoA:retinol acyltransferase (ARAT).

The water-soluble vitamins (see Ch. 10) are absorbed by specific transport proteins. Vitamin C is present in the intestinal lumen as both reduced ascorbic acid and oxidised dehydroascorbic acid. Ascorbic acid is absorbed by a sodium-dependent transporter (SVCT1), while dehydroascorbic acid is absorbed by the sodium-independent glucose transporters GLUT1 and GLUT3. Phosphorylated derivatives of vitamins B_1, B_2 and B_6 are dephosphorylated in the intestinal lumen, absorbed by facilitated (passive) transporters, then trapped inside the cells by rephosphorylation (see Ch. 10). Vitamin B_{12} is absorbed bound to intrinsic factor, a glycoprotein that is secreted by the parietal cells of the gastric mucosa (see Ch. 10).

Water and electrolytes

The human small intestine absorbs 6.5 to 7.5 litres of water each day (see Fig. CD 3.12). This comes from several sources as indicated in Figure 3.1. How this gets across the membrane is still a mystery because the lipid bilayer that surrounds each cell is impermeable to water, and the intestinal mucosal surface is rather hydrophobic. Before describing several hypotheses of water movement across the mucosa, it is worth summarising the known characteristics of the process. Water absorption is proportional to the amount of substrate and electrolyte that moves across the membrane; approximately 2 Na^+ ions and 210 water molecules accompany each molecule of glucose absorbed. The direction of water movement is governed by solute movement. In cholera, excessive secretion of chloride into the colon is accompanied by water secretion and diarrhoea, leading to dehydration and eventually death, unless treated. Therefore, stimulation of water uptake by glucose (and sodium) is the basis of oral rehydration therapy for the treatment of diarrhoea, which is the most important cause of infant death worldwide.

Although it is not known how water is transported, several hypotheses have been proposed (Spring 1999). Simple osmosis may account for some water uptake, but the osmolality difference is only 3–30 mosmol/kg, and this would mean that enterocytes replaced their entire fluid volume every few seconds. While some water is co-transported with solutes such as glucose through the transporter itself, enterocytes do not have enough transporters to account for all the water absorbed. Specific water transporters (aquaporins) occur in the cells of secretory epithelia, and studies in gene knockout mice suggest they may be quantitatively the most important factor in water absorption. The colon acts as an organ of water and electrolyte salvage, but its capacity is limited. Rapid infusion of 500 ml or more of water into the colon will provoke diarrhoea through reflex defecation and this is the basis of rectally administered enemas.

Sugar alcohols, used as sweeteners, such as xylitol, lactitol and sorbitol, are poorly absorbed and will enter the colon with sufficient water to maintain luminal isotonicity before fermentation and the absorption of SCFAs, water and Na^+. If the colonic fermentation capacity is exceeded then osmotic diarrhoea ensues because the excess water cannot be absorbed.

Clinically the synthetic disaccharide lactulose (which is not hydrolysed in the small intestine) and the sugar alcohol lactitol are used as laxatives. Other causes of osmotic diarrhoea include dietary fibre such as guar gum, probiotics such as fructose oligosaccharide and beans that contain large quantities of stachyose, all of which are good substrates for bacterial fermentation. The laxative threshold (where gastrointestinal symptoms are unacceptable) for most non-absorbed carbohydrates is about 70 g/day, but most people will notice the effects of 40 g/day.

Most minerals are absorbed by carrier-mediated diffusion, and are then accumulated by binding to intracellular binding proteins, followed by sodium-dependent transport from the enterocyte into the villous microcirculation. Genetic defects of either the intracellular binding proteins or the active transport systems at the basal membrane of the enterocyte can result in minerals deficiency despite an apparently adequate intake. As discussed in Chapter 11, the enterocyte calcium binding protein is induced by vitamin D, and vitamin D deficiency results in much reduced absorption of calcium.

3.5 THE ROLE OF THE GASTROINTESTINAL TRACT IN THE REGULATION OF FEEDING

As discussed in Chapter 5, there are both long-term and short-term mechanisms to regulate food intake and energy expenditure, so as to maintain energy balance. Short-term control of appetite is regulated by the gastrointestinal tract as well as by the metabolic response to ingested nutrients. There are three ways in which the gastrointestinal tract provides regulatory feedback signals. These signals arise from direct effects of absorbed nutrients in the circulation, from neural signals from the gut and liver and from hormonal signals (Rehfeld 1998).

Although the existence of more than 100 gastrointestinal peptide hormones complicates this, one investigative approach has been to predict the properties of an ideal short-term 'satiety hormone'. It would be secreted in response to feeding, and have receptors in both the gut and the central nervous system that will result in a decrease in the size of a single meal. Its effect will decrease quickly, to be followed by a compensatory increase in feeding (see Fig. CD 3.13A).

At least two hormones secreted by the gastrointestinal tract meet these criteria: cholecystokinin (CCK), secreted by the duodenum (which also stimulates secretion of bile and pancreatic juice, and regulates intestinal motility), and leptin, secreted by the stomach, although the main source of leptin is adipose tissue, and its main function is to regulate long-term food intake and energy expenditure in response to the state of fat reserves (see Ch. 5 and Fig. CD 3.13B).

The mouth

The taste of food, as well as the smell before eating, stimulates secretion of gastric juice and intestinal motility. There are five families of receptors on the tongue, for sweet, salty or meaty/savoury (umami) flavours, which are generally pleasurable, and for sour or bitter tastes, which are generally aversive. In addition, the tongue can sense the fatty acids liberated from triacylglycerols by lingual lipase. Combinations of taste and sensation may have additive effects, for example sugar mixed with fat is particularly pleasurable, and salt may be useful in masking bitter flavours that are taste-aversive. The importance of taste in controlling sensations of hunger and satiety is seen in patients receiving long-term tube-feeding who experience constant feelings of hunger although nutritionally replete.

The taste of food provides a strong signal to stimulate eating. However, this process operates only when there are sensations of hunger and is suppressed when sensations of satiety become strong. This is known as sensory-specific or conditioned satiety. It is thought that a dominant factor in this process is the action of dopamine on the hypothalamus in response to absorbed fat.

The stomach

During eating, food stretches the stomach and induces a complex series of signals that lead to cessation of eating. The importance of this can be illustrated by taking a glass of water with a meal to induce feelings of satiety whilst eating, but not afterwards. Conversely, in rats in which gastric contents are continuously removed during the meal through a fistula ('shamfeeding'), the amount of food eaten each meal is greatly increased. The mechanism is due to stretch, not gastric pressure, and works through direct inhibition of the stimulating effect of pleasurable tastes on eating. Signals from taste receptors in the mouth and from gastric stretch receptors are integrated in the parabrachial nucleus of the pons in the brainstem so that one signal will downregulate the other (see Fig. CD 3.14).

The small intestine

In addition to stretch receptors, the intestinal mucosa possesses an abundance of receptors for acid and for fatty acids and glucose and amino acids, which will provide information about the contents of the lumen that the brainstem will integrate and use to control eating behaviour. Cholecystokinin, released in response to luminal fat, leads to powerful inhibition of eating.

Absorbed nutrients are also potent signals that modulate eating behaviour. For example, in adequately nourished subjects, the intravenous infusion of lipid stimulates dopamine activity (which acts as a feeding inhibitor) and increases satiety ratings, feelings of fullness and reduces the desire to select particular foodstuffs. In contrast, studies in the hospital population (which experience 40–50% malnutrition) have shown that fortification of hospital food with fat actually stimulates energy intake. This mechanism thus depends on sensations of hunger that are related to nutritional status. However, these mechanisms can be overridden centrally. An example of this would be the inability to resist the unexpected offer of a plate of strawberries and cream after a particularly heavy meal.

⤷ Key points

- ⤷ The gastrointestinal tract provides a linear sequence of events resulting in the hydrolysis of dietary carbohydrates, triacylglycerols and proteins, and the absorption of the products of digestion.

- ⤷ Salivary and gastric secretions are stimulated before eating, then the presence of food in the mouth and stomach stimulates further secretion.

- ⤷ Gastric emptying is controlled by both the amount of food eaten during a meal, and also nutrients present in the food and the progress made in liquidising it within the stomach.

- ⤷ Pancreatic and intestinal secretion are stimulated by hormones secreted in response to the presence of food in the stomach.

- ⤷ The monosaccharides resulting from carbohydrate digestion, and free amino acids from protein digestion, are absorbed into the hepatic portal vein, and the liver regulates the entry into the peripheral circulation of the products of digestion.

- ⤷ Amylases in saliva and pancreatic juice catalyse hydrolysis of starch to disaccharides and limit dextrins; disaccharides are hydrolysed by intestinal brush-border enzymes, and monosaccharides are absorbed by active transport (glucose and galactose) or passive transport (other monosaccharides and sugar alcohols).

- ⤷ Lipases secreted by the tongue, in gastric juice and pancreatic juice catalyse the progressive hydrolysis of triacylglycerol until dietary lipid is emulsified into micelles small enough to be absorbed across the small intestinal lumen. Most absorbed fatty acids are re-esterified in the mucosal cells and absorbed into the lymphatic system in chylomicrons, but medium-chain fatty acids are absorbed into the hepatic portal vein.

⟳ Proteolytic enzymes are secreted as inactive zymogens. Pepsinogen in the gastric juice is activated by gastric acid and autocatalysis; trypsinogen in the pancreatic juice is activated by intestinal enteropeptidase. Trypsin then activates the other intestinal zymogens.

⟳ Protein digestion begins with the action of endopeptidases, which hydrolyse proteins at specific sites within the molecule, resulting in the formation of a large number of oligopeptides. Exopeptidases then remove amino and carboxy terminal amino acids, resulting in free amino acids and di- and tripeptides.

⟳ Free amino acids are absorbed by a variety of group-specific transporters; di- and tripeptides are absorbed by non-specific transporters, and hydrolysed within the intestinal mucosal cells

References and further reading

References

Atuma C, Strugala V, Allen A, Holm L 2001 The adherent gastrointestinal mucus gel layer: thickness and physical state in vivo. American Journal of Physiology (Gastrointestinal and Liver Physiology) 280(5):G922–G929

Pacha J 2000 Development of intestinal transport function in mammals. Physiological Reviews 80(4):1633–1667

Rehfeld J F 1998 The new biology of gastrointestinal hormones. Physiological Reviews 78(4):1087–1108

Rothman S, Liebow C, Isenman L 2002 Conservation of digestive enzymes. Physiological Reviews 82(1):1–18

Schultz S G 1998 A century of (epithelial) transport physiology: from vitalism to molecular cloning. American Journal of Physiology (Cell Physiology) 274(1):C13–C23

Spring K R 1999 Epithelial fluid transport – a century of investigation. News in Physiological Sciences 14:92–98

Further reading

Havel P J 2001 Peripheral signals conveying metabolic information to the brain: short-term and long-term regulation of food intake and energy homeostasis. Experimental Biology and Medicine (Maywood) 226(11):963–977

Lowe M E 1997 Molecular mechanisms of rat and human pancreatic triglyceride lipases. Journal of Nutrition 127(4):549–557

Spring K R 1999 Epithelial fluid transport – a century of investigation. News in Physiological Sciences 14:92–98

Stevens C E, Hume I D 1998 Contributions of microbes in vertebrate gastrointestinal tract to production and conservation of nutrients. Physiological Reviews 78(2):393–427

Website

http://arbl.cvmbs.colostate.edu/hbooks/pathphys/digestion/basics/index.html#top

CD-ROM contents

Tables

Table CD 3.1 Substrate transporters in the human intestine

Figures

Figure CD 3.1 The regulation of intestinal absorption and secretion by communication between intestinal cells

Figure CD 3.2A Size of the human intestine

Figure CD 3.2B Intestinal architecture

Figure CD 3.2C Relative locations of digestion and absorption of nutrients in the healthy gastrointestinal tract

Figure CD 3.3 The swallowing motor pattern

Figure CD 3.4 The depth of the mucus layer

Figure CD 3.5 Hydrolysis of lipid droplets by human gastric lipase

Figure CD 3.6 How a gastric hormone alters the stomach's response to a meal

Figure CD 3.7A Pressure waves in the colon and movement of a meal

Figure CD 3.7B Regional velocity of propagating pressure waves in the colon

Figure CD 3.8 Transporters and their classification

Figure CD 3.9 Intestinal epithelium and routes of solute transport

Figure CD 3.10 Glucose transport via the sodium glucose-linked transporter (SGLT1)

Figure CD 3.11A Distribution of a fatty acid transporter along the intestine

Figure CD 3.11B Resistant starch granules and their digestion in the colon

Figure CD 3.12 Water movements in the gut

Figure CD 3.13A Short-term signals regulating food intake and control of energy balance

Figure CD 3.13B Long-term signals regulating food intake and control of energy balance

Figure CD 3.14 How the taste of food and gastric distension have opposite effects on appetite

Further reading from the book

4

Body size and composition

John Garrow

Objectives

By the end of this chapter you should be able to:

- define terms for components of body composition
- describe their relative size and variation
- describe their main characteristics and functions
- summarise the use of composition information in nutrition
- describe the main methods for measurement of body fat, fat-free mass, lean body mass, body water and blood fractions.

4.1 INTRODUCTION

Nutrients in the diet are essential to provide: the elements from which the human body is built, the energy on which all metabolic activity depends, and cofactors (vitamins and trace elements) which cannot be synthesised within the body. This chapter is concerned with composition of the body, and the information that this gives us about the quality of the diet. For example, normal growth in children is impossible without an adequate intake of protein and energy, normal fat stores depend on balancing energy input and output, and synthesis of essential components such as haemoglobin or thyroid hormone depends on an adequate intake of iron, or iodine, respectively.

4.2 BODY COMPOSITION AND FUNCTION

Fat-free mass or lean body mass: definitions

The earliest measurements of body composition in living human subjects were made to discover if overweight individuals contained an unusually large amount of fat, or of muscle (see 'Body fat', below). The method used was to measure average body density, since fat has a density of $0.900\,g/cm^3$ and a typical mixture of non-fat tissues has a density of $1.100\,g/cm^3$. Therefore density, and other methods that have been calibrated against density (like skinfold thickness), yield estimates of *fat* and *fat-free mass*, which together make up total body weight.

Computer scanning methods recognise tissues, such as adipose tissue, by the amount of X-radiation they absorb. Adipose tissue is not pure fat, but approximately 79% fat, 3% protein and 18% water. Tissue other than adipose tissue is not totally fat-free, since there is lipid in cell membranes and in nervous tissue. Therefore scanning methods measure *adipose tissue* and *lean body mass*, which together make up total body weight. The terms fat-free mass and lean body mass are often used interchangeably, but this is not correct.

Human cadaver analysis

Our understanding of body composition in human subjects is based on the chemical analyses of six cadavers (five male and one female), performed between 1945 and 1956. First the fat in these bodies was separated by dissection and extraction with an ether-chloroform mixture, so what remained was fat-free mass. The fat-free body in adults has a fairly constant composition with respect to its water, protein and potassium content. Table 4.1 summarises these results. On average, fat-free tissue contains about 72.5% water, 20.5% protein and 69 mmol K/kg. In Section 4.4 there is further discussion about the methods by which estimates of whole body density, or water, or potassium, combined with the data in Table 4.1, can be used to calculate the fat-free mass of living people.

The concept of a fat-free mass of constant composition is a great help in estimating fat-free mass in living people, but Table 4.1 also shows that this assumption is an over-simplification. For example, skin and brain have very different chemical compositions. Skin has a very high protein content and low water content (30.0% and 69.4%, respectively) and

Table 4.1 **The contribution of water and protein to the fat-free weight of adult bodies and in some organs**

	Water (g/kg)	Protein (g/kg)	Remainder (g/kg)	Potassium (mmol/kg)	K:N ratio
Fat-free whole bodies					
Age (years)					
25	728	195	77	71.5	2.29
35	775	165	60	–	–
42	733	192	75	73.0	2.38
46	674	234	92	66.5	1.78
48	730	206	64	–	–
60	704	238	58	66.6	1.75
Mean	724	205	71	69.4	2.05
Selected organs					
Skin	694	300	6	23.7	0.45
Heart	827	143	30	66.5	2.90
Liver	711	176	113	75.0	2.66
Kidneys	810	153	37	57.0	2.33
Brain	774	107	119	84.6	4.96
Muscle	792	192	16	91.2	2.99

Data compiled from various sources.

very little K (23.7 mmol/kg). By contrast, brain has a very low protein and high water content (10.7% and 77.4%, respectively) and a high concentration of K (84.6 mmol/kg). This is because brain has a lot of intracellular water, which contains K, whereas skin has little water, and most of that is extracellular. This detailed information about the chemical composition of individual tissues and organs can only be obtained by chemical analysis of autopsy or biopsy samples.

Water and electrolytes: intracellular and extracellular

Using the data from cadaver analyses we can construct a diagram of the components of the body of a typical normal young adult who weighs 70 kg: this is shown in Figure 4.1.

For the sake of simplicity we will use rounded numbers, and assume a fat content of 12 kg (17%), so the fat-free mass is 58 kg. By far the largest component of fat-free mass is water (42 kg), which is 72.5% of fat-free weight. Approximately two-thirds of this water (28 kg) is inside cells, i.e. intracellular fluid (ICF), and the remaining third (14 kg) is extracellular, i.e. extracellular fluid (ECF).

The total amount of water in the body, and the partition of body water between ICF and ECF, is closely regulated. Body stores of protein, energy,

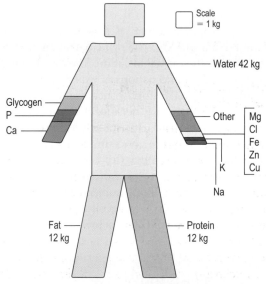

Figure 4.1   Diagrammatic representation of the body composition of a normal adult male weighing 70 kg. The contributions of the components to body weight are represented by their area in the diagram: only fat, protein and glycogen contribute to the energy stores of the body.

vitamins and minerals ensure survival for many weeks without dietary intake, but deprivation of water causes death in a few days (see 'Changes in hydration: diarrhoea, oedema, kwashiorkor, heart or kidney failure', below).

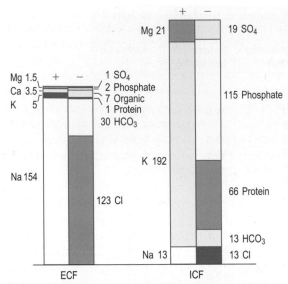

Figure 4.2 Electrolyte composition (mEq/kg water) of extracellular fluid (ECF) and intracellular fluid (ICF).

The electrolyte composition of ICF and ECF is shown in Figure 4.2.

The principal anion in ICF is K, with a small amount of Na and Mg. The principal anion in ECF is Na, and Cl is the principal cation. The total electrical charge of anions and cations is exactly balanced in ICF and in ECF. The total concentration of ions is greater in ICF than ECF, because ICF contains polyvalent cations, particularly proteins, but the osmolality (determined by the concentration of molecules, rather than ions) of the two fluids is identical.

Methods by which we can measure the total amount of water in a living subject, and the proportion of this water that is extracellular, are described in 'Total body water (TBW)', below.

Bone: composition, types, density, growth and turnover

Bone contains a matrix of fibrillar collagen that gives it tensile strength. Packed in an orderly manner around the collagen fibres is the mineral that gives the bone rigidity. This mineral is a complex crystalline calcium phosphate, called hydroxyapatite. Finally the bone is covered by a vascular fibrous sheath, the periosteum. An adult body contains approximately 1 kg of Ca, of which 99% is in bone. The skeleton also contains approximately 500 g of P, and more than half the collagen in the body, the remaining collagen being in skin, tendons and fascial sheaths.

Every bone has a dense outer osseous layer which is filled inside by spongy bone arranged with trabeculae of different direction and strength, depending on the stress to which the bone is subjected. The spaces between the trabeculae are filled with bone marrow which is highly vascular, and in which new blood cells are made.

Bone has two main functions: to provide a rigid frame for the body and protect certain organs from injury, and to afford attachments for muscles and their tendons. The shape of the bone depends on its function. The bones of the skull, shoulder blade and pelvis are flat, and have dense outer layers separated by a small amount of spongy bone. They provide protection to the brain, chest and pelvic organs, respectively, as well as attachment for muscles. The small bones of the hands and feet have a thin compact outer layer, and relatively large proportion of spongy bone; they provide attachments for the many small muscles that cause the intricate movements of fingers and toes. The long bones of the limbs are designed to resist twisting and bending stresses, for which their design is appropriate. The shaft of the long bones is a thick-walled tube of dense bone that has expanded ends to bear the articular surfaces of the shoulder, elbow, wrist, hip, knee or ankle joints, and to provide anchorage for the powerful muscles that move these joints. The spine is a column of short cylindrical vertebrae, separated by cartilaginous discs, that bear the weight of the body in the standing position. The body of the vertebra is filled with spongy bone, but the dorsal processes of compact bone provide both anchorage for the powerful spinal muscles, and a protective tunnel for the spinal cord.

Bone density is determined by the quantity of bone per unit volume. This in turn depends on the balance of activity between osteoblasts (cells that stimulate new bone formation) and osteoclasts (cells that cause resorption of bone). Factors that influence this balance are discussed in Chapter 24. It has become possible to measure the bone mineral content of selected bones since the development of quantitative radiological scanning techniques (see 'Body fat', below). Normally bone density reaches a maximum around the age of 30 years, and then declines. Peak bone density is greater in men than in women, so women are more liable than men to develop osteoporosis in later life. This is a condition in which the quantity of bone per unit volume is decreased, so the trabeculae become thinner and weaker, and the dense cortical bone becomes porous. (This should not be confused with osteomalacia (or rickets, in children), which is a defect of bone mineralisation, and causes deformities because the bones are unduly pliable.) Osteoporosis is a common and important disorder in the elderly, since it predisposes to fractures, especially of the vertebrae, femoral neck and forearm. (See Section 24.3 for further information.)

Bone growth does not progress at an equal rate in all parts of the skeleton. The brain (and therefore also the skull that encloses it) is proportionately very large in the fetus, but after birth the limbs grow more rapidly in both length and strength. At birth there are no ossification centres for the wrist bones, or for the ends of the humerus, radius, ulna or fibula. This is of importance for nutritional assessment, since a child who is chronically undernourished will show delayed development of these ossification centres. If the undernutrition is severe and prolonged the normal growth of long bones will not occur, and adult height will be stunted. The normal changes in body size and composition throughout the lifespan are described further in Section 4.3. The proportion of body weight as adipose tissue, muscle bone and skin is shown in Table CD 4.1.

The constituents of bone are not static: both the protein and mineral in bone are constantly exchanging with the amino acid and mineral metabolic pools in the body. Whereas most body proteins turn over with a half-life of days or weeks, the turnover of collagen is very slow. Enzymic hydrolysis of collagen yields a mixture of amino acids that have a low nutritional value, because, in the synthesis of collagen, proline is hydroxylated, and hydroxyproline cannot be used to synthesise new protein. The turnover rate of collagen can be estimated from the urinary excretion of hydroxyproline, which is typically about 20 mg per day in an adult. This is very little compared with the 10 g of urea nitrogen excreted daily from the catabolism of all the other body proteins in an adult on a normal diet.

Bone calcium also exchanges with calcium in other organs, especially kidney and gut. These fluxes are controlled by the action of parathyroid hormone, 1,25-dihydroxycholecalciferol (vitamin D, see Ch. 11) and calcitonin. It is essential for normal muscular and neurological function that plasma Ca is maintained in the range of 2.25–2.60 mmol/l. Disorders of bone metabolism are described further in Chapter 24.

Muscle: types, growth, repair, function

In a typical adult, skeletal muscle accounts for approximately 40% of body weight, and another 10%

is smooth muscle. The water, protein and potassium content of muscle is shown in Table 4.1. Since muscle makes up so much of fat-free weight, the composition of muscle is similar to that of the average of all fat-free tissues. However, skeletal muscle differs markedly from other tissues in an important respect: resting muscle has a lower energy consumption per unit weight than tissues such as heart, liver, kidneys or brain, but during vigorous physical exercise the energy consumption in muscle greatly exceeds the total of all other body tissues.

There are three types of muscle: skeletal, smooth and cardiac. Skeletal muscle consists of bundles of individual muscle fibres, each of which ranges from 10 to 80 μm in diameter. In most muscles these fibres extend the whole length of the muscle. Each fibre is activated by a single nerve ending, situated near the middle of the fibre. Each fibre contains several hundred to several thousand myofibrils. Each myofibril contains about 1500 myosin filaments and 3000 actin filaments arranged longitudinally with an overlapping zone between the two types of filament that shows as a darker band on electron micrographs, which causes a striated appearance on the whole muscle. When the muscle contracts the overlap between the actin and myosin fibres increases, and thus the two ends of the muscle, and the bones to which these ends are attached, are pulled towards each other. During muscle relaxation the actin and myosin units slide apart, but even at full relaxation they retain a degree of overlap.

Smooth muscle also consists of actin and myosin units sliding together and apart, but the muscle fibres are far smaller. Smooth muscle fibres are 2 to 5 μm in diameter, and only 50 to 200 μm in length, whereas the diameter of skeletal muscle fibres is up to 20 times greater, and they are thousands of times longer. Smooth muscle does not move joints, but lies in the walls of blood vessels, gut, bile ducts, ureters and uterus. Contraction and relaxation of the smooth muscle in the walls of these organs alters the diameter of the tubes, or may be organised in peristaltic waves so as to move forwards the contents of the tube.

Cardiac muscle, as its name implies, forms the chambers of the heart. Unlike skeletal muscle it is not organised as bundles of individually innervated muscle fibres, but is a syncytium of cells fused end-to-end in a latticework. The electrical potential that causes one cell to contract readily passes to adjacent cells, and the whole mass of muscle contracts and relaxes synchronously. Thus contraction expels the blood within the chamber through an exit valve, and then as it relaxes the chamber refills by permitting blood to flow in through an entry valve.

In skeletal muscle, physiologists distinguish two types of muscle cell: red and white fibres. In birds, for example, muscles in the breast are designed for the rapid movement required for flight, and breast muscle is white. However, the legs of birds contain mainly red muscle, since legs are required to sustain posture for long periods, but not to move as quickly as wings. In human subjects there is a less marked difference between the fibre types of muscles in different parts of the body, and most muscles in human beings contain a mixture of red and white fibres. The effect of different types of physical training on the size and proportions of red and white fibres is considered in Chapter 18, and fuel selection in muscle in Chapter 5.

Blood: serum, plasma, RBC, WBC, normal values, cell turnover

Blood consists of plasma and cells – red blood cells (RBC), white blood cells (WBC) and platelets. It is primarily a medium for the transport of oxygen, nutrients, and hormones to the tissues, and for the removal of carbon dioxide and other waste products from tissues. In a typical adult the volume of blood is approximately 5 litres, of which about 55% is plasma and 45% the volume of packed cells (the haematocrit). If a sample of blood is withdrawn from a peripheral vein and put in a glass test tube it will solidify as a web of fibrin forms. The fibrin then contracts and squeezes together the trapped cells, so after a few minutes there is a firm dark red mass at the bottom of the tube (a blood clot) and a clear yellowish supernatant fluid (serum). Serum is plasma from which the proteins involved in blood clotting have been removed. If we wish to obtain a sample of plasma it is necessary to put the fresh blood sample into a tube with an anticoagulant, and then to separate the cells by centrifugation.

If blood did not contain red cells (RBC) it would be able to transport only 0.3 ml of oxygen dissolved in 100 ml of plasma. This would be quite inadequate to meet the oxygen requirements of the body tissues, even under conditions of basal metabolism. RBCs are packets of haemoglobin in a rather tough bi-concave cell wall which is freely permeable to oxygen, so the presence of RBCs enables 100 ml of blood to transport up to 20 ml of oxygen.

Red blood cells develop in the bone marrow from stem cells to the reticulocyte stage in about 3 days. The reticulocyte is so called because, on staining, remnants of nucleic acid appear as a blue network in the cytoplasm. This is the most immature form of red cell normally seen in the peripheral circulation, but normally 99% of red blood cells are fully mature, with no nucleic acid or nucleus. The mature red blood cells survive in the circulation for about 120 days, after which they are destroyed in the reticuloendothelial system. The haemoglobin is broken down to bilirubin, and the iron is recycled for the synthesis of new haemoglobin for new red blood cells.

White cells are approximately a thousand times less common than red cells in the blood. The commonest type of white blood cell is the polymorph, or neutrophil granulocyte, which, like RBCs, is formed in bone marrow. The neutrophil count increases rapidly in response to infection or tissue injury. Neutrophils survive in the peripheral circulation for a very short time: their half-life is estimated at 6 to 8 hours. The next commonest white blood cell is the lymphocyte, which is formed in lymphoid tissue. This cell is involved in immune responses. The remaining white blood cells (monocytes, basophil and eosinophil granulocytes) occur still more rarely. Platelets are very small cells that are involved in blood clotting and the repair of damaged blood vessels.

Body fat: subcutaneous, intra-abdominal and intra-organ, and brown fat

Body fat has become unfashionable: in modern affluent communities it is desirable to be slim, but to our ancestors, and to those now living in subsistence economies, body fat is a valuable store of energy during times of famine, and a thermal insulator when the environment is cold. These valuable characteristics of fat still exist, but in affluent countries (and increasingly in developing countries) the need for protection from famine and cold is less often required, and excessive fatness is increasingly common.

The typical adult illustrated in Figure 4.1 contains 12 kg of fat, which is 17% of body weight. This degree of fatness is within the healthy range. Usually 90% of this fat is in a layer under the skin, but there is also fat within the abdominal cavity, and a small amount is in the fascial planes between muscles. Not all of body fat is available as an energy store: even in the bodies of people who have died of starvation there is still about 2 kg of fat remaining. A reserve of 10 kg of fat contains 375 MJ (90 000 kcal), equivalent to about 4 weeks of normal energy requirements. In fact, people of normal weight on total starvation survive for about 10 weeks, because energy expenditure decreases. In severely obese people the fat stores may reach 80 kg: such people can survive a year of starvation, but this is not appropriate treatment for severe obesity. See Chapters 5 and 20 for further discussion of this topic.

The distribution of body fat differs between men and women, and this has metabolic significance. At puberty, women tend to store fat around breast, hip and thigh regions, whereas men tend to accumulate fat in and on the abdomen. If adults become obese they may deposit the excess fat in female (or gynoid) pattern, or the male (android) pattern (see Fig. CD 4.1). This pattern is probably genetically determined: even when excess fat is lost the characteristic pattern is preserved. In vitro measurement of rates of lipolysis in biopsies of adipose tissue have shown similar basal rates of lipolysis in femoral and abdominal adipose tissue in non-pregnant women. However, lipolysis in femoral fat increases during lactation. It seems that femoral fat is conserved in the non-pregnant woman, but made available as an energy source in later stages of pregnancy and lactation.

It has been observed that obesity, and particularly fat deposited in the abdominal cavity (and hence associated with the android body shape), strongly predisposes to diabetes mellitus and heart disease. This is probably because the intra-abdominal fat is much more sensitive to lipolytic stimuli than subcutaneous fat, and this intra-abdominal lipolysis causes a rapid increase in the free fatty acid flow into the portal vein. This in turn predisposes to hyperinsulinaemia, hyperlipidaemia and hypertension. For further discussion of the risk factors associated with abdominal obesity see Chapter 20.

Body fat is synthesised by, and stored in, fat cells, or adipocytes. Adipocytes from subcutaneous white fat can be sampled by needle biopsy and studied in the laboratory. They have a nucleus in a thin rind of cytoplasm surrounding a large fat globule (see Fig. CD 4.2). A typical adipocyte in a biopsy sample from a normal-weight person contains about 0.6 µg of fat. If we assume that the 12 kg of fat in the man in Figure 4.1 is stored in adipocytes of this size we can calculate that he has 2.0×10^{10} fat cells in his body. If a biopsy sample is taken from an obese adult with, say, 60 kg of body fat, the average adipocyte is not five times the normal size, but only about 50% larger than normal, so there must be more adipocytes than normal in obese people. This reasoning led to the

hypothesis that if a child became obese before a certain age then proliferation of adipocytes was stimulated, and the child would be predisposed to obesity in later life.

We now know the hypothesis is not true, because new adipocytes can develop at any age if the amount of fat to be stored increases. However, the idea stimulated research into the metabolic activity of adipocytes, which has yielded valuable information. We now know that white adipose tissue has two important functions related to energy balance and reproductive function. Aromatase is an enzyme in adipose tissue that catalyses the conversion of androstenedione to oestrogen, and in postmenopausal women it is the only route of oestrogen production. This probably explains the association between obesity and abnormalities of sex steroid hormones, especially in conditions such as polycystic ovarian syndrome.

There is now intense research on the product of the *ob* gene, which is lacking in the obese mutant mouse. This is the hormone leptin. It was discovered in 1994, it is produced by adipocytes, and it is involved in the control of both food intake and energy expenditure. Obese mice are deficient in leptin and infertile, so there was great excitement when it was shown that administration of leptin cured both obesity and infertility in these animals. Unfortunately studies on obese human subjects showed that they had abnormally high, rather than low, leptin concentrations, and therapeutically the administration of leptin has not realised early expectations.

Unlike the white fat cell, the brown fat cell has small fat droplets in a cytoplasm rich in mitochondria in which heat can be generated (see Fig. CD 4.2). It is important to small mammals to be able to generate heat to maintain body temperature in cold environments. Hypothermia is particularly a problem in newborn mammals (including human babies) because their small body mass does not generate enough heat by normal metabolic processes to maintain body temperature, so some extra thermogenic source is required. A defect in thermogenesis is the cause of obesity in some animal models, so it was thought that defective brown fat might be a cause of human obesity. However, obese human beings have a higher (not lower) total heat production than lean people, and in mammals weighing more than 6 kg the heat generated in normal metabolism is sufficient to maintain body temperature in normal environments, so there is no need for additional thermogenesis.

4.3 CHANGES IN BODY SIZE AND COMPOSITION

Throughout the lifespan – normal growth and composition

On the first day after fertilisation the human embryo is a single cell, approximately 0.15 mm in diameter. After 2 months of intrauterine life it is about 30 mm long with recognisable head, trunk and limbs; at that stage the head accounts for half the total body length. By the end of normal gestation, at 9 months, the fetus is 500 mm in length and weighs about 3.5 kg: the head is then one-quarter of total length. After two decades of extrauterine life the average adult weighs about 70 kg, is 1.7–1.8 m tall, of which the head accounts for only one-eighth of total stature.

Changes in the ratio of head size to that of the whole body during growth are associated with changes in the chemical composition of the tissues. The embryo contains a very high percentage of water, but with maturation the proportion of water decreases, and there is a shift in the distribution of water from extracellular (with sodium, Na, as the chief anion) to intracellular (with potassium, K, as the chief anion). As the proportion of water decreases, protein and electrolytes, as a proportion of body weight, increase. Fat is deposited mainly during the last trimester of pregnancy and the first year of extrauterine life. These changes are shown in Table 4.2.

During childhood and adolescence the proportion of water in the body, and the proportion of extracellular to intracellular water, continues to decrease. Increase in total body K, Ca and P in fat-free tissue reflects the increase in intracellular water and growth in the skeleton. Fat-free mass remains fairly constant in both men and women between the ages of 20 and 65 years, but then decreases by about 15% in the next two decades (see Fig. CD 4.3). Throughout adult life there is a trend for fat mass to increase in both men and women, but the increase is more rapid in postmenopausal women. Changes in body composition with age are shown in Table CD 4.2 and changes in tissue protein content with age in Table CD 4.3.

Effects of diet and exercise on body size and composition

The laws of thermodynamics require that if over a given period the energy intake of an individual is 10 MJ (2400 kcal) less than energy output, then the energy stored in the body must be reduced by 10 MJ. That is invariably true. However, a decrease of 10 MJ in energy stores may be achieved by losing 0.27 kg of fat, or 2.4 kg of fat-free tissue, or (more probably) an intermediate amount of weight made up from a mixture of lean and fat tissue. But it does not follow that if the individual increases his energy output by 10 MJ (for example by exercising) and does not change his

Table 4.2 Effect of growth, malnutrition and obesity on the composition of the body and of fat-free tissue

	Fetus, 20–25 weeks	Premature baby	Full-term baby	Infant (1 year)	Adult man	Malnourished infant	Obese man
Body weight (kg)	0.3	1.5	3.5	20	70	5	100
Water (%)	88	83	69	62	60	74	47
Protein (%)	9.5	11.5	12	14	17	14	13
Fat (%)	0.5	3.5	16	20	17	10	35
Remainder (%)	2	2	3	4	6	2	5
Fat-free weight (kg)	0.30	1.45	2.94	8.0	58	4.5	65
Water (%)	88	85	82	76	72	82	73
Protein (%)	9.4	11.9	14.4	18	21	15	21
Na (mmol/kg)	100	100	82	81	80	88	82
K (mmol/kg)	43	50	53	60	66	48	64
Ca (g/kg)	4.2	7.0	9.6	14.5	22.4	9.0	20
Mg (g/kg)	0.18	0.24	0.26	3.5	0.5	0.25	0.5
P (g/kg)	3.0	3.8	5.6	9.0	12.0	5.0	12.0

Data compiled from various sources.

energy intake, the above losses will be achieved. As weight is lost, resting energy expenditure also decreases, so for a given energy intake the energy deficit, and hence the rate of weight loss, also decreases. This effect is quite small: about 70 kJ (16 kcal)/day/kg weight lost in men, and about 50 kJ (12 kcal)/day/kg weight lost in women.

A larger rate of weight loss was observed in a study of 108 obese women whose average starting weight was 100.8 kg (SD 23.6) (see Fig. CD 4.4). On a diet supplying 3.4 MJ (800 kcal)/day their average weight loss in 3 weeks was 5.0 kg, but it was significantly faster (330 g/day) during the first week than during the next 2 weeks (210 g/day). This is because during the first week on a diet, glycogen (and its associated water, see Ch. 6) is lost, with an energy density of 4.2 MJ/kg, but by the second week the tissue lost is a mixture of 75% fat and 25% fat-free mass (FFM), which has an energy density of 30 MJ (7000 kcal)/kg. Very low carbohydrate diets cause rapid initial weight loss because they cause early loss of glycogen and the attached water.

During total starvation weight loss is even more rapid, partly because the energy deficit is greater, and partly because a higher proportion of the weight loss is FFM (to provide amino acids for glucose synthesis; see Section 6.3, under 'Gluconeogenesis – the synthesis of glucose from non-carbohydrate precursors' and Section 8.4, under 'The metabolism of amino acid carbon skeletons'). Severely obese patients lose 300 to 500 g/day on prolonged starvation, but about 50% of the weight lost is FFM. Total starvation ceased to be an acceptable treatment for gross obesity because several patients died unexpectedly, due to damage to heart muscle.

The interaction between diet, exercise and muscle bulk is controversial. There is no doubt that strenuous isometric exercise causes muscle hypertrophy, and immobilisation causes atrophy of muscle (see Ch. 18). It is also true that exercise increases energy expenditure, so it is plausible that in obese people a combination of a low energy diet and exercise should achieve more fat loss, and less loss of FFM, than diet alone. There is no evidence from randomised controlled trials to support this view, because there are no such trials on obese people (BMI > 30), because they have too low an exercise tolerance to complete such trials. A meta-analysis of 28 publications reporting trials on overweight subjects (BMI 25–29) showed that aerobic exercise without dietary restriction caused a weight loss of 3 kg in 30 weeks in men, and 1.4 kg in 12 weeks in women, but had no effect on FFM. Resistance exercise had little effect on weight loss, but increased FFM by 2 kg in men and 1 kg in women. A combination of aerobic exercise and diet to cause a weight loss of 10 kg reduced the loss of FFM from 2.9 kg to 1.7 kg in men, and from 2.2 kg to 1.7 kg in women, compared with diet alone. In summary, a combination of diet and exercise causes a small reduction in loss of FFM in overweight subjects compared with diet alone, but data are not yet available for obese people.

The effect of diet and exercise on bone density is even more controversial. Studies have shown that calcium supplementation in the diet increases bone density, but bone density is high in African and other countries where people have a low calcium intake but a high level of physical activity. Bone density is clearly affected by diet, exercise and no doubt genetic and other factors not yet clarified. For further discussion see Chapter 24.

Changes in hydration: diarrhoea, oedema, kwashiorkor, heart or kidney failure

In the previous section, it has been assumed that there will be no change in the hydration of the body with diet and exercise, but if there is a change in hydration during changes in these factors, there will be weight changes that bear no simple relationship to energy balance.

Total body water is regulated to maintain an osmotic pressure in body fluids of 285 mosmol/kg. If the tonicity of these fluids increases then water intake is stimulated by thirst, and water losses are reduced by secretion of more concentrated urine. If the tonicity decreases, dilute urine is secreted to remove the excess water. Urine osmolality can vary from 50 to 1200 mmol/kg. This regulatory mechanism may be overwhelmed, and dehydration may occur if water losses are very high, as in severe diarrhoea, or with sweat loss in high ambient temperature or during prolonged vigorous exercise. Dehydration may also occur with abuse of diuretic drugs to achieve weight loss, or during the recovery phase of diabetic coma. In severe untreated diabetes mellitus (due to infection, or interruption of insulin administration in a diabetic), the patient becomes dehydrated by two mechanisms. First, the excretion of large amounts of glucose in urine causes an osmotic diuresis and hence excessive loss of water. Second, ketosis is associated with vomiting and further

Table 4.3 **Percentage body fat in men and women related to the sum of four skinfolds (biceps, triceps, subscapular and suprailiac)**

Skinfold (mm)	Men, age (years)				Women, age (years)			
	17–29	30–39	40–49	50+	17–29	30–39	40–49	50+
20	8.1	12.2	12.2	12.6	14.1	17.0	19.8	21.4
30	12.9	16.2	17.7	18.6	19.5	21.8	24.5	26.6
40	16.4	19.2	21.4	22.9	23.4	25.5	28.2	30.3
50	19.0	21.5	24.6	26.5	26.5	28.2	31.0	33.4
60	21.2	23.5	27.1	29.2	29.1	30.6	33.2	35.7
70	23.1	25.1	29.3	31.6	31.2	32.5	35.0	37.7
80	24.8	26.6	31.2	33.8	33.1	34.3	36.7	39.6
90	26.2	27.8	33.0	35.8	34.8	35.8	38.3	41.2
100	27.6	29.0	34.4	37.4	36.4	37.25	39.7	42.6
110	28.8	30.1	35.8	39.0	37.8	38.6	41.0	42.9
120	30.0	31.1	37.0	40.4	39.0	39.6	42.0	45.1
130	31.0	31.9	38.2	41.8	40.2	40.6	43.0	46.2
140	32.0	32.7	39.2	43.0	41.3	41.6	44.0	47.2
150	32.9	33.5	40.2	44.1	42.3	42.6	45.0	48.2
160	33.7	34.3	41.2	45.1	43.3	43.6	45.8	49.2
170	34.5	34.8	42.0	46.1	44.1	44.4	46.6	50.0

Source: from data reported by Durnin & Womersley (1974).

Mid-upper arm circumference is a useful tool for assessing the nutritional status of both adults and children in famine conditions. The technique of measurement and calculation is given in Chapter 31.

It has been recognised in the last decade that intra-abdominal fat has a greater influence on the risk of heart disease and diabetes than an equal weight of fat in subcutaneous sites (see Chs 19 and 21). Attempts have therefore been made to estimate intra-abdominal fat by measurements of waist circumference, or sagittal diameter. However, these measurement are difficult to make accurately, and computerised scanning techniques are now generally used to assess intra-abdominal fat.

Body fat

There is no 'best' method for measuring body composition in living subjects: every method has errors, and some methods require expensive laboratory equipment that would be impossible to use in the field, for example during famine relief. The first three methods described below estimate FFM and so, by subtraction from total body weight, fat mass (FM). They all require expensive laboratory equipment and cooperative subjects. They are used (preferably in combination) to provide reference values with which simpler methods can be compared and calibrated. They all depend on an assumption, based on the data in Table 4.1, that the fat-free body has a constant density, water content and potassium content.

Body density

Human fat at body temperature has a density of $0.900\,g/cm^3$. The remainder of the body (the fat-free mass) is a mixture of water, protein, bone mineral, glycogen, and minor components such as nucleic acids and electrolytes. This mixture has a density of approximately $1.100\,g/cm^3$ (Keys & Brozek 1953). Therefore if we know the average density of all the tissues of the body we can calculate the ratio of fat to fat-free mass: for example, if the average density was $1.00\,g/cm^3$ then that person must be 50% fat and 50% FFM. The body shown in Figure 4.1 weighs 70 kg and has 12 kg fat, so his fat content is 17% and his total body density would be $1.06\,g/cm^3$.

It is easy to measure the weight of a subject accurately, but difficult to measure tissue volume with similar accuracy. For example, the 70 kg subject who is 50% fat will have a volume of 70 litres, but if he had only 17% fat his volume would be 66.05 litres. The usual method for measuring body volume is to compare body weight in air and totally immersed in water: the decrease in weight on immersion shows the volume of water displaced. However, some of the water is displaced by air trapped in the subject's lungs and gut, and if allowance is not made for this the fat content of the subject will be overestimated. It is difficult to measure this trapped air, so other methods for measuring FFM that do not require total immersion have been developed, such as the 'bod pod', but they require complicated apparatus and a cooperative subject (Garrow et al 1979, Fields et al 2002).

Total body water (TBW)

The total amount of water in the body can be measured quite accurately by isotope dilution. The subject is given a known dose of water labelled with deuterium (^2H), the stable heavy isotope of hydrogen, and this is allowed to equilibrate with total body water, which takes about 3 hours. Then the dilution of ^2H in a sample representative of body water, such as blood plasma, is measured, and TBW is calculated. Fat (by definition) does not contain any water. If we assume that the fat-free tissues contain 73% of water, then FFM is TBW/0.73. By subtraction of FFM from body weight, the weight of fat in the body is estimated.

The limitations of this approach are that it requires a high-precision isotope-ratio mass spectrometer with a competent operator to measure the concentration of ^2H in the equilibrated body water sample, and that in many conditions the assumption that FFM is 73% water is not valid. In patients with oedema caused by heart or kidney disease, in severely obese people, and in severely malnourished people, the assumption that FFM is TBW/0.73 will overestimate FFM and hence underestimate fat. In dehydrated subjects the same assumption will overestimate fat.

It is possible to measure subcompartments of total body water using a similar dilution principle. Instead of using deuterated water as a tracer, a tracer that distributes only in the vascular space (such as radiolabelled red cells) can be used to measure blood volume. Various compounds (such as thiocyanate or inulin) that distribute in the extracellular water can be used to measure the volume of extracellular water. These measurements are rarely made in clinical practice. The situation in which it is dangerous to life to have an excessive volume of extracellular water is congestive heart failure, leading to overfilling of the venous circulation, pulmonary oedema and death. In this case central venous pressure is easier, quicker and more relevant to measure.

Total body potassium (TBK)

All potassium (K), including that in the human body, contains a natural radioactive isotope (^{40}K), so each gram of K emits 3 gamma rays per second. This radiation is of high energy (1.46 MeV) so most of it emerges from the tissues and can be counted by high sensitivity detectors. However, this level of radiation is low compared with the normal background, which arises mainly from cosmic rays, so the subject being measured, and the detectors, must be screened by a massive shield of lead and steel. With this cumbersome and expensive 'whole body counter' it is possible to measure total body potassium and, assuming a constant K content in FFM, to calculate FFM, and hence fat mass.

The value of this technique is mainly that the errors in estimates of body composition by TBK and TBW, arising from oedema or dehydration are in opposite directions. With oedema TBK overestimates fat, while TBW underestimates fat; with dehydration the converse applies.

A 'gold standard' for measurement of fat and fat-free mass

For research purposes it is useful to have a best, or 'gold standard', estimate of fat and FFM in living subjects against which simpler methods can be compared. The two-compartment models regard body weight as the sum of fat and FFM, and make assumptions about density, water or potassium content for FFM. If the assumptions are wrong, then the estimate is wrong. To try to avoid this source of error the four-compartment models measure water (see 'Total body water (TBW)', above) and bone mineral by DEXA (see 'Dual-energy X-ray absorptiometry (DEXA)', below) and density (see 'Body density', above). Knowing the water and bone mineral content of the body, the remainder must be either fat or non-mineral, non-water FFM, which means essentially protein. Thus by combining the results of three measurements (water, density and bone mineral) it is not necessary to assume that FFM has a density of 1.100 or a water content of 73%. The relation of body weight to body fat, measured by these three methods, is shown in Figure CD 4.5. Over a wide range of weight (42–132 kg) and fat (9–75 kg) the relationship is linear ($r = 0.960$) with a slope of 1.27. This shows that for every 1 kg extra fat by which an obese woman exceeds a normal-weight control, body weight is (on average) increased by 1.27 kg. The

To get round this difficulty some researchers have measured segmental BIA, using electrodes placed so as to measure the impedance of the limb and truncal sections separately. Also, the frequency of the alternating current affects the ability of the current to penetrate from extracellular to intracellular water, but it is not yet clear if these developments improve the clinical utility of the measurement.

Estimating change in body composition

Body composition measurements may be made to find out if a given patient, or population, has an abnormal amount of some component, such as fat, or bone mineral. The techniques described above will usually provide a reliable answer to this question. But the problem may be more difficult. For example, two treatments for weight loss may be compared (say diet versus exercise) and both treatment groups lose the same amount of weight (say 5 kg). The question is: 'Does the composition of the weight lost by dieting differ from that lost by exercise?' At the start, and again at the completion of treatment, the body composition of participants is measured by DEXA. The standard deviation (SD) of estimates of fat mass measured by DEXA is about 1 kg, but if there are 16 in each group the standard error of the mean (SEM) of

the group will be only 0.25 kg (SEM $= SD/n^{-2}$). If there is a clinically significant difference in the mean fat lost (say 1 kg) it should be possible to show this at a statistically significant level. However, it is not possible to calculate from two DEXA measurements an answer to the question: 'What is the proportion of fat in the weight lost by an individual within either group?' The combined error of the first and second DEXA measurements is greater than the probable contribution of fat to a total loss of 5 kg, so no reliable estimate of the composition of weight loss can be made.

If it is important to measure in individuals the composition of small changes in body fat (or any other component of body weight), this cannot be done by serial measurements of body composition using techniques described above. The alternative is to perform metabolic balance studies to measure the total intake and output of the element of interest – for example N balance for protein, Ca balance for bone mineral.

Bone density

Measurement of bone density is a facility offered by the DEXA instrument, described above. Usually measurements are made specifically on vertebral body, forearm or femoral neck, since these are the sites most liable to fracture.

⊃ Key points

- ⊃ There are remarkably few data on the chemical composition of the body from analysis of cadavers; a healthy adult male contains about 60% water, 17% protein and 17% fat.

- ⊃ Total body water, and the partition between intracellular and extracellular water, and its electrolyte composition is normally tightly regulated.

- ⊃ The skeleton accounts for 14% of total body weight. Bone contains 99% of total body calcium, which acts as a reservoir to maintain an appropriate plasma concentration of calcium. Bone turnover can be estimated from the urinary excretion of hydroxyproline.

- ⊃ Skeletal muscle accounts for 40% of body weight, and smooth muscle 10%, but resting muscle accounts for only 22% of basal metabolic rate.

- ⊃ Total blood volume is about 5 litres, of which 55% is plasma and 45% packed cells.

- ⊃ In a lean male fat amounts to 17% of body weight, of which about 80% can be considered to be energy reserves.

- ⊃ Fat reserves are in white adipose tissue. White adipocytes contain about 80% triacylglycerol, as a single central droplet surrounded by a thin layer of cytoplasm containing the nucleus.

- ⊃ Males tend to accumulate fat in the abdomen, while women accumulate subcutaneous fat stores around the breast, hip and thigh. In obesity, people may accumulate fat in the male or female pattern; this is probably genetically determined. Abdominal adipose tissue is more closely related to diabetes and heart disease than is total body fat.

- ⊃ In addition to being a storage organ, adipose tissue has endocrine functions concerned with fertility and regulation of food intake and energy balance.

⟳ Brown adipose tissue cells contain small droplets of triacylglycerol in a cytoplasm rich in mitochondria. Its main function is thermogenesis, especially in infants.

⟳ Body composition changes throughout life. The water content of the body decreases, and the content of protein and fat increases, through gestation, infancy and into adolescence.

⟳ Fat-free mass remains relatively constant from age 20 to 65, but then decreases; fat mass increases throughout adult life.

⟳ Food restriction and starvation result in loss of fat-free mass as well as adipose tissue.

⟳ Excessive water losses can lead to dehydration.

⟳ A variety of conditions can lead to excessive accumulation of body water, resulting in oedema. Even severely wasted undernourished people may be oedematous.

⟳ Assessment of body composition can be used to assess current nutritional status; serial measurements assess changes in status.

⟳ Most of the methods available to assess body composition are research methods that are not suitable for use in the field or clinic; they are used to validate simpler methods that are applicable to field and clinic use.

⟳ The two most common methods of assessing body fat are skinfold thickness and (becoming increasingly applicable outside research laboratories) dual-energy X-ray absorptiometry (DEXA).

References and further reading

References

Durnin J V G A, Womersley J 1974 Body fat assessed from total body density and its estimation from skinfold thickness: measurements on 481 men and women aged from 16 to 72 years. British Journal of Nutrition 23:77–97

Fields D A, Goran M I, McCrory M A 2002 Body-composition assessment via air-displacement plethysmography in adults and children: a review. American Journal of Clinical Nutrition 75:453–467

Garrow J S, Stalley S, Diethelm R et al 1979 A new method for measuring body density of obese adults. British Journal of Nutrition 42:173–183

Genton L, Hans D, Kyle U G et al 2002 Dual-energy X-ray absorptiometry and body composition: differences between devices and comparison with reference methods. Nutrition 18:66–70

Heitman B L 1990 Evaluation of body fat estimated from body mass index, skinfolds and impedance: a comparative study. European Journal of Clinical Nutrition 44:831–837

Keys A, Brozek J 1953 Body fat in adult man. Physiological Reviews 33:245–325

Further reading

Demerath E W, Guo S S, Chumlea W C et al 2002 Comparison of percent body fat estimates using air displacement plethysmography and hydrodensitometry in adults and children. International Journal of Obesity and Related Metabolic Disorders 26:389–397

Heitman B L 1990 Evaluation of body fat estimated from body mass index, skinfolds and impedance: a comparative study. European Journal of Clinical Nutrition 44:831–837

Keys A, Brozek J 1953 Body fat in adult man. Physiological Reviews 33:245–325

Rogalla P, Meii N, Hoksch B et al 1998 Low-dose spiral computed tomography for measuring abdominal fat volume and distribution in a clinical setting. European Journal of Clinical Nutrition 52:597–602

Webster J D, Hesp R, Garrow J S 1984 The composition of excess weight in obese women estimated by body density, total body water and total body potassium. Human Nutrition: Clinical Nutrition 38C:299–306.

CD-ROM contents

Figure CD 4.2 Diagram to illustrate chief
morphological differences between white
and brown fat cells

Figure CD 4.3 Percentile changes in fat-free mass
and fat mass of Caucasian men and women
with advancing age

Figure CD 4.4 Average cumulative weight loss
in 108 obese women on a reducing diet

Figure CD 4.5 Relation of body weight to total
body fat in a series of 104 women

**Additional references related to CD tables
and figures**

Further reading from the book

5

Energy balance and body weight regulation

Abdul G. Dulloo and Yves Schutz

Objectives

By the end of this chapter you should be able to:

- define types and units of energy
- explain the laws of thermodynamics
- identify and quantify the food sources of energy
- describe the main factors affecting energy intake
- describe the assessment of energy needs and approximate values throughout the life cycle
- explain the components of energy expenditure, their relative size and variability
- describe the methods of measurement of energy expenditure and their validity for different purposes
- identify the main types of signals in relation to hunger and satiety
- describe the changes in energy expenditure that occur in response to undernutrition and overnutrition
- summarise the components of models of energy intake and energy expenditure.

5.1 INTRODUCTION

Understanding how body weight is regulated is still a challenging issue for human research today. It is likely that long-term constancy of body weight is achieved through a highly complex network of regulatory systems through which changes in food intake, body composition and energy expenditure are interlinked. Failure of this regulation leads either to obesity and its co-morbidities (see Ch. 20) or to protein-energy malnutrition and cachexia in disease states such as anorexia, cancer and infections. Between these disorders attributed to 'failure of regulation' lie those due to chronic undernutrition because of poverty, war and famine. Achieving energy balance and weight homeostasis is central to the quality of life. An understanding of how they are achieved requires an appreciation of the following:

- the basic concepts and principles concerning the flux of energy transformations through which body weight is regulated
- an appraisal of factors affecting food intake and energy expenditure, which represent the entry and exit in this flux of energy transformations
- the methods for assessing energy expenditure and energy requirements, and
- a number of models that have been proposed to explain the regulation of body weight and body composition in humans.

5.2 BASIC CONCEPTS AND PRINCIPLES IN HUMAN ENERGETICS

Energy balance and the laws of thermodynamics

Energy represents the capacity of a system to perform work. It can appear in various forms – light, chemical, mechanical, electrical – all of which can be completely converted to heat. According to the *first law of thermodynamics*, energy cannot be created or destroyed but can only be transformed from one form into another. Biological systems, like machines, depend on the transformation of some form of energy in order to perform work. Whereas plants depend on light energy captured from the sun to synthesise molecules like carbohydrates, proteins and fats, animals meet their energy needs from chemical energy stored in plants or in other animals. The chemical energy obtained from foods (plant or animal in origin) is used to perform a variety of work, such as the synthesis of new macromolecules (*chemical work*), in muscular contraction (*mechanical work*) or in the maintenance of ionic gradients across membranes (*electrical work*). Overall energy balance is given by the following equation:

$$\text{energy intake} = \text{energy expenditure} + \Delta \text{ energy stores}$$

Thus, if the total energy contained in the body (as fat, protein and glycogen) is not altered (i.e. Δ energy stores = 0), then energy expenditure must be equal to energy intake. In this case, the individual is said to be in a state of *energy balance*. If the intake and expenditure of energy are not equal, then a change in body energy content will occur, with *negative energy balance* resulting in the utilisation of the body's energy stores (glycogen, fat and protein) or *positive energy balance* resulting in an increase in body energy stores, primarily as fat. There are, however, interrelationships between energy intake and energy expenditure. Voluntary energy intake may rise with intense physical activity (lumberjacks eat more than clerks), energy expenditure may increase in response to increased food intake, and both energy intake and expenditure can be influenced by changes in body energy stores (body fat depletion may lead to increased hunger and reduced energy expenditure).

The *second law of thermodynamics*, in biological terms, makes a subtle distinction between the potential energy of food, useful work and heat. It states that when food is utilised in the body, whether for muscle contraction, synthesis of new tissues or for maintenance of electrolyte equilibrium across membranes, these processes must be accompanied inevitably by a loss of heat. In thermodynamic terms, some energy is degraded, and such heat energy, which is no longer available for work, is termed 'entropy'. In other words, the conversion of available food energy is not a perfectly efficient process, and about 75% of the chemical energy contained in foods may be ultimately dissipated as heat because of the inefficiency of intermediary metabolism in transforming food energy into a form (e.g. adenosine triphosphate, ATP) which can be used for useful work, whether it be the internal work required to maintain structure and function or external physical work.

Units of energy

Since all the energy used by the body at rest is ultimately lost as heat, and physical (external) work will also be eventually degraded as heat, the energy that is consumed, stored and expended is expressed as its heat equivalent. The calorie was originally adopted as the unit of energy in nutrition; it is defined as the amount of heat required to raise the temperature of 1 gram of water by 1°C (from 14.5 to 15.5°C); nutritionally the kilocalorie (=1000 calories) is used. With the introduction of the SI system, energy is expressed as joule (J). One joule is the energy used when a mass of 1 kilogram (kg) is moved through 1 metre (m) by a force of 1 newton (N). Because one joule is a very small unit of energy, it is more convenient to use kilojoule (kJ), or megajoule (MJ) in nutrition. Rates of energy expenditure (often referred to as metabolic rate) are expressed in kJ or MJ per unit time (kJ/min or MJ/day), which correspond to 10^3 J and 10^6 J, respectively. The conversion of calorie to joules is: 1 calorie = 4.18 J, or 1 kilocalorie (kcal) = 4.18 kilojoule (kJ).

Sources of energy and macronutrient balance

The macronutrients (carbohydrate, fat, protein and alcohol) are the sources of energy, so it makes sense to consider energy balance and macronutrient balance together. There is a strong relationship between energy balance and macronutrient balance, and the sum of individual substrate balance (expressed as energy) must be equivalent to the overall energy balance. Thus, it follows that:

exogenous carbohydrate
  − carbohydrate oxidation
  = carbohydrate balance
exogenous protein − protein oxidation
  = protein balance

Table 5.1 Macronutrient storage in the body, its energy density and its degree of autoregulation

Substrate	Form of storage	Pool size	Tissues	Energy density[a] (kJ/g)	Autoregulation
Carbohydrate	Glycogen	Small	Liver, muscle	~4	Accurate
Fat	Triglycerides	Moderate-large (unlimited)	Adipose tissue	~33	Poor
Protein	Protein	Moderate (limited)	Lean tissue	~4	Accurate

[a]As stored in tissues.

exogenous lipid − lipid oxidation
   = lipid balance
total energy intake − total oxidation
   = energy balance

Unlike the size of the fat stores, which can increase very considerably, there is a limited capacity for storing protein in fat-free mass and carbohydrate as glycogen in liver and muscles (Table 5.1). It is therefore not surprising that protein and glucose tend to be oxidised more readily than fat, and that alcohol, which is not stored in the body, is oxidised rapidly (sparing fat).

5.3 ENERGY INTAKE

Energy value of foods and Atwater factors

The traditional way of measuring the energy content of foodstuffs is to use a 'bomb calorimeter' in which the heat produced when a sample of food is combusted (in presence of oxygen) is measured. When the food is combusted, it is completely oxidised to water, carbon dioxide and oxides of other elements such as sulphur and nitrogen. The total heat liberated (expressed in kilocalories or kilojoules) represents the *gross energy* value or *heat of combustion* of the food. The heat of combustion differs between carbohydrates, proteins and fats. There are also important differences within each category of macronutrient. The gross energy yield of sucrose, for example, is 16.5 kJ/g, whereas starch yields 17.7 kJ/g. The energy yield of butterfat is 38.5 kJ/g and of lard, 39.6 kJ/g. These values have been rounded off to give 17.3 kJ/g for carbohydrates rich in starch and poor in sugar, 39.3 kJ/g for average fat and 23.6 kJ/g for mixtures of animal and vegetable proteins. The heat of combustion of alcohol is 29 kJ/g.

The gross energy value of foodstuffs, however, does not represent the energy actually available to the body, since no potentially oxidisable substrate can be considered available until it is presented to the cell for oxidation. None of the foodstuffs is completely absorbed; some energy therefore never enters the body and is excreted in faeces. Digestibility of the major foodstuffs, however, is high; on average, 97% of ingested carbohydrates, 95% of fats, and 92% of proteins are absorbed from the intestinal lumen. There is a difference between the true and apparent digestibility – the latter includes energy which is excreted in the faeces from sources such as bacteria in the gut and enzyme secretions.

In the body, the tissues are able to oxidise carbohydrate and fat completely to carbon dioxide and water, but the oxidation of protein is not complete, and results in the formation of urea and other nitrogenous compounds which are excreted in the urine. Determination of both the heat of combustion and the nitrogen content of urine indicates that approximately 33.0 kJ/g of urine nitrogen is equivalent to 5.3 kJ/g of protein since 1 g urinary N arises from ~6.25 g protein. This energy represents metabolic loss and must be subtracted from the 'digestible' energy of protein. From these considerations, the 'Atwater factors' for available energy (or metabolisable energy) of the three macronutrients have been derived (Fig. 5.1). It is the metabolisable energy value that is quoted in food composition tables (Southgate & Durnin 1970). It is important to remember that these factors make allowance for the energy in the food lost in faeces and urine. They are physiological *approximations* based on experiments on a limited number of subjects on one kind of diet.

Pattern of food intake

Human beings eat food in a discontinuous manner, even under conditions of nibbling, and the amount of food eaten can range from zero to up to 21 MJ/day in highly active individuals or during acute episodes of hyperphagia. This contrasts with energy expenditure, which is continuous irrespective of the conditions encountered. This irregularity of food behaviour occurs both within-day and between-days, which explains why there is a 2–3 times greater coefficient of variation for energy intake (15–20%) than for energy expenditure (5–8%). It also explains the difficulty in assessing food intake in order to obtain a representative picture of 'habitual' food (energy) intake. The physiological control of food intake is highly complex (see Section 5.6). There is a wide variety of food behaviour. This makes it extremely difficult to interpret data on food intake, the measurement of which has plagued nutritionists for more than a century. The various methods used to assess energy intake are described in Chapter 31, including factors leading to

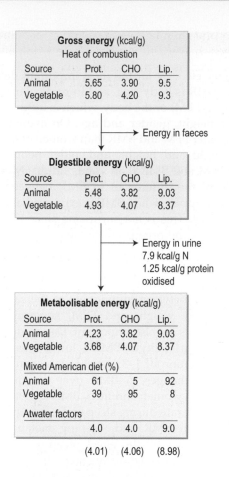

Figure 5.1 diagram content:

Gross energy (kcal/g)
Heat of combustion

Source	Prot.	CHO	Lip.
Animal	5.65	3.90	9.5
Vegetable	5.80	4.20	9.3

→ Energy in faeces

Digestible energy (kcal/g)

Source	Prot.	CHO	Lip.
Animal	5.48	3.82	9.03
Vegetable	4.93	4.07	8.37

→ Energy in urine
7.9 kcal/g N
1.25 kcal/g protein
oxidised

Metabolisable energy (kcal/g)

Source	Prot.	CHO	Lip.
Animal	4.23	3.82	9.03
Vegetable	3.68	4.07	8.37
Mixed American diet (%)			
Animal	61	5	92
Vegetable	39	95	8
Atwater factors			
	4.0	4.0	9.0

(4.01) (4.06) (8.98)

Coefficient of apparent digestibility

	Animal	Vegetable
Protein	97	85
CHO	98	97
Lipid	95	90

Figure 5.1 Physiological energy value of energy-yielding nutrients obtained in humans. CHO, carbohydrate.

Table 5.2 Exogenous factors, typically encountered in affluent societies, contributing to a poor control of food intake in humans

1. Large food diversity and high palatability diets
2. Profuse availability of food
3. Television watching (reduced activity, pressure of food advertising)
4. Snacking rather than meal eating
5. Fast rate of eating ('fast foods')
6. High energy density diets (e.g. high fat diet)
7. Eating outside home and unsociable eating
8. Technological developments, less activity
9. Reduced physical activity level
10. Urbanisation: more access to energy-dense food, less need to walk

underestimation or overestimation of energy intake, and hence leading to a bias in the estimation of energy balance.

Factors affecting patterns of food intake and energy intake

Since the ultimate function of energy intake is the provision of energy for metabolic processes and performance of work, body size and physical activity are important factors influencing energy intake. However, eating is a pleasure which fulfils not only nutritional but also social, cultural, emotional and psychological needs. The increasing buying power in industrialised society, combined with the intense marketing from food companies, has led to a progressive change in eating behaviour over the past two decades. Food technologists are constantly inventing new foods and flavours, which may not be compatible with sound nutritional guidelines. Many processed foods and snacks are rich in refined sugars and fats, and their high energy density and palatability are conducive to overeating. Apart from snacking and quick eating, a non-exhaustive list of the exogenous factors contributing to a poor control of food intake is given in Table 5.2. Among these factors, it has long been known that the nutrient composition of the diet has marked effects on food intake. Diets which are either very low or very high in protein, as well as those with an unbalanced amino acid mixture, tend to depress food intake. Similarly, low fat diets cause a reduction in food intake, in part because they are bland and difficult to swallow, and also because of their low energy density; the total bulk may limit energy intake through greater gastric distension and delayed gastric emptying. Furthermore, carbohydrates, and specifically glucose, have been directly implicated in the control of food intake, and it is well established that low blood glucose (hypoglycaemia) stimulates hunger and feeding. By contrast, high fat diets, in addition to adding palatability to foods, have high energy density and low bulk, which leads to diminished gastric distension and gastric emptying, so retarding the feeling of fullness and the cessation of eating.

5.4 ENERGY EXPENDITURE

Components of energy expenditure

It is customary to consider energy expenditure as being made up of three components: the energy spent for basal metabolism (or basal metabolic rate), the energy spent on physical activity, and the increase in resting energy expenditure in response to a variety of stimuli (including food, cold, stress and drugs). These three components are depicted in Figure 5.2 (model A), and are described below.

Basal metabolic rate (BMR)

This is the largest component of energy expenditure for most individuals. Typically in developed countries, BMR accounts between 60–75% of daily energy expenditure, and reflects the energy needed for the work of vital functions (maintaining electrolyte equilibrium across cell membranes, cell and protein turnover, respiratory and cardiovascular

functions, etc.). By far the most important determinant of BMR is body size, and in particular the fat-free mass (FFM) of the body, which is influenced by weight, height, gender and age. On average, men have greater FFM and BMR than women of the same age, weight and height, and, older people have lower FFM and BMR than young adults. Most, but not all, of the differences in BMR between these groups disappear when BMR is expressed as a function of FFM. This is not surprising since FFM contains tissues and organs which have high metabolic activities such as liver, kidneys, heart, and to a lesser extent the resting muscles. In contrast, the contribution of adipose tissue to BMR is small. BMR can vary up to ±10% between individuals of the same age, gender, body weight and FFM, suggesting that genetic factors are also important. Day-to-day intra-individual variability in BMR is low in men (coefficient of variation of 1–3%) but is larger in women because of changes in BMR over the menstrual cycle. In both women and men, BMR is greater than the metabolic rate during sleep by 5–20%, the difference between BMR and sleeping metabolic rate being explained by the effect of arousal. BMR is known to be depressed during starvation. Although this is to a large extent explained by the loss in body weight and lean tissues, the fall of BMR is often reported to be lower than predicted from the reduction in body weight or FFM. During rapid overfeeding, the evidence that BMR is increased is equivocal, and when it is found to be increased, it is within 5–10% of the excess energy intake.

Energy expenditure due to physical activity

The energy spent on physical activity depends on the type and intensity of the physical activity and on the time spent in different activities. Physical activity is often considered to be synonymous with 'muscular work', which has a strict definition in physics – force × distance, when external work is performed on the environment. During muscular work (muscle contraction), the muscle produces 3–4 times more heat than mechanical energy, so that useful work costs more than muscle work. There is a wide variation in the energy cost of any activity both within and between individuals. The latter variation is due to differences in body size and in the speed and dexterity with which an activity is performed. In order

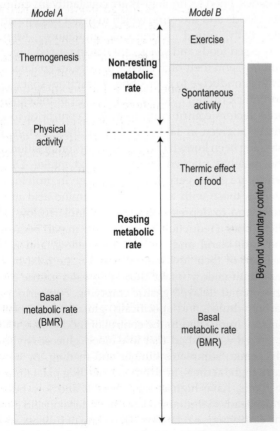

Figure 5.2 Components of energy expenditure.

to adjust for differences in body size, the energy cost of physical activities is expressed as multiples of BMR (see 'Estimations of energy requirements', below). These generally range from 1 to 5 for most activities, but can reach values between 10 and 14 during intense exercise. In terms of daily energy expenditure, physical activity can represent up to 70% of daily energy expenditure in an individual involved in heavy manual work or competition athletics. For most people in industrialised societies, however, the contribution of physical activity to daily energy expenditure is relatively small (10–15%). In a hospitalised patient in bed, it is still lower.

Energy expenditure in response to various thermogenic stimuli

This component of energy expenditure – often referred to as 'thermogenesis' – is best described by the various forms in which it can exist. These have been described by Miller (1982) as follows:

1. *Isometric thermogenesis*: This is due to increased muscle tension; no physical work is done. The differences in energy expenditure in a person who is lying, sitting or standing are due mainly to changes in muscle tone.

2. *Dynamic thermogenesis*: The term 'negative work' is used to describe heat production of stretched muscle, with heat being again produced without any work. For example, when someone goes down a ladder, heat production increases but no work is done. In the physical sense of work, contracting muscles produce heat because of their inefficiency, but tensed and stretched muscles are simply thermogenic.

3. *Psychological thermogenesis*: The psychological state may affect energy expenditure, as anxiety, anticipation and stress stimulate adrenaline secretion, leading to increased heat production. A two-fold difference can be found in the energy cost of sitting at ease and sitting playing chess, a difference that cannot entirely be attributed to muscular movement. The best evidence comes from a study on pilots whose energy expenditure increased when they were under air traffic control, with the rise being inversely related to their level of experience.

4. *Cold-induced thermogenesis*: Human beings rarely need to increase heat production for the purpose of thermal regulation because they are able to seek an equitable environment or wear suitable clothing. At low temperatures, resting metabolic rate (and hence heat production) increases. For example, normal weight women maintained in identical clothing in a room calorimeter adjusted their 24-hour heat production by about 7% when the temperature in the calorimeter room was lowered from 28 to 22°C. It is customary to distinguish between two forms of cold-induced thermogenesis – shivering and non-shivering thermogenesis. Shivering is rhythmic muscle contraction. Non-shivering thermogenesis is increased heat production not associated with muscle contraction, and is due to increased sympathetic nervous system activity, particularly in brown adipose tissue in small mammals. Non-shivering thermogenesis is inversely correlated with body size, age and ambient temperature and has been demonstrated in adult human beings chronically exposed to low temperatures.

5. *Diet-induced thermogenesis*: Heat production increases following the consumption of a meal, and this thermic effect of food was classically termed 'specific dynamic action'. Heat production also increases on a high plane of nutrition, the so-called 'luxusconsumption'. These two forms of thermogenesis related to food have been regrouped under the term 'diet-induced thermogenesis' or DIT, and are often divided into an *obligatory* component (related to the energy costs of absorption and metabolic processing of nutrients or the energy cost of tissue synthesis during overfeeding) and a *facultative* component which in part results from the sensory aspects of foods (smell and taste) and in part from stimulation of the sympathetic nervous system.

6. *Drug-induced thermogenesis*: The consumption of caffeine, nicotine and alcohol may form an integral part of daily life for many people, and all three of these drugs stimulate thermogenesis. A cup of coffee (containing 60–80 mg caffeine) can increase BMR by 5–10% over an hour or two. Oral intake of 100 mg caffeine every 2 hours during the day or smoking a packet of 20 cigarettes increases energy expenditure by 5% and 15%, respectively. Furthermore the thermogenic effect of nicotine is potentiated by caffeine. The cessation of elevated thermogenesis induced by nicotine or nicotine and caffeine may be a factor that contributes to the average weight gain of 7 kg after cessation of smoking.

Alternative compartmentalisation of energy expenditure

Another way to look at the components of energy expenditure is shown in Figure 5.2, model B, where energy expenditure is divided into resting and non-resting expenditure. Resting expenditure comprises all measurements of energy expenditure made at rest – BMR, and the thermic effects of food (and other food ingredients or drugs). Non-resting energy expenditure is divided into exercise (voluntary) and low level of involuntary physical activity which is spontaneous and subconscious. Involuntary activity is often referred to as thermogenesis due to fidgeting, or non-exercise activity thermogenesis (NEAT). The potential importance of variations in this involuntary energy expenditure in body weight regulation is discussed in Section 5.7 under 'Thermogenesis associated with physical activity'.

Fuel metabolism at the level of organs and tissues

The energy supplied by the diet is in the form of macronutrients (also called substrates or metabolic fuels): carbohydrates, proteins and fat. These macromolecules cannot be directly utilised by the tissues as such but must be first broken down into smaller molecules: carbohydrates into monosaccharides (see Ch. 6), triacylglycerols into free fatty acids (see Ch. 7) and proteins into amino acids (see Ch. 8). Ethanol (alcohol) is not usually considered a macronutrient, but also constitutes a source of energy utilised by the body (see Ch. 9) The major substrates, which circulate in the blood and are taken up by the tissues to serve as fuels, are shown in Table 5.3. The amount stored in the tissues, the level of exogenous supply and the metabolic state of the individual determine the relative importance of the utilisation of each fuel, with synthesis and utilisation of body reserves controlled by hormones.

Metabolic rate at the level of organs and tissues

The heat production of individual tissues and organs can be calculated from the oxygen consumption by measuring blood flow and the arteriovenous difference in oxygen concentration across tissues and organs. Normalised for body mass, adipose tissue has the lowest metabolic rate (approximately 18.8 kJ/kg/day for subcutaneous abdominal adipose tissue). Note that there are regional differences in

Table 5.3 **Substances that circulate in the blood and are used to supply energy (from Elia 2000)**

Fuel	Source
Glucose	Dietary carbohydrate; glycogen stores; gluconeogenesis in liver and kidney from lactate, amino acids and glycerol
Free fatty acids (FFA)	Dietary fats; triglyceride stores (especially in adipose tissue); synthesised from carbohydrate in liver and adipose tissue, especially after feeding on low fat diets
Amino acids	Dietary protein; tissue protein stores; synthesised from carbohydrates
Ketone bodies (acetacetate, 3-hydroxybutyrate)	Produced from FFA and some amino acids in liver
Glycerol	Produced from triglyceride breakdown
Lactate	Anaerobic glycolysis
Acetate	Gut fermentation of carbohydrates; produced from FFA in liver and muscle, and from ethanol in liver
Ethanol	Dietary intake; gut fermentation
Fructose	Dietary sucrose
Galactose	Dietary intake, especially as milk lactose

the lipolytic activity of different anatomical sites of adipose tissue with intra-abdominal depot having the greatest metabolic activity and gluteal fat the lowest. In a non-obese subject, adipose tissue contributes to 3–5% of the total resting energy expenditure, although it represents 20–30% of body weight. The majority of the heat production (about 60%) comes from active organs such as the liver, kidney, heart and brain, although they account for only 5–6% of total body weight (Table 5.4). The heat production of muscles per unit mass (42 to 63 kJ/kg) is 15–40 times lower than that of metabolically active organs, but because of its large size (more than half of the total fat-free mass) it contributes about 20% of total heat production.

The heat production or metabolic rate per kilogram of organ seems to change little during growth

Table 5.4 Contribution of different tissues and organs to basal metabolic rate (BMR) of a reference man (from Elia 2000)

	Weight of tissue		Organ/tissue metabolic rate		
	kg	% body weight	MJ/kg/day	MJ/day	% BMR (7.03 MJ/day)
Liver	1.8	2.6	0.84	1.51	21
Brain	1.4	2.0	1.00	1.41	20
Heart	0.33	0.5	1.84	0.61	9
Kidney	0.31	0.4	1.84	0.57	8
Muscle	28.0	40	0.054	1.52	22
Adipose tissue	15	21.4	0.019	0.28	4
Miscellaneous by difference, e.g. skin, intestine, bone	23.16	33.1	0.049	1.13	16
Whole body	70	100	0.1	7.03	100

and development. However, the metabolic rate per kilogram body weight (or per kilogram fat-free mass) is much greater in young children than in adults. The reduction of metabolic rate with increasing age is mostly due to a change in the proportion of different tissues, and to a lesser extent to a reduction in the metabolic rate per kilogram of individual (Elia 2000). The larger proportion of metabolically active tissues (brain, liver, heart, kidneys) in infants and children explains their higher metabolic rates compared with adults when expressed in relation to fat-free mass). The contribution of different tissues to body weight and BMR in a 'reference male' is shown in Table 5.4.

Fuels used by different tissues and fuel selection

The main fuels available to tissues are glucose, triacylglycerol, free fatty acids and ketone bodies; Table 5.5 shows the fuels that can be used by different tissues. Red blood cells are wholly reliant on anaerobic metabolism of glucose, releasing lactate, and the brain is largely reliant on glucose; it cannot utilise fatty acids, but in prolonged fasting and starvation ketone bodies can meet about 20% of its energy needs. Other tissues can utilise a variety of fuels, depending on their availability in the circulation, and hormonal control.

Measurements of energy expenditure

Principles of energy expenditure measurements

The energy expended by an individual can be assessed by two different techniques: *direct* and

Table 5.5 Important fuels utilised by various tissues (adapted from Elia 2000)

Brain	Glucose, ketone bodies
Muscle	Glucose, NEFA, ketone bodies (starvation), acetate (after alcohol ingestion), triacylglycerol, branched-chain amino acids
Liver	Amino acids, fatty acids including short-chain fatty acids, glucose, alcohol
Kidney:	
Cortex	Glucose, NEFA, ketone bodies
Medulla	Glucose (glycolysis)
Brown adipose tissue	NEFA, glucose
White adipose tissue	Glucose, NEFA
Gastrointestinal tract:	
Small intestine	Glutamine, ketone bodies (starvation), a variety of other fuels in smaller amounts
Large intestine	Short-chain fatty acids, glutamine, glucose, and other fuels in smaller amounts
Red blood cells	Glucose (glycolysis)
Lymphocytes/ macrophages	Glutamine, glucose, ? NEFA/ketones

NEFA, non-esterified fatty acid.

indirect calorimetry. Direct calorimetry is the direct measurement of heat output; indirect calorimetry depends on the fact that the heat released by metabolic processes can be calculated from the rate of oxygen consumption (VO_2). This is because energy expenditure to maintain electrochemical gradients, support biosynthetic processes, and generate muscular contraction utilises ATP (adenosine triphosphate), which is formed by oxidative phosphorylation, directly linked to the oxidation of substrates and reduction of oxygen to water. It is the rate of ATP utilisation that determines the rate of substrate oxidation and therefore oxygen consumption.

The energy expenditure per mole of ATP formed can be calculated from the heat of combustion of 1 mole of substrate, divided by the total number of moles of ATP generated in its oxidation. Each mole of ATP formed is accompanied by the release of about the same amount of heat (~75 kJ/mol ATP) during the oxidation of carbohydrates, fats or proteins and the consumption of 1 litre of oxygen is equivalent to about 20.3 kJ energy expenditure. Direct calorimetry consists of the measurement of heat dissipated by the body through radiation, convection, conduction and evaporation. Under conditions of thermal equilibrium in a subject at rest and in post-absorptive conditions, heat production, measured by indirect calorimetry, is identical to heat dissipation, measured by direct calorimetry. This is an obvious confirmation of the first law of thermodynamics, which states that the energy released is ultimately transformed into heat (and external work during exercise), and validates the use of indirect calorimetry.

Energy metabolism and nutrient utilisation

Open-circuit indirect calorimeters permit measurement of oxygen consumption and carbon dioxide production both at rest, when a ventilated hood is placed over the subject, and over 24 hours, by confining the subject to a respiration chamber (fitted with furniture, bed, washbasin, TV, etc.) and analysing O_2 and CO_2 in the air entering and leaving the chamber together with the air flow. Descriptions of available equipment and techniques are given by Murgatroyd et al (1993).

Metabolic rate (M), which corresponds to energy expenditure per unit of time, can be calculated from oxygen consumption (VO_2 in litres, at standard temperature (0°C), pressure (760 mmHg) and dry (STPD – standard temperature and pressure for dry air) per minute, according to the Weir formula as follows:

$$M \text{ (kJ/min)} = 20.3 \times VO_2$$

The value of 20.3 is a mean value (in kJ/l) of the energy equivalent for the consumption of 1 litre (STPD) of oxygen (Table 5.6) and is practically independent of the respiratory quotient (RQ) because the error involved is less than 1%. To estimate the contribution of the three macronutrients (carbohydrates, fats and proteins) to metabolic rate, three measurements must be carried out: oxygen consumption (VO_2), carbon dioxide production (VCO_2) and urinary nitrogen excretion (N). Metabolic rate is then:

$$M = aVO_2 + bVCO_2 - cN$$

The factors a, b and c (which are the coefficients of regression) depend on the respective constants for the amount of O_2 used and the amount of CO_2 produced during oxidation of the three classes of nutrients (Table 5.6). An example of such a formula is given below.

$$M = 16.18VO_2 + 5.02VCO_2 - 5.99N$$

Where M is in kilojoules, VO_2 and VCO_2 are in litres STPD, and N is in grams, per unit time. As an

Table 5.6 Energy yields from oxidation of substrates						
Substrates	O_2 consumed[a]	CO_2 produced[a]	RQ	Heat released	Energy equivalent	Energy equivalent
				per gram kJ	KJ per l CO_2	KJ per l CO_2
Starch	0.829	0.829	1.00	17.6	21.2	21.2
Saccharose	0.786	0.786	1.00	16.6	21.1	21.1
Glucose	0.746	0.746	1.00	15.6	21.0	21.0
Lipid	2.019	1.427	0.71	39.6	18.6	27.7
Protein	1.010	0.844	0.83	19.7	18.9	23.3
Lactic acid	0.746	0.746	1.00	15.1	20.3	20.3

[a]In litres per gram of substrate oxidised.
RQ, respiratory quotient.
Source: Livesey & Elia (1988).

example, if $VO_2 = 600$ litres per day, $VCO_2 = 500$ litres per day (respiratory quotient or RQ = 0.83), and N = 25 g per day, then M = 12068 kJ per day.

Indirect calorimetry also allows calculation of the nutrient oxidation rates in the whole body. An index of protein oxidation is obtained from the total amount of nitrogen excreted in the urine during the test period. Because 1 g urinary nitrogen arises from approximately 6.25 g protein, the protein oxidation rate (P in grams per minute) is given by the equation:

P = 6.25N

An index of carbohydrate oxidation (c) and of fat oxidation (f) is given below:

$c = 4.59VCO_2 - 3.25VO_2 - 3.68n$

$f = 1.69VO_2 - 1.69VCO_2 - 1.72n$

where c, f and n (urinary nitrogen secretion) are in grams per minute.

Assessment of BMR and energy cost of activity

The measurement of BMR is made under standardised conditions – i.e. in an awake subject lying in the supine position, in a state of physical and mental rest in a comfortable warm environment, and in the morning in the post-absorptive state, usually 10–12 hours after the last meal. Under these conditions, the expired air (collected in a Douglas bag over a certain period of time or coming from a ventilated hood system at a constant flow rate) is analysed for changes in O_2 and CO_2 concentrations. The energy cost of activities is measured by a portable indirect calorimeter. Nowadays, new technologies have permitted the development of a small size (<1 kg) computerised calorimeter, plugged to the trunk and connected to a comfortable face mask which continuously measures pulmonary ventilation. Breath-to-breath analysis can be performed on systems, which makes it possible to track the minute-by-minute profile of energy expenditure up to the time when steady state is reached.

Assessment of energy expenditure in free-living conditions

Various indirect methods have been used to assess total energy expenditure in humans under natural conditions of life. As shown in Table 5.7, they have been based on physiological measurements, human observations and records, kinematic recordings, or more recently isotopic dilution techniques. Early studies estimated energy expenditure using an activity diary, but today the two most commonly employed non-calorimetric methods are the heart rate and the doubly labelled water technique.

Heart rate

As far back as 1914, the pioneer American investigators Benedict and Talbot suggested that in infants 'heart rate may be considered a very fair index of energy metabolism'. The method involves establishing individual regression lines between heart rate and energy expenditure within a range of activities that bracket the habitual heart rate observed in normal life. By monitoring heart rate minute-by-minute throughout the day, using portable heart rate integrators, a frequency histogram can be obtained giving the number of minutes spent at each heart rate. By referring this value to the individual regression line, the energy expenditure at a given heart rate can be calculated and integrated throughout the day. Unfortunately, the relationship between heart rate and energy expenditure is not linear within the sedentary range of measurements. This is primarily due to the confounding effects of variations in stroke volume, which substantially increases in a non-linear fashion up to 40% of the maximal aerobic capacity. As a result, the measurement of cardiac output (i.e. heart rate × stroke volume) would predict

Table 5.7 Non-calorimetric methods for estimating energy expenditure or physical activity in humans

Physiological measurements
  Pulmonary ventilation volume
  Heart rate
  Electromyography
  Energy intake/body composition

Human observations and records
  Time and motion studies
  Activity diary
  Activity recall (i.e. questionnaire and interview)

Kinematic recordings
  Radar
  Cine photography
  Activity monitors meters (i.e. accelerometers, pedometers, satellites, global positioning system)

Isotope dilution methods
  Doubly labelled water ($^2H_2{}^{18}O$) or triple labelled water ($^2H^3H^{18}O$)
  Bicarbonate method

energy expenditure with more accuracy and precision than heart rate itself, but the non-invasive monitoring of cardiac output in free-living conditions is not yet possible. In addition, a variety of confounding factors (such as eating meals, variations in posture, and cigarette smoking) affect heart rate more than energy expenditure. The development of respiration chambers has allowed the validation of the heart rate method for estimating energy expenditure (Schutz et al 1981). At the group level, the average accuracy in four studies involving 8 to 22 subjects ranged from 1 to 3%. However, the standard deviation of the error is much greater, suggesting that the heart rate method is much less reliable for an individual than for a group.

Doubly labelled water

The stable (non-radioactive) isotope method for estimating energy expenditure using the doubly labelled water ($^2H_2$ and ^{18}O) can simultaneously provide an estimation of total body water (and hence body composition) and of water intake (and hence milk intake in studies of infants), as well as an estimate of energy expenditure. The method is based on the difference in the rates of turnover of ^2H_2O and $H_2^{18}O$ in body water, which is used to estimate CO_2 production rate and hence the rate of energy expenditure. Briefly, a subject is given a single oral dose of $^2H_2^{18}O$ so that body water is labelled by both isotopes. After equilibrium is reached, ^{18}O will be lost as both $C^{18}O_2$ and $H_2^{18}O$, because of the rapid exchange of ^{18}O between water and carbon dioxide. The loss of the isotope as water is determined by measuring the rate of disappearance of ^2H_2O. The rate of CO_2 production is calculated from the difference in rates of loss of the oxygen and hydrogen labels. The disappearance rates can be measured in urine (blood or saliva) for a period equivalent to 2 to 3 biological half-lives, i.e. about one week in adults. Under controlled conditions, studies have compared the energy expenditure obtained by using the doubly labelled water method with that measured by indirect calorimetry in a respiration chamber or with a ventilated hood system. These studies have demonstrated that the error at the group level ranged from 2 to 5%. However, greater errors are expected for a given individual. The accuracy and precision of the doubly labelled water method in free-living conditions is probably not constant and depends on the physiological and nutritional state of the subject as well as the environmental conditions.

Estimations of energy requirements

The energy requirement of an individual is defined by the World Health Organization (WHO) as 'the level of energy intake that will balance energy expenditure when the individual has a body size and composition, and a level of physical activity, consistent with long-term good health' (FAO/WHO/UNU 1985). The energy requirement should also allow the maintenance of economically necessary and socially desirable physical activity. In children and pregnant or lactating women, the energy requirement includes the energy needs associated with the deposition of tissues or the secretion of milk at rates consistent with good health. There are two approaches to assessing the energy requirements of people of different age, sex, and physical activity:

1. assessment of food intake followed by the calculation of energy intake
2. assessment of total energy expenditure.

The energy needs of a group represent – in contrast to protein and micronutrient needs – the *average* value of the individuals making up that group. When possible, energy requirement should be based on estimates of energy expenditure rather than energy intake. The term 'requirements' refers to the 'habitual' or 'usual' requirements over a certain period. From one day to the next, individuals are not expected to maintain energy balance precisely, and hence energy intake and energy expenditure measurements may not give the same values. Because the variability of energy intake is greater than the variability of expenditure, the habitual energy requirements can best be determined from expenditure rather than intake measurements. In addition, it is difficult to measure energy intake accurately without influencing the subject's ingestive behaviour.

In the estimation of daily energy expenditure by the so-called 'factorial' approach, the BMR is first calculated (Durnin 1991). The physical activities are broken down into occupational activities (work) and discretionary (i.e. desirable) activities. Occupational activities include salaried and non-salaried chores (such as housework). The energy expenditure for occupational activities will depend on the type of occupation, the time spent in performing the work and the physical characteristics of the individuals. These activities are classified into *light* (1.7 × BMR), *moderate* (2.2 × BMR for women and 2.7 × BMR for men) and *heavy* (2.8 × BMR for women and

3.8 × BMR for men). Discretionary activities include socially desirable activities (such as the exploratory activities of children and the participation in tasks implying social improvement), exercise for physical and cardiovascular fitness, and optional household tasks. In addition, the BMR is used to estimate the energy cost of sleeping. Finally, the residual time during which there is no clear definition of activity has been taken as BMR × 1.4. (There is a program on the CD – Energy balance program) that permits you to calculate energy requirements by this factorial method, using an activity diary.)

Once the separate components of energy expenditure (sleep, physical activity and residual time) have been calculated, the total energy requirement can be calculated by summation. It should be realised that when the energy expenditure is calculated *over 24 hours* and categorised into 'light', 'moderate' and 'heavy' work, the value expressed in multiples of BMR is obviously much lower than that calculated during a working task. For example, a group with occupational work classified as 'moderate' activity will have an energy requirement calculated over 24 hours of 1.78 × BMR in men and 1.64 × BMR in women because it includes sleeping hours and residual time, whereas during the actual performance of

the given task, the energy expended will be 2.7 × BMR for men and 2.2 × BMR for women.

The rate of total energy expenditure (TEE), directly assessed in a respiration chamber or by doubly labelled water, can be expressed as a multiple of some baseline value such as BMR. This approach has been used by an international expert committee (James & Schofield 1990) for calculating the energy requirement in the 'factorial' method. The ratio of TEE and BMR provides a rough index of physical activity (referred to as 'physical activity level' or PAL) but the contribution of the thermic effect of foods represents a small confounding factor. Since the energy cost of a given activity is proportional to body weight, especially for weight-bearing activities, the absolute energy expenditure during weight-bearing activity will be linearly related to body weight. In non-obese subjects the ratio TEE/BMR ranged from 1.64 to 1.98, based on doubly labelled water measurements of energy expenditure. In the confined condition of a respiratory chamber (without prescribed exercise on a treadmill or bicycle, etc.) the ratio is 1.3 to 1.35, indicating that small discontinuous activities of daily life (washing, moving around, studying, TV, etc.) increased basal energy expenditure by one-third.

5.5 TIMESCALE OF ENERGY BALANCE AND BODY WEIGHT VARIABILITY

Any regulated function varies within limits that are largely determined by the limits for survival. These are clearly much narrower for body temperature and blood pH than for body weight and body fat. Because large variations in body fat can be observed both between and within individuals, it could therefore be argued that body weight is a poorly regulated variable. By contrast, the fact that in many individuals, body weight remains relatively constant over years and decades in spite of large day-to-day variations in the amount of food consumed might instead suggest that body weight is precisely regulated in these individuals. But, constancy of body weight per se is not evidence for regulation. In fact, a critical feature of any regulated system is that disturbance of the regulated variable results in compensatory responses that tend to attenuate the disturbance and to restore the system to its 'set' or 'preferred' value. The direct application of this approach to test whether body weight is regulated in human beings is difficult because of ethical and

practical considerations, but observations on adults recovering from food shortages during post-war famine or from experimental starvation indicate that a return to normal body weight is eventually achieved. Conversely, excess weight gained during experimental overeating or during pregnancy is subsequently lost, and most individuals return to their initial body weight. There is therefore little doubt that regulation of body weight occurs (albeit with varying degrees of precision), although the timescale over which it occurs is not clear. In this context, it is important to emphasise three cardinal features of energy balance and weight regulation:

1. Human beings do not balance energy intake and energy expenditure on a day-to-day basis nor is positive energy balance one day spontaneously compensated by negative energy balance the next day. Near equality of intake and expenditure most often appear over 1–2 weeks. Longer measurements are difficult to conduct and impractical

because of cumulative errors, but there is no doubt that over months and years, total energy intake and expenditure must be very close in any individual whose body weight and body composition have remained relatively constant.

2. This matching of long-term energy intake and energy expenditure must be extremely precise since a theoretical error of only 1% between input and output of energy, if persistent, will lead to a gain or loss of about 10 kg per decade. But this does not occur for most individuals, whose weight remains constant within a few kilograms over several decades.

3. Even in adults who apparently maintain a stable body weight over months, years and decades, there is in reality no 'absolute' constancy of body weight. Instead, body weight tends to fluctuate or oscillate around a constant mean value, with small or large deviations from a 'set' or 'preferred'

value being triggered by events that are seasonal and/or cultural (weekend parties, holiday seasons), psychological (stress, depression, anxiety or emotions) and pathophysiological (ranging from minor health perturbations to serious diseases). According to Garrow (1974), very short-term day-to-day changes in body weight have a standard deviation of about 0.5% of body weight, while longitudinal observations over periods of between 10 and 30 years indicate that individuals experience slow trends and reversal of body weight amounting to between 7 and 20% of mean weight. In the town of Framingham, in the USA, after 10 examinations spanning 18 years among both men and women, the average peak-to-peak fluctuation in body weight was 10 kg (Gordon & Kannel 1973). Figure CD 5.1 shows the day-to-day variation in body weight over a 4-year period in a non-obese male.

5.6 CONTROL OF FOOD INTAKE

Hunger and satiety

Research into the control of energy intake is very difficult, primarily because habitual intake is not easy to measure (see 'Pattern of food intake', above) and because the intake of foods is altered by the experiments themselves. Because of these difficulties, much of the work carried out in human beings has been concerned with short-term hunger and appetite studies or with short-term satiety and satiation. It is important to differentiate between these terms. Hunger may be defined as a 'demand for energy' (e.g. after starvation), while appetite refers to 'a demand for a particular food'. In rodents, kept in cages and fed ad libitum on standard laboratory chow, energy intake is controlled mainly by the sensations of hunger and satiety. If (like human beings) the laboratory rat has access to a variety of palatable foods rather than to a monotonous diet, it may be stimulated to eat by appetite rather than by hunger. The physiological mechanisms which control energy intake in rats certainly exist in humans. If a person is deprived of food, he becomes hungry, and if he has eaten a lot, he becomes satiated. *Satiation* refers to processes involved in the termination of a meal, and is studied by providing individuals with test meals and measuring the amount consumed when the food is freely available. *Satiety* refers to the

inhibition of further intake of a food and meal after eating has ended. However, lifestyle factors ensure that appetite is a powerful but poorly controlled stimulus to eat even when not hungry. Thus, the total energy ingested in a day is determined by the interaction of many exogenous and endogenous factors.

Psychosocial factors and sensory specific satiety

It is common experience that feeding patterns are influenced strongly by psychological, economic and social factors. Even though subjects may feel satiated by one particular food, they will continue to eat when a new food is presented – a phenomenon that is referred to as 'sensory specific satiety'. Conversely, when subjects are presented with a monotonous diet, their intakes are usually low. In many parts of the developing world, the major part of energy intake derives from one staple food, which together with low fat intakes, constitutes a bland and monotonous diet, so that even when supplies are adequate, obesity is rarely seen. These observations suggest that when the psychosocial incentives to eat are removed, human beings (like the laboratory rat fed chow diet) can control food intake quite precisely.

Hunger–satiety control centres in the brain

Much of our understanding about centres in the brain that are involved with the control of food intake derives from studies conducted in laboratory animals. As a result of numerous experiments involving ablation, electrical and chemical stimulation of specific areas in the brain, it has been proposed that 'centres' in the hypothalamus are involved in the control of feeding behaviour. People with damage in the hypothalamus, due to trauma or tumour, often show abnormalities in feeding behaviour and weight regulation. However, many other extra-hypothalamic areas also play a role in the control of food intake (see Section CD 5.6(a)).

Hunger–satiety signals from the periphery

The sensations of hunger and satiety result from the central integration of numerous signals originating from a variety of peripheral tissues and organs, including the gastrointestinal tract, liver, adipose tissue, and perhaps also skeletal muscle. The putative hunger–satiety signalling systems that have generated the most interest are outlined below.

Signals from the gastrointestinal tract

The progression of food through the stomach and small intestine – which can be considered as a short-term nutrient reservoir – initiates a number of sequential peripheral satiety signals that are thought to be important in influencing meal-to-meal feeding responses. Signals from stretch- and mechano-receptors or from chemoreceptors that respond to the products of digestion (sugars, fatty acids, amino acids and peptides), are transmitted via vagal afferent nerves to the hindbrain, where integration of this visceral output occurs. This provides a pathway whereby the physical and chemical properties of food can have a major role in the short-term regulation of food intake by limiting the size of a single meal. These signals may also affect energy intake in a subsequent meal. Among the gastrointestinal signals that are believed to be important influences on food intake are: cholecystokinin (CCK) which decreases meal size; pancreatic glucagon, which appears to exert its satiety effects via the liver; bombesin-like peptides, which delay gastric emptying and reduce appetite, and the hormone ghrelin, whose concentration increases after food deprivation and decreases in response to the presence of nutrients in the stomach (see Section CD 5.6(b)).

Aminostatic or protein-static signals

A link between fluctuations in serum amino acids and food intake was proposed nearly 50 years ago. Dietary protein induces satiety in the short term, and consumption of low protein diets leads to increased appetite for protein-containing foods. Administration of amino acids such as phenylalanine and tryptophan that are precursors of monoamine neurotransmitters leads to reduced food intake, and the ratio of plasma tryptophan to other amino acids affects brain serotonin, which is known to have an inhibitory influence on food intake. These observations lead to an aminostatic theory, which states that food intake is determined by the level of plasma amino acids, and that this could be related to the regulation of lean body mass, which is known to be rigorously defended against experimental or dietary manipulation. A 'protein-stat' mechanism for the regulation of lean body mass has been proposed by Millward (1995). In fact, food intake during growth is known to be dominated by the impetus for gaining lean tissue (see Ch. 8).

Glucostatic and glycogenostatic signals

A glucostatic theory for the regulation of feeding behaviour was proposed by Mayer some 50 years ago. It proposes that there are chemoreceptors in the hypothalamic satiety centre which would be sensitive to the arteriovenous difference in glucose or to the availability and utilisation of glucose. The arguments in favour of this hypothesis include: (a) the small decreases of blood glucose observed prior to spontaneous meal consumption, (b) the suppression of food intake induced by infusion of glucose, and (c) the spontaneous decrease in total energy intake observed when dietary carbohydrate content is increased. These same arguments in support of the glucostatic theory of food intake also form the basis of the proposal of Flatt (1995) that the control of food intake, via the prevention of hypoglycaemia and maintenance of adequate glycogen levels, primarily serves the maintenance of the carbohydrate balance (see 'Integrated models of food intake control', below).

Lipostatic or adipostat signals

A lipostatic theory of food intake control, first proposed by Kennedy in the early 1950s, postulates that substances released from the fat stores function as satiety signals. This theory is based on a set-point control system with body fat (rather than body weight) acting as the regulated variable and energy intake as the controlled variable. Body fat is thus maintained at a set value, and any deviation from this value is detected by the hypothalamus via a circulating metabolite (the error signal), which is related to the size of the fat stores. Having detected such a deviation, the hypothalamus elicits compensatory changes in energy intake and hence restores the system to its pre-set or preferred level. The lipostatic hypothesis is perhaps the one that provides the most plausible explanation for long-term regulation of the fat stores. Many experiments support this theory, leading to the suggestion that people who are predisposed to obesity may have a homeostatic mechanism in which the set-point for weight regulation is set at a higher level than in those who are more resistant to obesity.

The nature of the various components, such as the set-point and feedback signal(s), involved in the lipostatic theory remains unclear. A major advance came in 1995 following the cloning of the *ob* gene, whose protein product (leptin) is primarily produced by adipocytes, is released into the circulation and acts on hypothalamic receptors to induce satiety (see Section CD 5.6(c)). The blood concentration of leptin is proportional to the adipose mass, and its elevation in obese individuals has led to the hypothesis that resistance to the action of leptin is a factor in obesity. People with rare mutations causing complete leptin deficiency show marked hyperphagia and severe obesity – which can be reversed by administration of small doses of leptin. People with rare mutations affecting the leptin receptor mechanism also showed hyperphagia and severe obesity, but do not respond to administration of leptin. However, although circulating leptin is diminished during starvation and restored during refeeding, its rapid fall in starvation and rapid restoration on refeeding suggest that changes in circulating leptin are independent of acute changes in body fat content, and that changes in leptin are a function of changes in the flux of energy intake rather than a 'lipostatic' signal whose level is altered as a function of depletion and repletion of the fat stores. Both the feedback signal on food intake, and the nature of the set-point (if it exists) remain elusive.

Integrated models of food intake control

These various signals from the periphery can be integrated in a model (see Fig. CD 5.2) in which the control of food intake is considered in three phases, each with a distinct goal. These are summarised below; for further details see Section CD 5.6(d):

- *short-term* (hour to hour) blood glucose homeostasis
- *medium-term* (day-to-day) maintenance of adequate hepatic stores of glycogen, and
- *long-term* (weeks, months or years) maintenance of the body's fat and protein compartments, i.e. fat mass and fat-free mass.

Nutrient balance model

The long-term stability of body weight and body composition requires not only that energy expenditure is equal to energy intake, but also that the composition of the fuel mix which is oxidised follows that which is ingested. Since, as shown in Table 5.1, the protein and carbohydrate stores in the body are limited, they tend to be modulated by an autoregulatory process, allowing an increase in their own oxidation in response to an increase in their exogenous supply. In contrast, the stores of fat are not well regulated by fat oxidation since an increase in dietary fat does not promote its oxidation. Hence (unlike carbohydrate and protein), fat balance is not precisely regulated. The failure to adjust fat oxidation in response to excess intake will contribute to depletion of glycogen stores by increasing carbohydrate oxidation, with consequent negative feedback on total energy intake. In other words, the size of carbohydrate stores exerts negative feedback on total energy intake, so that high fat diets (containing little carbohydrate) will promote excess energy intake to reach an appropriate level of carbohydrate intake. This energy imbalance would persist until the fat stores build up sufficiently to provide a greater supply for fat oxidation. When the higher fat oxidation matches the higher intake, the individual would then be both in fat balance and in energy balance, but at a higher percentage of body fat. Obese individuals have a significantly lower respiratory quotient (RQ) than lean people (Schutz 1995) and hence a greater proportion of their elevated energy expenditure is met by fat oxidation. The interpretation of this concept of nutrient balance is that the control of food intake can be viewed as both glycogenic (short term) and lipostatic (long term) and tends to integrate control of food intake via glycogenostatic and lipostatic signalling.

5.7 AUTOREGULATORY ADJUSTMENTS IN ENERGY EXPENDITURE

A brief summary follows; for further information see Section CD 5.7.

Whatever mechanisms operate for the control of food intake, this control is not by itself sufficient to explain long-term regulation of body weight and body composition. There is also ample evidence that autoregulatory adjustments in energy expenditure play an important role in correcting deviations in body weight and body composition.

The dynamic equilibrium model

There is a built-in stabilising mechanism in the overall homeostatic system for body weight regulation. Any imbalance between energy intake and energy requirements would result in a change in body weight which, in turn, will alter the maintenance energy requirements in a direction that will tend to counter the original imbalance and hence be stabilising. There is a built-in negative feedback and the system thus exhibits *dynamic equilibrium*.

Role of adaptive thermogenesis

Subjects maintaining body weight 10% above their initial weight show an increase in daily energy expenditure even after adjusting for changes in body weight and composition. Similarly, in subjects maintaining weight 10% below their initial weight, daily energy expenditure is lower after adjusting for losses in weight and lean tissues. These compensatory changes in energy expenditure (about 15% above or below predicted values) reflect changes in metabolic efficiency (i.e. thermogenesis) that oppose the maintenance of a body weight that is above or below the 'set' or 'preferred' body weight.

The most striking feature of virtually all experiments of overfeeding is the wide range of individual variability in the amount of weight gained per unit of excess energy consumed. These differences in the efficiency of weight gain are mostly attributed to (a) variability in the ability to convert excess calories to heat, i.e. in the large inter-individual capacity for diet-induced thermogenesis (DIT), and (b) differences in body composition for the same change in body weight. In addition to the control of food intake, changes in efficiency of energy utilisation (via adaptive thermogenesis) play an important role in the regulation of body weight and composition, and the magnitude of adaptive changes in thermogenesis is strongly influenced by the genetic make-up of the individual.

Thermogenesis associated with physical activity

A main cause of controversy about the importance of adaptive thermogenesis in the aetiology of human obesity is the difficulty of identifying which component(s) of energy expenditure could contribute to the changes in metabolic efficiency and hence adaptive thermogenesis. Changes in resting energy expenditure that are not accounted for by changes in body weight and composition reflect changes in metabolic efficiency. By contrast, the heat production from non-resting energy expenditure is more difficult to quantify. The efficiency of muscular contraction during exercise is low (~25%), but that of spontaneous physical activity (SPA) (including fidgeting, muscle tone and posture maintenance, and other low-level physical activities of everyday life) is even lower since these essentially involuntary (subconscious) activities comprise a larger proportion of isometric work. A change in the *level* or *amount* of such involuntary SPA activity in a direction that defends a 'preferred' body weight constitutes autoregulatory mechanisms that contribute to the overall changes in metabolic efficiency. In this context, an increase in the amount of SPA in response to overfeeding, or a decrease during starvation, also constitute adaptive behavioural changes in thermogenesis.

Even under conditions where subjects are confined to a metabolic chamber, the 24-hour energy expenditure attributed to SPA (as assessed by radar systems) was found to vary between 400 and

3000 kJ/day, and to be a predictor of subsequent weight gain. Levine et al (1999) found that more than 60% of the increase in total daily energy expenditure in response to overfeeding was associated with SPA, and that inter-individual variability in energy expenditure associated with SPA – which they referred to as non-exercise-activity thermogenesis (NEAT) – was the most significant predictor of the resistance or susceptibility to obesity.

Model of adaptive thermogenesis in body composition regulation

Any change in metabolic efficiency (ME) in resting or non-resting state that would tend to *attenuate energy imbalance* or to *restore body weight and body composition* towards its 'set' or 'preferred' value constitutes adaptive changes in thermogenesis. The available evidence suggests the existence of two distinct control systems underlying adaptive thermogenesis (Dulloo et al 2002). One control system is a direct function of energy imbalance and responds *rapidly* to attenuate the impact of changes in food intake on changes in body weight; it is suppressed during starvation and increased during overfeeding. The other control system has a much *slower* time-course since it operates as a feedback loop between the size of the fat stores and thermogenesis (i.e. a lipostatic or adipose-specific control of thermogenesis). Its suppression during weight (and fat) loss acts to reduce the overall rate of fuel utilisation during starvation, while its sustained suppression until body fat is recovered during refeeding serves to accelerate the replenishment of the fat stores. Conversely during periods of excess fat gain, its activation will serve to oppose the maintenance of the excess fat and hence to restore body fat to its 'set' or 'preferred' level.

5.8 INTEGRATING INTAKE AND EXPENDITURE

In attempting to explain the responses in energy balance and weight regulation in real life, it is important to recognise that several factors may be operating simultaneously on both sides of the energy balance equation. In order to achieve long-term constancy of body weight, compensatory adjustments occur in both energy intake and energy expenditure, so that unravelling the importance of one or other is difficult, if not impossible. Models of body weight regulation have primarily focused on physiologically-induced *autoregulatory* adjustments in energy intake and in energy expenditure, i.e. those beyond voluntary control. However, the range of variation in body weight (see Section 5.5) is large enough to be detected consciously and there is certainly some degree of cognitive control. As pointed out by Garrow (1974), a change of several kilograms in body weight can hardly be ignored since clothes which formerly would fit will no longer do so, and there will be changes in appearance, exercise tolerance, and general well-being. When such chronic energy imbalance occurs during adolescent or adult life, it is also corrected by more or less conscious effort when the individual decides – for efficient survival, cultural or health reasons – that the change in body weight is no longer acceptable. In response, they control or attempt to control food intake or energy expenditure via changes in physical activity. In many individuals, the importance of such cognitive (conscious) controls over food intake and energy expenditure can be as important as non-conscious physiological regulations.

⊃ Key points

⊃ Energy in foods is provided by the macronutrients (carbohydrate, proteins, fats) and alcohol. In the transformation of the chemical energy in food (i.e. gross energy) to energy available for the body (i.e. metabolisable energy), 5–10% is lost through faeces and urine. The metabolisable energy is on average 16 kJ/g of carbohydrate, 17 kJ/g of protein, 37 kJ/g of fat and 29 kJ/g of alcohol.

⊃ Energy balance is the difference between metabolisable energy intake and total energy expenditure. It is strongly related to macronutrient balance, and the sum of individual substrate balances, expressed as energy, is equivalent to the overall energy balance.

⊃ The matching between energy intake and expenditure is poor over the short term, but (in most people) it is accurate over the long term. Because day-to-day variability in energy intake is much greater than that of energy expenditure, the habitual energy requirements are best determined from total energy expenditure.

- The mechanisms underlying long-term energy balance and weight regulation are unknown, but involve both involuntary controls as well as conscious alterations in lifestyle to correct unwanted changes in body weight.

- Modern lifestyles have led to considerable changes in what food is eaten and in the amount of time spent on physical activity, leading to an environment when the matching between energy intake and energy expenditure is more difficult to achieve.

- A high fat (energy-dense) diet promotes weight gain because it promotes increased energy intake. However, there is a large inter-individual variability in susceptibility to overconsume high fat diets or for the ability to oxidise excess fat; part of this variability is genetically determined.

- Undernutrition leads to a decrease in energy expenditure, in part because of the loss in body weight (and metabolically active tissues) and in part because of energy conservation resulting from increased efficiency of metabolism.

- Overnutrition leads to gain in body weight which is often less than predicted because of compensatory increases in energy expenditure – the magnitude of which is determined by the composition of the diet, the proportion of lean to fat tissue in the extra weight gained and by capacity of the individual to burn off excess calories through diet-induced thermogenesis.

References and further reading

References

Dulloo A G, Jacquet J, Montani J P 2002 Pathways from weight fluctuations to metabolic diseases: focus on maladaptive thermogenesis during catch-up fat. International Journal of Obesity 26(suppl 2):S46–S57

Durnin J V G A 1991 Practical estimates of energy requirements. Journal of Nutrition 121:1907–1913

Elia M 2000 Fuels of the tissues. In: Garrow J S, James W P T, Ralph A (eds) Human nutrition and dietetics, 10th edn. Churchill Livingstone, Edinburgh, p 37–59

FAO/WHO/UNU 1985 Energy and protein requirements. WHO Technical Report Series No. 724. World Health Organization, Geneva

Flatt J P 1995 Diet, lifestyle and weight maintenance. American Journal of Clinical Nutrition 62: 820–836

Garrow J S 1974 Energy balance and obesity in man. North-Holland Publishing, Amsterdam

Gordon T, Kannel W B 1973 The effects of overweight on cardiovascular disease. Geriatrics 28:80–88

James W P T, Schofield E C 1990 Human energy requirements. A manual for planners and nutritionists. Published by arrangement with the Food and Agricultural Organization of the United Nations. Oxford University Press, Oxford, p 25–34

Levine J A, Eberhardt N L, Jensen M D 1999 Role of nonexercise activity thermogenesis in resistance to fat gain in humans. Science 283:212–214

Livesey G, Elia M 1988 Estimation of energy expenditure, net carbohydrate utilisation and net fat oxidation and synthesis by indirect calorimetry: evaluation of errors with special reference to detailed composition of fuels. American Journal of Clinical Nutrition 47:608–628

Miller D S 1982 Factors affecting energy expenditure. Proceedings of the Nutrition Society 41:193–202

Millward D J 1995 A protein-stat mechanism for the regulation of growth and maintenance of the lean body mass. Nutrition Research Reviews 8:93–120

Murgatroyd P R, Shetty P S, Prentice A M 1993 Techniques for the measurement of human energy expenditure: a practical guide. International Journal of Obesity 17:549–568

Schutz Y 1995 Macronutrients and energy balance in obesity. Metabolism 44 (suppl 3):7–11

Schutz Y, Bray G A, Margen S 1981 Effect of a meal on the oxygen consumption-heart rate relationship. American Journal of Clinical Nutrition 34:965–966

Southgate D A T, Durnin J V G A 1970 Calorie conversion factors. An experimental reassessment of the factors used in the calculation of the energy value of human diets. British Journal of Nutrition 24:517–535

Further reading

Blundell J E, Lawton C L, Cotton J R, Macdiarmid J I 1996 Control of human appetite: implications for the intake of dietary fat. Annual Review of Nutrition 16:285–319

Dulloo A G, Jacquet J, Girardier 1998 Poststarvation hyperphagia and body fat overshooting in humans: a role for feedback signals from lean and fat tissues. American Journal of Clinical Nutrition 65:717–723

Keys A, Brozek J, Hanschel A et al 1950 The biology of human starvation. University of Minnesota Press, Minneapolis

Schutz Y, Garrow J S 1996 Energy and substrate balance, and weight regulation. In: Garrow J S, James W P T, Ralph A (eds) Human nutrition and dietetics, 10th edn. Churchill Livingstone, Edinburgh, p 137–148

Stock M J 1999 Gluttony and thermogenesis revisited. International Journal of Obesity 23:1105–1117

Stubbs F J 1998 Appetite, feeding behaviour and energy balance in humans. Proceedings of the Nutrition Society 57:341–356

CD-ROM contents

Expanded material
Section CD 5.6(a) Hypothalamic neurons

Section CD 5.6(b) Hypothalamic mechanisms of action of ghrelin

Section CD 5.6(c) Hypothalamic mechanisms of action of leptin

Section CD 5.6(d) Integrated models of food intake control

Section CD 5.7 Autoregulatory adjustment in energy expenditure

Figures
Figure CD 5.1 Day-to-day fluctuations in body weight over a 4-year period in a lean man

Figure CD 5.2 Sequence of events in food intake control

Figure CD 5.3 Patterns of changes in body weight, food intake and adaptive changes in thermogenesis of men subjected to experimental starvation and refeeding in the Minnesota experiment

Energy balance program

Additional references related to CD-ROM material

Further reading

Further reading from the book

6
Carbohydrate metabolism

Nils-Georg Asp and David A. Bender

Objectives

By the end of this chapter you should be able to:

- classify the dietary carbohydrates
- explain the importance of the glycaemic index
- describe the main functions of carbohydrates
- describe the pathway of glycolysis, and how it can operate under aerobic or anaerobic conditions
- describe the Cori cycle of anaerobic glycolysis and gluconeogenesis
- describe the metabolic importance of pyruvate and the principal factors that determine its metabolic fate
- describe the complete oxidation of acetyl CoA through the citric acid cycle
- describe the role of glycogen as a carbohydrate reserve and explain how its synthesis and utilisation are regulated
- explain the importance of gluconeogenesis and describe the pathway
- explain how carbohydrate utilisation in tissues is controlled by hormones and by the products of fatty acid metabolism
- describe the main factors involved in the control of carbohydrate metabolism in muscle
- describe the main types of dietary fibre (non-starch polysaccharides, resistant starch, resistant oligosaccharides), and their effects on health, including intestinal bacterial fermentation and effects on digestion and absorption of other nutrients.

6.1 INTRODUCTION

In average Western diets carbohydrates provide somewhat over 40% of energy intake, with a desirable level of around 55%; in developing countries, where fat is scarce, 75% or more of energy may come from carbohydrates.

As discussed in Section 2.2 under 'Carbohydrates', and shown in Table 6.1, dietary carbohydrates can be divided into three groups: polysaccharides with 10 or more monomeric residues, oligosaccharides with 3–9, and sugars that can be either free monosaccharides or disaccharides. Polysaccharides can be further divided into two groups: starch, and non-starch polysaccharides. Although this classification according to molecular size is important for the chemist, other properties determine the nutritional effects of the various food carbohydrates.

Table 6.1 **Classification of main food carbohydrates**

Class (DP[a])	Subgroup	Components	Monomers	Digestibility[b]
Sugars (1–2)	Monosaccharides	Glucose		+
		Galactose		+
		Fructose		+
	Disaccharides	Sucrose	Glu, Fru	+
		Lactose	Glu, Gal	+ (−)
		Trehalose	Glu	+
Oligosaccharides (3–9)	Malto-oligosaccharides	Maltodextrins	Glu	+
	Other oligosaccharides	α-Galactosides	Gal, Glu	−
		Fructo-oligosaccharides	Fru, Glu	−
Polysaccharides (>9)	Starch	Amylose	Glu	+ (−)
		Amylopectin	Glu	+ (−)
		Modified starch	Glu	+ −
	Non-starch polysaccharides	Cellulose	Glu	−
		Hemicelluloses	Variable	−
		Pectins	Uronic acids	−
		Hydrocolloids, e.g. gums and mucilages	Variable	−

[a] DP, Degree of polymerisation.
[b] Denotes digestibility in the small intestine: + digestible, − indigestible, + − partly digestible, + (−) mainly digestible.
Adapted from Asp N-G 1996 Dietary carbohydrates: classification by chemistry and physiology. Food Chemistry 57:9–14.

The classification into 'simple' and 'complex' carbohydrates stems from the perception that 'complex', i.e. high molecular weight, carbohydrates are more slowly absorbed than simple sugars, but as described below, properties other than the molecular weight determine the glycaemic index of carbohydrate foods. Another classification used in terms of health promotion is two separate groups of sugars: intrinsic sugars that are contained within cell walls of plants, and extrinsic sugars, which are free in solution, added as purified sugars, which may promote dental caries (see Ch. 25). Because lactose in milk is not cariogenic (except at extreme continuous breastfeeding practices), and because milk is an important source of vitamin B_2, calcium and protein, lactose is considered separately from other sugars in free solution, which are known as non-milk extrinsic sugars. The main extrinsic sugar in most diets is sucrose, and according to recent international recommendations (WHO 2003) it is desirable that added free sugars (including sugars in fruit juices) should provide no more than 10% of energy intake (the current average in UK is about 14%).

Fruits also provide fructose, and small amounts of pentose (5-carbon) and other sugars, as well as sugar alcohols (polyols). Fructose is 40% sweeter-tasting than sucrose, and 75% sweeter than glucose.

High-fructose syrups prepared by hydrolysis of corn starch and isomerisation of about half the glucose to fructose are now widely used in food manufacture, but since this replaces sucrose it has no great impact on the glucose/fructose ratio of the diet.

Various sugar alcohols are 50–100% as sweet as sucrose; they are poorly absorbed, so have an energy yield about half that of sugars, and provoke a lower insulinaemic response than sugars, so they are widely used as bulk sweeteners in foods suitable for diabetics and weight-reducing diets.

Nutritionally, the most important classification is by differentiation between two broad categories of carbohydrates: (1) carbohydrates that are digested and absorbed in the small intestine, and thus provide carbohydrates for metabolism in various body tissues, and (2) carbohydrates that pass to the large intestine providing substrate for the colonic microflora. Already in the 1920s McCance and Widdowson made such a differentiation and classified carbohydrates as 'available' or 'unavailable'. Later on the term 'dietary fibre' was introduced and used increasingly as more or less synonymous with 'unavailable carbohydrates'. The latest FAO/WHO Expert Consultation on Carbohydrates in Human Nutrition (FAO Food and Nutrition Paper 66, 1998) recommended the term 'glycaemic carbohydrate' for absorbable/available/metabolisable carbohydrates.

Table 6.2 **Food factors influencing the glycaemic index of foods**

Structural properties	Properties of the starch	Other factors
Gross structure, e.g. whole cereal grains	Degree of gelatinisation	Soluble, viscous types of dietary fibre, e.g. guar gum, pectin
Cellular structures, e.g. leguminous seeds	Amylose/amylopectin ratio	Organic acids, e.g. lactate, propionate
Starch granular structure	Crystallinity	Amylase inhibitors
	Retrogradation, i.e. recrystallisation	Disaccharidase inhibitors

Glycaemic carbohydrates

The main glycaemic carbohydrates are glucose and fructose (monosaccharides), sucrose and lactose (disaccharides), and starch. There is one group of glycaemic oligosaccharides, dextrins, which are fragments of starch with 1–4 or 1–6 α-glycosidic linkages hydrolysed by digestive amylase and disaccharidases.

An increasingly important way to classify dietary carbohydrates is by their glycaemic index (GI) – the extent to which they raise blood glucose concentration compared with an equivalent amount of a reference carbohydrate (glucose or white bread). The GI is calculated as the area under the blood glucose response curve after a 50 g glycaemic carbohydrate portion of a food/the response after the standard. GI values obtained with the glucose standard are generally lower by a factor of about 0.7 compared to a white bread standard. Carbohydrates with a high glycaemic index generally provoke a higher secretion of insulin than those with a low glycaemic index, and both the glycaemic index of, and insulinaemic response to, dietary carbohydrates are important in the maintenance of glycaemic control in diabetes mellitus (see Section 21.5). Other possible health benefits related to the GI are discussed further in Section 6.6 under 'Importance of the glycaemic index'. Milk products provoke a prominent insulin response due to specific proteins or amino acid composition, in spite of a low glycaemic index. The importance of this effect is not known. Food factors important for the glycaemic index are listed in Table 6.2.

Intact kernels in cereal products hinder starch digestion with a resulting low GI. A proportion of the starch in foods may be enclosed by plant cell walls, which are composed of indigestible non-starch polysaccharides, and so is protected against digestion. For that reason, leguminous seeds have a high content of resistant starch and low GI (see next section). Similarly, intrinsic sugars may have a lower glycaemic index than would be expected, because they are within intact cells. Other factors lowering the GI are viscous types of non-starch polysaccharides (which hinder diffusion), organic acids (which inhibit gastric emptying and interact with starch) and amylase inhibitors.

Uncooked starch is resistant to amylase action, because it is present as small insoluble, partly crystalline granules. The process of cooking swells the starch granules, resulting in a gel on which amylase can act. The swelling and dissolution of starch by cooking is called gelatinisation. Thus, uncooked starches have very low GI, which increases with the degree of gelatinisation. Because of the high activity of amylase in the small intestine, fully gelatinised and dissolved starch may have a GI as high as glucose.

Dietary fibre

The main constituent of dietary fibre is non-starch polysaccharides (NSP) from plant cell walls, and it was first defined as the skeletal remnants of plant cell-walls resisting digestion in the human small intestine. The term dietary fibre used to be synonymous with non-digestible carbohydrates, but it includes lignin and other non-carbohydrate substances. There are three classes of non-digestible carbohydrate in dietary fibre: NSP, resistant starch (RS) and resistant oligosaccharides (ROS).

NSP consists of cellulose, a glucose polymer, and other polysaccharides with variable properties in terms of monomeric composition, molecular size and structure. They are often classified as hemicellulose, pectins, gums etc., or according to main monomeric constituents, e.g. galactans, arabinoxylans etc. The physico-chemical properties of NSPs vary widely, as do their physiological effects. Soluble, viscous types of dietary fibre affect digestion and absorption in the small intestine, attenuating postprandial rises in blood glucose and lipids. In the large intestine, dietary fibre is subject to anaerobic bacterial fermentation, leading to increased bacterial cell mass and metabolites that affect both the colon and the peripheral metabolism. Insoluble and especially lignified NSPs are more resistant to fermentation and bind water in the distal large bowel, providing, together with the increased bacterial mass, faecal bulk.

RS is starch that escapes digestion in the small intestine, and it may be a substantial fraction of the total carbohydrate delivered to the colon. Four types of RS can be defined, based on the reason for resistance to digestion:

1. physically enclosed starch due to intact cell walls (RS1)
2. ungelatinised starch granules, as in green bananas and high-amylose corn starch (RS2)

3. retrograded starch: as cooked starch cools, a proportion undergoes crystallisation (retrogradation) to a form that is again resistant to amylase action – this is part of the process of staling of starchy foods (RS3)
4. chemically modified starches used as food additives may be partially resistant (RS4).

Foods with a low GI also often have a high content of RS, e.g. beans, but in bread and corn flakes, there is a substantial RS content in spite of a high GI for the digestible starch.

Resistant oligosaccharides include polymers of fructose (fructo-oligosaccharides, from onions and artichokes, as well as added inulin and oligofructose), and galacto-oligosaccharides from leguminous seeds.

6.2 FUNCTIONS OF GLYCAEMIC CARBOHYDRATES

The most obvious function of glycaemic carbohydrates is as an energy source; in the fed state most tissues metabolise glucose as their main metabolic fuel. In addition, liver and muscle synthesise the polysaccharide glycogen in the fed state, as a reserve of carbohydrate for use in the fasting state between meals.

Carbohydrate in excess of requirements for immediate metabolism and synthesis of glycogen provides the acetyl CoA required for fatty acid synthesis, as well as the glycerol phosphate required for esterification of fatty acids to form triacylglycerols (see Section 7.4).

Amino acid synthesis from carbohydrates

The carbon skeletons of the non-essential amino acids (Ch. 8, Fig. 8.1) are derived from intermediates of carbohydrate metabolism. As shown in Figure 6.1, several amino acids are synthesised from pyruvate, the end-product of glycolysis, and others are synthesised from intermediates of the citric acid cycle.

Synthesis of other sugars with specific functions

The main carbohydrate entering the bloodstream from carbohydrate digestion is glucose, with small amounts of fructose and galactose, and traces of other monosaccharides. A number of sugars are required for specific purposes, and these can all be synthesised from glucose. Glycerol phosphate, which is required for esterification of fatty acids to triacylglycerol and phospholipids, arises from dihydroxyacetone phosphate, an intermediate in glycolysis (see Section 6.3).

There is a requirement for relatively large amounts of two pentoses, ribose and deoxyribose, for synthesis of RNA (ribose) and DNA (deoxyribose). In addition, ribose is required for the synthesis of ATP and GTP, as well as the coenzymes NAD and NADP, and its sugar alcohol, ribitol, is required for the synthesis of the flavin coenzymes derived from vitamin B_2. Ribose is an intermediate in, and can be a product of, the pentose phosphate pathway of glucose metabolism (see 'The pentose phosphate pathway – an alternative to glycolysis', below, and Fig. CD 6.3); deoxyribose and ribitol are synthesised by reduction of ribose.

Glucuronic acid is required for the conjugation of bile salts, steroid hormone metabolites and the metabolites of a variety of xenobiotics, including compounds ingested in the diet and taken as drugs, in order to render them water-soluble for excretion in bile or urine. It is synthesised from glucose, by the oxidation of uridine diphosphate glucose. In animals for which vitamin C is not a dietary essential, glucuronic acid is metabolised onwards to ascorbate; in human beings and other animals for which ascorbate is a dietary essential, glucuronic acid is

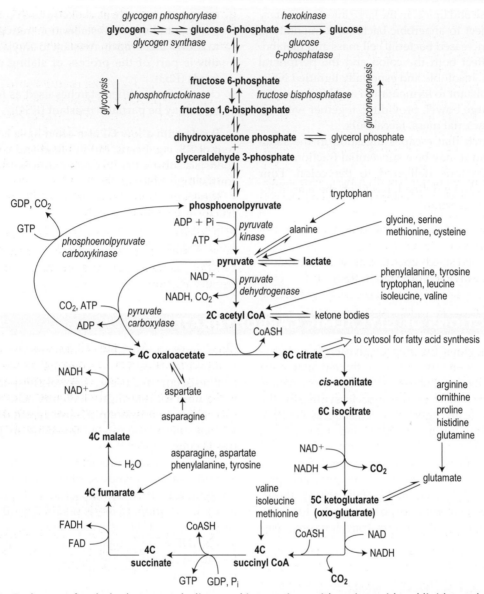

Figure 6.1 Pathways of carbohydrate metabolism, and interactions with amino acid and lipid metabolism.

metabolised to yield the pentose sugar xylulose and its alcohol xylitol, which is further metabolised via the pentose phosphate pathways (see Section 6.3). Genetic lack of the enzyme that reduces xylulose to xylitol results in the harmless condition of pentosuria – urinary excretion of relatively large amounts of xylulose. Xylulose is a reducing sugar, and gives a positive result when urine is tested with copper reagents (Clinitest) for monitoring glycaemic control in diabetes mellitus, although it does not react with glucose oxidase, which is the basis of the Clinistix test for urine glucose.

Complex carbohydrates with special functions

The amino derivative of glucose, glucosamine, is synthesised from fructose 6-phosphate (an intermediate in glycolysis, see 'Glycolysis – the (anaerobic) metabolism of glucose', below), and is the precursor for synthesis of other amino sugars, including *N*-acetyl-glucosamine, *N*-acetyl-galactosamine and the 9-carbon sialic acid *N*-acetyl-neuraminic acid. These amino sugars are important for the synthesis of glycoproteins, glycosaminoglycans and glycolipids.

Glycoproteins

Glycoproteins are proteins that are esterified to one or more oligosaccharides containing various sugars and amino sugars; the carbohydrate content of different glycoproteins ranges between 1 and 85% of the mass. They include albumin and other serum proteins, collagen in connective tissue, mucins secreted to protect the intestinal mucosa, immunoglobulins, peptide hormones and enzymes. In addition, glycoproteins at cell surfaces are important in cell recognition, including the major blood group determinants, and intracellular glycoproteins are involved in targeting of proteins to intracellular organelles.

Lectins are proteins that recognise, and bind to, cell surface glycoproteins, and may cause cell agglutination. A number of lectins occur in legumes and other foods, and if not denatured by adequate cooking can cause severe intestinal disorder by binding to intestinal mucosal cell surface glycoproteins.

Glycosaminoglycans and proteoglycans

Glycosaminoglycans are unbranched polysaccharides made up of repeating disaccharide units; one component of the disaccharide is an amino sugar (glucosamine or galactosamine), and the other is normally glucuronic acid or one of its isomers. Most glycosaminoglycans are also sulphated, and apart from hyaluronic acid they all occur as proteoglycans, linked to proteins. Major glycosaminoglycans include:

- hyaluronic acid, an important constituent of synovial fluid, cartilage and loose connective tissue
- chondroitin sulphates, which occur both in cartilage and at the sites of calcification in bone
- keratan and dermatan sulphates, which also occur in cartilage, and have a critical role in maintaining the transparency of the cornea
- heparin, a proteoglycan secreted by the liver that acts as an anticoagulant.

A number of proteoglycans are found at the outer surface of cell membranes, where they may function as receptors and mediators of cell–cell communication.

Glycolipids

Glycolipids are found in cell membranes, especially in the nervous system. The major glycolipids consist of a fatty acid esterified to sphingosine with covalently bound glucose, galactose, N-acetyl-neuraminic acid and other amino sugars. Like glycoproteins and proteoglycans, they act as receptors and cell-surface recognition compounds.

6.3 THE METABOLISM OF GLYCAEMIC CARBOHYDRATES

Figure 6.1 shows an overview of carbohydrate metabolism. The first stage is glycolysis, which results in the cleavage of glucose to yield 2 mol of the 3-carbon compound pyruvate and a net yield of $6 \times$ ATP. Glycolysis is (indirectly) reversible, so that glucose can be synthesised from non-carbohydrate precursors that yield pyruvate – the pathway of gluconeogenesis (see under 'Gluconeogenesis', below). Glycolysis can also proceed under anaerobic conditions; anaerobic glycolysis is especially important in muscle under conditions of maximum exertion.

Pyruvate arising from glycolysis enters the mitochondria and is oxidised and decarboxylated to yield $3 \times$ ATP per pyruvate (and hence 6 per glucose) and acetyl CoA, which may undergo one of two fates:

- complete oxidation in the citric acid cycle, yielding $12 \times$ ATP per acetyl CoA (and hence 24 per glucose);

- utilisation as the precursor for synthesis of fatty acids and cholesterol (and hence other steroid hormones and the bile acids).

Glycolysis – the (anaerobic) metabolism of glucose

Glycolysis occurs in the cytosol; overall it results in cleavage of the 6-carbon glucose molecule into two 3-carbon units. The key steps in the pathway are:

- two phosphorylation reactions to form fructose-bisphosphate
- cleavage of fructose-bisphosphate to yield two molecules of triose (3-carbon sugar) phosphate
- two steps in which phosphate is transferred from a substrate onto ADP, forming ATP
- one step in which NAD^+ is reduced to NADH
- formation of 2 mol of pyruvate per mol of glucose metabolised.

The immediate substrate for glycolysis is glucose 6-phosphate; this may arise from two sources:

- by phosphorylation of glucose, catalysed by hexokinase (also by glucokinase in the liver in the fed state)
- by phosphorolysis of glycogen in liver and muscle to yield glucose 1-phosphate, catalysed by glycogen phosphorylase. Glucose 1-phosphate is readily isomerised to glucose 6-phosphate.

The pathway of glycolysis is shown in Figure CD 6.1. Although the aim of glucose oxidation is to form ATP from the phosphorylation of ADP, the pathway involves two steps in which ATP is used, one to form glucose 6-phosphate when glucose is the substrate, and the other to form fructose bisphosphate. In other words, there is a modest cost of ATP to initiate the metabolism of glucose.

Glucose 6-phosphate undergoes isomerisation to fructose 6-phosphate, which is then phosphorylated to fructose bisphosphate. The formation of fructose bisphosphate, catalysed by phosphofructokinase, is an important step for the regulation of glucose metabolism. Once it has been formed, fructose bisphosphate is cleaved into two 3-carbon compounds, dihydroxyacetone phosphate and glyceraldehyde 3-phosphate, which are interconvertible. The onward metabolism of these 3-carbon sugars is linked to both the reduction of NAD^+ to NADH, and direct (substrate-level) phosphorylation of ADP to form ATP. The result is the formation of 2 mol of pyruvate from each mol of glucose.

As discussed below in 'Gluconeogenesis', the reverse of the glycolytic pathway is important as a means of glucose synthesis – the process of gluconeogenesis. Most of the reactions of glycolysis are readily reversible, but at three points (the reactions catalysed by hexokinase, phosphofructokinase and pyruvate kinase) there are separate enzymes involved in glycolysis and gluconeogenesis. For all of these reactions, the equilibrium is strongly in the direction of glycolysis.

The glycolytic pathway also provides a route for the metabolism of fructose, galactose (which undergoes phosphorylation to galactose 1-phosphate and isomerisation to glucose 1-phosphate) and glycerol. Some fructose is phosphorylated directly to fructose 6-phosphate by hexokinase, but most is phosphorylated to fructose 1-phosphate by a specific enzyme, fructokinase. Fructose 1-phosphate is then cleaved to yield dihydroxyacetone phosphate and glyceraldehyde; the glyceraldehyde can be phosphorylated to glyceraldehyde 3-phosphate by triose kinase. The metabolism of galactose and fructose occurs in the intestinal mucosa and liver, so little fructose or galactose reaches the peripheral circulation. Ethanol, however, inhibits the metabolism of galactose, leading to increased plasma levels and galactosuria.

Glycerol, arising from the hydrolysis of triacylglycerols, can be phosphorylated and oxidised to dihydroxyacetone phosphate. Important to triacylglycerol synthesis, glycerol phosphate is formed from dihydroxyacetone phosphate.

Glycolysis under aerobic conditions

Glycolysis occurs in the cytosol, but the oxidation of NADH linked to phosphorylation of ADP to form ATP occurs inside the mitochondria. The mitochondrial inner membrane is impermeable to NAD, and two substrate shuttles are used to oxidise cytosolic NADH, transport reduced substrates into the mitochondrion and reoxidise them at the expense of mitochondrial coenzymes that are then reoxidised by the electron transport chain, linked to phosphorylation of ADP to ATP. The two substrate shuttles are:

1. The malate acetate shuttle, which involves reduction of oxaloacetate in the cytosol to form malate (with the oxidation of NADH). Malate then enters the mitochondria and is reduced back to oxaloacetate (and NADH is reformed).

2. The glycerol phosphate shuttle, which involves the reduction of dihydroxyacetone phosphate in the cytosol to form glycerol 3-phosphate (with the oxidation of NADH). Once inside the mitochondrion the glycerol 3-phosphate is oxidised back to dihydroxyacetone phosphate (and NADH is reformed).

Glycolysis under anaerobic conditions – the Cori cycle

In red blood cells, which lack mitochondria, reoxidation of NADH formed in glycolysis cannot be by way of the substrate shuttles discussed above and the electron transport chain. Similarly, under conditions of maximum exertion, for example in sprinting, the rate at which oxygen can be taken up into the muscle is not great enough to allow for the reoxidation of all the NADH that is being formed in glycolysis. In order to maintain the oxidation of glucose, and the yield of ATP, NADH is oxidised to NAD^+ by the reduction of pyruvate to lactate, catalysed by lactate dehydrogenase.

The resultant lactate is exported from the muscle and red blood cells, and taken up by the liver, where it is used for the resynthesis of glucose. This is the Cori cycle (see Fig. CD 6.2), an inter-organ cycle of glycolysis in muscle and gluconeogenesis in liver. The synthesis of glucose from lactate is an ATP (and GTP) requiring process. The 'oxygen debt' after strenuous physical activity is due to an increased rate of energy-yielding metabolism to provide the ATP and GTP that are required for gluconeogenesis from lactate. While most of the lactate will be used for gluconeogenesis, a proportion will have to undergo oxidation to CO_2 in order to provide the ATP and GTP required for gluconeogenesis.

Lactate may also be taken up by other tissues, where oxygen availability is not a limiting factor, such as the heart. Here it is oxidised to pyruvate, which is then a substrate for complete oxidation to carbon dioxide and water, via the citric acid cycle (see 'Oxidation of acetyl CoA', above).

Many tumours have a poor blood supply and hence a low capacity for oxidative metabolism, so that much of their energy-yielding metabolism in the tumour is anaerobic. Lactate produced by anaerobic glycolysis in tumours is exported to the liver for gluconeogenesis. The energy cost of this increased cycling of glucose between anaerobic glycolysis in the tumour and gluconeogenesis in the liver may account for much of the weight loss (cachexia) that is seen in patients with advanced cancer.

The pentose phosphate pathway – an alternative to glycolysis

There is an alternative pathway for the conversion of glucose 6-phosphate to fructose 6-phosphate, the pentose phosphate pathway (sometimes known as the hexose monophosphate shunt), shown in Figure CD 6.3.

Overall, the pentose phosphate pathway produces 2 mol of fructose 6-phosphate, 1 mol of glyceraldehyde 3-phosphate and 3 mol of carbon dioxide from 3 mol of glucose 6-phosphate, linked to the reduction of 6 mol of $NADP^+$ to NADPH. The sequence of reactions is as follows:

- 3 mol of glucose are oxidised to yield 3 mol of the 5-carbon sugar ribulose 5-phosphate + 3 mol of carbon dioxide
- 2 mol of ribulose 5-phosphate are isomerised to yield 2 mol of xylulose 5-phosphate

- 1 mol of ribulose 5-phosphate is isomerised to ribose 5-phosphate
- 1 mol of xylulose 5-phosphate reacts with the ribose 5-phosphate, yielding (ultimately) fructose-6-phosphate and erythrose 4-phosphate
- The other mol of xylulose-5-phosphate reacts with the erythrose 4-phosphate, yielding fructose 6-phosphate and glyceraldehyde 3-phosphate.

This is also the pathway for the synthesis of ribose for nucleotide synthesis, and the source of about half the NADPH required for fatty acid synthesis. Tissues that synthesise large amounts of fatty acids have a high activity of the pentose phosphate pathway. It is also important in the respiratory burst of macrophages that are activated in response to infection.

The pentose phosphate pathway in red blood cells – favism

The pentose phosphate pathway is also important in the red blood cell, where NADPH is required to maintain an adequate pool of reduced glutathione, which is used to remove hydrogen peroxide.

The tripeptide glutathione (γ-glutamyl-cysteinyl-glycine) is the reducing agent for glutathione peroxidase, which reduces H_2O_2 to H_2O and O_2. Oxidised glutathione (GSSG) is reduced back to active GSH by glutathione reductase, which uses NADPH as the reducing agent. Glutathione reductase is a flavin-dependent enzyme, and its activity can be used as an index of vitamin B_2 status (see Ch. 10, Section 10.2).

Partial or total lack of glucose-6-phosphate dehydrogenase (and hence impaired activity of the pentose phosphate pathway) is the cause of favism, an acute haemolytic anaemia with fever and haemoglobinuria, precipitated in genetically susceptible people by the consumption of broad beans (fava beans) and a variety of drugs, all of which, like the toxins in fava beans, undergo redox cycling, producing hydrogen peroxide. Infection can also precipitate an attack, because of the increased production of oxygen radicals as part of the macrophage respiratory burst. Favism is one of the commonest genetic defects; an estimated 200 million people worldwide are affected. It is an X-linked condition, and female carriers are resistant to malaria; this advantage presumably explains why defects in the gene are so widespread.

glycogen has been depleted the rapid loss of water (and weight) will cease.

Glycogen synthesis

In the fed state, glycogen is synthesised from glucose in both liver and muscle. The reaction is a stepwise addition of glucose units onto the glycogen that is already present. The pathway is shown in Figure CD 6.8.

Glycogen synthesis involves the intermediate formation of UDP-glucose (uridine diphosphate glucose) by reaction between glucose 1-phosphate and UTP (uridine triphosphate). As each glucose unit is added to the growing glycogen chain, so UDP is released, and must be rephosphorylated to UTP by reaction with ATP. There is thus a significant cost of ATP in the synthesis of glycogen: 2 mol of ATP are converted to ADP + phosphate for each glucose unit added, and overall the energy cost of glycogen synthesis may account for 5% of the energy yield of the carbohydrate stored.

Glycogen synthetase forms only the $\alpha 1 \rightarrow 4$ links that form the straight chains of glycogen. The branch points are introduced by the transfer of 6–10 glucose units in a chain from carbon-4 to carbon-6 of the glucose unit at the branch point.

Endurance athletes require a slow release of glucose from glycogen over a period of hours, rather than a rapid release. There is some evidence that this is achieved better from glycogen that is less branched, and therefore has fewer points at which glycogen phosphorylase can act. The formation of branch points in glycogen synthesis is slower than the formation of $\alpha 1 \rightarrow 4$ links, and this has been exploited in the process of 'carbohydrate loading' in preparation for endurance athletic events. The athlete exercises to exhaustion, when muscle glycogen is more or less completely depleted, then consumes a high carbohydrate meal, which stimulates rapid synthesis of glycogen, with fewer branch points than normal. There is little evidence to show whether this improves endurance performance or not; such improvement as has been reported may be the result of knowing that one has made an effort to improve.

Glycogen utilisation

In the fasting state, glycogen is broken down by the removal of glucose units one at a time from the many ends of the molecule. The reaction is a phosphorolysis – cleavage of the glycoside link between two glucose molecules by the introduction of phosphate. The product is glucose 1-phosphate, which is then isomerised to glucose 6-phosphate. In the liver glucose 6-phosphatase catalyses the hydrolysis of glucose 6-phosphate to free glucose, which is exported for use, especially by the brain and red blood cells.

Muscle cannot release free glucose from the breakdown of glycogen, since it lacks glucose 6-phosphatase. However, muscle glycogen can be an indirect source of blood glucose in the fasting state. Glucose 6-phosphate from muscle glycogen undergoes glycolysis to pyruvate, which is then transaminated to alanine. Alanine is exported from muscle, and taken up by the liver for use as a substrate for gluconeogenesis (see 'Gluconeogenesis', below).

Glycogen phosphorylase stops cleaving $\alpha 1 \rightarrow 4$ links four glucose residues from a branch point, and a debranching enzyme catalyses the transfer of a three glucosyl unit from one chain to the free end of another chain. The $\alpha 1 \rightarrow 6$ link is then hydrolysed by a glucosidase, releasing glucose.

The branched structure of glycogen means that there are a great many points at which glycogen phosphorylase can act; in response to stimulation by adrenaline there can be a very rapid release of glucose 1-phosphate from glycogen.

Gluconeogenesis – the synthesis of glucose from non-carbohydrate precursors

The pathway of gluconeogenesis is essentially the reverse of the pathway of glycolysis (see 'Glycolysis – the (anaerobic) metabolism of glucose', above). However, at three steps there are separate enzymes involved in the breakdown of glucose (glycolysis) and gluconeogenesis. The reactions of pyruvate kinase, phosphofructokinase and hexokinase cannot readily be reversed (i.e. they have equilibria that are strongly in the direction of the formation of pyruvate, fructose bisphosphate and glucose 6-phosphate respectively).

There are therefore separate enzymes, under distinct metabolic control, for the reverse of each of these reactions in gluconeogenesis:

1. Pyruvate is converted to phosphoenolpyruvate for glucose synthesis by a two step reaction, with the intermediate formation of oxaloacetate. Pyruvate is carboxylated to oxaloacetate in an ATP-dependent reaction in which the vitamin biotin is the coenzyme. This reaction can also be used to replenish oxaloacetate in the citric acid cycle

when intermediates have been withdrawn for use in other pathways. Oxaloacetate then undergoes a phosphorylation reaction, in which it also loses carbon dioxide, to form phosphoenolpyruvate. The phosphate donor for this reaction is GTP; this prevents the withdrawal of oxaloacetate for gluconeogenesis if citric acid cycle activity would be impaired.

2. Fructose bisphosphate is hydrolysed to fructose 6-phosphate by a simple hydrolysis reaction catalysed by the enzyme fructose bisphosphatase.

3. Glucose 6-phosphate is hydrolysed to free glucose and phosphate by the action of glucose 6-phosphatase.

The other reactions of glycolysis are readily reversible, and the overall direction of metabolism, either glycolysis or gluconeogenesis, depends mainly on the relative activities of phosphofructokinase and fructose bisphosphatase.

Many of the products of amino acid metabolism can also be used for gluconeogenesis, since they are sources of pyruvate or intermediates in the citric acid cycle, and hence provide increased oxaloacetate. The requirement for gluconeogenesis from amino acids in order to maintain a supply of glucose for the nervous system and red blood cells explains why there is often a considerable loss of muscle in prolonged fasting or starvation, even if there are apparently adequate reserves of adipose tissue to meet energy needs.

Substrates that give rise to acetyl CoA directly (alcohol, fatty acids, ketone bodies and ketogenic amino acids) cannot be substrates for gluconeogenesis since the two carbons added in the reaction to yield citrate are lost in the citric acid cycle, and acetyl CoA cannot provide an increase in the pool of oxaloacetate to act as a precursor for gluconeogenesis. However, the glycerol that arises from the hydrolysis of triacylglycerol in the fasting state can be a substrate for gluconeogenesis, since it is interconvertible with dihydroxyacetone phosphate, an intermediate of glycolysis.

6.4 THE CONTROL OF CARBOHYDRATE METABOLISM AND INTEGRATION WITH LIPID AND PROTEIN METABOLISM

Energy expenditure is relatively constant throughout the day, but most of the food intake normally occurs in two or three meals. There is therefore a need for metabolic regulation to ensure that there is a more or less constant supply of metabolic fuel to tissues, regardless of the variation in intake.

There is a particular need to regulate carbohydrate metabolism since the nervous system is largely reliant on glucose as its metabolic fuel, and red blood cells are entirely so. The plasma concentration of glucose must be regulated within strict limits, between 3 and 5.5 mmol/l. If it falls below about 2 mmol/l there is loss of consciousness – hypoglycaemic coma; similarly an excessively high concentration can cause hyperglycaemic coma. Prolonged moderate hyperglycaemia leads to the complications of poorly controlled diabetes mellitus (see Ch. 21).

The plasma concentration of glucose is maintained in short-term fasting by the use of glycogen, and by releasing free fatty acids from adipose tissues, and later ketone bodies from the liver, which are preferentially used by muscle, so sparing such glucose as is available, for use by the brain and red blood cells. However, the total body content of glycogen would be exhausted within 12–18 hours of fasting if there were no other source of glucose, and in more prolonged fasting gluconeogenesis from amino acids and the glycerol of triacylglycerol is important. The regulation of blood glucose is achieved largely by changes in the rates of glycolysis and gluconeogenesis, as well as changes in the rates of glycogen synthesis and breakdown. Both hormonal control (mainly insulin and glucagon) and regulation of carbohydrate metabolism by intermediates of fatty acid metabolism are important. In response to muscle stimulation there needs to be a very rapid increase in the rate of glycolysis.

Hormonal control of carbohydrate metabolism in the fed state

During the 3–4 hours after a meal, there is an ample supply of metabolic fuel entering the circulation from the gut. Glucose from carbohydrate digestion and amino acids from protein digestion are absorbed into the portal circulation, and to a considerable extent the liver controls the amounts that enter the peripheral circulation. Under these conditions, when there is a plentiful supply of glucose, it is the main metabolic fuel for most tissues, and after a meal the RQ (respiratory quotient: the ratio of the volume of carbon dioxide formed to volume of oxygen consumed in metabolism) is close to 1.0, indicating that it is mainly glucose that is being oxidised.

The increased concentration of glucose and amino acids in the portal blood stimulates the β-cells of the pancreas to secrete insulin, and suppresses the secretion of glucagon by the β-cells of the pancreas. Insulin has four main actions:

1. Increased uptake of glucose into muscle and adipose tissue. This is effected by recruitment to the cell surface of glucose transporters that are in intracellular vesicles in the fasting state.
2. Stimulation of the synthesis of glycogen from glucose in both liver and muscle, by activation of glycogen synthetase.
3. Stimulation of fatty acid synthesis in adipose tissue by activation of acetyl CoA carboxylase and parallel inactivation of hormone-sensitive lipase.
4. Stimulation of amino acid uptake into tissues, leading to an increased rate of protein synthesis.

In the liver, glucose uptake is by carrier-mediated diffusion and metabolic trapping as glucose 6-phosphate, and is independent of insulin. The uptake of glucose into the liver increases very significantly as the concentration of glucose in the portal vein increases, and the liver has a major role in controlling the amount of glucose that reaches peripheral tissues after a meal. There are two isoenzymes that catalyse the formation of glucose 6-phosphate in liver:

1. Hexokinase has a K_m of approximately 0.15 mmol/l. This enzyme is saturated, and therefore acting at its V_{max}, under all conditions. It acts mainly to ensure an adequate uptake of glucose into the liver to meet the demands for liver metabolism.
2. Glucokinase has a K_m of approximately 20 mmol/l. This enzyme will have very low activity in the fasting state, when the concentration of glucose in the portal blood is between 3 and 4 mmol/l. However, after a meal the portal concentration of glucose may well reach 20 mmol/l or higher, and under these conditions glucokinase has significant activity, and there is increased formation of glucose 6-phosphate in the liver. Most of this will be used

for synthesis of glycogen, although some will also be used for synthesis of fatty acids that will be exported in very low density lipoprotein.

Hormonal control of carbohydrate metabolism in the fasting state

In the fasting state (sometimes known as the post-absorptive state, since it begins about 4–5 hours after a meal, when the products of digestion have been absorbed) metabolic fuels enter the circulation from the reserves of glycogen, triacylglycerol and protein laid down in the fed state. The metabolic problem in the fasting state is that the brain is largely dependent on glucose as its metabolic fuel, and red blood cells (which lack mitochondria) cannot utilise any metabolic fuel other than glucose. Therefore those tissues that can utilise other fuels do so, in order to spare glucose for the brain and red blood cells.

As the concentration of glucose and amino acids in the portal blood falls, so the secretion of insulin by the β-cells of the pancreas decreases. The most important reason for the reversed metabolic events in the post-absorptive state is the decreased plasma insulin level. Furthermore, the secretion of glucagon by the β-cells increases. Glucagon has two main actions:

- stimulation of the breakdown of liver glycogen to glucose 1-phosphate, resulting in the release of glucose into the circulation
- stimulation of the synthesis of glucose from amino acids in liver and kidney (gluconeogenesis, see Section 6.3, under 'Gluconeogenesis').

At the same time, the reduced secretion of insulin results in:

- a reduced rate of glucose uptake into muscle
- a reduced rate of protein synthesis, so that the amino acids arising from protein catabolism are available for gluconeogenesis
- relief of the inhibition of hormone-sensitive lipase in adipose tissue, leading to release of non-esterified fatty acids.

Three additional hormones are important for glucose homeostasis. Adrenaline (epinephrine) stimulates glycogenolysis and gluconeogenesis. Its lipolytic effect also stimulates lipolysis, making fatty acids available as an alternative fuel. Cortisol and growth hormone stimulate both gluconeogenesis and lipolysis, and inhibit glucose uptake with a resulting blood glucose elevating effect.

Control of glycogen synthesis and utilisation

In response to insulin (secreted in the fed state) there is increased synthesis of glycogen, and inactivation of glycogen phosphorylase. In response to glucagon (secreted in the fasting state) or adrenaline (secreted in response to fear or fright) there is inactivation of glycogen synthase, and activation of glycogen phosphorylase, permitting utilisation of glycogen reserves. Both effects are mediated by protein phosphorylation and dephosphorylation:

- In response to glucagon or adrenaline, protein kinase is activated, and catalyses phosphorylation of both glycogen synthase, resulting in loss of activity, and glycogen phosphorylase, resulting in activation of the inactive enzyme.
- In response to insulin, phosphoprotein phosphatase is activated, and catalyses dephosphorylation of both phosphorylated glycogen synthase, restoring its activity, and of phosphorylated glycogen phosphorylase resulting in loss of activity.

There is also control by intracellular metabolites which can override this hormonal regulation. Inactive glycogen synthase is allosterically activated by high concentrations of its substrate, glucose 6-phosphate. Active glycogen phosphorylase is allosterically inhibited by ATP, glucose and glucose 6-phosphate, all of which signal that there is an ample supply of glucose available. (See also Fig. CD 6.9.)

Control of glycolysis – the regulation of phosphofructokinase

The reaction catalysed by phosphofructokinase in glycolysis, the phosphorylation of fructose 6-phosphate to fructose 1,6-bisphosphate, is essentially irreversible. In gluconeogenesis the hydrolysis of fructose 1,6-bisphosphate is catalysed by a separate enzyme, fructose bisphosphatase. Regulation of the activities of these two enzymes determines whether the overall metabolic flux is in the direction of glycolysis or gluconeogenesis.

Inhibition of phosphofructokinase leads to an accumulation of glucose 6-phosphate in the cell, and this results in inhibition of hexokinase, which has an inhibitory binding site for its product. The result of this is a decreased rate of entry of glucose into the glycolytic pathway.

Feedback control of phosphofructokinase

Phosphofructokinase is inhibited by ATP binding at a regulatory site that is distinct from the substrate-binding site for ATP (allosteric inhibition). At physiological intracellular concentrations of ATP, phosphofructokinase has very low activity, and a more markedly sigmoid dependency on the concentration of its substrate. This can be considered to be end-product inhibition, since ATP can be considered to be an end-product of glycolysis.

When there is a requirement for increased glycolysis, and hence increased ATP production, this inhibition is relieved, and there may be a 1000-fold or higher increase in glycolytic flux in response to increased demand for ATP. However, there is less than a 10% change in the intracellular concentration of ATP, which would not have a significant effect on the activity of the enzyme. What happens is that as the concentration of ADP begins to increase, so adenylate kinase catalyses the reaction:

$$2 \times ADP \rightleftharpoons ATP + AMP$$

AMP acts as an intracellular signal that energy reserves are low, and ATP formation must be increased. It binds to phosphofructokinase and both reverses the inhibition caused by ATP and also increases the cooperativity between the subunits, so that the enzyme has greater affinity for fructose 6-phosphate. AMP also binds to fructose 1,6-bisphosphatase, reducing its activity.

Citrate, which can also be considered to be an end-product of glycolysis, also inhibits phosphofructokinase, by enhancing the inhibition by ATP. Phosphoenolpyruvate, which is synthesised in increased amounts for gluconeogenesis, also inhibits phosphofructokinase.

Feed-forward control of phosphofructokinase

High intracellular concentrations of fructose 6-phosphate activate a second enzyme, phosphofructokinase-2, which catalyses the synthesis of fructose 2,6-bisphosphate from fructose 6-phosphate. Fructose 2,6-bisphosphate is an allosteric activator of phosphofructokinase and an allosteric inhibitor of fructose 1,6-bisphosphatase. It thus acts both to increase glycolysis and inhibit gluconeogenesis. This is feed-forward control – allosteric activation of phosphofructokinase – because there is an increased concentration of substrate available.

Substrate cycling

A priori it would seem sensible that the activities of opposing enzymes such as phosphofructokinase and fructose 1,6-bisphosphatase should be regulated in such a way that one is active and the other inactive at any time. If both were active at the same time then there would be cycling between fructose 6-phosphate and fructose 1,6-bisphosphate, with hydrolysis of ATP – a so-called futile cycle.

What is observed is that both enzymes are indeed active to some extent at the same time, although the activity of one is greater than the other, so there is a net metabolic flux. One function of such substrate cycling is thermogenesis – hydrolysis of ATP for heat production.

Substrate cycling also provides a means of increasing the sensitivity and speed of metabolic regulation. The increased rate of glycolysis in response to need for ATP for muscle contraction would imply a more or less instantaneous 1000-fold increase in phosphofructokinase activity if phosphofructokinase were inactive and fructose 1,6-bisphosphatase active. If there is moderate activity of phosphofructokinase, but greater activity of fructose 1,6-bisphosphatase, so that the metabolic flux is in the direction of gluconeogenesis, then a more modest increase in phosphofructokinase activity and decrease in fructose 1,6-bisphosphatase activity will achieve the same reversal of the direction of flux.

Control of the utilisation of pyruvate

Pyruvate is at a metabolic crossroads, and in the liver and kidney it can either undergo decarboxylation to acetyl CoA, and hence oxidation in the citric acid cycle, or be carboxylated to provide oxaloacetate for gluconeogenesis. Its metabolic fate is largely determined by the oxidation of fatty acids.

Pyruvate dehydrogenase is inhibited in response to increased acetyl CoA, and also an increase in the $NADH:NAD^+$ ratio in the mitochondrion. The concentration of acetyl CoA will be high when β-oxidation of fatty acids is occurring, and there is no need to utilise pyruvate as a metabolic fuel. Similarly, the $NADH:NAD^+$ ratio will be high when there is an adequate amount of metabolic fuel being oxidised in the mitochondrion, so that again pyruvate is not required as a source of acetyl CoA. Under these conditions it will mainly be carboxylated to oxaloacetate for gluconeogenesis.

The regulation of pyruvate dehydrogenase is the result of phosphorylation. Pyruvate dehydrogenase kinase is activated by acetyl CoA and NADH, and catalyses the phosphorylation of the enzyme to an inactive form. Pyruvate dehydrogenase phosphatase acts constantly to dephosphorylate the inactive enzyme, so restoring its activity, and maintaining sensitivity to changes in the concentrations of acetyl CoA and NADH.

Control of glucose utilisation in muscle

Muscle can use a variety of fuels: plasma glucose; its own reserves of glycogen; triacylglycerol from plasma lipoproteins; plasma non-esterified fatty acids; plasma ketone bodies; triacylglycerol from adipose tissue reserves within the muscle. The selection of metabolic fuel depends on both the intensity of work being performed and also whether the individual is in the fed or fasting state.

The effect of work intensity on muscle fuel selection

Skeletal muscle contains two types of fibres:

1. Type I (red muscle) fibres. These are also known as slow-twitch muscle fibres. They are relatively rich in mitochondria and myoglobin (hence their colour), and have a high rate of citric acid cycle metabolism, with a low rate of glycolysis. These are the fibres used mainly in prolonged, relatively moderate, work.

2. Type II (white muscle) fibres. These are also known as fast-twitch fibres. They are relatively poor in mitochondria and myoglobin, and have a high rate of glycolysis. Type IIA fibres also have a high rate of aerobic (citric acid cycle) metabolism, while type IIB have a low rate of citric acid cycle activity, and are mainly glycolytic. White muscle fibres are used mainly in high intensity work of short duration (e.g. sprinting and weight-lifting).

Intense physical activity requires rapid generation of ATP, usually for a relatively short time. At the very beginning of a strenuous muscle activity, creatine phosphate is used to regenerate ATP. This is the basis for use of dietary supplements with creatine phosphate hoping to increase tissue levels of this compound. Initially, substrates and oxygen cannot enter the muscle at an adequate rate to meet the demand, and muscle depends on anaerobic glycolysis of its glycogen reserves. As discussed above in 'Glycolysis under anaerobic conditions – the Cori cycle', this leads to the release of lactate into the bloodstream, which is used as a substrate for gluconeogenesis in the liver, mainly after the exercise has finished. Less intense physical activity is often referred to as aerobic exercise, because it involves mainly red muscle fibres (and type IIA white fibres), and there is less accumulation of lactate.

The increased rate of glycolysis for exercise is achieved in three ways:

1. As ADP begins to accumulate in muscle, it undergoes a reaction catalysed by adenylate kinase: $2 \times \text{ADP} \leftrightarrow \text{ATP} + \text{AMP}$. AMP is a potent activator of phosphofructokinase, reversing the inhibition of this key regulatory enzyme by ATP, and so increasing the rate of glycolysis.

2. Nerve stimulation of muscle results in an increased cytosolic concentration of calcium ions, and hence activation of calmodulin. Calcium-calmodulin activates glycogen phosphorylase, so increasing the rate of formation of glucose 1-phosphate, and providing an increased amount of substrate for glycolysis.

3. Adrenaline, released from the adrenal glands in response to fear or fright, acts on cell surface receptors, leading to the formation of cAMP, which leads to increased activity of protein kinase, and increased activity of glycogen phosphorylase.

In prolonged aerobic exercise at a relatively high intensity (e.g. cross-country or marathon running), muscle glycogen and endogenous triacylglycerol are the major fuels with a gradual switch from glucose to fatty acid oxidation, with a modest contribution from plasma non-esterified fatty acids and glucose. As the exercise continues, and muscle glycogen and triacylglycerol begin to be depleted, so plasma non-esterified fatty acids become more important (see Ch. 18 for further consideration of this topic).

Muscle fuel utilisation in the fed and fasting states

As discussed, glucose is the main fuel for muscle in the fed state, but in the fasting state glucose is spared for use by the brain and red blood cells; glycogen, fatty acids and ketone bodies are now the main fuels for muscle. There are four mechanisms involved in the control of glucose utilisation by muscle:

1. The uptake of glucose into muscle is dependent on insulin. This means that in the fasting state, when insulin secretion is low, there will be little uptake of glucose into muscle.

2. Hexokinase inhibited by its product, glucose 6-phosphate, which may arise either as a result of the action of hexokinase on glucose or by isomerisation of glucose 1-phosphate from glycogen breakdown. The activity of glycogen phosphorylase is increased in response to glucagon in the fasting state and the resultant glucose 6-phosphate inhibits utilisation of glucose.

3. The activity of pyruvate dehydrogenase is reduced in response to increasing concentrations of both NADH and acetyl CoA. This means that the oxidation of fatty acids and ketones will inhibit the decarboxylation of pyruvate. Under these conditions the pyruvate that is formed from muscle glycogen by glycolysis will undergo transamination to form alanine, which is used for gluconeogenesis in the liver.

4. ATP is an inhibitor of pyruvate kinase, and at high concentrations acts to inhibit the enzyme. More importantly, ATP acts as an allosteric inhibitor of phosphofructokinase. This means that under conditions where the supply of ATP (which can be regarded as the end-product of all energy-yielding metabolic pathways) is more than adequate to meet requirements, the metabolism of glucose is inhibited.

Specific features of dietary fructose metabolism

High intakes of fructose causes increased plasma concentrations of triacylglycerol. Hepatic fructose metabolism begins with phosphorylation by fructokinase to fructose-1-P, which then enters the glycolytic pathway at the triose phosphate level. Fructose thus bypasses phosphofructokinase, which is the major control point for glycolysis, so that more enters the pathway than is required for energy-yielding metabolism. The resultant acetyl CoA is used for lipogenesis.

6.5 FUNCTIONS AND METABOLISM OF NON-DIGESTIBLE CARBOHYDRATES (DIETARY FIBRE)

Non-digestible carbohydrates may influence digestive and absorptive events in the small intestine and provide bulk and substrate for the endogenous microflora of the large intestine. The importance of fermentation products, mainly short-chain fatty acids, for the function and health of the colon as well as effects on host metabolism and immune functions, is increasingly being recognised.

Fermentation in the large intestine and laxation

Carbohydrates that are not digested in the small intestine are subject to anaerobic fermentation by the colonic microflora. The rate, extent and site of fermentation in the colon are dependent on both the substrate and host factors. The molecular structure and physical form of the dietary fibre constituents, and the bacterial flora and transit time are main determinants of fermentation.

Short-chain fatty acids (SCFAs) such as acetate, propionate and butyrate, and gases, notably hydrogen and methane, are the main fermentation products (Fig. 6.2). The decrease in pH of the colonic content may be protective through reduced formation of bile salt metabolites that have been implicated in carcinogenesis. A low pH may also promote colonic absorption of calcium. Butyrate is a major source of energy for colonocytes with effects on cell differentiation and apoptosis that may be protective. Absorbed acetate and propionate may have systemic effects on carbohydrate and lipid metabolism. Propionate inhibits liver cholesterol synthesis in experimental animals, but the importance in human beings is not clear. The pattern of SCFA formation differs with the fermentation substrate, and resistant starch and oat fibre are types of dietary fibre that yield high proportions of butyrate.

The large intestinal microflora contains several hundred different bacteria in a delicate balance that affects, and is affected by, the fermentation substrate. *Probiotics* are generally regarded as live microbial food ingredients that are beneficial to health and *prebiotics* have been defined as non-digestible food components that beneficially affect the host by selectively stimulating the growth and/or activity of one or a limited number of bacteria in the colon that have the potential to improve host health. Fructo-oligosaccharides (FOS, inulin and shorter oligosaccharides) as well as other oligosaccharides, (galacto-oligosaccharides, GOS, resistant types of malto-oligosaccharides, MOS) and resistant starch have prebiotic effects in increasing the count of *Bifidobacteria*. Oligosaccharides are fermented rapidly in the proximal colon, and gas formation leads to side effects in many individuals if the intake exceeds some 20 g/day. Resistant starch on the other hand is fermented more slowly and does not cause flatulence.

Lactose similarly may cause intolerance symptoms in some people with low intestinal lactase activity if the intake exceeds 5–10 g/day. Otherwise, unabsorbed lactose can also be regarded as a prebiotic carbohydrate with potential beneficial effects in stimulating what is perceived as a 'healthy' intestinal microflora dominated by *Bifidobacteria* and lactobacilli. Breast milk contains a host of different oligosaccharides known as 'bifidus factors'.

Insoluble, especially lignified types of fibre, such as in wheat bran, are largely resistant to fermentation. They have the most prominent laxation effects due to binding water in the distal colon. More easily fermented fibre also contributes to the faecal bulk through an increased bacterial mass. The increase in

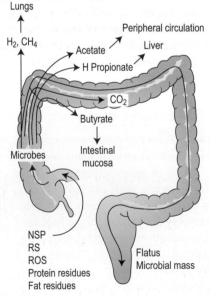

Figure 6.2 Fermentation of carbohydrates in the large intestine.

faecal bulk ranges from 1 g per gram of ingested pectin to 6 g per gram of wheat bran fibre.

Effects of dietary fibre in the upper gastrointestinal tract

Viscous types of soluble fibre that have a high water-binding capacity may inhibit gastric emptying, and also have beneficial effects on both lipid and carbohydrate metabolism.

Total and LDL cholesterol levels in the blood are reduced by soluble viscous polysaccharides, such as pectins and gums, notably guar gum which is a galactomannan. These effects are related to reduced cholesterol and/or bile acid absorption, helping to lower the body pool of cholesterol. Fasting triacylglycerol levels are generally not affected, but attenuation of the postprandial rise in triacylglycerol may be important. Resistant starch and resistant oligosaccharide have effects on lipid metabolism in experimental animals, but the importance of such effects for humans is unclear.

Viscous soluble fibre has also been demonstrated to diminish postprandial blood glucose and insulin responses, and thus contribute to a low glycaemic index of foods. The mechanisms involve diffusion barriers due to increased viscosity of the intestinal contents, hindering both amylase action in the lumen and the absorption of monosaccharides. Inhibition of gastric emptying may also contribute.

The inhibiting effect of dietary fibre on the absorption of minerals such as iron, zinc and calcium is due to phytate (inositol hexaphosphate) associated with the dietary fibre in cereal brans and legumes, and can be abolished by the degradation of phytate. There is no evidence that the dietary fibre per se affects mineral absorption.

Carbohydrate malabsorption

In certain individuals malabsorption of other dietary carbohydrates may cause excessive delivery of fermentation substrate to the large intestine, causing intolerance. Congenital sucrase deficiency is a rare cause of sucrose malabsorption, which can cause gastrointestinal complaints, including diarrhoea, when an increasing amount of sucrose is introduced in the diet. Similarly, congenital lactase deficiency is a rare condition causing severe diarrhoea and malnutrition in the newborn. Breast milk has a high content (7%) of lactose, providing about half of its energy content.

The common reason for lactose intolerance in adults is a genetically determined downregulation of lactase in most people in the world, usually at the age of 2–15 years. This causes more or less pronounced limitation of the lactose absorption capacity; some, but not all, individuals with low lactase activity experience symptoms due to fermentation of malabsorbed lactose in the large intestine. Most adults can drink 1–200 ml of milk (containing 5–10 g of lactose) without symptoms. In fermented milk products much of the lactose has been fermented to lactic acid, and microbial enzymes in live yoghurt may help to hydrolyse more lactose in the small intestine, and cheese is practically lactose free. These products are therefore tolerated better than ordinary milk. Individual sensitivity is variable and should be tested. Gradual introduction of lactose may help to adapt the colonic microflora, and milk taken with meals is generally tolerated better. Reports of sensitivity to very small amounts of lactose, a few grams or less, have not been reproduced in controlled studies.

6.6 DIETARY CARBOHYDRATES AND DISEASE

Basic requirement for carbohydrate

Carbohydrates do not fulfil the definition of an essential nutrient since there is no absolute requirement for food carbohydrates to sustain life. This is provided that adequate amounts of protein for de novo synthesis of glucose, and fat are consumed. Only red blood cells and some other cells that are dependent on anaerobic glycolysis have an absolute requirement for glucose. The central nervous system

is largely dependent on glucose, but can meet a proportion of its energy needs from ketone bodies (see Section 7.4). A very low carbohydrate diet, however, results in a chronically increased production and plasma concentrations of the ketone bodies of these acids, referred to as ketosis, and absence of glycogen stores, with adverse effects on high-intensity work by muscles. Other possible adverse effects of diets very low in carbohydrates are bone mineral loss, hypercholesterolaemia and increased risk of urolithiasis.

The average requirement of (glycaemic) carbohydrate was estimated by Food and Nutrition Board, USA, to be 100 g/day for children as well as adults, based mainly on data regarding carbohydrate utilisation by the brain. As shown below, however, there are advantages with considerably higher intake of carbohydrates.

Importance of the glycaemic index

The blood glucose concentration is determined by three main factors: the rate of intestinal carbohydrate absorption, the net liver uptake or output, and peripheral glucose uptake, which in turn depends upon the insulin level and the sensitivity of tissues to insulin. With a constant dietary carbohydrate load, there is a range of blood glucose responses between individuals, from low responses with a continuum to what is defined as 'impaired glucose tolerance, IGT' and 'diabetes' (see Ch. 21, Section 21.3).

It has for long been regarded as important for the control of diabetes to avoid excessive rises in blood glucose and concomitant high postprandial insulin levels with rapid decline and the risk of a fall of the blood glucose below the fasting level. A stable blood glucose level has also been considered advantageous in relation to satiety and mood, and recent epidemiological studies have lent support to hypotheses that a low glycaemic load would help to diminish the risk for developing both maturity onset diabetes and cardiovascular disease.

The blood glucose response after a meal is determined by both the glycaemic index (GI) and the amount of carbohydrate in a normal portion of the food. Therefore, the concept of glycaemic load (GL) was introduced to quantify the overall glycaemic effect of a portion of food. GL is the product of the amount of available carbohydrate in a typical serving of a food × the GI of the food/100. Protein and fat may also influence the glycaemic response to a meal, as well as the amount of drink taken with the meal. However, the glycaemic response to a meal can be predicted from properly determined GI of the constituent foods. GI values published in international tables, however, may be less appropriate due to the many factors influencing the glycaemic index of a particular food product.

The glycaemic response to for example a morning meal may influence the metabolic response to a subsequent meal. Such 'second-meal effects' on blood glucose and insulin levels have been demonstrated after a lunch following a low-GI breakfast.

An improved glucose tolerance in the morning has also been demonstrated after a late evening meal with low GI and high dietary fibre content, or containing slowly released carbohydrates from raw maize starch. The colonic fermentation of dietary fibre may be partly responsible for such effects.

Some intervention studies, mainly in diabetic subjects but also in healthy people, have lent support to a total and LDL-cholesterol-lowering effect of low GI diets, which are also associated with a higher HDL cholesterol level.

There are some epidemiological studies suggesting that excessive postprandial glycaemia may be related to increased all-cause mortality in diabetics as well as in people with normal fasting blood glucose concentration. This could be related to effects on established risk factors such as LDL and HDL cholesterol, triglycerides and blood coagulation and fibrinolysis, as well as protein glycation and possibly increased oxidative stress.

More long-term intervention studies are needed to establish the role of low GI foods and diets for maintenance of health and prevention of chronic disease. In order to perform such studies in a realistic way, a variety of low GI foods are needed.

Glycaemic carbohydrates and plasma lipids

Possible unfavourable effects of plasma lipids have been a concern when recommending high carbohydrate diets. A number of short- to medium-term studies have shown increased fasting triglyceride and decreased HDL cholesterol levels after introduction of high-carbohydrate diets, i.e. >50–55 energy per cent (E%). The overall lipid profile, however, is usually favourable in relation to cardiovascular risk when comparing a recommended high-carbohydrate diet with current Western diets.

A specific triacylglycerol-elevating effect of fructose, and hence sucrose, has been demonstrated in animal experiments, but is questionable in human beings at normal intakes. A well-controlled study with 17% of the energy as fructose did show increased fasting and day-long triacylglycerol in men but not in women. On the other hand, a 3-month multicentre study did not show any adverse effects on plasma lipids of high-carbohydrate diets (with 51–56 E% carbohydrates) either with predominantly sugars, including fructose, or predominantly starch.

In summary, effects on plasma lipids do not motivate specific restrictions in sucrose (being half fructose) or fructose for the general population, in addition to those based on general nutritional considerations. The recommendation to limit added refined sugars to maximum 10 E% is made mainly to ensure the intake of micronutrients and other essential nutrients, as well as dietary fibre.

Dietary fibre and chronic disease

The reduced transit time, increased faecal weight with dilution of the intestinal content and improved laxation, were factors behind the early hypotheses that an appropriate intake of dietary fibre would reduce the risk of both colonic cancer and diverticular disease. Indeed, epidemiological evidence supports a protective effect, but more refined case control studies and intervention studies with alternative end-points such as precancerous polyps, have so far been unsuccessful in substantiating the relationship.

There is evidence from both epidemiological studies and intervention studies that dietary fibre may be an important factor in combating obesity. A number of epidemiological studies have consistently shown a lower risk of coronary heart disease (CHD) with increased intake of whole grain cereals. There is also epidemiological evidence for a protective effect against type 2 diabetes. Correlations with whole grain are consistently stronger than with dietary fibre or cereal fibre. There is also increasing epidemiological evidence for a protective effect of fruits and vegetables on CHD, whereas protective effects against cancers are less clear. As mentioned above, viscous types of dietary fibre, such as pectin, guar gum and oat α-glucans lower serum cholesterol, but it is not known to what extent the protective effects of whole grain cereals and fruits are due to dietary fibre, to other constituents of these foods, or to other diet or lifestyle related factors associated with the consumption of whole grain foods and fruits and vegetables.

The possible protective effects of dietary fibre against breast cancer, diabetes (in addition to the well-documented effects of viscous types of fibre on glycaemic response), duodenal ulcer, and gastric cancer need further substantiation, as do the possible effects of fermentation and specific probiotic micro-organisms on immune functions.

⮑ Key points

⮑ Carbohydrates, i.e. glycaemic carbohydrates, and especially starch, provide the main energy source in the diet, and after a meal it is mainly carbohydrate that provides metabolic fuel to all tissues.

⮑ Dietary glucose and other monosaccharides are also the precursors for synthesis of ribose, deoxyribose, glucuronic acid, and the carbohydrate moieties of complex carbohydrates, including glycoproteins and glycolipids, which have important structural and cell signalling and recognition functions.

⮑ The main monosaccharides are all metabolised by the same pathway, glycolysis, leading to the formation of pyruvate. Fructose bypasses a main control point in glycolysis.

⮑ Glycolysis can operate ether aerobically or anaerobically; under anaerobic conditions lactate is formed and used in the liver for resynthesis of glucose.

⮑ Under aerobic conditions pyruvate arising from glycolysis is oxidised to acetyl CoA, which can either be a precursor for fatty acid synthesis or undergo complete oxidation in the citric acid cycle.

⮑ Pyruvate and intermediates of the citric acid cycle can be used for synthesis of non-essential amino acids, and can also be formed by the metabolism of amino acids.

⮑ A net increase in citric acid cycle intermediates permits utilisation of oxaloacetate for gluconeogenesis to maintain a supply of glucose in the fasting state and starvation. Acetyl CoA arising from fatty acids and ketone bodies cannot provide a source of oxaloacetate for gluconeogenesis.

⮑ The main storage carbohydrate in the body is glycogen in liver and muscle; its synthesis in the fed state and utilisation in the fasting state are closely regulated by insulin and glucagon.

⮑ In the fasting state glucose is spared for the brain and red blood cells by regulation of its uptake into, and utilisation by, muscle and other tissues. This is achieved by both hormonal control and also inhibition of glucose metabolism by products of fatty acid and ketone body metabolism.

⊃ The plasma concentration of glucose is regulated within strict limits; failure of this regulation, and poor glycaemic control, leads to the complications of diabetes mellitus.

⊃ The glycaemic index denotes the blood glucose elevating potential of a food. Low glycaemic index foods may confer benefits in metabolic control of diabetes and may help to reduce risk factors for chronic diseases.

⊃ Dietary fibre consists of carbohydrates that are not digested in the small intestine. It is the main energy substrate for the colonic microbiota.

⊃ Dietary fibre increases faecal bulk through water binding by unfermented fibre and through an increased microbial mass.

⊃ Fermentation products, notably the short-chain fatty acids acetate, propionate and butyrate, are important sources of energy for the colonic epithelial cells and may influence peripheral metabolism.

References and further reading

Reference

WHO 2003 Diet, nutrition and the prevention of chronic diseases. Report from a joint WHO/FAO Expert Consultation. WHO Technical Report Series 916. World Health Organization, Geneva

Further reading

Bender D A 2002 Introduction to nutrition and metabolism, 3rd edn. Taylor and Francis, London

Cummings J H, Rombeau J, Sakata T (eds) 1995 Physiological and clinical aspects of short-chain fatty acids. Cambridge University Press, Cambridge

Frayn K N 2003 Metabolic regulation: a human perspective, 2nd edn. Blackwell Science, Oxford

Joint FAO/WHO Expert Consultation 1998 Carbohydrates in human nutrition. Food and Agriculture Organization. World Health Organization. FAO Food and Nutrition Paper 66. Rome

Mittendorfer B, Klein S 2003 Physiological factors that regulate the use of endogenous fat and carbohydrate fuels during endurance exercise. Nutrition Research Reviews 16(1):97–108

National Academy of Sciences 2002 Dietary reference intakes for energy, carbohydrates, fiber, fat, protein and amino acids (macronutrients). The National Academy of Sciences, USA

WHO 2003 Diet, nutrition and the prevention of chronic diseases. Report from a joint WHO/FAO Expert Consultation. WHO Technical Report Series 916. World Health Organization, Geneva

CD-ROM contents

Figures

Figure CD 6.1 The glycolytic pathway

Figure CD 6.2 The Cori cycle: anaerobic glycolysis in muscle and gluconeogenesis in the liver

Figure CD 6.3 The pentose phosphate pathway

Figure CD 6.4 The reaction of pyruvate dehydrogenase

Figure CD 6.5 Overview of the citric acid cycle

Figure CD 6.6 The citric acid cycle

Figure CD 6.7 The citric acid cycle in gluconeogenesis

Figure CD 6.8 Glycogen synthesis

Figure CD 6.9 Hormonal control of glycogen synthesis and utilisation

Further reading from the book

7

Fat metabolism

Parveen Yaqoob, Anne Marie Minihane and Christine Williams

7.2 FUNCTIONS OF DIETARY FAT

Fats perform a range of essential functions within the body, including the provision of energy, structural and specific functional roles in cell membranes and hormone-like activities.

Energy storage

Due to its energy density, fat, as triacylglycerol (Fig 7.1), is the nutrient of choice to act as a long-term fuel reserve for the organism. The majority of fat is stored as triacylglycerols. Although some fat reserve is also found in other cells in the body, such as liver and muscle cells, (where excessive accumulation has pathological consequences), the majority of fat is stored in specially adapted adipose tissue cells, adipocytes (see Section 4.2). Although there is a relationship between the fatty acid composition of the adipose tissue and long-term dietary intake (e.g. an individual eating polyunsaturated fatty acids will have a greater proportion in their adipose tissue), fatty acids stored in the adipocyte as triacylglycerol tend to be more saturated than the fatty acids in cell membrane phospholipids.

Following a meal, ingested fat which is not required by the body tissues for immediate use is transported to the adipose tissue in lipoproteins (Section 7.3). The fatty acids are hydrolysed from the triacylglycerols in circulating lipoproteins by the enzyme lipoprotein lipase (LPL), taken up by the adipose tissue and re-esterified into triacylglycerols. When dietary energy is limited (e.g. after an overnight fast), the fat is mobilised and fatty acids are released from the adipocyte into the circulation, bound to serum albumin. This tightly controlled dynamic process is regulated by the concentration of metabolites (glucose, fatty acids, triacylglycerols) in the blood and by hormones (insulin, glucagon, adrenaline), which are themselves responsive to diet (Section 7.5).

In addition to its role as an energy reserve, subcutaneous adipose tissue is important in the maintenance of body temperature, whereas internal fat (visceral fat) protects the vital organs such as the kidney and spleen. Accumulation of excessive visceral fat (abdominal obesity), is a risk factor for heart disease and diabetes and is linked with insulin resistance (see Ch. 20).

Structural functions: as components of cell membranes

Fats form an integral part of cell membranes, which form a barrier between the cell and the external environment. Intracellular membranes compartmentalise different areas within the cell. The basic structural unit of most biological membranes is phospholipids, which, like triacylglycerols, have fatty acids esterified at carbons-1 and -2 of glycerol. Carbon-3 is esterified to a phosphate group, which in turn is esterified to one of a variety of bases (choline, ethanolamine, serine, inositol); this contributes to the amphiphilic nature of membrane lipids providing both hydrophobic (fat-soluble) and hydrophilic (water-soluble) regions. In mammalian tissues the most common base is choline, and phosphatidylcholine is the main membrane phospholipid (Fig 7.1).

Lipids based on a sphingosine rather than a glycerol backbone (sphingolipids) are also widespread in membranes, and are particularly abundant in the brain and nervous system (see Fig. CD 7.1). In sphingomyelin the amino group of the long unsaturated hydrocarbon chain of sphingosine is linked to a fatty acid and the hydroxyl group is esterified to phosphoryl choline, yielding a molecule with a similar conformation to phosphatidylcholine. Glycolipids, as their name implies, contain carbohydrate (see Section 6.2, under 'Glycolipids'). They consist of a sphingomyelin backbone and a fatty acid unit bound to the amino group, with one or more sugars attached to the hydroxyl group. The simplest is cerebroside, which contains a single sugar, either glucose or galactose.

In the membrane, phospholipids and sphingolipids arrange themselves in a lipid bilayer with the hydrophobic fatty acid tails facing inwards and the hydrophilic head interacting with the aqueous environment of the cytosol (at the inner face) and the extracellular fluid at the outer face (see Fig. CD 7.2). The chain length and degree of unsaturation of the fatty acids within the bilayer has a large impact on the physical properties of the membrane, altering membrane fluidity and therefore function. Dietary fatty acid intake affects membrane composition to a limited extent. The presence of lipid-soluble antioxidants such as α-tocopherol within the membrane serves to minimise oxidation of the unsaturated fatty acids.

Cholesterol, which is almost entirely absent from plant tissues, is the most common sterol found in animal tissues. It inserts itself into the lipid bilayer where its hydrophobic interactions with fatty acids are essential to maintain membrane structure and fluidity. On a diet rich in polyunsaturated fatty acids, an increase in the cholesterol to phospholipid ratio serves to maintain membrane fluidity.

In addition to lipids, membranes contain a variety of proteins: enzymes, receptors or transporters (see Fig. CD 7.2). The protein content is variable and reflects the function of the cell. Myelin, the function of which is mainly to provide electrical insulation in nerve fibres, contains only about 18% protein, whereas highly active membranes such as mitochondrial membranes have the highest protein content, typically 75%.

Specific functions in membranes

In addition to their relatively non-specific function in membrane structure, membrane lipids have a wide variety of specific roles such as a lung (pulmonary) surfactant, in cell signalling and as precursors of a diverse range of the metabolically active eicosanoids.

Pulmonary surfactant

Each time we exhale, our lungs are prevented from collapsing by a protein–lipid mixture known as pulmonary surfactant. It contains about 85% lipid, dominated by a single compound, dipalmitoylphosphatidylcholine. Surfactant forms a solid film on the alveolar surface as we breathe out, reducing the surface tension and preventing lung collapse. Its importance is evident in newborn infants with acute respiratory distress, an often fatal condition, resulting from an inability to synthesise pulmonary surfactant leading to respiratory dysfunction.

Cell signalling

Various lipids are involved in cell signalling and the conversion of extracellular signals into intracellular ones. The discovery of the phosphatidylinositol cycle indicated that membrane inositol phospholipids are important mediators of hormone and neurotransmitter action (see Fig. CD 7.3). The binding of a hormone to membrane receptor proteins activates the enzyme phospholipase C, which hydrolyses the phosphatidylinositol molecule to diacylglycerol and inositol-1,4,5-triphosphate (IP_3). Both products activate protein kinases and act as secondary messengers involved in regulation of cellular processes such as smooth muscle contraction, glycogen metabolism (see Section 6.3, under 'Glycogen as a carbohydrate reserve') and cell proliferation and differentiation.

In addition to inositol phospholipids, sphingolipids are important modulators of membrane receptor activity in all stages of the cell cycle including apoptosis (cell death) and in inflammation. Intact membrane sphingolipids act as a ligand for receptors on nearby cells, and modulate the activity of receptors and membrane-associated proteins in the same cell. Hydrolysis of sphingolipids can give rise to a variety of second messengers such as ceramide, lactosylceramide, glycosylceramide and sphingosine, via the sphingomyelin cycle (see Fig. CD 7.4). Ceramide is the best known of the sphingoid signalling molecules. Activation of membrane-bound sphingomyelinase releases ceramide from membrane sphingolipids. Ceramide activates protein kinases involved in various metabolic processes within the cell, including cell growth and death, and inflammatory responses (see Fig. CD 7.4).

The eicosanoids

See also Sections CD 7.2.3.3(a) and CD 7.2.3.3(b).

Membrane unsaturated fatty acids, in particular the C20 and C22 PUFA, are the precursors of a variety of hormone-like compounds known collectively as eicosanoids, which mediate a variety of cellular functions including smooth muscle contraction and blood clotting. They act locally to their site of synthesis and are metabolised very rapidly. It is largely this role of fatty acids as precursors of eicosanoids that underlies the essentiality of linoleic and α-linolenic acids, since these two fatty acids, which cannot be synthesised in the body, are the precursors of the C20 and C22 PUFA.

The main precursor for the synthesis of eicosanoids is arachidonic acid (20:4 n-6), which can be released from membrane phospholipids by phospholipase A following an appropriate stimulus and metabolised by lipoxygenases or by cyclo-oxygenase, as illustrated in Figure CD 7.5. Metabolism by lipoxygenases gives rise to leukotrienes, lipoxins and hydroxy fatty acids, while metabolism by cyclo-oxygenase gives rise to prostaglandins, thromboxanes and prostacyclin.

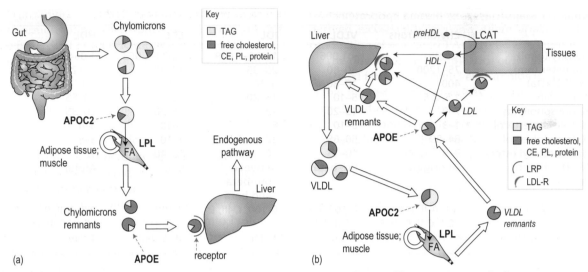

Figure 7.2 Pathways of lipoprotein metabolism. (a) Exogenous pathway of lipoprotein metabolism. Chylomicrons may pass through the tissue capillary beds several times where they are hydrolysed by lipoprotein lipase, resulting in a chylomicron remnant which has lost a large portion of its original TAG content (see Fig. CD 7.14). The resultant particle is taken up by the liver by receptor-mediated endocytosis. (b) Endogenous pathway of lipoprotein metabolism. VLDL may pass through the tissue capillary beds several times where they are hydrolysed by lipoprotein lipase (LPL), resulting in a VLDL remnant which has lost a large portion of its original TAG content (see Fig. CD 7.14). The remnant particle has two possible metabolic fates: (a) it can be further hydrolysed to LDL, which is the main transporter of cholesterol to the target tissue; (b) the remnant particle is taken up by the liver by receptor-mediated endocytosis. Excess tissue cholesterol is returned to the liver by reverse cholesterol transport mediated by HDL and lecithin cholesterol acyltransferase. *Abbreviations:* LDL-R, LDL receptor; LRP, LDL-R-related protein; LPL, lipoprotein lipase; CE, cholesterol esters; PL, phospholipids; LCAT, lecithin-cholesterol acyltransferase.

bloodstream. Following a number of cycles through the tissues and the eventual removal of a large fraction of the triacylglycerol and a portion of cholesterol, and the surface phospholipids and apoproteins (to HDL), a smaller, more cholesterol ester enriched particle remains. This contains the original apoB48 and the majority of the fat-soluble vitamins. ApoE is acquired from HDL upon arrival at the liver, and the liver cell takes up the chylomicron remnant by a receptor-mediated process with the primary receptors. These are thought to be the LDL-receptor (LDL-R, also known as the apoB/apoE receptor) and the LDL-R related protein (LRP).

The endogenous lipoprotein pathway: VLDL metabolism

VLDL distributes triacylglycerols from the liver to the tissues via the endogenous lipoprotein pathway. The sources of fatty acids for liver triacylglycerol synthesis include fatty acids returned to the liver by chylomicron remnants, LDL or HDL, fatty acids

delivered bound to albumin, and fatty acids formed by de novo lipogenesis in the liver. This latter source is thought to be small on a typical Western diet, but may become more significant on a high-carbohydrate diet. ApoB100 is the main structural and functional protein of VLDL. Upon secretion into the bloodstream VLDL acquires apoC2 from HDL, then VLDL triacylglycerols are hydrolysed by LPL and the fatty acids are accumulated by tissues in a similar manner to those from chylomicrons (see previous section). However, mainly due to their greater surface area, chylomicrons are thought to provide a better substrate for LPL and are hydrolysed preferentially when both particles are present in the postprandial (fed) state. In the fasting state, as no chylomicrons are present, the VLDL is hydrolysed more rapidly.

VLDL remnants, known as intermediate density lipoproteins (IDL), have two metabolic fates. Approximately 40–50% are taken up by the liver by receptor-mediated endocytosis, with both the apoB100 and apoE acting as ligands. The remaining 50–60% lose all surface components except for a layer of phospholipids, free cholesterol and apoB100 and become LDL, the major carrier of cholesterol in the blood. An increased secretion or delayed clearance of triacylglycerol-rich lipoproteins (VLDL and chylomicrons) is a significant risk factor for coronary heart disease (see Ch. 19).

The endogenous lipoprotein pathway: LDL metabolism

The role of LDL formed from VLDL is to transport cholesterol to the peripheral tissues and regulate de novo synthesis of cholesterol at these sites. On arrival at the cell surface, the apoB100 component of LDL is recognised by the LDL-receptor. Following internalisation of the LDL-receptor complex, the vesicle fuses with lysosomes, which contain a variety of degradative enzymes. The apoB100 protein is hydrolysed to free amino acids and the cholesterol esters to free cholesterol. The majority of the LDL-receptor is returned to the cell surface unaltered, with a round trip time of approximately 10 minutes; the receptor is thought to have a lifespan of approximately 1 day. The released cholesterol can be used immediately for incorporation into cell membranes or synthesis of steroid hormones. Alternatively, the cholesterol can be re-esterified and stored within the cell. Cellular cholesterol is derived from both extracellular sources (LDL) and synthesised in the cell. The process of cellular cholesterol metabolism is tightly regulated.

The physiological importance of the LDL-receptor in cholesterol homeostasis is demonstrated in the condition familial hypercholesterolaemia (FH) (see Section CD 7.3(b)), in which there is an absence or deficiency of functional LDL-receptors. Marked elevations in circulating LDL levels are evident, which leads to deposition of cholesterol in a variety of tissues, including the artery walls, thus contributing to atherogenesis.

A number of additional receptors which recognise LDL, one class of which is known as the scavenger receptors, have been identified. These receptors, which are present in large numbers on the surface of macrophages, do not bind to native LDL, but only LDL that has been chemically modified, e.g. oxidised. Unlike the LDL-receptor, scavenger receptors are not subject to downregulation and therefore macrophages can take up LDL indefinitely until they become lipid laden, when they are known as foam cells. This process forms the basis of the lipid accumulation which occurs in the development of atherosclerosis and the process is accelerated in people with high circulating LDL levels (see Ch. 19).

Reverse cholesterol transport: HDL metabolism

Excessive accumulation of cholesterol in tissues is toxic as the cell cannot break down cholesterol and in the artery wall it leads to the development of atherosclerosis. This excess cholesterol is transported in HDL back to the liver, where it can be excreted in the bile, or be transported to other cells, where it is needed via the VLDL–LDL pathway. More than 40% of individuals who have a myocardial infarction (heart attack) have low HDL levels.

Pre-β-HDL is synthesised in the intestine and liver and secreted into the bloodstream as a discoidal pre-HDL particle containing apoA1 and a small amount of phospholipid. The emerging HDL particles gather some surface material (phospholipids and free cholesterol) released following the hydrolysis of chylomicrons and VLDL by LPL. Nascent HDL particles bind to cell surface receptors and avidly absorb cholesterol from the cell membrane. Lecithin-cholesterol acyltransferase (LCAT) present in HDL esterifies the cholesterol, allowing it to move to the core of the particle and freeing up space on the surface for further cholesterol absorption. This enzyme, which is activated by apoA1, ensures a unidirectional movement of cholesterol from the cell to the HDL particle. Gradually the HDL accumulates cholesterol and becomes a mature spherical α-HDL particle (HDL$_2$).

Subsequent movement of this excess cholesterol in HDL back to the liver is mediated by either a direct or an indirect pathway. In the direct pathway, HDL itself takes the cholesterol to the liver, although quantitatively this is not the most important route. The majority of cholesterol delivery is achieved via the indirect route, where HDL transfers its cholesterol to chylomicrons and VLDL remnants, which subsequently transport the cholesterol to the liver. In addition to its role in reverse cholesterol transport, HDL may also have some additional benefits with respect to the development of atherosclerosis. For example, it inhibits the movement of macrophages (cells which accumulate cholesterol) into the artery wall, it is important for maintaining endothelial (cells lining the blood vessels) health and it inhibits LDL oxidation.

7.4 THE ROUTES OF INTRACELLULAR FAT METABOLISM

Fatty acid uptake and activation

Fatty acids can be oxidised to form ATP by many tissues. They are delivered to tissues either in the form of non-esterified fatty acids (NEFAs), bound to serum albumin, or by the hydrolysis of the triacyl-glycerol component of circulating lipoproteins. The mechanism by which NEFAs are taken up by cells has often been controversial, but it is possible that both carrier-mediated transport (i.e. involving proteins) and diffusion are involved. The proteins implicated in fatty acid transport are fatty acid binding proteins (FABPs), fatty acid translocase (FAT) and the fatty acid transport protein (FATP). In addition to their roles in fatty acid uptake by cells, FABPs are also important intracellular carriers of fatty acids, delivering them to subcellular organelles, such as mitochondria, where they can be oxidised.

Before fatty acids can take part in metabolic reactions, whether they are anabolic or catabolic, they are esterified to coenzyme A (CoA), forming the thiol ester acyl CoA. The formation of acyl CoAs is catalysed by several acyl CoA synthetases, which differ in their subcellular location and their specificity for fatty acids of different chain length (see further details in Section CD 7.4.1). Esterification of fatty acids to CoA involves hydrolysis of ATP to AMP and pyrophosphate, and hence a cost equivalent to 2 × ATP per mol of fatty acid esterified.

Fatty acid synthesis

De novo fatty acid synthesis usually signifies an excess of energy-yielding substrates; carbon for fatty acid synthesis is supplied by carbohydrate, or, in some cases, amino acids. As discussed in Section 6.3 under 'The oxidation of pyruvate to acetyl CoA', these precursors are metabolised to acetyl CoA in the mitochondria. There are three major steps in the pathway leading to the synthesis of fatty acids: (i) the transport of acetyl CoA to the cytoplasm, (ii) the formation of malonyl CoA and (iii) elongation of the fatty acid chain.

Under conditions which favour fatty acid synthesis, citrate that has been formed in the mitochondrion by condensation of acetyl CoA and oxaloacetate (see Fig. 6.2) is transported into the cytosol where it is cleaved by ATP citrate lyase to yield acetyl CoA and oxaloacetate. This compartmentalisation separates fatty acid synthesis, which occurs in the cytosol, from fatty acid oxidation, which occurs exclusively in mitochondria, and the transport step is therefore crucial in control of fatty acid synthesis. The oxaloacetate re-enters the mitochondria as pyruvate (see Fig. CD 7.7), yielding about half the NADPH required for fatty acid synthesis in the process; the other half comes from the pentose phosphate pathway (see Section 6.3, under 'The pentose phosphate pathway – an alternative to glycolysis').

Fatty acids are synthesised by the successive addition of two-carbon units from acetyl CoA, followed by reduction. Two key multi-enzyme complexes are responsible for the synthesis of fatty acids from acetyl CoA. The first is acetyl CoA carboxylase, which catalyses the carboxylation of acetyl CoA to malonyl CoA, a 3-carbon unit. Its activity is regulated in response to insulin and glucagon. Malonyl CoA is not only the substrate for fatty acid synthesis, but also a potent inhibitor of carnitine palmitoyl transferase (see Section 7.4 'Oxidation of fatty acids', below), so inhibiting the uptake of fatty acids into the mitochondrion for β-oxidation.

The second enzyme complex to take part in fatty acid synthesis is fatty acid synthase (FAS), which catalyses a series of reactions involving the successive addition of 2-carbon units to a growing fatty acid chain, using malonyl CoA as the donor of each 2-carbon unit (see Fig. CD 7.8). The enzymes required for fatty acid synthesis form a multi-enzyme complex, arranged in a series of concentric rings around a central acyl carrier protein (ACP), which carries the growing fatty acid chain from one enzyme to the next. As the chain grows in length, so the middle, then outermost ring of enzymes are used. Short- and medium-chain fatty acids are not released from one set of enzymes to bind to the next.

The malonyl group formed by acetyl CoA carboxylase is transferred onto an acyl carrier protein, and then reacts with the growing fatty acid chain, bound to the central acyl carrier protein of the fatty acid synthase complex. The carbon dioxide that was added to form malonyl CoA is lost in this reaction. For the first cycle of reactions, the central acyl carrier protein carries an acetyl group, and the product of reaction with malonyl CoA is acetoacetyl ACP; in subsequent reaction cycles, it is the growing fatty acid chain that occupies the central ACP, and the product of reaction with malonyl CoA is a keto-acyl ACP.

This intermediate is then reduced to yield a hydroxyl group. In turn, this is dehydrated to yield a carbon–carbon double bond, which is reduced to yield a saturated fatty acid chain. Thus, the sequence of chemical reactions is the reverse of that in β-oxidation (see 'Oxidation of fatty acids', below). For both reduction reactions in fatty acid synthesis, NADPH is the hydrogen donor.

The normal end-product of FAS action is palmitic acid, a saturated, 16-carbon fatty acid, which is cleaved from the complex by an integral thioesterase. However, many tissues contain longer-chain fatty acids, which may be unsaturated, in their membranes. This is achieved by elongation and/or desaturation of fatty acids after palmitic acid has been cleaved from the FAS complex.

Elongation and desaturation of fatty acids

Elongases are enzymes that add carbon atoms to preformed fatty acids that either have been synthesised de novo or originate from the diet. Two elongation systems exist in many tissues, one in the mitochondria and the other in the endoplasmic reticulum. The mitochondrial system involves the addition of 2-carbon units from acetyl CoA, whereas elongation in the endoplasmic reticulum employs malonyl CoA as the donor.

One of the most important roles of the elongases and desaturases is the conversion of the essential fatty acids, linoleic acid and α-linolenic acid, to their longer-chain derivatives. Thus, linoleoyl-CoA undergoes sequential desaturation and elongation to form intermediates of the n-6 family of polyunsaturated fatty acids, the key end-product of which is arachidonic acid. As a result of the sequential nature of these reactions, polyunsaturated fatty acids usually contain methylene-interrupted double bonds. A similar series of desaturations and elongations generate the n-3 family of polyunsaturated fatty acids. Although they are not essential fatty acids by the true definition, the derivatives of linoleic and α-linolenic acid are often termed 'conditionally essential', since their synthesis is determined by the presence of the essential fatty acid precursors. The extent and regulation of conversion of α-linolenic acid to EPA, DPA and DHA remains unclear. It appears that in human beings, α-linolenic acid can be converted to EPA and DPA, but only very low levels of DHA are synthesised. This needs to be borne

in mind when considering the theoretical pathway for metabolism depicted in Figure CD 7.9, which has been proposed on the basis of in vitro experiments.

Importantly, the elongation and desaturation pathways for linoleic and α-linolenic acid share one set of desaturase and elongase enzymes, which means that there is competition between the n-6 and n-3 families of fatty acids. The elongation and desaturation of oleic acid, although possible, does not occur to a significant degree in mammalian tissues, probably because the Δ6 desaturase has a preference for the essential fatty acids. However, if essential fatty acid deficiency occurs, oleic acid is desaturated and elongated, usually to mead acid (C20:3 n-9). The presence of mead acid in biological samples is interpreted as a sign of essential fatty acid deficiency.

Oxidation of fatty acids

Fatty acids can undergo oxidation starting at the α-, β- or ω-carbon; β-oxidation is the most physiologically important pathway – see Figure CD 7.10 and also Section CD 7.4(b).

In β-oxidation, fatty acids are degraded by the sequential liberation of acetyl CoA units. Although mitochondria are the major site for β-oxidation, the peroxisomes also contain the enzymes for this pathway. This additional site is particularly important in the liver, serving to oxidise very long-chain fatty acids to medium-chain products, which are subsequently transported to the mitochondria for complete oxidation. In addition to partial oxidation of long-chain fatty acids, peroxisomes are also the site for the degradation of xenobiotics and eicosanoids.

Once it has entered the mitochondria, fatty acyl CoA undergoes a repeating series of four reactions, as shown in Figure CD 7.10, which results in the cleavage of the fatty acid molecule to give acetyl CoA and a new fatty acyl CoA which is two carbons shorter than the initial substrate. This new, shorter, fatty acyl CoA is then a substrate for the same sequence of reactions, which is repeated until the final result is cleavage to yield two molecules of acetyl CoA. The reactions of β-oxidation are chemically the same as those in the conversion of succinate to oxaloacetate in the citric acid cycle, and the reverse of those in fatty acid synthesis (see 'Fatty acid synthesis', above):

1. Removal of two hydrogens from the fatty acid forms a carbon–carbon double bond – an oxidation reaction which yields a reduced flavin, so for

each double bond formed in this way there is a yield of ~2 × ATP.

2. The newly formed double bond in the fatty acyl CoA then reacts with water, yielding a hydroxyl group – a hydration reaction.

3. The hydroxylated fatty acyl CoA undergoes a second oxidation in which the hydroxyl group is oxidized to an oxo group, yielding NADH (equivalent to ~3 × ATP).

4. The oxo-acyl CoA is then cleaved by reaction with CoA, to form acetyl CoA and the shorter fatty acyl CoA, which undergoes the same sequence of reactions.

Regulation of the rate of β-oxidation

See also Section CD 7.4(b).

The rate of β-oxidation is regulated by two mechanisms, the availability of fatty acids and the rate of utilisation of β-oxidation products. The availability of fatty acids in turn is dictated by the insulin: glucagon ratio, which, when high, inhibits the breakdown of triacylglycerols from adipose tissue and therefore the release of NEFAs from adipose stores. The insulin:glucagon ratio will be high in the fed state, when there is adequate availability of fuel from the ingested food and the release of NEFAs from adipose tissue is therefore not required. In muscle, the rate of β-oxidation is dependent on the plasma NEFA concentration and the energy demand of the tissue. A reduction in energy demand (e.g. when physical activity is low) will lead to accumulation of NADH (which will inhibit the citric acid cycle) and acetyl CoA.

The role of carnitine in fatty acid uptake for oxidation

Fatty acyl CoA cannot cross the mitochondrial membranes to enter the matrix. On the outer face of the outer mitochondrial membrane, the fatty acid is transferred from CoA onto carnitine, forming acylcarnitine, which enters the inter-membrane space through an acylcarnitine transporter.

Acylcarnitine can cross only the inner mitochondrial membrane on a counter-transport system which takes in acylcarnitine in exchange for free carnitine being returned to the inter-membrane space. Once inside the mitochondrial inner membrane, acylcarnitine transfers the acyl group onto CoA ready to undergo β-oxidation. This counter-transport system provides regulation of the uptake of fatty acids into the mitochondrion for oxidation. As long as

there is free CoA available in the mitochondrial matrix, fatty acids can be taken up, and the carnitine returned to the outer membrane for uptake of more fatty acids. However, if most of the CoA in the mitochondrion is acylated, then there is no need for further fatty acid uptake immediately, and indeed, it is not possible.

This carnitine shuttle also serves to prevent uptake into the mitochondrion (and hence oxidation) of fatty acids synthesised in the cytosol in the fed state; malonyl CoA (the precursor for fatty acid synthesis; see 'Fatty acid synthesis', above) is a potent inhibitor of carnitine palmitoyl transferase I in the outer mitochondrial membrane.

Synthesis of ketone bodies

In the liver, the acetyl CoA formed by β-oxidation is positioned at a crossroad for two important metabolic fates. It can react with either oxaloacetate to form citrate (and hence undergo complete oxidation) or with acetoacetyl CoA to form ketone bodies (ketogenesis). Its fate is determined chiefly by the rate of β-oxidation and the availability of oxaloacetate. If the rate of β-oxidation is high (as in fasting), then oxaloacetate will be diverted towards gluconeogenesis, so reducing the amount of acetyl CoA entering the citric acid cycle. In this situation, acetyl CoA will be directed towards ketogenesis.

Under conditions that favour ketone body synthesis (i.e. extended starvation), plasma insulin levels are low and fatty acid oxidation to acetyl CoA predominates in the liver and other tissues that are able to oxidise fatty acids. As the liver oxidises fatty acids to acetyl CoA, the citric acid cycle becomes progressively less able fully to oxidise the acetyl CoA formed, partly because high amounts of ATP begin to inhibit the activity of the cycle and partly because oxaloacetate is diverted towards gluconeogenesis (see Section 6.3) and so becomes limiting for citric acid cycle activity. This is a situation specific to the liver because of its important role in synthesising and secreting glucose during starvation. Acetyl CoA that does not undergo further oxidation is condensed to form the four-carbon compound acetoacetyl CoA, which is further metabolised to form the ketone bodies acetoacetate and β-hydroxybutyrate (see Fig. CD 7.11).

Most ketone bodies are converted back into acetyl CoA by muscle and other tissues that are able to use ketone bodies as a fuel (see Fig. CD 7.12), and the acetyl CoA is oxidised in the citric acid cycle.

The formation of ketone bodies from fatty acids released by adipose tissue during starvation is extremely important because ketone bodies provide a water-soluble fuel to meet part of the energy requirements of the brain, which cannot oxidise fatty acids, so sparing glucose. Normal levels of circulating ketone bodies in the fed state are approximately 0.01 mmol/l, but they can rise to 0.1 mmol/l after an overnight fast and 6–8 mmol/l following several days of starvation. Excessively high concentrations of ketone bodies (which are acidic) can cause acidosis, inducing coma or death if untreated. This usually only occurs in uncontrolled type 1 diabetes mellitus, when it is termed diabetic ketoacidosis (see Ch. 21).

Synthesis of cholesterol

Cholesterol can be obtained through the diet, but all nucleated cells have the capacity to synthesise cholesterol, with the liver being quantitatively the most important site. An important function of cholesterol is its structural role in membranes, but it is also important as a precursor for the synthesis of bile acids and steroid hormones. The precursor for the synthesis of cholesterol is cytosolic acetyl CoA (for details of the metabolic pathway, refer to Section CD 7.4(c)). Since high levels of unesterified cholesterol are likely to be undesirable for cells, and cells (other than the liver) are unable to oxidise cholesterol, excess cholesterol is converted into cholesteryl esters by the enzyme acyl CoA cholesterol acyltransferase, which is located on the endoplasmic reticulum. The cholesteryl esters can be stored in lipid droplets within the cytosol; these are commonly observed in steroidogenic tissues.

Synthesis and utilisation of triacylglycerols

See also Section CD 7.4(d).

Triacylglycerols (TAGs) are both the chief form of dietary fat, and also the main form of fat stored in the body. TAG provides a highly reduced, anhydrous form of metabolic fuel, which can potentially be stored in very large amounts. Whenever energy supply from the diet exceeds the energy expenditure of the body, TAG is deposited in adipose tissue.

As discussed in Section 4.2, white adipose tissue is distributed throughout the body, surrounding many internal organs, and provides a protective subcutaneous layer. The cells within adipose tissue are adipocytes, which are bound together by connective tissue and are supplied by an extensive network of blood vessels. When a fat-containing meal is consumed, adipocytes acquire fat from circulating lipoproteins by hydrolytic breakdown of TAG by lipoprotein lipase, releasing fatty acids (see 'Triacylglycerol', below). In the reverse situation, when there is a demand for fatty acids for metabolism, TAG is mobilised by the enzyme hormone-sensitive lipase (HSL). These phases are integrated and controlled by the nutritional status of the individual through a number of hormones, the most important of which is insulin (see 'Integration of fat metabolism from the fasted to the fed state at the whole body level', below).

Biosynthesis of triacylglycerol involves the esterification of three fatty acids (acyl groups) to a glycerol backbone. It can occur in a number of tissues, the most predominant of which are adipose tissue, liver, enterocytes and the mammary gland during lactation.

Under conditions where the demand for mobilisation of fuel reserves increases, usually signalled by low concentrations of insulin, biosynthetic pathways are inhibited and hormone-sensitive lipase is activated within adipocytes (for more detailed description of both TAG synthesis and breakdown, refer to Section CD 7.4(d)). Once released, the NEFAs are bound to plasma albumin and may be taken up by tissues that are able to utilise fatty acids as a fuel source.

7.5 INTEGRATION, CONTROL AND DYNAMICS OF FAT METABOLISM

Coordinated regulation of fatty acid synthesis and oxidation

In the fed state, when carbohydrate may be converted to fatty acids, the level of malonyl CoA is raised and this results in inhibition of carnitine palmitoyl transferase 1 (CPT1), which controls the uptake of acyl CoA into mitochondria for oxidation and hence inhibits β-oxidation of fatty acids (see 'Fatty acid synthesis', above). In the fasting state, the reverse situation occurs and CPT1 activity is high, stimulating β-oxidation and ketogenesis. Coinciding with this, in the fasting state, a low insulin:glucagon ratio and/or the release of adrenaline inhibits acetyl CoA carboxylase activity, reducing the synthesis of malonyl CoA and relieving the inhibition of CPT (for details of this regulation, see Section CD 7.5).

Tissues such as muscle, that oxidise fatty acids but do not synthesise them, also have acetyl CoA carboxylase, and produce malonyl CoA in order to control the activity of carnitine palmitoyl transferase I, and thus control the mitochondrial uptake and β-oxidation of fatty acids. Tissues also have malonyl CoA decarboxylase, which acts to remove malonyl CoA and so reduce the inhibition of carnitine palmitoyl transferase I. The two enzymes are regulated in opposite directions in response to insulin, which stimulates fatty acid synthesis and reduces β-oxidation, and glucagon, which reduces fatty acid synthesis and increases β-oxidation.

Fatty acids are the major fuel for red muscle fibres, which are the main type involved in moderate exercise. Children who lack one or other of the enzymes required for carnitine synthesis, and are therefore reliant on a dietary intake, have poor exercise tolerance, because they have an impaired ability to transport fatty acids into the mitochondria for β-oxidation. Provision of supplements of carnitine to the affected children overcomes the problem.

Integration of fat metabolism with the metabolism of carbohydrate and protein

As described above, fats can circulate in the blood in the form of NEFAs, as triacylglycerols in lipoproteins and as ketone bodies in prolonged starvation. In addition to these fat-derived fuels, carbohydrates circulate as glucose, lactate, pyruvate or glycerol and proteins as amino acids. What determines which of these fuels are oxidised by a tissue at any given time? This question is best answered by considering:

- The ability of tissue to oxidise the fuel; some tissues are anaerobic, or lack mitochondria, and therefore cannot oxidise fatty acids or ketone bodies.
- The availability of fuel; this will be determined by the prevailing conditions. If an individual has been fasting for 18 hours, it is likely that the liver glycogen stores will be depleted and the circulating concentration of fatty acids will be high.

In summary, fatty acids are the preferred fuel for oxidation whenever their circulating concentrations

are high and glucose is spared whenever necessary (see Fig. CD 7.13). When the energy provided by the diet exceeds immediate requirements, excess carbohydrate is preferentially used to replenish liver glycogen stores (see Section 6.3). Excess amino acids will be oxidised only after satisfying the needs for protein synthesis (see Section 8.5). Any remaining excess of fuel will be used for fatty acid and triacylglycerol synthesis for storage in adipose tissue (see Fig. CD 7.13). All of these processes will be coordinated by changes in the circulating levels of hormones, the most important of which are insulin and glucagon.

Interconversion of fuels and the energy paradox

The following rules regarding interconversion of fuels are absolutely central to understanding the integration of metabolic pathways.

- Fatty acids can be made from carbohydrates and amino acids, but cannot be converted to either.
- Carbohydrates can be made from amino acids and can be used to make triacylglycerols.

The inability to convert fatty acids to glucose gives rise to what is known as the 'energy paradox'. The basis of this paradox is that the brain requires 500 kcal of water-soluble fuel (usually glucose) per day, yet the chief energy store in the body is fat, not glycogen, and fatty acids cannot be converted to glucose. The energy paradox is dealt with in four ways:

1. The oxidation of fatty acids (especially by muscle) spares glucose.
2. Lipolysis of TAG during starvation releases glycerol as well as fatty acids and the glycerol can be used as a substrate for gluconeogenesis. Thus glucose can be synthesised from the glycerol component of TAG.
3. Fatty acid oxidation in the liver provides the ATP required for gluconeogenesis.
4. Fatty acids can be converted to ketone bodies, a water-soluble fuel which can be used by the brain to meet perhaps one-fifth of its energy needs in starvation.

Mechanisms for integration of fat and carbohydrate metabolism
Control of phosphofructokinase (PFK) activity

As discussed in Chapter 6, phosphofructokinase catalyses a key irreversible and controlling step in glycolysis. Control of this enzyme is key to the integration of the metabolism of fat and carbohydrate. High levels of ATP inhibit PFK and therefore inhibit glycolysis. In tissues that are oxidising fatty acids (e.g. during starvation or exercise), large amounts of ATP are generated. As a result, the oxidation of fatty acids will prevent oxidation of glucose by inhibiting glycolysis and glucose will be spared for other tissues. This regulatory mechanism is termed the 'glucose–fatty acid cycle'.

Control of pyruvate dehydrogenase (PDH) activity

Pyruvate dehydrogenase catalyses the irreversible oxidation of pyruvate to acetyl CoA. When glucose is freely available, PDH is active and acetyl CoA does not accumulate because it is rapidly used for synthesis of citrate and either complete oxidation in the citric acid cycle or fatty acid synthesis (if carbohydrate is in excess). However, when glucose supplies are diminished and plasma NEFA levels increase as a result of lipolysis in adipose tissue, the oxidation of fatty acids in tissues results in an increase in intracellular acetyl CoA, ATP and NADH. These inhibit PDH activity, reinforcing the glucose–fatty acid cycle. Thus, oxidising fatty acids will conserve glucose by inhibiting both PFK and PDH.

Integration of fat metabolism from the fasted to the fed state at the whole body level

Non-esterified fatty acids

Following an overnight fast, the plasma NEFA concentration is normally about 0.5 mmol/l and the TAG concentration about 1 mmol/l (largely contributed by VLDL). The NEFAs are released by lipolysis of adipose tissue TAG by hormone-sensitive lipase, and they are taken up by a number of tissues, including skeletal muscle and liver. The regulatory mechanisms which lead to the activation of hormone-sensitive lipase and of the reverse process, the esterification of fatty acids in adipose tissue, are key determinants of the plasma concentration of NEFA. The rate of oxidation of NEFA by tissues depends mainly on the plasma concentration, so that the higher the concentration, the greater the rate of utilisation. Hence, the plasma concentration of NEFA is directly related to rate of release

from adipose tissue (and therefore activation of hormone-sensitive lipase versus esterification). Since the key regulatory signal for activation of hormone-sensitive lipase is a fall in insulin concentration, the plasma NEFA concentration over the course of a day is normally an inverse reflection of the plasma concentrations of glucose and insulin. In the fasting state the concentrations of glucose and insulin are at their lowest and those of NEFA highest. The plasma concentration of NEFA has an upper limit of approximately 2 mmol/l, because above this concentration, the relative proportion of NEFAs which are not bound to albumin increases; NEFAs not bound to albumin will cause significant haemolysis and may also have adverse effects on other tissues, particularly the heart.

Following consumption of a meal (the absorptive phase), the rise in blood glucose concentration stimulates insulin secretion, which suppresses hormone-sensitive lipase activity, and the plasma concentration of NEFA will subsequently fall to <0.1 mmol/l. The concentration at which insulin inhibits the activity of hormone-sensitive lipase is much lower than the concentration at which it stimulates glucose metabolism. This means that NEFA falls very rapidly and dramatically very soon after food ingestion. Nevertheless the activity of this enzyme is never completely suppressed, even at very high concentrations of insulin. However, the increase in plasma glucose and insulin concentrations will also increase the uptake of glucose and of glycolysis within the adipocyte, and, as a result, glycerol-3-phosphate will become available for re-esterification of fatty acids, so any NEFA released by the action of hormone sensitive lipase will be re-esterified. After a meal, therefore, release of NEFA from adipose tissue will be almost completely suppressed.

As a result of the fall in NEFA concentration, tissues that were oxidising fatty acids in the fasted state (and so sparing glucose) will reduce their uptake and oxidation of fatty acids and utilise glucose once more. The increased insulin:glucagon ratio on feeding also leads to a reduction in the synthesis of ketone bodies by the liver, so that plasma levels of ketone bodies fall from overnight fasted values of 0.1–0.2 mmol/l to levels that are almost undetectable. The absorptive phase finally begins to decline after about 5 hours, the exact time depending on the composition of the meal, allowing insulin concentrations to decline and relaxing the restraint on fat mobilisation. In general, a meal containing a significant amount of fat slows absorption.

Triacylglycerol

After an overnight fast, the plasma triacylglycerol concentration is normally about 1 mmol/l, almost all in the endogenous triacylglycerol-rich lipoprotein particles (VLDL). Consumption of a meal containing fat results in the formation of chylomicrons in the enterocyte and their entry into the bloodstream (as described in 'The exogenous lipoprotein pathway', above) approximately 3–5 hours after a meal. The postprandial plasma concentration of triacylglycerol can rise to between 1.5 mmol/l and 3.0 mmol/l, depending on the amount of fat in the meal and the metabolic capacity of the individual. The magnitude and duration of the postprandial lipaemic response will depend on the efficiency of the regulatory mechanisms for the disposal and storage of the triacylglycerol. Lipoprotein lipase is activated by insulin and will therefore be most active following a meal; in adipose tissue its activity reaches a peak approximately 3–4 hours after a meal, coinciding with the peak in postprandial plasma triacylglycerol. Insulin clearly plays a key role in the coordination of all aspects of fat metabolism, since both the hydrolysis of chylomicron-triacylglycerol by lipoprotein lipase and the subsequent uptake of the liberated fatty acids are facilitated by the fact that the activity of hormone-sensitive lipase is suppressed. Furthermore, insulin also promotes the re-esterification of fatty acids to form triacylglycerol for storage. However, adipose tissue is not the only tissue able to utilise the fatty acids released from chylomicron-triacylglycerol by the action of lipoprotein lipase. Skeletal muscle, for example, uses fatty acids from chylomicrons (or VLDL) as a source of energy.

During the postprandial period, chylomicron-triacylglycerol represents only a proportion of the total plasma triacylglycerol (perhaps 0.3–0.4 mmol/l after a very fatty meal). This is because the endogenous pathway (VLDL synthesis) is always active and after a meal the hydrolysis of VLDL is suppressed in favour of hydrolysis of chylomicrons. In addition, not all the NEFA released from chylomicrons is taken up and re-esterified in adipose tissue; much remains in the circulation and is taken up by liver, where it is used as substrate to drive synthesis of VLDL. Thus, a significant proportion of the postprandial lipaemic response is, in fact, contributed by VLDL. It should also be noted that the duration of elevation of triacylglycerols following a fat-containing meal is quite prolonged. It may be 6–8 hours before concentrations return towards the fasted values and because most people eat fat-containing meals throughout the day, postprandial lipaemia is the normal state. Once chylomicrons have been completely hydrolysed and their remnants removed by the liver, the exogenous pathway ceases and the endogenous pathway once again becomes the dominant route of triacylglycerol metabolism in the body.

⇌ Key points

- ⇌ Fats perform a range of essential functions in the body; they can be stored for later release of energy, they are important structural components of cell membranes, they play roles in cell signalling, are essential for the absorption of fat-soluble vitamins and are precursors for the synthesis of hormones and other physiological mediators.

- ⇌ Dietary fats are packaged into chylomicrons in enterocytes within the small intestine and enter the exogenous lipoprotein pathway via the lymph system. The TAG they carry is hydrolysed by the enzyme lipoprotein lipase, which is found on the surface of endothelial cells lining capillaries. The NEFAs released are taken up for use by the tissues.

- ⇌ The endogenous pathway of lipoprotein metabolism involves the synthesis of VLDL by the liver and its subsequent metabolism to LDL. Chylomicrons and VLDL are carriers of TAG, while LDL and HDL transport cholesterol.

- ⇌ Linoleic and α-linolenic acids are essential because they cannot be synthesised by animal cells. These essential fatty acids give rise to the n-6 and n-3 polyunsaturated fatty acids respectively through the action of desaturases and elongases. The metabolism of the essential fatty acids is competitive because the same set of enzymes is shared by the n-6 and n-3 pathways.

- ⇌ The oxidation of fatty acids is regulated by their availability and their rate of utilisation. Fatty acids are stored as TAG in adipose tissue, which can be mobilised by the action of hormone-sensitive lipase during fasting. Fats can circulate as TAG in lipoproteins, NEFA or ketone bodies (in prolonged starvation). Fatty acids are the preferred fuel for oxidation whenever their circulating concentrations are high and glucose is spared whenever necessary.

Further reading

Key papers

Brown M S, Kovanen P T, Goldstein J L 1981 Regulation of plasma cholesterol by lipoprotein receptors. Science 212:628–635

Hussain M M, Strickland D K, Bakillah A 1999 The mammalian low-density lipoprotein receptor family. Annual Review of Nutrition 19:141–172

Sethi S, Gibney M J, Williams C M 1993 Postprandial lipoprotein metabolism. Nutrition Research 6:161–183

Key textbooks

Assmann G (ed) 1993 Lipoprotein metabolism disorders and coronary heart disease. MMV Medizin Verlag, Munich

Betteridge D J, Illingworth D R, Shepherd J 1999 Lipoproteins in health and disease. Arnold, London

British Nutrition Foundation 1992 Unsaturated fatty acids: nutritional and physiological significance. Report of the British Nutrition Foundation's Task Force. Chapman and Hall, London

Frayn K N 2003 Metabolic regulation, a human perspective, 2nd edn. Frontiers in Metabolism series, Blackwell Science, Oxford

Gunstone F D, Harwood J L, Padley F B 1994 The lipid handbook, 2nd edn. Chapman and Hall, London

Gurr M I 1992 Role of fats in food and nutrition. Elsevier Applied Science Publishers, London

Gurr M I, Harwood J L, Frayn K N 2002 Lipid biochemistry – an introduction, 5th edn. Blackwell Science, Oxford

Vance D E, Vance J E 1996 Biochemistry of lipids, lipoproteins and membranes. Elsevier, Amsterdam

CD-ROM contents

Expanded material

Section CD 7.2(a) Tissue distribution and biological activity of cyclo-oxygenase and lipoxygenases

Section CD 7.2(b) Biological activities of eicosanoids

Section CD 7.3(a) Polymorphisms and lipoprotein metabolism

Section CD 7.3(b) Disturbed lipoprotein metabolism

Section CD 7.4(a) Acyl CoA synthetases

Section CD 7.4(b) Degradation of fatty acids

Section CD 7.4(c) Synthesis and regulation of intracellular cholesterol

Section CD 7.4(d) Synthesis and degradation of triacylglycerols

Section CD 7.5 Regulation of acetyl CoA carboxylase and FAS

Figures

Figure CD 7.1 Structure of sphingomyelin

Figure CD 7.2 Cell membrane structure

Figure CD 7.3 Phosphatidylinositol cycle

Figure CD 7.4 Sphingomyelin cycle and ceramide

Figure CD 7.5 Synthesis and functions of eicosanoids

Figure CD 7.6 General structure of a lipoprotein particle

Figure CD 7.7 Source of acetyl CoA for fatty acid synthesis

Figure CD 7.8 The pathway of fatty acid synthesis

Figure CD 7.9 Metabolism of unsaturated fatty acids

Figure CD 7.10 The β-oxidation pathway

Figure CD 7.11 Pathway for ketone body formation in the liver

Figure CD 7.12 Oxidation of ketone bodies

Figure CD 7.13 Integration of carbohydrate and fat metabolism in the fed and fasted states

Figure CD 7.14 Hydrolysis of chylomicrons and VLDL in tissues

Figure CD 7.15 Neutral lipid exchange

Figure CD 7.16 Entry of fatty acids into mitochondria for β-oxidation

Figure CD 7.17 Pathway for β-oxidation of linoleic acid

Figure CD 7.18 Pathway for the synthesis of cholesterol

Figure CD 7.19 Esterification of fatty acids to form triacylglycerol

Figure CD 7.20 Regulation of the activity of hormone-sensitive lipase

Figure CD 7.21 Regulation of the activity of acetyl CoA carboxylase

Additional references related to CD-ROM material

Further reading from the book

8

Protein metabolism and requirements

David A. Bender and D. Joe Millward

Objectives

By the end of this chapter you should be able to:

- describe the key features of protein structure, and the main functions of proteins
- explain what is meant by nitrogen balance, and describe how it can be used to determine protein requirements
- explain what is meant by dynamic equilibrium, and explain the energy cost of protein turnover and describe how it is controlled
- explain what is meant by dispensable and indispensable amino acids, the problem of unavailable amino acids
- describe the metabolism of amino acids
- explain the difficulty of determining amino acid and protein requirements
- describe the effects of physical activity and special needs on protein requirements
- explain what is meant by protein quality and describe the different ways of expressing it
- describe the stable isotope methods of determining protein and amino acid requirements, and explain the problems inherent in each.

8.1 INTRODUCTION

Protein is the most complex of the macronutrients. Indeed, dietary protein is not a single entity, but rather a complex mixture of many different proteins, each with its own amino acid composition. Any individual protein may contain between 50 and 1000 amino acids; the sequence of these amino acids is specific for that protein.

The need for protein in the diet was demonstrated early in the nineteenth century, when it was shown that animals which were fed only on fats, carbohydrates and mineral salts were unable to maintain their body weight, and showed severe wasting of muscle and other tissues. It was known that proteins contain nitrogen (mainly in the amino groups of their constituent amino acids), and methods of measuring total amounts of nitrogenous compounds in foods and excreta were soon developed.

The nutritional requirement is not only for total protein intake, but for the various amino acids, in the proportions that are required to maintain turnover of the complex mixture of body proteins. There are some 30 000 to 50 000 different proteins in the human body, and they are broken down and replaced at different rates.

8.2 PROTEIN STRUCTURE AND FUNCTION

Proteins are composed of linear chains of amino acids, joined by condensation of the carboxyl group of one with the amino group of another, to form a peptide bond. Chains of amino acids linked in this way are known as polypeptides.

The amino acids

Twenty-one amino acids are involved in the synthesis of proteins, together with a number that occur in proteins as a result of chemical modification after the protein has been synthesised. In addition, a number of amino acids occur as metabolic intermediates, but are not involved in proteins.

Chemically the amino acids all have the same basic structure – an amino group ($-NH_3^+$) and a carboxylic acid group ($-COO^-$) attached to the same carbon atom (the α-carbon). As shown in Figure 8.1, what differs between them is the nature of the other group that is attached to the α-carbon. In the simplest amino acid, glycine, there are two hydrogen atoms, while in all other amino acids there is one hydrogen atom and a side-chain. Figure 8.1 does not show the structure of the 21st amino acid, the selenium analogue of cysteine, selenocysteine (see Ch. 12, Section 12.2).

The amino acids can be classified according to the chemical nature of the side-chain: whether it is hydrophobic (on the left of Fig. 8.1) or hydrophilic (on the right of Fig. 8.1); and the chemical nature of the group: hydrophobic, branched chain, aromatic, S-containing, neutral hydrophilic, acidic or basic.

The sequence of amino acids in a protein is its primary structure. It is different for each protein, although proteins that are closely related to each other often have similar primary structures. The primary structure of a protein is determined by the gene containing the information for that protein (see Section 8.3 under 'Protein synthesis').

Folding of the protein chain

The linear chain of amino acids in a polypeptide chain folds in a variety of ways to form secondary and tertiary levels of structure. As a result of this, amino acids that may be far apart in the primary sequence come close together to form reactive regions that bind ligands (in receptor and transport proteins, and enzymes) and catalyse chemical reactions (in enzymes). Two main types of chemical interaction are responsible for the folding of the polypeptide chain: hydrogen bonds between the oxygen of one peptide bond and the nitrogen of another, and interactions between the side-chains of the amino acids.

The folding of the protein chain also provides proteins with physical properties: most soluble proteins have a relatively compact globular structure; structural proteins such as collagen (in bone and connective tissue) and keratin (in skin and hair) have a fibrous structure, with considerable cross-linkage between adjacent fibres, so that they are flexible, but resist stretching. Elastin, the structural protein of elastic connective tissue, as in the arteries, has multiple cross-links between three or four adjacent chains, forming a three-dimensional network that is both flexible and elastic.

Having formed regions of secondary structure (regular helices and pleated sheets), the whole protein molecule then folds up into a compact shape. This is the third (tertiary) level of structure, and is largely the result of interactions between the side-chains of the amino acids, with each other and with the environment.

Two further interactions between amino acid side-chains may be involved in tertiary structure, forming covalent links between regions of the peptide chain:

- The ε-amino group on the side-chain of lysine can form a peptide bond with the carboxyl group on the side-chain of aspartate or glutamate. This is nutritionally important, since the side-chain peptide bond is not hydrolysed by digestive enzymes, and the lysine, which is an indispensable amino acid, is not available for absorption (see Section 8.4 under 'Unavailable amino acids').
- The sulphydryl (-SH) groups of two cysteine molecules may be oxidised, to form a disulphide bridge between two parts of the protein chain.

Some proteins consist of more than one polypeptide chain; the way in which the chains interact with each other after they have separately formed their secondary and tertiary structures is the quaternary structure of the protein. Interactions between the subunits of multi-subunit proteins, involving changes in quaternary structure and the conformation of the protein, affecting activity, are important in a number of regulatory enzymes.

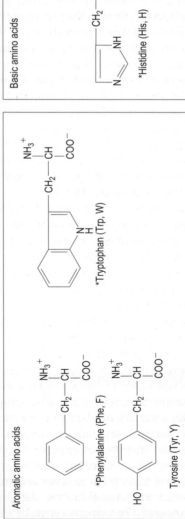

Figure 8.1 The amino acids; left, hydrophobic; right, hydrophilic.

Denaturation of proteins

Because of their compact structures, most proteins are resistant to digestion; few bonds are accessible to proteolytic enzymes. However, the native structure of proteins is maintained by relatively weak non-covalent forces that are disrupted by heat and acid. When this happens, proteins become insoluble (the process of denaturation), and most of the peptide bonds are accessible to digestive enzymes. Gastric acid is also important, since relatively strong acid will also disrupt hydrogen bonds and denature proteins.

8.3 NITROGEN BALANCE AND PROTEIN TURNOVER

The average dietary intake of protein is around 80 g/day, and about the same amount of endogenous protein is secreted into the intestinal lumen in digestive enzymes, protective mucus secreted by intestinal mucosal goblet cells and shed intestinal epithelial cells, so that the total flux of protein through the intestinal tract is about twice the dietary intake.

There is a small faecal loss equivalent to about 10 g of protein/day; the remainder is hydrolysed to free amino acids and small peptides, and absorbed. The faecal loss of nitrogen is partly composed of undigested dietary protein, but the main contributors are intestinal bacteria and shed mucosal cells that are only partially broken down, and mucus. Mucus is especially resistant to enzymic hydrolysis, and contributes a considerable proportion of obligatory nitrogen losses.

There is only a small pool of free amino acids in the body, in equilibrium with proteins that are being catabolised and synthesised. Part of this is used for synthesis of a variety of specialised metabolites (including hormones and neurotransmitters, purines and pyrimidines). An amount of amino acids equivalent to that absorbed is oxidised, with the carbon skeletons being used as metabolic fuels or for gluconeogenesis (see Section 6.3), and the nitrogen being excreted mainly as urea.

The state of protein nutrition, and the overall state of body protein metabolism, can be determined by measuring the dietary intake of nitrogenous compounds and the output of nitrogenous compounds from the body. Nitrogen constitutes 16% of most proteins, and the protein content of foods is calculated on the basis of mg N × 6.25, although for some foods with an unusual amino acid composition other factors are used.

The output of N from the body is largely in the urine and faeces, but significant amounts may also be lost in sweat and shed skin cells. Although the intake of nitrogenous compounds is mainly protein, the output is mainly urea, although small amounts of a number of other products of amino acid metabolism are also excreted.

The difference between intake and output of nitrogenous compounds is nitrogen balance. Three states can be defined:

- An adult in good health and with an adequate intake of protein excretes the same amount of nitrogen each day as is taken in from the diet. This is nitrogen balance or nitrogen equilibrium: intake = output, and there is no change in the total body content of protein.
- In a growing child, a pregnant woman or someone recovering from protein loss, the excretion of nitrogenous compounds is less than the dietary intake – there is a net retention of nitrogen in the body, and an increase in the body content of protein. This is positive nitrogen balance: intake > output, and there is a net gain in total body protein.
- In response to trauma or infection, or if the intake of protein is inadequate to meet requirements, there is net a loss of nitrogen from the body – the output is greater than the intake. This is negative nitrogen balance: intake < output, and there is a loss of body protein.

Dynamic equilibrium

The proteins of the body are continually being broken down and replaced. Some proteins (especially enzymes that control metabolic pathways) may turn over within minutes or hours; others last for days or weeks before they are broken down. This is dynamic equilibrium. An adult catabolises and replaces some 3–6 g of protein/kg body weight/day, with no change in total body protein content. However, if an isotopically-labelled amino acid is given, the process of turnover can be followed.

Protein breakdown occurs at a more or less constant rate throughout the day. Replacement synthesis is greater than breakdown after a meal, when there is an abundant supply of amino acids and metabolic fuels, and less than breakdown in the fasting state, when amino acids are being used as substrates for gluconeogenesis.

Protein turnover also occurs in growing children, who synthesise considerably more protein per day than their net increase in body protein. Even children recovering from severe protein energy malnutrition, who are increasing their body protein rapidly, still synthesise two to three times more protein each day than the net increase.

Although an adult may be in overall N balance, this is the average of periods of negative balance in the fasting state, and positive balance in the fed state. As discussed in Section 8.3 under 'The energy cost of protein synthesis', protein synthesis is energy expensive, and in the fasting state the rate of synthesis is lower than that of protein catabolism. There is a loss of tissue protein, which provides amino acids for gluconeogenesis. In the fed state, when there is an abundant supply of amino acids and metabolic fuel, the rate of protein synthesis increases, and exceeds that of break-down, so that what is observed is an increase in tissue protein, replacing that which was lost in the fasting state.

Even in severe undernutrition, the rate of protein breakdown remains more or less constant, while the rate of replacement synthesis falls, as a result of the low availability of metabolic fuels. It is only in cachexia that there is increased protein catabolism as well as reduced replacement synthesis.

Tissue protein catabolism

The catabolism of tissue proteins is a highly regulated process; different proteins are catabolised (and replaced) at very different rates. Three different mechanisms are involved in the process: lysosomal cathepsins, the cytosolic protease calpain, and the ubiquitin-proteasome system. Ubiquitin is a small peptide is attached to the ε-amino groups of lysine residues in target proteins in an ATP-dependent process.

It is the continual catabolism of tissue proteins that creates the requirement for dietary protein. Although some of the amino acids released by breakdown of tissue proteins can be reused, most are metabolised to intermediates that can be used as metabolic fuels and for gluconeogenesis; the nitrogen is metabolised to urea, which is excreted.

Protein synthesis

The information for the amino acid sequence of each of the 30 000–50 000 different proteins in the body is contained in the DNA in the nucleus of each cell. As required, a working copy of the information for an individual protein (the gene for that protein) is transcribed, as messenger RNA (mRNA), and this is then translated during protein synthesis on the ribosomes. Both DNA and RNA are linear polymers of nucleotides. In RNA the sugar is ribose, while in DNA it is deoxyribose.

The structure and information content of DNA

DNA is a linear polymer of nucleotides. It consists of a backbone of deoxyribose linked by phosphate diester bonds from carbon-3 of one sugar to carbon-5 of the next (see Fig. CD 8.1). The bases of the nucleotides project from this sugar phosphate backbone. There are two strands of deoxyribonucleotides, held together by hydrogen bonds between a purine (adenine or guanine) and a pyrimidine (thymine or cytosine): adenine forms two hydrogen bonds to thymine, and guanine forms three hydrogen bonds to cytosine. The DNA double strand coils into a helix, the double helix.

It is difficult at first sight to understand how a code made up of only four letters (A, G, C and T) can carry the information which must be contained in the nucleus of the cell, for the 21 different amino acids which make up the 30 000–50 000 different proteins that are to be synthesised. The answer is that the bases are read in groups of three, not singly. Since each group of three (known as a codon) can contain any one of the four bases in each position, there are 64 possible combinations. This means that four bases give a code consisting of 64 words, while there is a need for only 21 for amino acids, plus a code for the end of the message. Each group of three nucleotides is a codon – a single unit of the genetic code.

As can be seen from the genetic code (transcribed to RNA) in Table CD 8.1, most amino acids are coded for by more than one codon. This provides a measure of protection against mutations – in many cases a single base change in a codon will not affect the amino acid that is incorporated into the protein, and therefore will have no functional significance.

Ribonucleic acid (RNA)

In RNA the sugar is ribose, rather than deoxyribose as in DNA, and RNA contains the pyrimidine uracil where DNA contains thymine. There are three main types of RNA in the cell: messenger RNA (mRNA), synthesised in the nucleus, as a copy of one strand of DNA; ribosomal RNA (rRNA), which forms the ribosomes on which protein is synthesised; and transfer RNA (tRNA), which provides the link between mRNA and the amino acids for protein synthesis on the ribosome (see below).

In the transcription of DNA to form mRNA a part of the desired region of DNA is uncoiled, and the two strands of the double helix are separated. A copy of one DNA strand is then synthesised by binding the complementary nucleotide triphosphate to each base of DNA in turn, followed by condensation to form the phospho-diester link between ribose moieties.

Transcription control sites in DNA include start and stop messages, and promoter and enhancer sequences. The main promoter region for any gene is about 25 bases before (upstream of) the beginning of the gene to be transcribed. It acts as a signal that what follows is a gene to be transcribed.

Enhancer and promoter regions may be found further upstream of the message, downstream or sometimes even in the middle of the message. The function of these regions, and of hormone response elements, is to increase the rate at which the gene is transcribed.

Translation of mRNA – the process of protein synthesis

The process of protein synthesis consists of translating the message carried by the sequence of bases on mRNA into amino acids, and then forming peptide bonds between the amino acids to form a protein. This occurs on the ribosome, and requires a variety of enzymes, as well as specific transfer RNA (tRNA) molecules for each amino acid. Amino acids bind to activating enzymes (amino acyl-tRNA synthetases), which recognise both the amino acid and the appropriate tRNA species, forming amino acyl tRNA.

The subcellular organelle concerned with protein synthesis is the ribosome, which assembles on mRNA, permitting the binding of the anti-codon region of amino acyl tRNA to the codon on mRNA, and aligning the amino acids for formation of peptide bonds. The peptide chain grows as the ribosome moves along the mRNA – and each mRNA is being translated by a number of ribosomes at the same time.

The energy cost of protein synthesis

The minimum estimate of the energy cost of protein synthesis is 4 ATP equivalents per peptide bond formed, or 2.8 kJ/gram of protein synthesised; if allowance is made for the energy cost of active transport of amino acids into cells, the cost of protein synthesis is increased to 3.6 kJ/gram. Allowing for the nucleoside triphosphates required for mRNA synthesis gives a total cost of 4.2 kJ/gram of protein synthesised.

In the fasting state, when the rate of protein synthesis is relatively low, about 8% of total energy expenditure (i.e. about 12% of the basal metabolic rate) is accounted for by protein synthesis. After a meal, when the rate of protein synthesis increases, it may account for 12–20% of total energy expenditure.

Hormonal control of protein turnover

Insulin, secreted in the fed state, increases the rate of protein synthesis, both by direct actions and also by stimulating the uptake of glucose and amino acids into cells. In addition, the amino acid leucine has a specific role in increasing the rate of overall protein synthesis.

Vitamins A and D and steroid hormones act to regulate the synthesis of specific proteins, by binding, via nuclear receptor proteins, to hormone response elements that regulate the expression of genes (see Ch. 11). In some cases there is increased synthesis of the proteins (induction); in others there is reduced synthesis (repression).

The glucocorticoid hormone cortisol acts at a whole body level to increase the rate of muscle protein catabolism and gluconeogenesis in the liver. It achieves this by inducing key regulatory enzymes of gluconeogenesis, and two liver enzymes that initiate the catabolism of two essential amino acids: tryptophan dioxygenase and tyrosine transaminase. As a result of increased catabolism of tryptophan and tyrosine, there is a lack of these two amino acids, leading to reduced protein synthesis, and a surplus of the other amino acids that cannot be used for protein synthesis, but are used as metabolic fuel or for gluconeogenesis.

8.4 AMINO ACID METABOLISM

Dispensable and indispensable amino acids

Early studies of nitrogen balance showed that not all proteins are nutritionally equivalent. More of some is needed to maintain nitrogen balance than others. This is because different proteins contain different amounts of the various amino acids. The body's requirement is not simply for protein, but for the amino acids that make up proteins, in the correct proportions to replace the body proteins.

As shown in Table 8.1, the amino acids can be divided into indispensable and dispensable groups:

- The nine indispensable or essential amino acids, which cannot be synthesised in the body. If one of these is provided in inadequate amount, then regardless of the total intake of protein, it will not be possible to maintain nitrogen balance, since there will not be an adequate amount of the amino acid for protein synthesis.
  - Two amino acids, cysteine and tyrosine, can be synthesised in the body, but only from essential amino acid precursors – cysteine from methionine and tyrosine from phenylalanine.
  - For premature infants, and possibly also for full-term infants, a tenth amino acid is essential – arginine. The capacity for arginine synthesis is low in infants, and may not be adequate to meet the requirements for growth.
- The non-essential or dispensable amino acids, which can be synthesised from metabolic intermediates, as long as there is enough total protein in the diet. If one of these amino acids is

omitted from the diet, nitrogen balance can still be maintained.
  - Only three amino acids, alanine, aspartate and glutamate, can be considered to be truly dispensable; they are synthesised from common metabolic intermediates (pyruvate, oxaloacetate and α-ketoglutarate, respectively).
  - The remaining amino acids are generally considered as non-essential, but under some circumstances the requirement may outstrip the capacity for synthesis.

Unavailable amino acids

Chemical analysis of the amino acid content of dietary proteins does not reflect their nutritional value, since some of the essential amino acids in dietary proteins are not released by digestive enzymes, i.e. they are biologically unavailable. Nutritionally, it is unavailable lysine that is most important, since in many proteins lysine is the limiting amino acid – it is present in the lowest amount compared with requirements. Lysine may be unavailable because of inter-chain peptide bonds from the ε-amino group to the side-chain carboxyl group of glutamic or aspartic acid, or as a result of reaction of the ε-amino group with a reducing sugar – the Maillard or non-enzymic browning reaction that occurs during cooking and storage of foods. Not only is the lysine that has undergone reaction unavailable, since the ε-amino bonds are not susceptible to digestive enzymes, but several amino acids either side of the reacted lysine will also be unavailable, because the side-chain links impair the activity of intestinal proteolytic enzymes.

Table 8.1 Indispensable and dispensable – essential amino acids

Indispensable	Indispensable precursor	Dispensable	Partially dispensable
Histidine		Alanine	Arginine
Isoleucine		Aspartate	Asparagine
Leucine		Glutamate	Glutamine
Lysine			Glycine
Methionine	Cysteine		Proline
Phenylalanine	Tyrosine		Serine
Threonine			
Tryptophan			
Valine			

Utilisation of amino acids other than for protein synthesis

An adult has a requirement for a dietary intake of protein because there is continual oxidation of amino acids as a source of metabolic fuel and for gluconeogenesis in the fasting state. In the fed state, amino acids in excess of immediate requirements for protein synthesis are oxidised. Overall, for an adult in nitrogen balance, the total amount of amino acids being metabolised will be equal to the total intake of amino acids in dietary proteins.

Amino acids are also required for the synthesis of a variety of metabolic products, including:

- purines and pyrimidines for nucleic acid synthesis
- haem, synthesised from glycine
- the catecholamine neurotransmitters, dopamine, noradrenaline and adrenaline, synthesised from tyrosine
- the thyroid hormones thyroxine and tri-iodothyronine, synthesised from tyrosine
- melanin, the pigment of skin and hair, synthesised from tyrosine
- the nicotinamide ring of the coenzymes NAD and NADP, synthesised from tryptophan (see also Ch. 10, Fig. CD 10.3)
- the neurotransmitter serotonin (5-hydroxytryptamine), synthesised from tryptophan
- the neurotransmitter histamine, synthesised from histidine
- the neurotransmitter GABA (γ-aminobutyrate) synthesised from glutamate
- carnitine, synthesised from lysine and methionine
- creatine, synthesised from arginine, glycine and methionine
- the phospholipid bases ethanolamine and choline, synthesised from serine and methionine; acetyl choline functions as a neurotransmitter
- taurine, synthesised from cysteine.

In general, the amounts of amino acids required for synthesis of these products are small compared with the requirement for maintenance of nitrogen balance and protein turnover.

Metabolism of the amino group nitrogen

The initial step in the metabolism of amino acids is the removal of the amino group ($-NH_2$), leaving the carbon skeleton of the amino acid. Chemically, these carbon skeletons are ketoacids (more correctly, they are oxoacids). A ketoacid has a $-C{=}O$ group in place of the $HC-NH_2$ group of an amino acid.

Some amino acids can be directly oxidised to their corresponding ketoacids, releasing ammonia: the process of deamination (see Fig. CD 8.2). There is a general amino acid oxidase that catalyses this reaction, but it has a low activity. Four amino acids (glycine, glutamate, serine and threonine) are deaminated by specific enzymes.

Most amino acids are not deaminated, but undergo the process of transamination, in which the amino group is transferred onto the enzyme, leaving the ketoacid; then in the second half of the reaction, the enzyme transfers the amino group onto an acceptor, which is a different ketoacid, so forming the amino acid corresponding to that ketoacid. The acceptor for the amino group at the active site of the enzyme is pyridoxal phosphate, the metabolically active coenzyme derived from vitamin B_6 (see Ch. 10, Fig. 10.4).

Transamination is a reversible reaction, so that if the ketoacid can be synthesised in the body, so can the amino acid. The essential amino acids are those for which the only source of the ketoacid is the amino acid itself. Three of the ketoacids are common metabolic intermediates; they are the precursors of the three amino acids that can be considered to be completely dispensable, in that there is no requirement for them in the diet: pyruvate (forming alanine), α-ketoglutarate (forming glutamate) and oxaloacetate (forming aspartate). See Figure CD 8.3.

If the acceptor ketoacid in a transamination reaction is α-ketoglutarate, then glutamate is formed, and glutamate can readily be oxidised back to α-ketoglutarate, catalysed by glutamate dehydrogenase, with the release of ammonia. Similarly, if the acceptor ketoacid is glyoxylate, then the product is glycine, which can be oxidised back to glyoxylate and ammonia, catalysed by glycine oxidase. Thus, by means of a variety of transaminases, and using the reactions of glutamate dehydrogenase and glycine oxidase, all of the amino acids can, indirectly, be converted to their ketoacids and ammonia (see also Fig. CD 8.4).

The metabolism of ammonia

The deamination of amino acids (and a number of other reactions in the body) results in the formation of ammonium ions. Ammonium is highly toxic, and is rapidly metabolised, by the formation of glutamate, then glutamine, from α-ketoglutarate (see Fig. CD 8.5).

In the liver, ammonium arising from the hydrolysis of glutamine and other reactions is used to synthesise urea, the main nitrogenous excretion product (see Fig. CD 8.6).

The total amount of urea synthesised each day is several-fold higher than the amount that is excreted. Urea diffuses readily from the bloodstream into the large intestine, where it is hydrolysed by bacterial urease to carbon dioxide and ammonium. Much of the ammonium is reabsorbed, and used in the liver for the synthesis of glutamate and glutamine, and then a variety of other nitrogenous compounds.

The metabolism of amino acid carbon skeletons

Acetyl CoA and acetoacetate arising from the carbon skeletons of amino acids may be used for fatty acid synthesis or be oxidised as metabolic fuel, but cannot be utilised for the synthesis of glucose (gluconeogenesis). Amino acids that yield acetyl CoA or acetoacetate are termed ketogenic.

By contrast, those amino acids that yield intermediates that can be used for gluconeogenesis are termed glucogenic. As shown in Table CD 8.2, only two amino acids are purely ketogenic: leucine and lysine. Three others yield both glucogenic fragments and either acetyl CoA or acetoacetate: tryptophan, isoleucine and phenylalanine. Figure CD 6.7 shows the ways in which amino acid carbon skeletons enter central metabolic pathways.

8.5 PROTEIN AND AMINO ACID REQUIREMENTS (*D. JOE MILLWARD*)

An inherently difficult problem

Defining minimum amino acid and protein requirements is inherently difficult and none of the recent advances in biology provides a solution. Human adults are exposed to a very wide range of protein intakes, which enable full expression of their genotypical lean body mass throughout the range. The intractable problem is that of identifying the lower limits of this range. There are several major difficulties. Firstly, for protein there are no unequivocal biochemical or physiological deficiency symptoms, apart from growth failure and tissue wasting which marks a severe deficiency. Thus protein or amino acid deficiency can only be identified as an intake that is below the requirement. This means that the extent of protein deficiency goes up or down as requirement values change. Secondly the long recognised problem of adaptation makes for great difficulties in defining protein requirements, because our derivation of RNI values assumes that there is no relationship between intakes and requirements. With adaptation, where intakes can influence apparent requirements, a more difficult model is required.

Another difficulty relates to the balance method. Without biochemical indicators, protein and amino acid requirements can only be defined in terms of maintenance of body protein, requiring balance methods of one sort or another. Such methods are inherently imprecise and logistically difficult, as discussed below in 'Nitrogen balance and factorial models'. Stable isotope techniques were expected

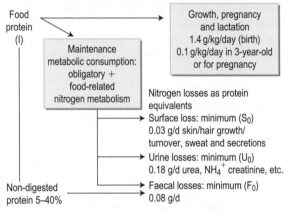

Protein: metabolic demands and utilisation

Food protein (I) → Growth, pregnancy and lactation
1.4 g/kg/day (birth)
0.1 g/kg/day in 3-year-old or for pregnancy

Maintenance metabolic consumption: obligatory + food-related nitrogen metabolism

Nitrogen losses as protein equivalents
Surface loss: minimum (S_0) 0.03 g/d skin/hair growth/turnover, sweat and secretions
Urine losses: minimum (U_0) 0.18 g/d urea, NH_4^+ creatinine, etc.
Faecal losses: minimum (F_0) 0.08 g/d

Non-digested protein 5–40%

Requirement = metabolic demand/efficiency of utilisation

Metabolic demand:
minimum
= total obligatory N losses, ONL
= losses on protein-free diet
= $S_0 + U_0 + F_0$
= 46 mgN/kg ≡ 0.29 g body protein/kg/d

Utilisation = digestibility × biological value
Digestibility
(D, faecal losses) = $(I-F)/I$
true digestibility = $(I-(F-F_0))/I$
Biological value
(BV, urinary losses) = retained N/absorbed N
= $(I-F-U-S)/(I-F)$
true BV = $(I-(F-F_0)-(U-U_0)-(S-S_0))/(I-(F-F_0))$
Net protein utilisation
(NPU) = digestibility × biological value
= (intake$-F-U-S$)/intake
true NPU = $(I-(F-F_0)-(U-U_0)-(S-S_0))/I$

Figure 8.2 Metabolic demands for protein and factors influencing utilisation.

to remedy such inadequacies, but in fact they bring their own problems. Indeed all current stable isotope methods based on amino acid oxidation are variants of the balance study, measuring the relationship between amino acid intake and some function of losses as amino acid oxidation rates, and, like the N balance method, they also suffer from the problem of a poorly defined end-point around equilibrium.

Protein requirements are best discussed in terms of *metabolic demand*, *dietary requirement* and *dietary allowances*.

Metabolic demand

This is determined by the nature and extent of those metabolic pathways which consume amino acids, and which vary with the phenotype and the developmental and physiological state of the individual.

As shown in Figure 8.2, *demands* are conventionally identified as *maintenance* and *special needs* such as growth, rehabilitation, pregnancy and lactation.

Maintenance comprises all those processes that consume amino acids and give rise to urinary, faecal and other losses; net protein synthesis is only a very small part. Minimum metabolic demands, measured in subjects adapted to a protein-free diet when body protein provides for them, are quite low, amounting to about 46 mg N/kg/day, equivalent to 0.29 g/kg/day of body protein.

Dietary requirement

This is the amount of protein and/or its constituent amino acids that must be supplied in the diet in order to satisfy the metabolic demand and achieve nitrogen equilibrium. The requirement will in most cases be greater than the metabolic demand because of those factors which influence the efficiency of protein utilisation, i.e. *net protein utilisation*. These are factors associated with digestion and absorption, which influence the *digestibility* and consequent amount of dietary nitrogen lost in the faeces, and the cellular bioavailability of the absorbed amino acids in relation to needs, which influences the *biological value*.

Dietary allowances

These are a range of intakes derived from estimates of individual requirements taking into account the variability between individuals.

8.6 METHODS OF DETERMINING PROTEIN REQUIREMENTS

The first estimates of protein requirements were made in the second part of the nineteenth century, with recommendations based on measurements of protein intakes of populations assumed to be healthy. The modern era began in 1957 with the first UN Food and Agriculture Organization (FAO) report, which derived estimates from nitrogen balance. These human studies have been supplemented with information about protein quality from animal studies.

Nitrogen balance and factorial models

The metabolic demands can be estimated from measurement of all losses of nitrogen in subjects adapted to a protein-free diet. This is the obligatory nitrogen loss (ONL). When losses are measured over a range of intakes, balance is calculated at each intake as intake minus losses, and the equation of the balance curve calculated to predict the requirement. As shown in Figure CD 8.7, which represents all published N balance studies up to 2001 (Rand et al 2003), a linear regression of balance against intake will allow prediction of the ONL as the zero intake intercept. The slope of the curve will indicate the efficiency of utilisation and the maintenance requirement, i.e. the amount that must be fed to balance losses and produce equilibrium, ONL/efficiency of utilisation. From these data the currently accepted maintenance requirement is 0.66 g/kg body weight/day.

Inherent difficulties with nitrogen balance studies

This apparently simple, but laborious, approach is beset with a large number of quite serious problems, as listed in Table 8.2.

Balance is the small difference between two large amounts and can seldom be precisely measured. Because of systematic errors (an overestimation of intake because subjects might eat less than the test meals, and an underestimation of the losses)

8.8 EXPRESSION OF REQUIREMENTS: NUTRIENT BASED (G/KG/DAY) OR NUTRIENT DENSITY (PROTEIN:ENERGY RATIOS)?

In the past, protein requirements have been expressed as amounts per person or more precisely per kilogram body weight. Whilst this is adequate in calculating recommended intakes for an individual, it is less useful when advice is given about the types of diets and foods to be recommended and in assessing the adequacy of intakes. Energy expenditure determines overall energy and nutrient intakes, so that food-based guidelines, especially the use of nutrient density, can result in a better definition of nutritional priorities for specific populations. The calculation of the protein:energy (P:E) ratio of requirements is shown in Figure CD 8.12. The changes with age in the RNI for protein and the energy requirements are shown at the top and the resultant P:E ratio in the bottom figure; i.e.:

$$PE\% = (RNI\ protein\ (g/kg/day)$$
$$* 4\ kcal/g)/(energy\ requirements$$
$$kcal/kg/day) * 100$$

Because the very high energy requirements during infancy and childhood decrease with age at a greater rate than the fall in the protein requirement, the P:E ratio of the requirements for infants is low and increases with age. This means that a diet which can meet both energy and protein needs of the infant can satisfy energy needs of older children or adults while failing to meet their protein needs.

Importance of physical activity for nutrient intakes and risk of deficiency

Protein requirements are generally not considered to vary with energy expenditure (but see 'N balance at varying levels of physical activity', above) and protein requirements are usually provided by the increased food energy intakes. With energy requirements predicted from BMR × physical activity level, energy requirements per kilogram will vary markedly with age (falling), with gender (women < men), with body weight (large < small) and with physical activity. The calculations in Figure CD 8.12 are for women weighing 58 kg, and a sedentary lifestyle (an energy requirement based on 1.5 × predicted BMR). Clearly as energy requirements increase, the P:E ratio of the protein requirements will fall, so that for adults and the elderly, increased physical activity reduces the P:E ratio of the protein requirement.

Protein energy ratios: key implications

- Protein dense foods are more important for adults, especially the elderly, than for infants and children.
- Energy dense foods are more important for children than for adults.
- Protein deficiency is more likely in the elderly than in children.
- Protein deficiency at any age is less likely as physical activity increases.

8.9 METHODS OF EVALUATING PROTEIN QUALITY AND ASSESSING AMINO ACID REQUIREMENTS

The nutritional importance of protein quality was established very early in the twentieth century, from N balance studies in human beings and growth studies in rats. The identification of separate metabolic demands for amino acids for maintenance and growth was an early discovery; as shown in Figure CD 8.13, rats fed zein, the main protein in maize, were unable to maintain weight and died. Various amino acids were added but only tryptophan allowed weight maintenance, lysine did not. However, when lysine was added with tryptophan, normal growth

occurred. This established not only that zein was deficient in both tryptophan and lysine, but that the metabolic demands for amino acids include growth (net protein synthesis) and maintenance, as indicated in Figure 8.2. Zein is inadequate for either maintenance, through tryptophan deficiency, or growth, through tryptophan plus lysine deficiency. W. C. Rose showed that rats could grow maximally on purified amino acid mixtures and then, with others, quantified the maintenance requirement of the essential amino acids with N balance studies in men and women. These data represent a major source of our understanding of amino acid requirements.

Protein quality evaluation in animals

The rat growth assay for protein quality was developed from the early studies of Osborne and Mendel, and is still in use to day.

Protein efficiency ratio (PER) is the simplest measure: g weight gain/g protein intake from a diet containing 9–10% of protein. Very marked differences are apparent, with values of 3.8, 2.0 and 0.3 for whole egg, soya and wheat gluten. It does not reveal why differences in weight gain might occur in terms of digestibility, and biological value (see Fig. 8.2).

Digestibility can vary through restriction of digestion by plant cell walls and the presence in plant foods of anti-nutritional factors. Values range from 60 to 80% in legumes and cereals with tough cell walls such as millet and sorghum to 97% for egg (see Table CD 8.3). Anti-nutritional factors in legumes and seeds include amylase and trypsin inhibitors, tannins in most legumes and cyanogens in lima beans. *Biological value (BV)* varies mainly through the composition of the absorbed amino acid mixture in relation to the pattern of the metabolic demand for maintenance and net protein deposition. Chemical modification of amino acids in food protein during processing can also reduce their bioavailability even though they are absorbed. The rat growth assay of BV shows marked differences between proteins when they are assessed individually in line with amounts of indispensable amino acids in the protein compared with tissue protein composition. In general, the overall amino acid composition is influenced by the number of different codons assigned to each amino acid in the genetic code (see Table CD 8.1), with high levels of leucine and serine and low levels of methionine, and tryptophan. However, since this is the same for both dietary and tissue proteins, it need not necessarily pose a nutritional problem. BV is low for cereal and legume proteins, because of low levels of lysine and tryptophan in cereals, and of the sulphur-containing amino acids in legumes in relation to metabolic demands. However, because the limiting amino acids differ between types of plant proteins, when they are combined they complement each other, so that mixed plant protein diets exhibit much higher BV values and may be similar to animal proteins.

Net protein utilisation (NPU, see Fig. 8.2) represents a specific measure of protein utilisation. It can be measured by means of N balance studies allowing separate evaluation of both digestibility and BV.

Because faecal and urinary losses include endogenous losses which occur on a protein-free diet (the ONL) the measurements need to differentiate between these and exogenous losses due to poor utilisation of food protein.

Endogenous losses $(S_0 + U_0 + F_0)$ (see Fig. 8.2) indicate metabolic demands and are measured in response to a protein-free diet.

Food-related losses $(S + U + F - (S_0 + U_0 + F_0))$ determine efficiency of utilisation.

Direct measurements of N retention

In practice, N balance studies are very laborious and Bender & Miller devised a simplified, more accurate method based on direct measurement of N retention in the rat carcass, as shown in Figure CD 8.14. Food protein intake and total carcass N are measured after 10 days on either the test diet or on a protein-free diet. NPU for both maintenance and growth is calculated from the difference in carcass N content between the two diets. With this approach, digestibility and BV are not separately indicated.

Protein quality evaluation in human nutrition

Protein quality assessment in rat growth assays measures mainly the needs for rapid tissue growth. It is this work with animals that has resulted in the concept of first and second class proteins. However, this concept is much less relevant in human nutrition.

For human beings, as shown in Figure CD 8.10, metabolic demands for growth fall rapidly during the first year of life, so that amino acid needs are for maintenance, and we know from extensive work in farm animals and rats that the amino acid pattern of these demands is quite different from the metabolic demands for growth. In particular, there is a much lower proportion of indispensable amino acids. Consistent with this is the difficulty of demonstrating differences in protein quality in human nutrition, especially with mixed plant food diets. N balance studies in adults indicate very small differences when comparisons are made between single

Table 8.4 Amino acid requirement values from FAO/WHO/UNU (1985), recalculated to allow for miscellaneous losses (Millward 1999), and as published in the DRI report (see text)

	FAO/WHO (1985) N balance (mg/day)	Recalculated N balance (mg/kg/day)	DRI values (stable isotopes) (mg/kg/day)
Histidine	–	–	11
Isoleucine	10	18	15
Leucine	14	26	34
Lysine	12	19	31
Methionine + cysteine	13	16	15
Phenylalanine + tyrosine	14	20	27
Threonine	7	16	16
Tryptophan	3.5	3.7	4
Valine	10	14	19
Total	84	133	172

Indicator amino acid oxidation studies

This approach to estimating amino acid requirements is, in principle, free from some of the problems associated with tracer balance studies. It was developed to study rapidly growing animals and rather than estimate balance, the end-point in this case is a change, or breakpoint, in amino acid oxidation when the intake supports growth or net protein synthesis. A fixed amount of an amino acid mixture is fed with varying amounts of the amino acid under test (e.g. lysine), below and above the likely requirement. The oxidation of a second 'indicator' labelled amino acid is measured. When the intake of the test amino acid is too low to support net protein synthesis, the rest of the amino acid intake is oxidised, including the indicator amino acid. As the test requirement intake is approached or exceeded, all of the amino acid intake, including the indicator, will be utilised, so that indicator oxidation falls. Typical results are shown in Figure CD 8.16. The indicator amino acid oxidation method works best with rapidly growing animals such as the piglet, where the method gives a clear breakpoint. However, in human studies, with net protein synthesis during feeding measured, as with the PPU method, this does not seem to result in such a clear end-point, and the exact intake for the breakpoint is model dependent.

In some studies an indirect measure of amino acid oxidation is reported ($^{13}CO_2$ production uncorrected for precursor enrichment). The main feature of these studies is the use of breakpoint analysis (two phase linear regression after assuming zero slope for the higher intakes). The value shown in Figure CD 8.11 is obtained by this analysis but it is clear that a lower

value between 20 and 30 could be identified by an alternative analysis, since none of the mean values above an intake of 20 mg/kg/day are different. This would fit with the changes in plasma lysine concentrations with intake, where increases occurred between 20 and 30 mg/kg/day. The fact that the breakpoint is so difficult to identify means that there is a great deal of variability in the results. In a study of tryptophan requirements with this approach values ranged from 1.7 to 5.4 mg/kg/day.

Twenty-four-hour ^{13}C leucine oxidation studies

These represent the limits of development of tracer methodologies with a 24-hour infusion of tracer during periods of feeding and fasting, and continuous collection of expired $^{13}CO_2$. ^{13}C Leucine balance studies have been conducted in subjects fed amino acid mixtures with varying levels of leucine, lysine and threonine, with up to 2 weeks on the diets. Because the studies are so logistically difficult, the number of different intakes tested is limited, with those aimed at identifying lysine requirements testing four different levels of intake. These studies have proved difficult to interpret, as shown in Figure CD 8.17. However, in subjects fed amino acid mixtures supplying about 1 g/kg/day with variable lysine, 24-hour leucine balances are dependent on both the lysine intake, as expected, but also on the leucine intake, so that 24-hour leucine equilibrium has proved an inadequate criterion of adequacy. Thus rather than use leucine balance, breakpoint analysis has been adopted, identifying about 30 mg lysine/kg/day as the requirement in each study.

8.10 DEFINITION OF REFERENCE AMINO ACID PATTERNS

It is clear that there is much uncertainty about the actual values for amino acid requirements from which scoring patterns can be constructed but there is agreement on the principles. For infants the amino acid composition of breast milk is assumed to represent an optimum pattern. Since it is quite clear that after the first year of life growth is relatively slow, there is no reason to expect amino acid requirements to vary much between the preschool child and the adult. This means that once an agreed maintenance pattern has been defined, a factorial calculation of amino acid requirements can be derived from maintenance and the composition and amount of tissue protein gain. In the DRI report, the values shown in Figure CD 8.18 are reported, based on amino acid requirements of maintenance or maintenance plus growth (corrected for 58% efficiency of utilisation of dietary protein), assuming EAR protein values of 0.88 and 0.66 g/kg/day for 1–3-year-olds and adults. Since these two patterns are so similar this report recommends that the 1–3-year-old pattern be used for all ages >1 year old.

Quality of animal and plant proteins

Table CD 8.5 shows PDCAAS values and adjusted P:E ratios of dietary protein sources. The important measure is available protein in foods, the adjusted P:E ratio, which is determined by both protein content and quality.

Animal foods generally perform well on both counts. Lysine is the limiting amino acid for cereal proteins, yam and cassava. Maize also contains less than the reference tryptophan level, but at 71% of reference, compared with lysine at 57%, lysine is limiting, and adjusting intake to supply lysine needs will supply more than enough tryptophan. The improved maize variety, opaque maize, with a higher ratio of cytoplasmic proteins to storage protein (zein), has adequate tryptophan and 80% of the reference lysine. Soya, in common with all legumes, has low levels of sulphur amino acids, but with this scoring pattern, is just sufficient.

Potatoes provide sufficient of all amino acids. It is interesting that even after correcting for digestibility the adjusted P:E ratio of potato at 8.2% is higher than that of breast milk. The idea that the potato is a high protein food compared with breast milk may seem incredible and in fact the growth of a newborn could not be supported on mashed potato, but the reason for this is energy density, not protein content. The P:E ratio of requirements for young adults shown in Figure CD 8.12 is 9.4% calories for a sedentary person (physical activity level (PAL) = 1.5) and this would fall to 8% or 7% calories with PAL = 1.75 and 2 respectively.

The high protein level in wheat means that it provides a much higher level of utilisable protein (PDCAAS-adjusted P:E ratio) than yam or cassava, even though wheat has the lowest lysine level of any staple. Clearly cassava does badly mainly due to its low protein content so that only 1.7% of its energy is utilisable protein.

8.11 THE GREAT DEBATE: 1. ARE THE DEVELOPING COUNTRIES PROTEIN DEFICIENT BECAUSE OF LYSINE DEFICIENCY?

Stable isotope studies have advanced our understanding of amino acid homeostasis but their initial promise of providing an alternative to nitrogen balance has yet to be fully realised. All methods published to date have serious methodological problems of one sort or another, and none can provide answers to the problem at the core of the protein quality debate: are minimally supplemented cereal-based diets as consumed in the developing world adequate?

It is the case that long-term studies (published in the 1960s–1970s) showed that wheat-based diets, providing 18–20 mg lysine/kg, enabled maintenance of body weight, N balance and fitness, but such studies tend to be ignored.

The US DRI report (Food and Nutrition Board 2002) has embraced the values from stable isotope studies to derive its age-related requirement values used to derive scoring patterns, arguing that the 1–3-year-old pattern be used for everyone. The outcome of this for protein quality assessment is shown in Table CD 8.5, which scores foods as discussed above. In Table CD 8.6, diets in the UK and India are scored with lysine values based on either recalculated N balance FAO/WHO/UNU data for the lysine requirement or the DRI recommended value.

This means that cereal-based diets in India would be judged markedly lysine deficient with the higher of these two values but not with the lower. In order for adequacy to be achieved 22–23% energy would need to be replaced from soya as shown. In the 1960s there was a UN call for 'international action to avert the impending protein crisis', which proved a false alarm. Some have repeated that call, but we need to be sure about our facts and it is clear that at least in 2003 many believe there is insufficient convincing evidence (Millward & Jackson 2004). Clearly this important debate needs to continue.

8.12 THE GREAT DEBATE: 2. IMPLICATIONS OF ADAPTATION FOR NUTRITION POLICY

The use of dietary guidelines in public health nutrition has recently been reviewed (Institute of Medicine 2000). In general, protein requirement figures serve two purposes.

One is as a basis for prescription, i.e. advice on safe diets through recommending appropriate dietary intakes. The adaptive model shown in Figure CD 8.9b implies a much lower, but difficult to define, RNI. Formulation of policy will inevitably and correctly be most concerned with satisfying the upper range of demands for protein and, where there is uncertainty, including positive margins of error. In this case it may be unwise to adopt an adaptive model and reduce the RNI. Indeed an adaptive model does not mean that protein is an unimportant nutrient for the maintenance of human health and well-being, but that indicators other than balance need to be identified. There is growing experimental evidence for potential benefit of protein intakes considerably above the current RNI for bone health in the elderly, and epidemiological evidence for benefit with respect to hypertension and ischaemic heart disease. This results in a dilemma for those attempting to frame dietary guidelines. It is probably wise to retain current values until it becomes possible to quantify the benefits (and any risks) of protein intakes within the adaptive range.

The other purpose of requirement figures is as a diagnostic indicator of risk, in population groups rather than individuals. In this case indicators used to estimate prevalence of disease states, or deficit risk, are carefully chosen so as to strike an acceptable balance between false positives and false negatives. The main implication of adaptation for estimating risk of deficiency as intakes < requirements, is a dramatic reduction in the prevalence of risk for most populations compared with that assessed according to the current model. As in the prescriptive context, this low risk of deficiency applies only to that of being unable to maintain N balance after full adaptation with otherwise nutritionally adequate diets satisfying the energy demands. Whether such populations enjoy optimal protein-related health is a separate issue. It has been suggested that maintenance of N balance can no longer be used as a surrogate of adequate protein-related health and that current lack of quantifiable alternative indicators is no excuse for ignoring the issue of adaptation.

⮑ Key points

⮑ Proteins are large polymers of 21 different amino acids; the amino acid sequence of each protein is different, and is determined by the gene for that protein.

⮑ Folding of the protein chain produces proteins that act as receptors, transport proteins and enzymes, and serve structural functions

⮑ An adult is overall in nitrogen equilibrium, with intake of nitrogenous compounds (mainly protein) matched by excretion of nitrogenous metabolites.

⮑ In growth and recovery from loss there is positive nitrogen balance; in response to trauma, or an inadequate intake, there is negative nitrogen balance. There is continual catabolism of tissue proteins, and replacement synthesis, so there is a dynamic equilibrium – even in an adult who is not increasing the total body protein content.

⮑ In the fasting state protein catabolism exceeds synthesis, and in the fed state synthesis exceeds catabolism.

⮑ Both protein synthesis and catabolism are energy-requiring processes, and a significant proportion of total energy expenditure is accounted for by protein turnover.

- After synthesis on the ribosome, many proteins undergo post-synthetic modification, resulting in the formation of a number of amino acids that cannot be utilised for new protein synthesis, but are metabolised or excreted unchanged after protein catabolism.

- Nine amino acids cannot be synthesised in the body, but must be provided in the diet – these are the essential or indispensable amino acids.

- Although the remaining amino acids can be synthesised in the body, only three (alanine, aspartic and glutamic acids) can be considered to be wholly dispensable.

- In addition to the requirement for protein synthesis, a variety of other important compounds are synthesised from amino acids.

- The catabolism of amino acids leads to the formation of ammonium by transamination linked to deamination; this is transported in the body as glutamine, and metabolised in the liver to form urea, the main urinary nitrogenous compound.

- The carbon skeletons of amino acids may provide substrates for energy-yielding metabolism, fatty acid synthesis or gluconeogenesis.

- The determination of protein and amino acid requirements is inherently difficult, partly because of adaptation over a wide range of intakes.

- Protein requirements can be considered in terms of the metabolic demand for total protein and individual amino acids, and the dietary requirement, taking into account the digestibility and nutritional value of different proteins.

- Protein requirements can be determined by nitrogen balance studies and factorial calculation; there are inherent problems in this method.

- Protein requirements may be calculated on the basis of intake per kilogram body weight or on the basis of energy density.

- Various methods can be used to estimate protein quality, either in experimental animals or in human beings.

- Protein and amino acid requirements can be determined by a variety of stable isotope tracer studies; there are inherent problems in the various methods that have been used.

References and further reading

References

Department of Health 1991 Dietary reference values for food energy and nutrients for the United Kingdom. Report on Health and Social Subjects no. 41. HMSO, London

FAO/WHO/UNU 1985 Energy and protein requirements. 15. Report of a joint FAO/WHO/UNU expert consultation. Technical report series 724. WHO, Geneva

FAO/WHO 1991 Protein quality evaluation. Report of a joint FAO/WHO Expert Consultation. FAO, Rome

Food and Nutrition Board, Institute of Medicine 2002 Dietary reference intakes for energy, carbohydrate, fiber, fat, fatty acids, cholesterol, protein, and amino acids (macronutrients). National Academy Press, Washington DC

Institute of Medicine 2000 Dietary reference intakes: application in dietary assessment. Washington DC

Jones E M, Bauman C A, Reynolds M S 1956 Nitrogen balances in women maintained on various levels of lysine. Journal of Nutrition 60:549–559

Millward D J 1999 The nutritional value of plant based diets in relation to human amino acid and protein requirements. Proceedings of the Nutrition Society 58:249–260

Millward D J 2001 Workshop on 'Protein and Amino Acid Requirements and Recommendations' methodological considerations. Proceedings of the Nutrition Society 60:1–4

Millward D J 2003 An adaptive metabolic demand model for protein and amino acid requirements. British Journal of Nutrition 90:249–260

Millward D J, Jackson A A 2004 Protein/energy ratios of current diets in developed and developing countries compared with a safe protein/energy ratio: implications for recommended protein and amino acid intakes. Public Health Nutrition 7(3):387–405

Rand W M, Pellett P L, Young V R 2003 Meta-analysis of nitrogen balance studies for estimating protein requirements in healthy adults. American Journal of Clinical Nutrition 77:109–127

Further reading

Bolourchi S, Friedmann C M, Mickelsen O 1968 Wheat flour as a source of protein for human subjects. American Journal of Clinical Nutrition 21:827–835

Dewey K G, Beaton G, Fjeld C, Lonnerdal B, Reeds P 1996 Protein requirements of infants and children. European Journal of Clinical Nutrition 50:5119–5150

Edwards C H, Booker L K, Rumph C H et al 1971 Utilization of wheat by adult man: nitrogen metabolism, plasma amino acids and lipids. American Journal of Clinical Nutrition 24:181–193

Institute of Medicine 2000 Dietary reference intakes: application in dietary assessment. Washington DC

Millward D J 1999a Inherent difficulties in defining amino acid requirements. In: The role of protein and amino acids in sustaining and enhancing performance. Committee on Military Nutrition Research, Food and Nutrition Board, Institute of Medicine, National Academy Press, Washington DC, p 169–208

Millward D J 1999b Optimal intakes of dietary protein. Proceedings of the Nutrition Society 58:403–413

Millward D J, Pacy P J 1995 Postprandial protein utilisation and protein quality assessment in man. Clinical Science 88:597–606

Millward D J, Fereday A, Gibson N R, Pacy P J 2002 Efficiency of utilization and apparent requirements for wheat protein and lysine determined by a single meal [^{13}C-1] leucine balance comparison with milk protein in healthy adults. American Journal of Clinical Nutrition 76:1326–1334

Pellett P L, Young V R 1992 The effects of different levels of energy intake on protein metabolism and of different levels of protein intake on energy metabolism: a statistical evaluation from the published literature. In: Scrimshaw N S, Schurch B (eds) Protein Energy Interactions. IDECG, Waterville Valley, NH, p 81–136

Young V R, Scrimshaw N S, Pellett P L 1998 Significance of dietary protein source in human nutrition. Animal or plant protein? In: Waterlow J C, Armstrong D G, Fouden L, Riley R (eds) Feeding a world population of more than eight billion people. A challenge to science. Oxford University Press, in association with The Rank Prize Funds, Oxford, p 205–222

CD-ROM contents

Tables

Table CD 8.1 The genetic code, showing the codons in mRNA

Table CD 8.2 Metabolic fates of the carbon skeletons of amino acids

Table CD 8.3 Typical values for N balance studies of protein utilisation in growing rats

Table CD 8.4 ^{13}C leucine balance measurements of metabolic demands, efficiency of protein utilisation (PPU) and the apparent protein requirement

Table CD 8.5 Protein and amino acid content of animal and plant food sources

Table CD 8.6 Lysine content of diets and amino acid scores

Figures

Figure CD 8.1 The structure of DNA

Figure CD 8.2 Deamination of amino acids

Figure CD 8.3 The reaction of transamination

Figure CD 8.4 Transamination of amino acids linked to deamination

Figure CD 8.5 The synthesis of glutamate and glutamine from ammonium

Figure CD 8.6 The synthesis of urea

Figure CD 8.7 Meta-analysis of N balance studies

Figure CD 8.8 The problem posed by non-linearity of the balance curve

Figure CD 8.9 Distribution of reported values for the protein requirement and obligatory nitrogen loss, and calculation of risk of deficiency for an individual for current (top) and adaptive metabolic demands model (bottom) of protein requirements.

Figure CD 8.10 Components of the protein requirements throughout the life cycle

Figure CD 8.11 Protein intakes and calculated requirements for the breastfed infant

Figure CD 8.12 Changes with age in protein and the energy requirements and the P:E ratio

Figure CD 8.13 Demonstration of the importance of protein quality

Figure CD 8.14 Assessment of net protein utilisation

Figure CD 8.15 Postprandial protein utilisation measured in ^{13}C-1 leucine balance studies

Figure CD 8.16 Indicator amino acid oxidation studies

Figure CD 8.17 Twenty-four-hour ^{13}C leucine oxidation studies

Figure CD 8.18 Reference amino acid patterns

Additional references related to CD-ROM material

Further reading from the book

9

Alcohol metabolism: implications for nutrition and health

Victor R. Preedy, Ross Hunter and Timothy J. Peters

Objectives

By the end of this chapter, you should be able to:

- appreciate the varying intake of alcohol by different population groups and the contribution that alcohol makes to energy intake
- understand the main features of alcohol metabolism
- explain the basis of nutritional deficiencies in alcoholism
- understand how alcohol damages virtually all organs in the body, especially the liver.

9.1 INTRODUCTION

Alcohol is commonly used interchangeably with *ethanol* or ethyl alcohol and the term 'drinking' is often used to describe the consumption of beverages containing alcohol. Individuals will consume wide-ranging quantities of alcohol but some countries or communities expressly forbid the consumption of alcohol on religious, cultural or moral grounds. Individuals may gain pleasure from the psychopharmacological effects of alcohol whereas others may react quite badly, with flushing, nausea and palpitations due to a genetic variation in alcohol-metabolising enzymes. In excess, alcohol may cause malnutrition or act as a toxin and induce pathological changes in a variety of tissues. By contrast, a substantial proportion of individuals consume moderate amounts of alcohol, comprising up to 5% of total dietary energy, and some controversial data suggest that moderate alcohol consumption may be beneficial in reducing cardiovascular and other risk factors. Thus, it is important to take a balanced view of ethanol's effects.

The chemical nature of alcohol

Ethanol is produced from glucose via the fermentation of yeast to produce ethanol, carbon dioxide and ATP. As a consequence of its combined polar (OH group) and non-polar (C_2H_5 groups) properties, and because it is relatively uncharged, ethanol is miscible with water and can cross cell membranes by passive diffusion. It also has the ability to dissolve lipids, hence its disordering effects on biological membranes.

The immediate metabolite of ethanol oxidation, acetaldehyde (Fig. 9.1), is a highly toxic, and chemically reactive molecule that can bind irreversibly with proteins and nucleic acids. Acetate, the product of acetaldehyde metabolism, is either oxidised peripherally to CO_2 in the Krebs (citric acid) cycle or used for synthesis of fatty acids and triacylglycerols. Acetate per se also has some biological activity, e.g. it dilates blood vessels.

The contribution to the energy intake of different population groups

Energy content of alcoholic beverages and the Unit system

The chemical energy content of ethanol is 7.1 kcal/g. In the UK, an alcoholic drink or 'Unit of alcohol' containing 10 ml of ethanol by volume will contain

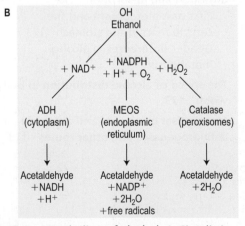

Figure 9.1 Metabolism of alcohol. A, Simplistic representation of conversion of alcohol to acetaldehyde and then acetate. B, Three major routes of ethanol oxidation.

8 g of ethanol (Table 9.1). However, there is a wide international variation in the amount of alcohol in a Unit: from 7 to 14 g ethanol (Table 9.1). The alcohol content of beverages can vary from 0.5% for low alcohol beers to 40–50% for distilled spirits such as vodka or whisky (Table 9.2).

The medical Royal Colleges have recommended either 21 Units (men) or 14 Units (women) per week as sensible limits and these are now generally accepted. The Department of Health (UK) also have guidelines that are based on daily amounts, namely 3–4 or 2–3 Units a day for men and women, respectively, and apply to whether consumption is daily, one or two times a week, or occasionally (Table 9.3). Despite these guidelines, the extent of alcohol misuse is considerable in the UK and there has been an increasing trend for women to drink excessively in recent years. Taking the adult population as a whole, about 27% of males and 12% of females drink more than 21 or 14 Units per week, respectively (see Table CD 9.1). The estimates for alcohol dependence in the UK are high at 7% and 2% of the adult male and female population, respectively (see Table CD 9.2). The problems of alcohol misuse are particularly evident in the young. There are a staggering number

Table 9.1 The Unit system

A. The Unit system of alcohol consumption
One Unit: Half a pint of beer
One glass of wine
One measure of fortified wine (sherry, port)
One measure of spirits (whisky, gin, vodka etc.)

B. Ethanol comprising one Unit
UK	8 g
Australia and New Zealand	10 g
USA	12 g
Japan	14 g

The Unit system of alcohol ingestion is a convenient way of abstracting the amount of ethanol consumed by individuals and offers a suitable means to give practical guidance. The amount of alcohol in each Unit will vary, for example depending on geographical location. Present day assessments may also take into account that some beers may also have widely different amounts of alcohol: for example, 0.3, 3.0, 5.0 or 9.0% alcohol by volume.

Table 9.2 Composition of alcoholic beverages

	Per 100 ml (all as g except energy)					
	kcal	kJ	Alcohol	Protein	Fat	Carbohydrate
Alcohol free lager	7	31	Trace	0.4	Trace	1.5
Low alcohol lager	10	41	0.5	0.2	0	1.5
Lager	29	131	4.0	0.3	Trace	Trace
Special strength lager	59	244	6.9	0.3	Trace	2.4
Bitter	30	124	2.9	0.3	Trace	2.2
Cider (dry)	36	152	3.8	Trace	0	2.6
Wine (red, dry)	68	283	9.6	0.1	0	0.2
Wine (white, dry)	66	275	9.1	0.1	0	0.6
Wine (white, sweet)	94	394	10.2	0.2	0	5.9
Sherry (dry)	116	481	15.7	0.2	0	1.4
Spirits (various; 40% proof)	222	919	31.7	Trace	0	Trace

	Per 100 ml (all as mg)									
	Na	K	Ca	Mg	P	Fe	Cu	Zn	Cl	Mn
Alcohol free lager	2	44	3	7	19	Trace	Trace	Trace	Trace	0.01
Low alcohol lager	12	56	8	12	10	Trace	Trace	Trace	Trace	0.01
Lager	7	39	5	7	19	Trace	Trace	Trace	20	0.01
Special strength lager	7	39	5	7	19	Trace	Trace	Trace	20	0.01
Bitter	6	32	8	7	14	0.1	0.001	0.1	24	0.03
Cider (dry)	7	72	8	3	3	0.5	0.04	Trace	6	Trace
Wine (red, dry)	7	110	7	11	13	0.9	0.06	0.1	11	0.10
Wine (white, dry)	4	61	9	8	6	0.5	0.01	Trace	10	0.10
Wine (white, sweet)	13	110	14	11	13	0.6	0.05	Trace	7	0.10
Sherry (dry)	10	57	7	13	11	0.4	0.03	N	14	Trace
Spirits (various; 40% proof)	Trace	Trace	Trace	Trace	Trace	Trace	Trace	Trace	Trace	Trace

(continued)

Table 9.2 **(continued)**

	Per 100 ml (all as g)							
	Riboflavin (mg)	Niacin (mg)	Trypt/60 (mg)	B$_6$ (mg)	B$_{12}$ (μg)	Folate (μg)	Pantothenate (mg)	Biotin (μg)
Alcohol free lager	0.02	0.6	0.4	0.03	Trace	5	0.09	Trace
Low alcohol lager	0.02	0.5	0.3	0.03	Trace	6	0.07	Trace
Lager	0.04	0.7	0.3	0.06	Trace	12	0.03	1
Special strength lager	0.04	0.7	0.3	0.06	Trace	12	0.03	1
Bitter	0.03	0.2	0.2	0.07	Trace	5	0.05	1
Cider (dry)	Trace	0	Trace	0.01	Trace	N	0.04	1
Wine (red, dry)	0.02	0.1	Trace	0.03	Trace	1	0.04	2
Wine (white, dry)	0.01	0.1	Trace	0.02	Trace	Trace	0.03	N
Wine (white, sweet)	0.01	0.1	Trace	0.01	Trace	Trace	0.03	N
Sherry (dry)	0.01	0.1	Trace	0.01	Trace	Trace	Trace	N
Spirits (various; 40% proof)	0	0	0	0	0	0	0	0

This table only gives an estimate of some of the compounds that will be present in alcoholic beverages. In addition, there will also be other compounds, which are not tabulated, such as fluoride, polyphenols and other organic and non-organic compounds that impart characteristics of taste and smell. Data from Foods Standards Agency (2002).

Table 9.3 **Categorisation of weekly alcohol consumption using Units**

	Men	Women
Low risk	0–21	0–14
Increasing risk	22–50	15–35
Harmful	>50	>35

Summary of Department of Health (UK) recommendations
Men:
Protection: 1–2 Units per day, possibly protection against heart disease (over 40)
Low risk: 3–4 Units a day (all ages)
Not advised: consistently drinking 4 or more Units a day

Women:
Protection: 1–2 Units day, possibly protection against heart disease (past menopause)
Low risk: 2–3 Units a day all ages
Not advised: consistently drinking 3 or more Units a day
Harmful: more than 1 or 2 Units of alcohol, once or twice a week, when pregnant or about to become pregnant

Guidelines are designed to limit harm (Royal Colleges 1995, Department of Health 1995). Whilst the Royal Colleges pertain to weekly consumption rates, the Department of Health's guidelines are more directed to daily rates.

Drinking in the young and gender susceptibility

The results of a UK survey showed that one-fifth of children aged 11–15 had drunk alcohol in the previous week (Department of Health 2001). There have been recent increases in the quantity of alcohol consumed by children in this age category, which presently averages 4 Units/week (see Table CD 9.3). Drinking by school children and adolescents has at least five serious consequences: (a) alcohol poisoning and fatalities; (b) drinking in formative years will predict the extent of alcohol misuse later on; (c) drinking may be compounded by polydrug and other substance misuse including tobacco; (d) total lifetime intake of alcohol, rather than recent intakes, is a good predicator of alcohol-related harm (Saunders & Devereaux 2002); (e) tissues in the young are particularly sensitive to alcohol.

Boys and men are more avid consumers of alcohol than girls (see Tables CD 9.1, CD 9.2, CD 9.3) but women are more susceptible to alcohol-induced injury such as cardiomyopathy, skeletal muscle myopathy, brain damage and liver disease. This may be related to lower clearance rates of alcohol on 'first-pass metabolism', as a consequence of smaller liver size, or gastric alcohol metabolising enzymes, endocrine factors, body fat composition or even psychosocial factors in reporting alcohol consumption. Compared with men, women also have higher blood acetaldehyde levels following the same amount of alcohol per unit body weight. It has been

of men and women in the UK who drink alcohol above either the daily (8.6 million) or weekly (9.1 million) guidelines. There are an estimated 2.8 million individuals classified as alcohol-dependent.

Table 9.4 **Ethanol consumption as dietary energy in the UK (mean daily intake)**

	Men					Women				
	19–24	25–34	35–49	50–64	All	19–24	25–34	35–49	50–64	All
All										
g/day	20.4	22.2	23.1	21.1	21.9	11.4	9.1	9.2	8.6	9.3
kcal/day	143	158	164	150	155	81	65	65	61	66
% total energy	6	6.6	6.8	6.4	6.5	4.6	4.0	3.9	3.7	3.9
Consumers only										
g/day	25.6	27.2	27.4	27.5	27.2	16.1	13.2	13.2	12.9	13.5
kcal/day	182	193	195	195	193	114	94	94	92	96
% total energy	7.6	8.1	8.1	8.3	8.1	6.4	5.8	5.6	5.4	5.7

Data adapted from Henderson et al (2003).
In the above calculations, it was assumed that the energy value of alcohol was 7.1 kcal/g. It should be recognised that specific dietary questionnaires which include alcohol as a constituent may give different answers to questionnaires designed specifically to investigate the intake of alcohol per se, especially in alcohol misusers or alcohol-dependent subjects where the reliability of such questionnaires has been called into question.

estimated that whilst men will show an increased chance of developing liver disease at an intake rate of 40–60 g ethanol/day, the threshold level for women is only 20 g/day.

Energy and micronutrient content of alcoholic beverages

Ten millilitres of ethanol will yield approximately 56 kcal. This underestimates the true energy content of alcoholic beverages as they also contain other constituents, such as carbohydrates, amino acids and fatty acids (see Table 9.2; Foods Standards Agency 2002). The energy composition of alcoholic beverages varies from about 30 to 220 kcal/100 ml. Low or zero alcohol beverages will of course have a lower energy content although usually they have higher carbohydrate content. Alcoholic beverages will also contain trace amounts of compounds that impart flavour or characteristics of taste and smell, e.g., aliphatic carbonyls, other alcohols, monocarboxylic acids, sulphur-containing compounds, tannins, polyphenols, inorganic salts or metals (Aceto 2003). Some of these compounds, such as fluoride, vitamins or polyphenols, are reported to have beneficial properties (see Ch. 13).

Proportion of ethanol calories in the diet

In the UK, the mean daily total energy intake excluding alcohol is 2110 and 1554 kcal for men and women, respectively, and 2310 and 1630 kcal including alcohol (Henderson & Gregory 2002). The mean daily intake of alcohol in all men (consumers and non-consumers) is 22 g (27 g for consumers only) and 9 g for all women (13 g for consumers only) (Table 9.4). Other recent estimates have shown similar data for overall consumption by all men and women, i.e. 18 g and 9 g of ethanol per day. Consideration must be taken of non-alcoholic energy contained within the beverages, for example carbohydrates or mixers that might accompany drinks.

Most of the consumption of alcohol in the UK is in the form of beer and wine (see Table CD 9.4). Overall (i.e. in alcohol consumers and non-consumers) the contribution of ethanol to total energy intake is 6.5% in men and 3.9% in women, respectively. In consumers, the contributions are 8.1% and 5.7%, respectively (Henderson & Gregory 2002). However, the contribution of ethanol-derived calories increases significantly in dependent alcoholics. In one recent study, patients attending an inner city Alcohol Misuse clinic in the UK consumed on average 160 g ethanol/day; contributing to about 60% of dietary energy intake. However, alcohol consumption may be under-reported in women and over-reported in men and no food frequency questionnaires have been unequivocally validated in alcohol misusers. Typical patients with chronic liver disease may consume 160–250 g ethanol/day (1140–1770 kcal/day). This has nutritional consequences as ethanol may be perceived as being 'empty,' i.e. having negligible or minor quantities of micro- or macronutrients. High ethanol loads also impair the normal functions of the liver (see next section).

Table 9.5 Systems and tissues affected by alcohol misuse

1. *Hepato-pancreatobiliary*
   Hepatomegaly – fatty liver, alcoholic hepatitis and fibrosis
   Cirrhosis and hepatocellular carcinoma
   Acute and chronic relapsing pancreatitis – malabsorptive syndrome

2. *Central, peripheral and autonomic nervous systems*
   Acute intoxication
   Progressive euphoria, incoordination, ataxia, stupor, coma and death
   Alcohol withdrawal symptoms including delirium tremens, morning nausea, retching and vomiting, nightmares and night terrors, blackouts and withdrawal seizures
   Nutritional deficiencies
      Wernicke–Korsakoff syndrome
      Pellagra
      Tobacco–alcohol amblyopia
   Others
   Cerebral dementia, cerebellar degeneration
   Demyelinating syndromes – central pontine myelinolysis
   Marchiafava–Bignami syndrome, associated with electrolyte disturbances
   Fetal alcohol syndrome – full-blown syndrome, mental impairment, attention deficit and hyperkinetic disorders, specific learning difficulties
   Peripheral nervous system
   Sensory, motor and mixed neuropathy
   Autonomic neuropathy

3. *Musculoskeletal*
   Proximal metabolic myopathy, principally affecting type II (white) fibres
   Neuromyopathy secondary to motor nerve damage
   Atrophy of smooth muscle of gastrointestinal tract, leading to motility disorders
   Osteopenia – impaired bone formation, degradation, nutritional deficiencies (e.g. calcium, magnesium, phosphate, vitamin D)
   Avascular necrosis (e.g. femoral head)
   Fractures – malunion

4. *Genitourinary*
   IgA nephropathy
   Renal tubular acidosis
   Renal tract infections
   Female and male hypogonadism, subfertility
   Impotence
   Spontaneous abortion
   Fetal alcohol syndrome

5. *Cardiovascular*
   Cardiomyopathy, including dysrhythmias
   Hypertension
   Binge strokes
   Cardiovascular disease (including stroke)
   Myocardial infarction

6. *Dermatological*
   Skin stigmata of liver disease – rosacea, spider naevi, palmar erythema, finger clubbing
   Skin infections – bacterial, fungal and viral
   Local cutaneous vascular effects
   Psoriasis
   Discoid eczema
   Nutritional deficiencies (including pellagra)

7. *Respiratory*
   Chronic bronchitis
   Respiratory tract malignancy
   Asthma
   Postoperative complications

8. *Oro-gastrointestinal*
   Periodontal disease and caries
   Oral infections, leukoplakia and malignancy
   Alcoholic gastritis and haemorrhage
   Alcoholic enteropathy and malabsorption
   Colonic malignancy

9. *Haematological*
   RBCs – macrocytosis, anaemia because of blood loss, folate deficiency and malabsorption, haemolysis (rarely)
   WBCs – neutropenia, lymphopenia
   Platelets – thrombocytopenia

This table is designed to show that diseases associated with alcohol misuse are not confined to only the liver and brain. Virtually all tissues and organs systems can be affected adversely but only some are life-threatening. However, not all individuals will get the diseases identified, perhaps due to inherent protective, dietary or genetic factors. (Compiled from Peters & Preedy 1998, 1999)

The serious negative consequences of chronic alcohol ingestion on health

There are at least 60–120 different alcohol-related pathologies (Table 9.5; Peters & Preedy 1999) and the myth that the most affected organs are the brain and liver should be dispelled. Many of the deleterious effects relate in some way to ethanol metabolism, altering cellular biochemistry because of either ethanol per se, or its immediate metabolite, acetaldehyde (Fig. 9.2). Approximately 10–20% of chronic alcohol misusers will have cirrhosis and 30% will have gastrointestinal pathologies (Table 9.6). Fatty liver will occur in 80% and 50% will have bone marrow changes (perturbing red blood cell morphology). Half of chronic

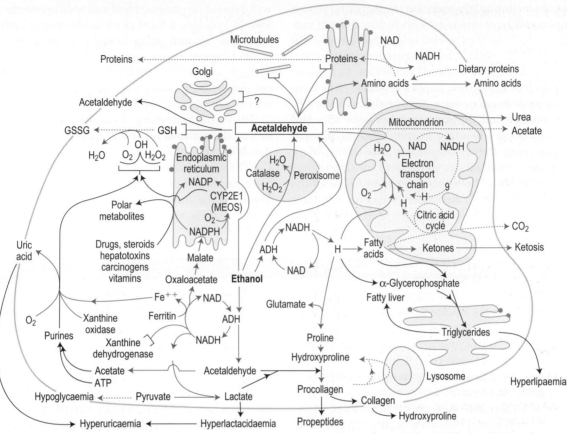

Figure 9.2 Metabolic effects of alcohol in liver cells. Illustration of the complexity of alcohol metabolism in hepatocytes. This figure only represents some of the changes occurring in this tissue. Broken lines signify alcohol-induced depression of pathways; lines with arrows signify activation or stimulation; square brackets signify metabolic interference or binding. Adapted from Lieber (1996), with permission.

Table 9.6 **Prevalence of alcohol-induced pathologies in chronic alcohol abusers**	
	(%)
Skin disorders	80
Alcoholic myopathy	50
Bone disorders	50
Gonadal dysfunction	50
Gastroenterological disorders	30
Cirrhosis	15
Neuropathy	15
Cardiomyopathy	10
Brain disease (organic)	10

The prevalence of alcohol-related disorders relate to chronic alcohol-dependent subjects.

alcoholics will have damaged skeletal tissue (osteoporosis, osteopenia, fractures including post-fracture malunion), and 20–30% will exhibit a spectrum of subclinical or clinical cardiac abnormalities (i.e. alcoholic cardiomyopathy) or other cardiovascular

Table 9.7 **Rule of thumb in alcohol misuse**

The five 'rules of thumb' for alcohol-induced pathologies

1. All tissues and organ systems have the potential to be affected by alcohol or its immediate metabolites
2. Alcohol or its immediate metabolites has the potential to affect all biochemical pathways, subcellular organelles and other cellular systems and/or structures
3. Not all individuals will suffer the consequences of alcohol ingestion due to cellular, nutritional or genetic protective systems
4. 50% of alcoholics will have one or more organ or tissue pathologies
5. 50% of alcoholics will have a deficiency of one or more micro- or macronutrients

The above rules of thumb are gross generalisations and one should take into account differences due to gender, socio-ethnicity, geographical and regional variations in alcohol ingestion.

diseases including hypertension. A staggering 80% of subjects will have skin lesions, including those of vascular, fungal, bacterial or viral origin, and 40–60% will have alcoholic myopathy. Abnormal gonadal function will occur in 50% of male alcoholics. As a rule of thumb, 50% of chronic alcohol misusers will have one or more organ or tissue abnormalities (Table 9.7).

In Europe and the Americas, between 15% and 55% of people attending hospital (as either inpatients or outpatients), or primary care centre attendees, are classified as dependent or hazardous alcohol abusers. However, fewer than 5% of adults have such misuse or dependency recorded in their medical records. Prevalence rates of alcohol misuse will depend on geographical and socioeconomic factors. In London, a third of all acute hospital admissions are alcohol related and the prevalence of alcohol misuse in inpatients in city hospitals may be as high as 30–50%. In fracture clinics, 40–70% of patients score positive for alcohol-related dependency or abuse syndromes.

There are numerous instruments designed to detect alcohol misuse and include the CAGE (Cut down, Annoyed, Guilty, Eye-opener), AUDIT (Alcohol Use Disorders Identification Test) and BMAST (Brief Michigan Alcoholism Screening Test) questionnaires. These can be more useful than laboratory tests on serum, plasma, urine or saliva.

9.2 ALCOHOL METABOLISM

Many of the pathologies associated with drinking alcoholic beverages are due to the effects of acetaldehyde, or the ensuing metabolic changes (e.g. redox state, antioxidant or endocrine status) that accompany ethanol oxidation (Fig. 9.2; Lieber 1996). All pathways and cell structures have the potential to be targeted by ethanol or its related metabolites (Table 9.7). Central to these effects is the liver, where 60–90% of ethanol metabolism occurs. Up to 90% of the substrates utilised in conventional metabolic pathways in liver may be displaced by ethanol oxidation. Ethanol ingestion can inhibit protein and fat oxidation in the body by approximately 40% and 75%, respectively. The 2.5-fold increases in oxidation of carbohydrate after a glucose load is also abolished by ethanol. Oxidation of ethanol by *gastric first-pass metabolism* (see below) will account for 5–25% of ethanol oxidation and 2–10% will appear in the breath, sweat or urine.

The metabolic fate of alcohol following digestion and absorption

Ethanol is rapidly absorbed, primarily in the upper gastrointestinal tract, and appears in the blood as quickly as 5 minutes after ingestion. Its distribution will approximate total body water. Its elimination thereafter will approximate to Michaelis–Menten kinetics, though zero-order elimination has also been described. Blood alcohol levels depend on pathophysiological factors, such as absorption rate, *first-pass metabolism*, the extent to which liver function has been altered and blood flow.

The rate at which alcohol is oxidised, or disappears from the blood, varies from 6 to 10 g per hour. This is reflected in plasma levels, which fall by 9–20 mg/100 ml/hour. In response to a moderate dose of alcohol of 0.6–0.9 g/kg body weight, the elimination rate from the blood is approximately 15 mg/100 ml blood/hour on an empty stomach, though there is considerable individual variation.

Food in the stomach will delay the absorption of alcohol and blunt the peak blood alcohol concentration. The peak blood levels are the points at which the rate of elimination equals the rate of absorption. Using a standard dose of ethanol/kg body weight, it has been shown that the peak is lower after a meal compared with an empty stomach. The time to metabolise the alcohol was 2 hours shorter in the fed state than the fasted state, indicative of a post-absorptive enhancement of ethanol oxidation which can be as much as 35–50%.

The type of food taken with alcoholic beverages will also alter the peak ethanol level: after a standard dose of ethanol of 0.3 g/kg, meals rich in fat, carbohydrate and protein result in peak ethanol levels of 16.6, 17.7 and 13.3 mg/100 ml, respectively. Part of this variation may be due to increased portal blood flow in response to feeding which will essentially deliver more ethanol to the liver for oxidation.

The concentrations of ethanol in beverages will also influence peak blood concentration. In the fed state, beer produces higher peak blood levels compared to whisky for a given alcohol load. In the fasted state, beer produces lower mean blood alcohol concentration and areas under the curve than whisky (Roine 2000). These differences are related to one of the primary determinants of alcohol metabolism: namely the rate of gastric emptying. In simple terms, the small intestine is the main site of ethanol absorption and food will have little effect on large volumes of ethanol-containing liquid (beer) compared to smaller volumes of high-ethanol containing liquids (whisky).

First-pass metabolism and the contribution of the stomach

First-pass metabolism is principally due to the liver (*hepatic first-pass metabolism*), but a small proportion of alcohol is also metabolised by the stomach (*gastric first-pass metabolism*). Stomach ADH (sigma-ADH) is a different isoform from the enzyme in the liver (Table 9.8). Physiological factors that influence gastric emptying will also influence the contribution of this pathway to ethanol elimination. In one study, where ethanol (0.3 g/kg body weight) was administered by different routes, it was calculated that the amount of ethanol absorbed (0.224 g/kg body weight) was 75% of the administered dose: the difference being ascribed to first-pass metabolism. The rate of gastric ethanol metabolism has been reported to be about 1.8 g of ethanol per hour (Haber 2000).

Reduced first-pass metabolism and/or reduced gastric ADH will occur in *Helicobacter pylori* infection and during histamine H2-receptor antagonist therapy. There are also ethnic differences: orientals have a lower stomach ADH/first-pass metabolism than do white Europeans. Chronic alcoholism reduces the capacity of this route of ethanol oxidation due to the development of gastritis.

Gender differences in alcohol metabolism

There are gender differences in the rate of ethanol elimination rates that have also been partially ascribed to first-pass metabolism. The activity of gastric ADH in women is lower than in men, though this is less apparent in women over 50 years old. Compared with men, women will have higher blood ethanol levels after an equivalent load. The lower first-pass metabolism activities account for the higher ethanol levels in women, rather than differences in gastric emptying or rate of ethanol oxidation in the liver. It has, however, been proposed that women and men have comparable peak blood alcohol concentrations when dosage is based on total body water.

The speed of alcohol distribution in body water

Alcohol is rapidly distributed around the body. After ingestion, alcohol that is not immediately absorbed traverses the gastrointestinal tract. Very high ethanol levels occur in the small intestine compared with serum. Effectively, there is a gradient down the gastrointestinal tract. For example, a dose of 0.8 g ethanol/kg body weight (equivalent to 56 g ethanol = 7 Units = 3.5 pints of ordinary beer, consumed by a 70 kg male) will result in blood ethanol levels of 100–200 mg/100 ml 15–120 minutes after dosage. Maximum blood concentrations occur after about 30–90 minutes. Gastric levels will peak at 8 g/100 ml, jejunal levels are approximately 4 g/100 ml compared to approximately 0.15 g/100 ml in the ileum. Levels in the ileum reflect serum levels, i.e. from the vascular space. After about 2 hours, ethanol concentrations in the stomach and jejunum will approximate levels in serum (Mezey 1985). In the post-absorption phase, the distribution of alcohol in the body will reflect body water to the extent that, for a given dose of alcohol, blood levels will reflect lean body mass. The solubility of ethanol in bone and lipid is negligible. Whole blood levels of ethanol are about 10% lower than plasma levels because red blood cells have less water than plasma.

Metabolism by alcohol and aldehyde dehydrogenases and other routes

Alcohol is oxidised to acetaldehyde by three routes (Fig. 9.1): (i) alcohol dehydrogenase (ADH; cystosolic; Table 9.8), (ii) MEOS (microsomal ethanol oxidising system; in endoplasmic reticulum) and (iii) catalase (in peroxisomes) (Fig. 9.1). There are at least six classes of ADH and oxidised substrates include steroids and some intermediates in the mevalonate pathway as well as fatty acid ω-oxidation and retinoids (Table 9.8; Lieber 2000).

There is an excess of reducing equivalents produced via ADH, so that the ratio of $NADH/NAD^+$ is increased, with a corresponding increase in the lactate/pyruvate ratio (Fig. 9.2). The conversion of acetaldehyde to acetate via aldehyde dehydrogenase (ALDH; principally in the mitochondria) will also generate NADH, so compounding the elevated ratio. Changes in the cellular (via ADH) or

Table 9.8 **Ethanol metabolising enzymes**

Class	Subunit	Location	K_m (mM)	V_{max}
Class I				
ADH1	α	Liver	4	54
ADH2	β	Liver, lung	0.05–34	–
ADH3	γ	Liver, stomach	0.6–1.0	–
Class II				
ADH4	π	Liver, cornea	34	40
Class III				
ADH5	χ	Most tissues	1000	–
Class IV				
ADH7	σ, μ	Stomach, oesophagus, other mucosae	20	1510
Class V				
ADH6	–	Liver, stomach	30	?
Class VI				
ADH8	–	None in humans; found in deer mouse and rats	–	?

From Kwo & Crabb (2002), with permission.

Table 9.9 **Aldehyde metabolising enzymes**

Class	Structure	Location	K_m (μM)[a]
Class 1			
ALDH1	α4	Many tissues: liver > kidney	30
Class 2			
ALDH2	α4	Low levels in most tissues: liver > kidney > muscle > heart	1
ALDH5	?	Low levels in most tissues: liver > kidney > muscle	?
Class 3			
ALDH3	α2	Stomach, liver, cornea	11
Other enzymes			
ALDH9	σ4	Liver	30
ALDH6-8	?	?	?

From Kwo & Crabb (2002), with permission.
[a] K_m for acetaldehyde (these enzymes also metabolise other substrates).

mitochondrial (via ALDH) redox state may explain such metabolic abnormalities in alcoholism as: hyper-lactacidaemia, hyperuricaemia, increased lipogenesis, decreased beta-oxidation of fatty acids in mitochondria, hypoglycaemia and disturbances in the tissue responsiveness to hormones.

The hypothesis that the altered $NADH/NAD^+$ ratio can explain most or all of the metabolic abnormalities in the liver is unproven, and many metabolic abnormalities are thought to be due to a number of processes, such as free radical damage, adduct formation, DNA damage and/or altered gene expression, apoptosis, perturbed proteolytic cascades, translational defects, membrane changes and alterations in cellular trafficking (Fig. 9.2; Lieber 1996). Extrahepatic tissues, e.g. mouth, oesophagus, duodenum, jejunum, rectum and muscle, also contain ethanol metabolising enzyme, leading to localised damage.

Peroxisomal catalase plays only a minor role in ethanol oxidation, and requires the concomitant presence of a hydrogen peroxide (H_2O_2) generating

system (Figs 9.1 and 9.2). When there is an increase in H_2O_2 generation, e.g. from the oxidation of long-chain fatty acids in the peroxisomes, there may also be an increase in catalase-mediated ethanol oxidation.

In simple terms, acetaldehyde is toxic and any situation that results in exposure of cells to this agent is harmful. Once acetaldehyde is formed, it is further oxidised to acetate via NAD^+-dependent aldehyde dehydrogenase (ALDH). As with ADH, there are several classes of ALDH (Table 9.9). The most important are ALDH2 and ALDH1, which are mitochondrial and cytosolic, respectively (Table 9.9). The location of ALDHs in extrahepatic tissues such as heart may be protective whereas lower levels in brain may explain the vulnerability of central nervous system tissues in alcoholism (Kwo & Crabb 2002).

Some acetaldehyde becomes bound to cellular constituents such as proteins, lipids and nucleic acids, generating harmful 'hybrid' molecules called adducts (Figs 9.1 and 9.2; Lieber 1996). Not only does adduct formation change the biochemical characteristic of the target molecule but the new structure may also be recognised as foreign (i.e. a neoantigen), thus initiating an immunological response.

Genetic or ethnic variations in ADH and ALDH may also explain some of the pathologies of alcoholism, and why some individuals will develop certain diseases when others do not. For example, many orientals (about 40%) will have a deficiency of ALDH2 activity due to a gene modification and this results in an elevation in acetaldehyde with a visible flushing of the skin after alcohol ingestion. The modified allele is designated ALDH2*2 whilst the normal is ALDH2*1. There are also genetic differences in ADH between populations and these contribute to variation in ethanol oxidation.

Formation of phosphatidylethanol and fatty acid ethyl esters (FAEEs) are two other important routes of ethanol metabolism albeit by non-oxidative pathway (Fig. 9.3; Laposata 1998). Phosphatidylethanol is formed when ethanol becomes the polar group of a phospholipid in a reaction catalysed by phospholipase D. It is found in blood of alcoholics and organs exposed to ethanol, including liver, intestines, stomach, lung, spleen and muscle, in a dose- and time-dependent manner. FAEEs are formed from fatty acids and ethanol in reactions catalysed by either cytosolic or microsomal FAEE synthase. In the former reaction, the immediate precursor is fatty acid, whereas the microsomal pathway utilises fatty acid CoA. The FAEEs are broken down by a cytosolic hydrolase or may traverse the membrane into the intravascular space. Both phosphatidylethanol and FAEEs are cytotoxic and may perturb cell-signalling and protein synthesis.

Induction of microsomal cytochromes following repeated ingestion of alcohol

With the MEOS, which utilises NADPH, there is free radical regeneration and induction of the cytochrome system (Figs 9.1 and 9.2; Lieber 1996). The MEOS is especially important in chronic ethanol ingestion as it is an inducible pathway of ethanol metabolism and is thus of particular significance in chronic ethanol misusers where the existing enzymes are unable to cope with the high ethanol load. The MEOS has a higher K_m for ethanol (8–10 mmol/l) compared with ADH (0.2 to 2.0 mmol/l) so that at low alcohol concentrations, the ADH isoenzymes are more important in oxidising ethanol. The purified protein of MEOS is commonly referred to as CYP2EI or 2EI (formally IIEI) and its induction is due to increases in mRNA levels and its rate of translation.

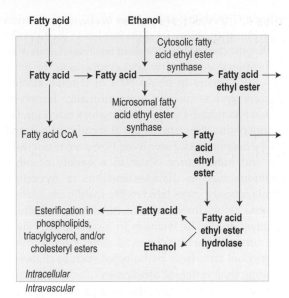

Figure 9.3 Non-oxidative routes of ethanol metabolism. Illustration of the formation of fatty acid ethyl esters in tissues. (Adapted from Laposata 1998.)

Uncoupling of metabolism from oxidative phosphorylation

Some subjects on alcohol feeding regimes have reduced weight, when compared with those on iso-caloric diets without alcohol, suggesting inadequate utilisation of metabolic fuels. Contributory factors responsible for the weight loss or energy deficits in ethanol consumers pertain to the induction of the MEOS, which is energetically wasteful, leads to inadequate coupling of ATP production and may involve increased hydrolysis of ATP via Na⁺-ATPase activities. Additionally, maldigestion or malabsorption, poor dietary intakes and defects in tissue protein turnover may also contribute to such weight loss in alcohol misusers.

Obesity is not apparent in all alcoholics but in some subjects who consume moderate to high amounts of alcohol, obesity may increase. The relationship between alcohol consumption and obesity is controversial and may relate to gender, genetic and dietary factors as well as the levels of alcohol consumed.

The metabolic basis for 'fatty liver' of chronic alcohol ingestion

Traditionally, alcohol-induced liver disease has been thought to have three stages, namely fatty liver (steatosis), alcoholic hepatitis with fibrosis, and cirrhosis, though fatty liver may progress directly to cirrhosis. The ability of the liver to develop steatosis in the presence of low fat diets has led to the hypothesis that the de novo synthesis of triacylglycerols may arise via increases in fatty acid synthesis in the liver. Fatty liver occurs in about 80% of chronic alcohol misusers and is usually asymptomatic. However, when it is combined with inflammatory reactions, i.e. steatohepatitis, the patients are at significant risk and may be hospitalised. Fatty liver, however, is not itself fatal and indeed may occur in a variety of other conditions such as diabetes mellitus or hyperlipidaemia/obesity associated with insulin resistance, oxidative stress/imbalance (i.e. NASH, non-alcoholic steatohepatitis). The changes in alcoholic fatty liver have some distinct biochemical differences to other non-alcohol fatty liver pathologies such as diabetes, reflecting their different aetiologies.

Increased fatty acids in the liver present a greater biochemical 'target' for the free radicals generated as a consequence of alcohol metabolism. This leads to peroxidation of fatty acids within the liver generating malondialdehyde, which in turn can form malondialdehyde-protein adducts. As with acetaldehyde-protein adducts, the malondialdehyde-protein adducts are immunogenic, increase inflammation and are cytotoxic; there are at least five different protein-adduct species formed in alcohol-exposed tissues.

The metabolic basis for fatty liver is still a matter of conjecture. The lipid in affected liver is largely triacylglycerol, which may increase between 10- and 50-fold; there is also a, less marked, increase in esterified cholesterol. Concomitant changes also include an increase in palmitic acid and a fall in arachidonic and linoleic acids in phospholipid. Contributing factors include some or all of the following (Bathgate & Simpson 2002).

(1) Increased NADH/NAD$^+$ ratio

Some groups consider this the driving force for the defects in triacylglycerol synthesis and fatty acid oxidation. Alternatively, H$^+$ derived from excess NADH may be transferred to NADPH, which provides reducing power for biosynthesis of fatty acids (Bathgate & Simpson 2002).

(2) Enhanced substrate supply, including glycerol-3-phosphate and fatty acyl CoA esters

Glycerol-3-phosphate is formed by reduction of dihydroxyacetone phosphate, in a reaction catalysed by glycerate-3-phosphate reductase, which is dependent on NADH, and the increased NADH

arising from alcohol or acetaldehyde oxidation may drive this reaction in favour of glyceraldehyde-3-phosphate. However, an increased NADH/NAD ratio is not necessarily associated with elevated triacylglycerol synthesis (Bathgate & Simpson 2002).

(3) Increased fatty acid uptake

Fatty acid uptake may increase in response to ethanol, possibly reflecting upregulation of intracellular fatty acid binding protein, or decreased peripheral clearance of chylomicrons. De novo synthesis of fatty acids may use ethanol-derived carbon, but acetate derived from ethanol is mainly metabolised in skeletal muscle.

Increased fatty acid synthesis (as a result of increased NADPH derived by transfer of H$^+$ from NADH) has been a favoured hypothesis. However, in human percutaneous liver biopsy samples, reduced fatty acid synthesis occurs and correlates with lipid content in the specimens. Furthermore, the activities of key enzymes in the hepatic synthesis of fatty acids (e.g. acetyl CoA carboxylase) are reduced in the livers of subjects with alcohol-induced steatosis.

Impairment in the rate of mitochondrial β-oxidation of fatty acids may also be another route whereby fatty liver occurs in alcoholism possibly via effects on specific enzymes such as carnitine palmitoyl transferase I or acyl CoA dehydrogenase. Esterification of free fatty acids may also be increased in alcoholic steatosis. Phosphatidate phosphohydrolase is a rate-limiting enzyme in triacylglycerol synthesis and increases in both human and animal liver exposed chronically to ethanol, correlated with the degree of steatosis in clinical samples. Diacylglycerol transferase activity also increases (Bathgate & Simpson 2002).

(4) Export from the liver

The impact of ethanol and/or acetaldehyde on the physiological export processes has been described previously with respect to albumin. The export of triacylglycerol-rich VLDL may also be impaired due to defects in the Golgi apparatus and/or microtubules via adduct formation with acetaldehyde (Bathgate & Simpson 2002).

Lactic acidosis resulting from alcohol ingestion

The increased tissue NADH levels because of alcohol and acetaldehyde metabolism also increase the lactate/pyruvate ratio leading to lactic acidosis which may also be combined with a β-hydroxybutyrate predominant ketoacidosis under some conditions. Blood pH may fall to 7.1 and hypoglycaemia may occur. In severe situations of ketoacidosis and hypoglycaemia, permanent brain damage may arise; in general the prognosis of alcoholic acidosis is good though it depends on liver function. These conditions may be exacerbated by thiamin deficiency and indeed thiamin deficiency per se may hasten acute episodes of lactic acidosis (see Ch. 10, Section 10.1, under 'Thiamin deficiency'). The high concentration of lactic acid also impairs the kidney's ability to excrete uric acid and consequently blood uric acid levels rise (hyperuricaemia), causing gout.

9.3 TOXIC EFFECTS OF CHRONIC ALCOHOL INGESTION

Alcohol ingestion leads to the release of catecholamines and steroid excess

Alcohol causes increased activation of the sympathetic nervous system, with increased circulating catecholamines secreted by the adrenal medulla. Increased circulating cortisol from the adrenal cortex can, very rarely, lead to a pseudo-Cushing's syndrome with typical symptoms of moon face, truncal obesity and muscle weakness, due to hypothalamic-pituitary stimulation. These changes in circulating catecholamines and cortisol have been considered to cause some of the pathology of alcoholism, but contribute little to the major complications such as myopathy, cardiomyopathy and alcoholic liver disease.

Alcoholism also affects the hypothalamic-pituitary-gonadal axis, and these effects are further exacerbated by alcoholic liver disease. There are conflicting data regarding the changes observed. Plasma testosterone is either normal or decreased in men, and increased in women, with oestradiol levels being increased in both men and women, and rising with worsening liver disease. The production of sex hormone-binding globulin is also perturbed by alcohol, complicating the picture further. Feminisation of males, with gynaecomastia and testicular atrophy, tends to occur only after cirrhosis begins, and is more severe in alcoholic compared to non-alcoholic cirrhosis. In women, these changes can cause decreased libido, disturbances in menstruation and early onset of menopause. Sexual dysfunction is also common in men, with reduced libido and impotence. Fertility may also be reduced, with decreased spermatozoa count and motility. It is worth remembering that alcohol misuse can affect virtually every endocrine axis.

Symptoms of excess alcohol intake

Perhaps the most obvious effects of alcohol are on the central nervous system. These are dose dependent and begin with the so-called social modulating effects of alcohol, including increasing cheerfulness, loss of inhibitions and impaired judgement. Heavier consumption leads to agitation, slurred speech, loss of memory, with double vision and staggering. This may then progress to a depressed level of consciousness. This is of particular concern in emergency departments as when people present drunk with a depressed level of consciousness and a head injury, it can be difficult to determine whether there is coexistent pathology such as an extradural haematoma or head injury. A good rule of thumb is not to assume that alcohol is solely responsible for any disturbance in consciousness. Ultimately loss of airway control may occur, with danger of suffocation or aspiration of vomitus and ultimately death. There is a great disparity in the effects of alcohol between individuals. This is due to varying effects of alcohol on the body, and differences in the metabolism of alcohol and waste products of its metabolism.

Acute effects of alcohol on the cardiovascular system involve both the heart and the peripheral vasculature. Peripheral vasodilation causes a sensation of warmth. Although this can be interpreted by the subject as being warmer, it can be dangerous, especially in cold weather or when swimming, as heat loss is rapid but lack of awareness leaves people vulnerable to hypothermia. Cardiac effects are usually in the form of arrhythmias, such as bradycardia, tachycardia (i.e. 'holiday heart' syndrome) or sometimes fatal atrial fibrillation, experienced as palpitations. These are usually self-limiting.

Effects of alcohol on muscle weakness

Alcoholic myopathy is common, affecting 40–60% of all chronic alcohol abusers, and is a major cause of morbidity. It is characterised by muscle weakness, myalgia, muscle cramps and loss of lean tissue; up to 30% of muscle may be lost. Histological assessment correlates well with symptoms, and shows selective atrophy of type II muscle fibres. Reductions in muscle protein and RNA, with reduced rate of protein synthesis, also occur. Rates of protein degradation appear either unaltered or reduced. Recently attention has focused on a role for free radicals in the pathogenesis of alcoholic myopathy. Cholesterol hydroperoxides are increased in alcohol-exposed muscle, implying membrane damage.

Effects of alcohol on facial flushing

Facial flushing with patchy erythematous rash on the trunk and arms is seen in approximately 40% of orientals and is thought to be due to a deficiency of ALDH2. This results in an accumulation of acetaldehyde, with plasma levels around 20 times higher in people with this deficiency. Acetaldehyde is thought to be chiefly responsible for many of the adverse effects of alcohol. Plasma and urinary catecholamine levels are greatly increased in people with aldehyde dehydrogenase deficiency after alcohol consumption. Flushing in Europeans (5%) is due to other mechanisms of unknown aetiology.

Acetaldehyde acts partially through catecholamines, although other mechanisms have also been implicated, including histamine, bradykinin, prostaglandin and endogenous opioids (as well as adduct formation). Administration of aspirin (which irreversibly acetylates and inactivates cyclooxygenase, preventing prostaglandin production) has been shown to block the facial flushing response in some people, implicating a role for prostaglandins. Use of naloxone (an opioid antagonist) has also been shown to reduce flushing in people in whom cyclooxygenase inhibitors had an effect, implicating an interaction between endogenous opioids and prostaglandins.

Effects of alcohol on dehydration

Ethanol affects hypothalamic osmoreceptors, reducing antidiuretic hormone release, so causing reduced salt and water reabsorption in the distal tubule. This results in polyuria and may cause dehydration, especially in spirit drinkers who do not consume much water with their alcoholic drinks. A loss of hypothalamic neurons secreting antidiuretic hormone has also been described in chronic alcoholics, suggesting long-term consequences for fluid balance. Increased plasma atrial natriuretic factor after alcohol consumption may also contribute to this diuresis and resultant dehydration.

Effects of alcohol on liver function

The pathological mechanisms by which cirrhosis occurs are complex, and are still the subject of intensive research. Induction of the MEOS and breakdown of ethanol by catalase results in free radical production. Glutathione (a free radical scavenger) is also reduced in alcoholics, decreasing the cell's ability to dispose of free radicals. Mitochondrial damage occurs, limiting their ability to oxidise fatty acids, which are then oxidised in peroxisomes, further increasing free radical production. These changes eventually result in hepatocyte necrosis, and inflammation and fibrosis then ensue. Acetaldehyde also contributes at this stage by promoting collagen synthesis and fibrosis.

Fatty changes are usually asymptomatic, but can be detected on ultrasound or CT, and are associated with abnormal liver function tests (e.g. raised activities of aminotransferases in serum). Progression to alcoholic hepatitis involves invasion of the liver by neutrophils with hepatocyte necrosis. Giant mitochondria are visible and dense cytoplasmic lesions, known as Mallory bodies, are seen. Alcoholic hepatitis can be asymptomatic but usually presents with abdominal pain, fever and jaundice, or, depending on the severity of disease, patients may have encephalopathy, ascites and ankle oedema, and mortality rates up to 50% have been reported. Continued alcohol consumption may lead to cirrhosis. There is increasing fibrocollagenous deposition, with scarring and disruption of surrounding hepatic architecture. There is ongoing necrosis with concurrent regeneration. This is classically said to be micronodular, but often a mixed pattern is present. Alcoholics usually present with one of the complications of cirrhosis such as gastrointestinal haemorrhage (often due to bleeding from oesophageal varices), ascites, encephalopathy or renal failure. It is uncertain why only a fraction of alcoholics go on to develop cirrhosis. It has been suggested that there may be genetic factors, and that differences in immune response may play a role. Dietary factors may also contribute. For example, with inadequate intake of cysteine and glycine, glutathione production may be impaired. Poor intake of vitamin A, C, E and β-carotene will also reduce the ability of the hepatocyte to cope with the oxidative stress imposed by alcoholism.

9.4 ALCOHOL AND NUTRITION

A variety of studies have shown that chronic ethanol misusers have impaired nutritional status due either to inadequate dietary intakes, persistent damage to the hepatointestinal system or the redirection of funds that would otherwise be used to purchase foods. Malnutrition frequently occurs in alcohol misuse and will further compromise alcohol-associated pathologies.

Chronic alcoholics frequently have deficient intakes of micronutrients (e.g. vitamins B_1, A, C, E and folate) and minerals (e.g. zinc and selenium). Ethanol-induced effects on digestion, absorption and storage will exaggerate these deficiencies. For example, hepatic stores of total retinoids (vitamin A) decrease in chronic ethanol misusers and correlate with severity of liver disease. In contrast, iron status may be adequate in some alcohol misusers due to increased absorption. In very severe cases of alcoholism, classical symptoms of beri-beri and pellagra arise, though these are less common.

A recent study of UK alcoholics attending an inner city alcohol misuse clinic showed that 95–100% had low (below UK RNIs) intakes of vitamin E, folate and selenium. Between 50% and 85% of all subjects had low intakes of calcium, zinc, vitamins A, B_1, B_2, B_6 and C. Reduced intakes of magnesium and iron were reported in about 45% of subjects. However, studies on middle-class alcoholics, free from major organ disease, suggest that when malnutrition is present it is only mild to moderate.

Alcohol will also affect the metabolism of a number of nutrients including thiamin and it has been suggested that about half of alcoholics with liver disease will have thiamin deficiency (see Section 10.1, under 'Thiamin deficiency'). A recent UK study showed that 45% of alcohol misusers without liver disease had either reduced activities of erythrocyte thiamin-dependent transketolase or a high activation ratio. This is of concern as Wernicke's encephalopathy/Wernicke–Korsakoff syndrome is a frequent manifestation of thiamin deficiency, particularly in alcohol misusers. Thiamin deficiency will arise from both inadequate intakes and alcohol-induced interference with active, transport of the vitamin in the gut. Formation of thiamin pyrophosphate may also be impaired by diseased hepatic tissue in alcoholism.

Acute or chronic alcohol impairs the absorption of galactose, glucose, other hexoses, amino acids, biotin, folate and vitamin C. There is no strong evidence that alcohol impairs the absorption of magnesium, riboflavin or pyridoxine so these deficiencies will arise as a result of poor intakes and/or excess loss. Hepato-gastrointestinal damage may have an important role in impairing the absorption of some nutrients such as the fat-soluble vitamins, due to villous injury, bacterial overgrowth of the intestine, pancreatic damage or cholestasis.

There is no association of muscle wasting with malnutrition; alcoholic myopathy arises directly as a consequence of the effect of alcohol or acetaldehyde on muscle. This implies that there is a fundamental problem in assessing malnutrition in chronic alcoholics using anthropometric measures such as muscle or limb circumference (see Ch. 4, Section 4.5, under 'Anthropometry') due to the presence of alcoholic myopathy.

A question arises as to whether the deleterious effects of alcohol on organs and tissues are the direct consequence of malnutrition. However, this belief is no longer held since the pioneering work of Charles Lieber in the 1960s showed that many pathologies, such as alcoholic hepatitis and cirrhosis, could be reproduced in laboratory animals fed an adequate diet. Nevertheless, the concomitant presence of alcoholism and malnutrition exacerbates organ damage and/or nutritional status.

9.5 LINKS BETWEEN ALCOHOL INTAKE AND RISK OF CARDIOVASCULAR DISEASE

A number of epidemiological studies have suggested that light–moderate amounts (1–6 Units per day) of alcohol are cardioprotective and reduce coronary heart disease, particularly in middle-aged men and postmenopausal women. This protective effect is not seen at higher levels of intake and indeed may increase incidence of cardiovascular disease including hypertension. In other words, there is a J- or U-shaped mortality curve. However, there is some uncertainty as to the exact shape of this curve and the point at which the putative protective effect of alcohol becomes harmful. Other studies have challenged any causal relationship between alcohol intake and the cardioprotective phenomena.

In one study, a decreased risk of coronary heart disease was seen at 0–20 g/day and evident up to 72 g/day, whilst consumption of greater than 89 g/day was associated with an increased risk of coronary heart disease. Increases in alcohol consumption from one drink per week or less to one to six drinks per week over 7 years is associated with a 29% fall in the risk of cardiovascular disease.

Some studies have shown that there is a linear relationship between alcohol consumption and blood pressure in men, but a J-shaped relationship in women. Moderate to heavy drinking is associated with an increased risk of stroke. Consumption of up to 3 Units/day, however, reduces ischaemic strokes but binge drinking increases the risk of all types of stroke.

However, when considering the public health consequences of such data, one must also take into account the other effects of alcohol. Consuming only one Unit of alcohol a day may increase the risk of death from some cancers, accidents and violence. Furthermore, there is a substantial body of evidence to support the notion that the total cumulative intake of ethanol (i.e. over a lifetime) will predict disease severity, particularly of the heart, muscle and liver.

The reported cardioprotective effects of alcohol may be due to antioxidants or other substances in the beverages such as polyphenols in red wine. Protective effects may also occur via clot formation and dissolution, reducing circulating levels of fibrinogen, factor VII and plasminogen activator. Platelet aggregability may also be reduced by alcohol. An effect of alcohol in increasing serum HDL cholesterol may be another mechanism.

⊃ Key points

- ⊃ Alcohol misuse is common: in the UK: about 9 million people drink more than recommended guidelines.

- ⊃ The young (school children and adolescents) and women are particularly vulnerable or susceptible to the deleterious effects of alcohol.

- ⊃ In the UK, the overall contribution of ethanol to total energy intake is 6.5% in men and 3.9% in women.

- ⊃ In alcohol misusers, the overall contribution of ethanol to total energy intake may rise to 60% or higher.

- ⊃ Alcohol absorption and metabolism is affected by a number of variables, including gastric alcohol-metabolising enzymes, ethnicity, gender, presence of different foods and body size.

- ⊃ It is a myth that the most affected organs are the brain and liver: organic brain disease and cirrhosis only occurs in about 10–15% of chronic alcoholics.

- ⊃ There are at least 60–120 different alcohol-related pathologies.

- ⊃ Fifty per cent of chronic alcohol misusers will have one or more organ or tissue abnormalities

- ⊃ Alcoholic myopathy is particularly prevalent, affecting 40–60% of chronic alcoholics.

- ⊃ The immediate metabolite of ethanol oxidation, acetaldehyde, is highly toxic.

- ⊃ The effects of alcohol or acetaldehyde on the body are due to many processes, such as adduct formation, changes in protein, carbohydrate and lipid metabolism, membrane dysfunction, altered cytokines and impaired immunological status, perturbations in gene expression, enhanced apoptosis, reactive oxygen species/oxidative stress and changes in intracellular signalling. Many of these will be exacerbated by malnutrition.

- ⊃ All pathways and cell structures have the potential to be targeted by ethanol or its related metabolites.

- ⊃ There are a number of routes of ethanol metabolism. The microsomal ethanol oxidising system (MEOS) is particularly important in chronic alcoholism.

- ⊃ The metabolic basis for 'fatty liver' in chronic alcohol ingestion is still a matter of conjecture and may reflect the fact that a number of processes are affected.

- ⊃ About 50% of alcoholics will have nutritional deficiencies and these can arise via a number of processes including poor dietary intakes, displacement of foods (empty calories theory), maldigestion and malabsorption.

- ⊃ Low to moderate amounts of alcohol may reduce cardiovascular disease, particularly in middle-aged men.

References and further reading

References

Aceto M 2003 Metals in wine. In: Preedy V R, Watson R R (eds) Reviews in food and nutrition toxicity, vol I. Taylor and Francis, London, p 169–203

Bathgate A J, Simpson K J 2002 Alcoholic fatty liver. In: Sherman D I N, Preedy V R, Watson R R (eds) Ethanol and the liver. Mechanisms and management. Taylor and Francis, London, p 3–20

Department of Health 1995 Sensible drinking: the report of an inter-departmental working group. Department of Health, London

Department of Health 2001 Statistical Bulletin. Statistics on alcohol: England, 1978 onwards. Department of Health, London

Foods Standards Agency 2002 McCance and Widdowson's The composition of foods. Royal Society of Chemistry, Cambridge

Haber P S 2000 Metabolism of alcohol by the human stomach. Alcoholism: Clinical & Experimental Research 24:407–408

Henderson L, Gregory J 2002 National diet and nutrition survey: adults aged 19 to 64 years. Volume 1. Types and quantities of foods consumed. HMSO, London

Henderson L, Gregory J, Irving K 2003 National diet and nutrition survey: adults aged 19 to 64 years. Volume 2. Energy, protein, carbohydrate, fat and alcohol intakes. HMSO, London

Kwo P Y, Crabb D W 2002 Genetics of ethanol metabolism and alcoholic liver disease. In: Sherman D I N, Preedy V R, Watson R R (eds) Ethanol and the liver. Mechanisms and management. Taylor and Francis, London, p 95–129

Laposata M 1998 Fatty acid ethyl esters: Nonoxidative metabolites of ethanol. Addiction Biology 3:5–14

Lieber C S 1996 The metabolism of alcohol and its implications for the pathogenesis of disease. In: Preedy V R, Watson R R (eds) Alcohol and the gastrointestinal tract. CRC Press, Boca Raton, p 19–39

Lieber C S 2000 Alcohol: Its metabolism and interaction with nutrients. Annual Review of Nutrition 20:395–430

Mezey E 1985 Effect of ethanol on intestinal morphology, metabolism and function. In: Seitz H K, Kommerell B (eds) Alcohol related diseases in gastroenterology. Springer-Verlag, Berlin, p 342–360

Peters T J, Preedy V R 1998 Metabolic consequences of alcohol ingestion. Novartis Foundation Symposium 216:19–24

Peters T J, Preedy V R 1999 Chronic alcohol abuse: effects on the body. Medicine 27:11–15

Royal Colleges 1995 Alcohol and the heart in perspective. Sensible limits reaffirmed. A Working Group of the Royal Colleges of Physicians, Psychiatrists and General Practitioners. Journal of the Royal College of Physicians of London 29:266–271

Saunders J B, Devereaux B M 2002 Epidemiology and comparative incidence of alcohol-induced liver disease. In: Sherman D I N, Preedy V R, Watson R R (eds) Ethanol and the liver. Mechanisms and management. Taylor and Francis, London, p 389–410

Further reading

Gluud C 2002 Endocrine system. In: Sherman D I N, Preedy V R, Watson R R (eds) Ethanol and the liver. Mechanisms and management. Taylor and Francis, London, p 472–494

Jones A W 2000 Aspects of in-vivo pharmacokinetics of ethanol. Alcoholism: Clinical & Experimental Research 24:400–402

Lader D, Meltzer H 2002 Drinking: Adults' behaviour and knowledge in 2002. Office for National Statistics, London

Roine R 2000 Interaction of prandial state and beverage concentration on alcohol absorption. Alcoholism – Clinical and Experimental Research 24:411–412

CD-ROM contents

Tables

Table CD 9.1 Alcohol consumption level (Units per week), by gender. England, 1988 to 1998

Table CD 9.2 Alcohol dependence of people living in private households, aged 16–64 years. Great Britain in last year

Table CD 9.3 Mean alcohol consumption of pupils in the last 7 days, by gender and age

Table CD 9.4 Consumption rates of different alcohol beverages in the UK

Further reading from the book

Part 3

Micronutrient function

Edited by David A. Bender

10

Water-soluble vitamins

David A. Bender

Objectives

By the end of this chapter you should be able to:

- identify the compounds classified as water-soluble vitamins
- identify good sources of each
- summarise the absorption and transport of each
- summarise the main metabolic functions of each
- describe the main effects of deficiency and excess of each
- be aware of the methods of assessment of status
- discuss the basis for dietary requirements
- appreciate the metabolic interactions between water-soluble vitamins and other nutrients.

10.1 VITAMIN B₁ – THIAMIN

The peripheral nervous system disease beriberi, due to thiamin deficiency, became a major problem of public health in the Far East in the nineteenth century with the introduction of the steam-powered rice mill, which resulted in more widespread consumption of highly milled (polished) rice. While now largely eradicated, beriberi remains a problem in some parts of the world among people whose diet is especially high in carbohydrate. A different condition, affecting the central rather than peripheral nervous system, the Wernicke-Korsakoff syndrome, is also due to thiamin deficiency. It occurs in developed countries, especially among alcoholics and narcotic addicts.

Forms of thiamin in foods, and food sources

In foods, most thiamin is present as the diphosphate (Fig. 10.1), also known as thiamin pyrophosphate; small amounts of mono- and triphosphate also occur. A number of biologically active allithiamins occur in plants. Pork is an especially rich source, but other meat and fish are good sources, as are potatoes, wheat, nuts and beans (see Table CD 10.1).

Thiamin is labile to sulphite, and sulphite treatment of foods results in more or less complete loss of the vitamin.

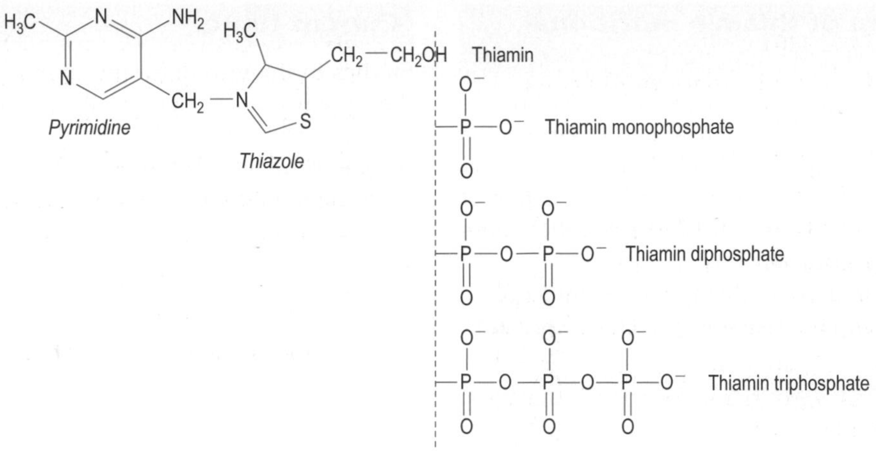

Figure 10.1   Thiamin and the thiamin coenzymes.

Absorption and transport of thiamin

Dietary thiamin phosphates are hydrolysed by intestinal phosphatases, and thiamin is absorbed by active transport in the duodenum and proximal jejunum. The transport system is saturated at relatively low concentrations, so limiting the amount that can be absorbed. There is active transport from the intestinal cells into the bloodstream; this is inhibited by alcohol, leading to thiamin deficiency in alcoholics.

Much of the absorbed thiamin is phosphorylated in the liver, and both free thiamin and thiamin monophosphate circulate in plasma, bound to albumin. All tissues can take up both thiamin and thiamin monophosphate, and are able to phosphorylate them to the active di- and triphosphates.

A small amount of thiamin is excreted in the urine unchanged; the major excretory product is thiochrome. Sweat may contain up to 30–56 nmol of thiamin/l, and in hot conditions this may represent a significant loss of the vitamin.

Metabolic functions of thiamin

Thiamin diphosphate is the coenzyme for three multi-enzyme complexes: pyruvate dehydrogenase (see Fig. CD 10.1) and 2-oxoglutarate dehydrogenase in central energy-yielding metabolic pathways and the branched-chain oxo-acid dehydrogenase in the catabolism of leucine, isoleucine and valine. It is also the coenzyme for transketolase in the pentose phosphate pathway of carbohydrate metabolism (see Fig. CD 10.2).

Thiamin also has a role in electrical conduction in nerve cells; thiamin triphosphate phosphorylates, and so activates, a chloride channel in nerve membranes.

Thiamin deficiency

The biological half-life of thiamin is 10–20 days, and deficiency can develop rapidly during depletion. Diuresis increases the excretion of the vitamin, and patients who are treated with diuretics are potentially at risk of thiamin deficiency.

In deficiency there is impaired entry of pyruvate into the citric acid cycle. Especially on a relatively high carbohydrate diet, this results in increased plasma concentrations of lactate and pyruvate, which may lead to life-threatening acidosis.

Thiamin deficiency can result in three distinct syndromes: a chronic peripheral neuritis, beriberi, which may or may not be associated with heart failure and oedema; acute pernicious (fulminating) beriberi (shoshin beriberi), in which heart failure and metabolic abnormalities predominate, with little evidence of peripheral neuritis; and Wernicke's encephalopathy with Korsakoff's psychosis, associated especially with alcoholism, narcotic abuse and HIV-AIDS. Results from post-mortem examination and brain imaging suggest that Wernicke's encephalopathy is significantly underdiagnosed.

In general, a relatively acute deficiency is involved in the central nervous system lesions of the Wernicke–Korsakoff syndrome. Dry beriberi is associated with a more prolonged, and presumably less severe, deficiency, with a generally low food intake, while higher carbohydrate intake and physical activity predispose to oedema and hence wet beriberi.

Assessment of thiamin nutritional status

The activation of apo-transketolase in erythrocyte lysate by thiamin diphosphate added in vitro is the most widely used index of thiamin nutritional status. An activation coefficient >1.25 is indicative of deficiency, and <1.15 is considered to reflect adequate thiamin nutrition.

Urinary excretion of thiamin plus thiochrome reflects intake, and has also been used to assess status.

The basis for setting dietary thiamin requirements

Thiamin requirements depend largely on carbohydrate intake. In practice, requirements are calculated on the basis of total energy intake, assuming that the average diet provides 40% of energy from fat. For diets that are lower in fat, and hence higher in carbohydrate and protein, thiamin requirements will be higher.

On the basis of depletion/repletion studies, an intake of 0.3 mg/1000 kcal is required for a normal transketolase activation coefficient. Reference intakes are based on 0.5 mg/1000 kcal (0.12 mg/MJ) for adults consuming more than 2000 kcal/day, with the proviso that even in fasting there is a requirement for 0.8 mg of thiamin/day to permit the metabolism of endogenous substrates.

There is no evidence of any toxic effect of high intakes of thiamin, although high parenteral doses have been reported to cause anaphylactic shock. The absorption of dietary thiamin is limited, and no more than about 2.5 mg (10 μmol) can be absorbed from a single dose; free thiamin is rapidly filtered by the kidneys and excreted.

Current topics

Studies in thiamin-deficient animals have revealed the presence of Alzheimer-like amyloid plaques in the brain, and although there is no evidence of similar plaque formation in the brains of patients with the Wernicke–Korsakoff syndrome, this has led to trials of thiamin for treatment of Alzheimer's disease. While some studies have shown beneficial effects, a systematic review has concluded that there is no evidence of beneficial effects of thiamin supplementation in Alzheimer's disease.

➲ Key points

- ➲ Thiamin functions as a coenzyme in energy-yielding metabolism, and in nervous system electrical activity.

- ➲ The classical thiamin deficiency disease, beriberi, affecting the peripheral nervous system, is now rare, although it is still a problem in some areas of the world.

- ➲ Thiamin deficiency, leading to central nervous system damage, is a significant, and underdiagnosed, problem among alcoholics and people with HIV-AIDS.

- ➲ Thiamin requirements depend largely on carbohydrate intake, and are generally calculated on the basis of energy intake or expenditure.

- ➲ Thiamin status is assessed by erythrocyte transketolase activation coefficient.

10.2 RIBOFLAVIN – VITAMIN B$_2$

Riboflavin has a central role as a coenzyme in energy-yielding metabolism, and a more recently discovered role as the prosthetic group of the cryptochromes, the blue-sensitive pigments in the eye that are responsible for day length sensitivity and setting circadian rhythms.

There is very efficient conservation and reutilisation of riboflavin in tissues in deficiency, so that while dietary deficiency is relatively widespread, it is never fatal.

Reoxidation of reduced flavin coenzymes is the major source of oxygen radicals in the body, and riboflavin is also capable of generating reactive oxygen species non-enzymically; as protection against this there is very strict control over the body content of riboflavin; absorption is limited, and any in excess of requirements is rapidly excreted.

Forms of riboflavin in food and dietary sources

The structure of riboflavin is shown in Figure 10.2. Apart from milk and eggs, which contain relatively large amounts of free riboflavin, most of the vitamin

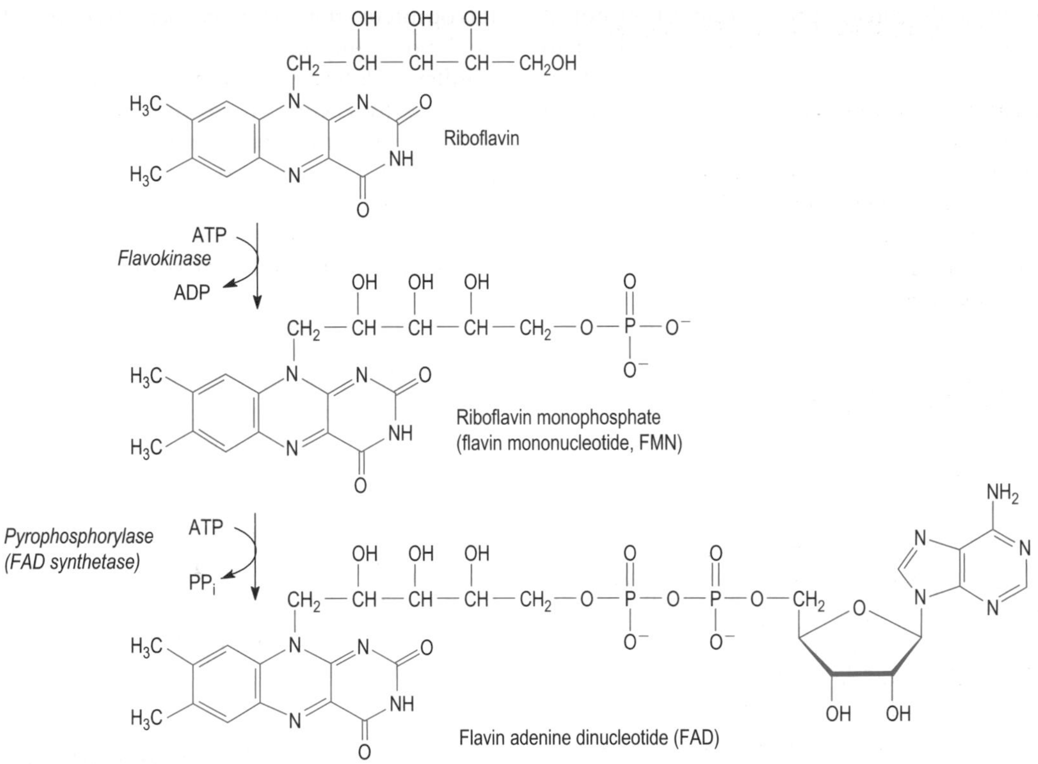

Figure 10.2   Riboflavin and the flavin coenzymes.

in foods is as flavin coenzymes (riboflavin phosphate and FAD, flavin adenine dinucleotide) bound to enzymes. Because of its intense yellow colour, riboflavin is used as a food colour (E-101). A small proportion of riboflavin in foods is covalently bound to enzymes and hence is not biologically available.

Liver, milk, meat and fish are good sources of riboflavin; some green leafy vegetables also provide significant amounts (see Table CD 10.3). In average Western diets some 25–30% of riboflavin comes from milk.

Absorption and transport of riboflavin

FAD and riboflavin phosphate in foods are hydrolysed in the intestinal lumen to yield free riboflavin, which is absorbed in the upper small intestine by a sodium-dependent mechanism that is readily saturated. Intestinal bacteria synthesise riboflavin, which may be absorbed in the colon. Much of the absorbed riboflavin is phosphorylated in the intestinal mucosa, and enters the bloodstream as riboflavin phosphate. Free riboflavin and FAD are the main transport forms in plasma, with a small amount of riboflavin phosphate.

Most riboflavin in tissues is as coenzymes, bound to enzymes; unbound coenzymes are rapidly hydrolysed and free riboflavin leaves cells. There is no evidence of any significant storage of riboflavin; surplus intake is excreted rapidly. In animals, the maximum growth response is achieved with intakes that give about 75% saturation of tissues, and the intake to achieve tissue saturation is that at which there is quantitative urinary excretion of the vitamin. Equally, there is very efficient conservation of tissue riboflavin in deficiency, with only a four-fold difference between the minimum tissue concentration seen in deficiency and saturation.

Metabolic functions of riboflavin

The metabolic function of the flavin coenzymes is as electron carriers in a wide variety of oxidation and reduction reactions central to all metabolic processes, including the mitochondrial electron transport chain.

Flavin oxidases make a significant contribution to the oxidant stress of the body, because the reoxidation of reduced flavins in oxidase reactions leads to the production of oxygen radicals. Overall, some

fruits and vegetables provide significant amounts, as does coffee (see Table CD 10.5).

Most of the niacin in cereals is biologically unavailable, since it is bound as niacytin–nicotinoyl esters to macromolecules. In calculation of niacin intakes, it is conventional to ignore the niacin content of cereals completely, although up to about 10% of niacytin may be labile to gastric acid and hence biologically available.

Quantitatively, synthesis from tryptophan is more important than dietary preformed niacin, and therefore foods that are good sources of protein are also good sources of niacin.

Total niacin intakes are calculated as mg niacin equivalents: the sum of preformed niacin plus 1/60 of tryptophan (the average equivalence of dietary tryptophan and niacin).

Absorption and transport of preformed niacin

Niacin is present in tissues, and therefore in foods, largely as the nicotinamide coenzymes; post-mortem hydrolysis is extremely rapid, so that much of the niacin of meat is free nicotinamide. Any remaining coenzymes in the intestine are also hydrolysed to nicotinamide. A significant proportion of dietary nicotinamide may be deamidated to nicotinic acid by intestinal bacteria. Both vitamers are absorbed from the small intestine by a sodium-dependent saturable process.

In the liver, NAD is synthesised from tryptophan, and then hydrolysed to release nicotinamide, which is exported to other tissues, which can take up both nicotinamide and nicotinic acid to synthesise coenzymes.

There is little or no urinary excretion of either nicotinamide or nicotinic acid, until the plasma concentration is so high that the renal transport mechanism is saturated. The principal metabolites of nicotinamide are N^1-methyl nicotinamide and its oxidation products, methyl pyridone carboxamides.

Metabolic functions of niacin

Nicotinamide is the reactive moiety of the nicotinamide nucleotide coenzymes NAD (nicotinamide adenine dinucleotide) and NADP (nicotinamide adenine dinucleotide phosphate), which are coenzymes in a wide variety of oxidation and reduction reactions in energy-yielding metabolism.

In general, NAD is involved as an electron acceptor in energy-yielding metabolism, and the resultant NADH is oxidised by the mitochondrial electron transport chain. The major coenzyme for reductive synthetic reactions is NADPH.

NAD is the source of ADP-ribose for the reversible modification of proteins by mono-ADP-ribosylation, catalysed by ADP-ribosyltransferases, and poly (ADP-ribosylation), catalysed by poly(ADP-ribose) polymerase. A variety of guanine nucleotide-binding proteins (G-proteins) involved with the regulation of adenylate cyclase activity are regulated by ADP-ribosylation, and poly(ADP-ribosylation) of nuclear proteins is an important step in the DNA repair mechanism.

NAD is also the precursor of two second messengers that act to increase the release of calcium from intracellular stores in response to hormones: cyclic ADP-ribose and nicotinic acid adenine dinucleotide phosphate (NAADP).

Effects of niacin deficiency and excess

Pellagra is the disease due to deficiency of tryptophan and niacin. It is characterised by a photosensitive dermatitis, like severe sunburn, affecting regions of the skin that are exposed to sunlight. Advanced pellagra is also accompanied by a 'dementia' or depressive psychosis, and there may be diarrhoea. Untreated pellagra is fatal.

Pellagra was a major problem of public health in the early part of the twentieth century, and continued to be a problem until the 1980s in some parts of the world. It is now rare, although there have been reports of outbreaks among refugees, and occasional cases are reported in alcoholics, and among people being treated with isoniazid.

The synthesis of NAD from tryptophan requires both riboflavin and vitamin B₆, and deficiency of either may lead to the development of secondary pellagra when intakes of tryptophan and preformed niacin are marginal. Similarly, an excessive intake of leucine, as occurs in parts of India where the dietary staple is jowar (*Sorghum vulgare*), inhibits tryptophan metabolism and may be a factor in the development of pellagra.

Assessment of niacin status

The two methods of assessing niacin nutritional status are measurement of blood nicotinamide nucleotides and the urinary excretion of niacin metabolites, neither of which is wholly satisfactory. Criteria of adequacy are shown in Table CD 10.6.

The basis of setting dietary requirements for niacin

Because of the central role of the nicotinamide nucleotides in energy-yielding metabolism, niacin requirements are conventionally expressed/unit of energy expenditure (i.e. /kcal or /MJ).

From depletion/repletion studies the average niacin requirement is 5.5 mg/1000 kcal (1.3 mg/MJ). Allowing for individual variation, reference intakes are set at 6.6 mg niacin equivalents (preformed niacin + 1/60 of the dietary tryptophan)/1000 kcal (1.6 mg/MJ). Even when energy intakes are very low, it must be assumed that energy expenditure will not fall below about 2000 kcal, and this is the basis for the calculation of reference intakes for subjects with very low energy intakes.

Upper levels of niacin intake

High intakes of niacin cause liver damage. Sustained release preparations are associated with more severe liver damage and clinical liver failure, because they permit more prolonged maintenance of high tissue concentrations of the vitamin. Nicotinic acid is used clinically to treat hyperlipidaemia. It causes a marked vasodilatation, with flushing, burning and itching of the skin and possibly also hypotension.

The tolerable upper limit of niacin intake is 35 mg/day for adults. The European Health Food Manufacturers' Federation restricts over-the-counter supplements to 500 mg/day. Where it is being used to treat hyperlipidaemia, and in trials for the prevention of type 1 diabetes mellitus, a tentative upper limit has been set at 3 g/day.

Current topics: nicotinamide for the prevention of type 1 diabetes mellitus

In experimental animals, nicotinamide protects against the destruction of pancreatic β-islet cells by diabetogenic agents. Type 1 diabetes mellitus is caused by autoimmune destruction of β-cells, and autoantibodies against β-cell proteins can be detected in the circulation several years before the onset of disease. It has been suggested that nicotinamide may delay the development of diabetes in susceptible subjects, although it has no effect once diabetes has developed. Preliminary studies in people at risk of developing type 1 diabetes are promising.

⊃ Key points

- ⊃ There are two niacin vitamers: nicotinic acid and nicotinamide.

- ⊃ Niacin is not strictly a vitamin; endogenous synthesis from tryptophan is more important than dietary intake of preformed niacin.

- ⊃ Niacin intake is calculated as mg niacin equivalents: preformed niacin + 1/60 tryptophan intake.

- ⊃ Deficiency of riboflavin or vitamin B_6 impairs tryptophan metabolism and may lead to the development of pellagra, as may a number of drugs that react with vitamin B_6.

- ⊃ Niacin functions as the nicotinamide ring of the coenzymes NAD and NADP in oxidation and reduction reactions.

- ⊃ NAD is the source of ADP-ribose for ADP-ribosylation of G-proteins and poly(ADP-ribosylation) of nuclear proteins for DNA repair.

- ⊃ NAD is the precursor for synthesis of second messengers that regulate intracellular calcium concentrations in response to hormones.

- ⊃ Current methods of assessing niacin status are unsatisfactory.

- ⊃ Niacin requirements are calculated on the basis of energy intake.

- ⊃ High intakes of niacin cause liver damage, and high intakes of nicotinic acid cause vasodilation.

- ⊃ Nicotinic acid is used in pharmacological doses to treat hyperlipidaemia.

- ⊃ Trials of high doses of nicotinamide to prevent the development of type 1 diabetes mellitus are promising.

10.4 VITAMIN B$_6$

Vitamin B$_6$ has a central role in the metabolism of amino acids, is the cofactor for glycogen phosphorylase, and has a role in the modulation of steroid hormone action and regulation of gene expression.

The vitamin is widely distributed in foods, and clinical deficiency is virtually unknown. However, marginal status, affecting amino acid metabolism and steroid hormone responsiveness, is relatively common.

Oestrogens cause abnormalities of tryptophan B$_6$ metabolism which resemble those seen in vitamin deficiency, and the vitamin is widely used to treat the side-effects of oestrogen administration and the premenstrual syndrome, although there is little evidence of efficacy. High doses of the vitamin, of the order of 100 times requirements, cause peripheral sensory neuropathy.

Forms of vitamin B$_6$ in foods and good food sources

The generic descriptor vitamin B$_6$ includes six vitamers: the alcohol pyridoxine, the aldehyde pyridoxal, the amine pyridoxamine and their 5'-phosphates (Fig. 10.4). The vitamers are metabolically interconvertible, and as far as is known, they have equal biological activity.

Meat, fish, potatoes and bananas are good sources of vitamin B$_6$; milk, nuts, beans and vegetables provide significant amounts (see Table CD 10.7). Up to 75% of the vitamin B$_6$ in plant foods is present as glycosides, which have limited availability.

A proportion of the vitamin B$_6$ in foods may be biologically unavailable after heating, as a result of the formation of (phospho)pyridoxyllysine by reduction of the bond by which the vitamin is bound to the ε-amino groups of lysine in proteins. Pyridoxyllysine is a vitamin B$_6$ antimetabolite, and formation of pyridoxyllysine may also affect the nutritional value of proteins in which lysine is the limiting amino acid (see Ch. 8, Table 8.1).

Absorption and transport of vitamin B$_6$

The phosphorylated vitamers are hydrolysed by alkaline phosphatase in the intestinal mucosa; pyridoxal, pyridoxamine and pyridoxine are all absorbed rapidly by carrier-mediated diffusion, and there is net accumulation by metabolic trapping as pyridoxal phosphate.

Liver exports both pyridoxal phosphate, bound to albumin, and pyridoxal, which circulates bound to both albumin and haemoglobin. Extrahepatic tissues take up pyridoxal after hydrolysis of pyridoxal phosphate in plasma by extracellular alkaline phosphatase, followed by phosphorylation to trap the vitamin in cells. In the liver, vitamin B$_6$ in excess of requirements is oxidised to 4-pyridoxic acid, which is the main excretory product.

Some 80% of the body's total vitamin B$_6$ is pyridoxal phosphate in muscle, bound to glycogen phosphorylase. This is not released from muscle in times of deficiency, but rather in starvation, as muscle glycogen reserves are exhausted. Under these conditions it is potentially available for redistribution to other tissues, and especially liver and kidney, to meet the requirement for gluconeogenesis from amino acids.

Metabolic functions of vitamin B$_6$

The metabolically active vitamer is pyridoxal phosphate, which is involved in many reactions of amino acid metabolism, in glycogen phosphorylase and in the recycling of steroid hormone receptors from tight nuclear binding.

Vitamin B$_6$-dependent enzymes catalyse four main types of reaction involving amino acids: transamination (permitting both utilisation of amino acid carbon skeletons for gluconeogenesis or ketogenesis and also the synthesis of non-essential amino acids); decarboxylation to form a variety of biologically

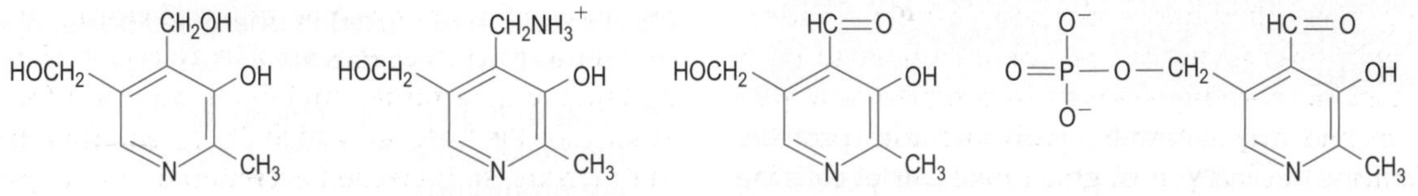

Figure 10.4 Vitamin B$_6$ vitamers.

active amines; racemisation; and a variety of side-chain reactions.

Steroid hormones act by binding to nuclear receptors that then bind to hormone response elements on DNA, altering the transcription of specific genes. Pyridoxal phosphate acts to release the hormone-receptor complex from DNA binding, so terminating the nuclear action of the hormone. In experimental animals, vitamin B$_6$ deficiency results in increased and prolonged nuclear uptake and retention of steroid hormones in target tissues, and enhanced end-organ responsiveness to low doses of hormones.

Effects of vitamin B$_6$ deficiency and excess

Clinical deficiency of vitamin B$_6$ is extremely rare. The vitamin is widely distributed in foods and it is synthesised by intestinal flora. However, several studies have shown that 10–20% of the population of developed countries have marginal or inadequate status.

Much of our knowledge of human vitamin B$_6$ deficiency is derived from an 'outbreak' in the early 1950s, which resulted from an infant milk preparation that had undergone severe heating in manufacture. The result was the formation of the antimetabolite pyridoxyllysine by reaction between pyridoxal phosphate and the ε-amino groups of lysine in proteins. In addition to a number of metabolic abnormalities, many of the affected infants convulsed. They responded to the administration of vitamin B$_6$.

Vitamin B$_6$ deficiency may result from the prolonged administration of drugs that are carbonyl trapping reagents and can form biologically inactive adducts with pyridoxal. Such compounds include penicillamine and isoniazid. Drug-induced vitamin B$_6$ deficiency frequently manifests as the tryptophan-niacin deficiency disease pellagra because synthesis of the nicotinamide nucleotide coenzymes from tryptophan is pyridoxal phosphate dependent.

Vitamin B$_6$ toxicity

Supplements of 50–200 mg vitamin B$_6$/day are widely prescribed and self-prescribed for a variety of conditions, including premenstrual syndrome, depression, morning sickness in pregnancy, hypertension and carpal tunnel syndrome, although the evidence of efficacy is slight. There are promising results from trials of pyridoxamine to prevent non-enzymic glycation of proteins in diabetic patients,

and hence slow the development of the adverse effects of poor glycaemic control.

Animal studies have shown that vitamin B$_6$ in gross excess is neurotoxic, causing peripheral neuropathy. Sensory neuropathy has been reported in patients who had been taking between 2000–7000 mg of pyridoxine/day for several months. On withdrawal of the supplements there was considerable recovery of neuronal function, although there was residual nerve damage in some patients.

There is little evidence that intakes up 200 mg vitamin B$_6$/day are associated with adverse effects. The US Food and Nutrition Board set a tolerable upper level for adults of 100 mg/day; the EU Scientific Committee on Food 25 mg/day.

The assessment of vitamin B$_6$ nutritional status

There are a number of indices of vitamin B$_6$ status available: plasma concentrations of the vitamin, urinary excretion of 4-pyridoxic acid, activation of erythrocyte aminotransferases by pyridoxal phosphate added in vitro, and the ability to metabolise test doses of tryptophan and methionine. None is wholly satisfactory, and where more than one index has been used in population studies there is poor agreement between different methods. Criteria of adequacy are shown in Table CD 10.8.

The oxidation of tryptophan (see Fig. CD 10.3) includes the vitamin B$_6$-dependent enzyme kynureninase and in deficiency, after a test dose of tryptophan, there is a considerable increase in the urinary excretion of xanthurenic and kynurenic acids. However, cortisol induces the first enzyme of the pathway, tryptophan dioxygenase, leading to a rate of metabolism that is greater than the capacity of kynureninase, so that people who are stressed will show results that falsely suggest vitamin B$_6$ deficiency. Similarly, oestrogen metabolites inhibit kynureninase and again give results that falsely suggest vitamin B$_6$ deficiency.

The conversion of homocysteine (arising from methionine) to cysteine (see Fig. CD 10.4) includes two pyridoxal phosphate dependent steps; in vitamin B$_6$ deficiency there is an increase in the urinary excretion of homocysteine after a loading dose of methionine. However, the metabolic fate of homocysteine is determined mainly by the need for cysteine and the rate at which it is remethylated to methionine, so increased excretion of homocysteine following a test dose of methionine cannot necessarily be regarded as evidence of vitamin B$_6$ deficiency.

The basis of setting dietary vitamin B₆ requirements

Early studies of vitamin B₆ requirements used the development of abnormalities of tryptophan or methionine metabolism during depletion, and normalisation during repletion. Abnormalities develop faster during depletion in subjects maintained on a high protein diet, and during repletion normalisation occurs faster in subjects maintained on a low protein diet. From such studies the average requirement was set at 13 μg/gram dietary protein, and reference intakes were based on 15–16 μg/g dietary protein.

More recent studies, using more sensitive indices of status, have shown average requirements of 15–16 μg/g of dietary protein, suggesting a reference intake of 18–20 μg/g protein.

In 1998 the reference intake in the USA and Canada was reduced from the previous RDA of 2 mg/day for men and 1.6 mg/day for women to 1.3 mg/day for both. The report cites six studies that demonstrated that this level of intake would maintain a plasma concentration of pyridoxal phosphate of at least 20 nmol/l, although, as shown in Table CD 10.8, the more generally accepted criterion of adequacy is 30 nmol/l.

Current topics: vitamin B₆ and hyperhomocysteinaemia, vitamin B₆ and hormone-dependent cancer

Epidemiological studies suggest that hyperhomocysteinaemia is most significantly correlated with low folate status, but there is also a significant association with low vitamin B₆ status. Supplementation trials have shown that while folate supplements lower fasting homocysteine in moderately hyperhomocysteinaemic subjects, supplements of 10 mg/day vitamin B₆ have no effect, although supplements do reduce the peak plasma concentration of homocysteine following a test dose of methionine. It thus seems unlikely that intakes of vitamin B₆ above amounts that are adequate to prevent metabolic signs of deficiency will be beneficial in lowering plasma concentrations of homocysteine.

The role of pyridoxal phosphate in attenuating the actions of steroid hormones suggests either that inadequate vitamin B₆ status may be a factor in the development of hormone-dependent cancer of the breast, uterus and prostate, or that supplements may be protective. There is no evidence as yet on which to base recommendations for higher intakes of the vitamin.

⮑ Key points

- ⮑ Vitamin B₆ functions as a coenzyme in a wide variety of reactions of amino acids, in glycogen phosphorylase and to regulate the actions of steroid hormones.

- ⮑ Clinical deficiency of vitamin B₆ is more or less unknown, but marginal status is widespread.

- ⮑ Inadequate vitamin B₆ status may be a factor in hyperhomocysteinaemia, and hence cardiovascular disease, and in steroid-dependent cancer.

- ⮑ A number of drugs react with vitamin B₆ and may cause deficiency that manifests as pellagra due to impaired synthesis of niacin from tryptophan.

- ⮑ Vitamin B₆ status can be assessed by measuring blood levels, excretion of 4-pyridoxic acid, erythrocyte aminotransferase activation coefficient or the metabolism of test doses of tryptophan or methionine.

- ⮑ Vitamin B₆ requirements are calculated per unit dietary protein intake.

- ⮑ Vitamin B₆ supplements are used to treat premenstrual syndrome and some other conditions (with little evidence of efficacy).

- ⮑ Very high doses of vitamin B₆ cause sensory nerve damage.

10.5 FOLATES

Folic acid derivatives function in the transfer of one-carbon fragments in a variety of reactions.

Although folate is widely distributed in foods, deficiency is not uncommon, and a number of commonly used drugs can cause folate depletion. Marginal folate status is a factor in the development of neural tube defects, and supplements of 400 μg/day periconceptionally reduce the incidence significantly.

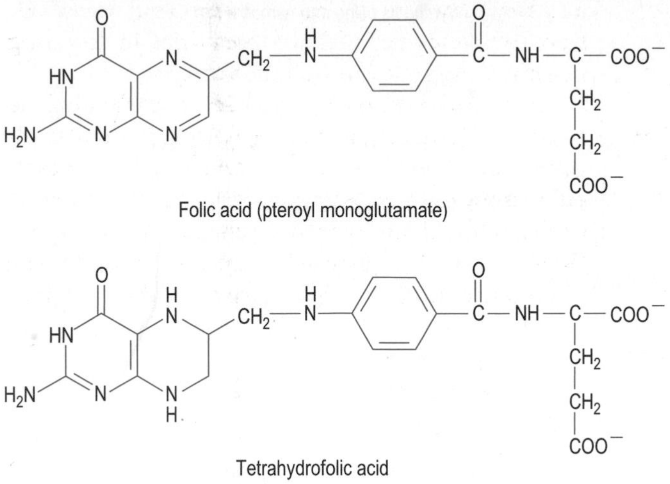

Figure 10.5 Folic acid.

Folic acid (pteroyl monoglutamate)

Tetrahydrofolic acid

High intakes of folate lower the plasma concentration of homocysteine in people genetically at risk of hyperhomocysteinemia, and may reduce the risk of cardiovascular disease. There is also evidence that low folate status is associated with increased risk of colorectal and other cancers. Mandatory enrichment of cereal products with folic acid has been introduced in the USA and elsewhere, and considered in other countries.

Forms in foods and good food sources

The structure of folic acid is shown in Figure 10.5. In the coenzymes the ring is fully reduced to tetrahydrofolate, and there are up to six additional glutamate residues, linked by γ-glutamyl peptide bonds. Although the terms 'folic acid' and 'folate' are often used interchangeably, correctly 'folic acid' refers to the oxidised compound, dihydrofolate monoglutamate, and the tetrahydrofolate derivatives are collectively known as 'folates'.

Tetrahydrofolate can carry one-carbon fragments attached to *N*-5 (formyl, formimino or methyl groups), *N*-10 (formyl) or bridging *N*-5-*N*-10 (methylene or methenyl groups) (see Fig. CD 10.5).

5-Formyl-tetrahydrofolate is more stable to atmospheric oxidation than folic acid, and is commonly used in pharmaceutical preparations; it is also known as folinic acid, and the synthetic (racemic) compound as leucovorin.

The folate in foods consists of a mixture of different one-carbon substituted derivatives, with varying numbers of conjugated glutamyl residues; their biological availability differs, but is consistently lower than that of folic acid, which is the compound used in studies to determine requirements, and in food fortification. In order to permit calculation of folate intakes in terms of both naturally occurring mixed food folates and added folic acid, 1 μg dietary folate equivalent has been defined as the sum of μg food folate + 1.7 × μg folic acid.

Liver is an especially rich source of folate; green leafy vegetables, beans, nuts and milk are good sources, as are some fruits (see Table CD 10.9).

Absorption and transport of folate

In the intestinal lumen, folate conjugates are hydrolysed by conjugase, a zinc-dependent enzyme, and folate is absorbed in the jejunum. The biological availability of folate from milk is considerably greater than that of unbound folate, because it is bound to a binding protein and the protein–folate complex is absorbed intact, from the ileum, by a different mechanism. The availability of folate from cereal foods, or of free folic acid taken with cereal foods, is lower.

Most of the folate undergoes reduction and methylation in the intestinal mucosa, so that what enters the bloodstream is mainly methyltetrahydrofolate, which circulates bound to albumin, and is the main vitamer for uptake by tissues. Small amounts of other one-carbon substituted folates also circulate, and are also available for tissue uptake.

Folate monoglutamates cross cell membranes readily, while polyglutamates do not, so formation of conjugates permits intracellular accumulation of folate. Rapid formation of at least a diglutamate is essential for tissue uptake and retention. Further conjugation to form the metabolically active coenzymes can proceed in a more leisurely fashion.

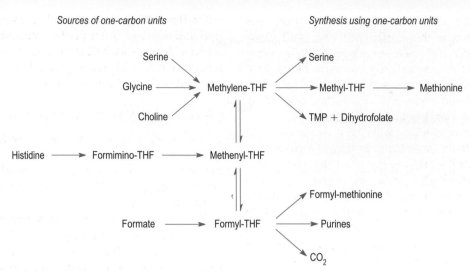

Figure 10.6 Sources and uses of one-carbon units bound to folate.

One-carbon substituted folates are poor substrates for conjugation; since the main form that is taken up into tissues is methyltetrahydrofolate, demethylation by the action of methionine synthetase is essential for tissue accumulation.

Metabolic functions of folate

The metabolic role of folate is as a carrier of one-carbon fragments, both in catabolism and biosynthetic reactions. The major sources of the one-carbon fragments, their uses, and interconversion of substituted folates, are shown in Figure 10.6.

The major point of entry for one-carbon fragments into substituted folates is methylene-tetrahydrofolate, which is formed by the catabolism of glycine, serine and choline. Serine is the major source of one-carbon substituted folates for biosynthetic reactions. The other sources of one-carbon-substituted folate are important for catabolism of the substrates rather than provision of one-carbon units for biosynthetic reactions.

Methylene, methenyl and 10-formyl tetrahydrofolates are freely interconvertible. This means that single carbon fragments entering the folate pool in any form other than methyltetrahydrofolate can readily be available for any of the biosynthetic reactions shown in Figure 10.6. When there is a greater entry of one-carbon units into the folate pool than is required for biosynthetic reactions, the surplus can be oxidised to CO_2 by way of 10-formyl-tetrahydrofolate, thus ensuring a continuing supply of free tetrahydrofolate for catabolic reactions.

The reduction of methylene tetrahydrofolate to methyltetrahydrofolate, catalysed by methylene tetrahydrofolate reductase, is irreversible and methyltetrahydrofolate, which is the main form of folate taken up into tissues, can only be utilised after demethylation catalysed by methionine synthetase.

Effects of folate deficiency and excess

Folate deficiency is relatively common; some 8–10% of the population of developed countries have low folate stores. Deficiency results in megaloblastic anaemia – the release into the circulation of immature red blood cell precursors due to a failure of the normal process of maturation in the bone marrow, because of impaired synthesis of purines and pyrimidines for DNA synthesis. There may also be a low white cell and platelet count, as well as more hyper-segmented neutrophils. Deficiency is frequently accompanied by depression, insomnia, forgetfulness and irritability, and sometimes cognitive impairment and dementia. Suboptimal folate status is also associated with increased incidence of neural tube defects, hyperhomocysteinaemia leading to increased risk of cardiovascular disease and altered methylation of DNA, which may increase cancer risk.

Folate deficiency and neural tube defects

The development of the brain and spinal cord begins around day 18 of gestation; closure begins about day 21 and is complete by day 24 – before the woman knows she is pregnant. The closed neural tube stimulates the development of the bony structures that will become the spinal cord and skull. Bone does not form over unclosed regions, leading to the congenital defects collectively known as neural tube defects, anencephaly and spina bifida, which affect between 0.5 and 8 per 1000 live births, depending on genetic and environmental factors.

A number of studies in the 1960s suggested that low folate status was a factor in neural tube defects, and in the 1990s intervention studies showed that supplements of 400 μg/day of folic acid, begun before conception, halved the incidence. It is unlikely that an increase in folate intake equivalent to 400 μg/day of folic acid could be achieved from unfortified foods, and women who are planning a pregnancy are advised to take supplements.

Drug-induced folate deficiency

A number of folate antimetabolites are used clinically, as cancer chemotherapy, and as antibacterial and antimalarial agents, and their prolonged use can result in iatrogenic folate deficiency. The older antiepileptic drugs, such as diphenylhydantoin (phenytoin), phenobarbital and primidone, can also cause folate deficiency.

Upper levels of folate intake

Although folic acid has low toxicity, two groups of people are at risk of adverse effects of high intakes that might result from widespread enrichment of foods or indiscriminate use of supplements:

1. High intakes of folic acid mask the development of megaloblastic anaemia due to vitamin B_{12} deficiency, so that irreversible nerve damage is the presenting sign. The elderly are especially vulnerable, because of atrophic gastritis. An intake of 1000 μg/day is considered unlikely to mask the development of megaloblastic anaemia in elderly people, and this can be considered to be an upper level of habitual intake.
2. Intakes of folic acid in excess of about 5000 μg/day antagonise the anticonvulsants used in treatment of epilepsy, leading to an increase in fit frequency.

The UK Department of Health considered the number of people aged over 50 who would be exposed to intakes greater than 1000 μg/day, and the number of neural tube defects that would be prevented, at various levels of folic acid enrichment of flour, and concluded that fortification at 240 μg/100 g flour would have a significant beneficial effect

without resulting in unacceptably high intakes by any population group. After public consultation in UK, it was decided in May 2002 not to require fortification of flour with folic acid pending surveillance of the effects of mandatory fortification in other countries.

Assessment of folate status

A number of methods have been developed to permit assessment of folate status and to differentiate between deficiency of folate or vitamin B_{12} as the cause of megaloblastic anaemia. Criteria of folate status are shown in Table CD 10.10.

The serum or erythrocyte concentration of folate can be measured by radioligand binding and microbiological assays. Folate is incorporated into erythrocytes during erythropoiesis, and does not enter the cells in the circulation to any significant extent; erythrocyte folate is generally considered to give an indication of folate status over 1–3 months (the lifespan of erythrocytes in the circulation is 120 days), and not to be subject to variations in recent intake.

The ability to metabolise a test dose of histidine provides a sensitive functional test of folate status; formiminoglutamate (FIGLU) is an intermediate in histidine catabolism, and is metabolised by a folate-dependent enzyme. In deficiency the activity of this enzyme is impaired, and FIGLU accumulates and is excreted in the urine.

The ability of deoxyuridine to suppress the incorporation of [³H]thymidine into DNA in rapidly dividing cells (bone marrow biopsy or transformed lymphocytes) also gives an index of folate status. Cells that have been pre-incubated with deoxyuridine then exposed to [³H]thymidine incorporate little or none of the labelled material into DNA, because of dilution by the larger pool of newly synthesised thymidine monophosphate (TMP). In normal cells the incorporation of [³H]thymidine into DNA after pre-incubation with dUMP is 1.4–1.8% of that without pre-incubation. By contrast, folate-deficient cells form little or no thymidine from dUMP, and hence incorporate as much of the [³H]thymidine after incubation with dUMP as they do without pre-incubation.

The basis of setting dietary requirements

At the time that the UK and EU reference intakes of folate shown in Appendix Table A13 were being discussed, the results of intervention trials for the prevention of neural tube defects were only just becoming available, and there was no information concerning the effects of folate status on hyper-homocysteinaemia. The US/Canadian report noted specifically that protective effects with respect to neural tube defects were not considered relevant to the determination of the dietary reference intake of folate, and there was insufficient evidence to associate higher intakes of folate with reduced risk of cardiovascular disease.

The total body pool of folate in adults is some 17 μmol (7.5 mg), with a biological half-life of 101 days, suggesting a minimum requirement for replacement of 85 nmol (37 μg) per day. Studies of the urinary excretion of folate metabolites in subjects maintained on folate-free diets suggest that there is catabolism of some 170 nmol (80 μg) of folate/day.

Depletion/repletion studies to determine folate requirements suggest a requirement of the order of 170–220 nmol (80–100 μg)/day. However, because of the problems of determining the availability of the mixed folates foods, reference intakes allow a wide margin of safety, and are generally based on an allowance of 3–6 μg (7–14 nmol)/kg body weight; 200–400 μg/day for adults.

Current topics: folic acid, hyperhomocysteinaemia, cardiovascular disease and colorectal cancer

A genetic polymorphism of methylene tetrahydrofolate reductase results in the enzyme being thermolabile (i.e. unstable to heating to about 40–45°C) (refer Section 29.5). The variant enzyme is also unstable in vivo; people who are homozygous for the thermolabile enzyme have about 50% of normal enzyme activity in tissues. A number of studies have shown that the thermolabile variant is two- to three-fold more common among people with atherosclerosis and coronary heart disease than among disease-free people of the same ethnic origin.

Being homozygous for the variant of the enzyme is a necessary, but not sufficient, condition for the development of hyperhomocysteinaemia. Homozygotes with a high folate intake have plasma concentrations of homocysteine as low as heterozygotes or people who are homozygous for the stable enzyme. Two possible mechanisms have been proposed to explain how a high intake of folate can mask the effect of being homozygous for the enzyme.

Most dietary folate is methylated to methyltetrahydrofolate in the intestinal mucosa. Intestinal mucosal cells have a rapid turnover, typically 48 hours from proliferation in the crypt to shedding at the tip of the villus. An unstable enzyme, which loses activity over a shorter time than normal, is irrelevant in cells that have a rapid turnover. A high intake of folate will therefore result in a high rate of supply of methyltetrahydrofolate to tissues, arising from newly absorbed folate, so that impaired turnover of folate within tissues would be less important.

Methylene tetrahydrofolate reductase may be more stable in the presence of its substrate. Hence it is possible that high tissue levels of methylene tetrahydrofolate (resulting from a high folate status) may protect the enzyme and enhance its stability.

A number of epidemiological studies during the 1990s identified elevation of plasma homocysteine as an independent risk factor for cardiovascular disease, and supplements of folate lower plasma homocysteine in many hyperhomocysteinaemic subjects. It remains to be demonstrated whether or not lowering homocysteine will reduce the risk of cardiovascular disease.

Epidemiological studies also suggest that low folate status is associated with an increased risk of colorectal and other cancers. It is difficult to determine the importance of folate per se, since the vegetables that are major sources of folate are also sources of a variety of other compounds that have potentially protective effects. There is, however, evidence that folate deficiency leads to aberrant methylation of DNA. Methylation is important in the silencing of genes during development and tissue differentiation, and altered methylation may well result in dedifferentiation and the development of cancer.

⊃ Key points

- ⊃ Folate functions as a coenzyme in one-carbon transfer reactions.

- ⊃ The availability of mixed food folates is lower than that of free folic acid.

- ⊃ Dietary folate deficiency is not uncommon; deficiency results in megaloblastic anaemia.

- ⊃ Low folate status is associated with neural tube defects, and periconceptional supplements reduce the incidence.

- ⊃ Low folate status is associated with hyperhomocysteinaemia and cardiovascular disease; high folate status overcomes the hyperhomocysteinaemia associated with the thermolabile variant of methylene tetrahydrofolate reductase.

➲ Low folate status is associated with altered methylation of DNA, and possibly cancer.

➲ Folate status can be assessed by measuring plasma or erythrocyte concentrations, metabolism of a test dose of histidine, or suppression of the incorporation in vitro of [^{3}H]thymidine into DNA by dUMP.

➲ Current estimates of folate requirements include a wide margin of safety because of the lack of information on the availability of mixed food folates. They do not take account of the higher intakes required to reduce neural tube defects or lower plasma homocysteine.

➲ High intakes of folate may mask the megaloblastic anaemia of vitamin B$_{12}$ deficiency due to atrophic gastritis in the elderly, and may antagonise antiepileptic medication.

10.6 VITAMIN B$_{12}$

Dietary deficiency of vitamin B$_{12}$ only occurs among strict vegans, but deficiency as a result of impaired absorption is not uncommon, especially among elderly people with atrophic gastritis. Deficiency results in the development of pernicious anaemia – megaloblastic anaemia (as seen in folate deficiency) with degeneration of the spinal cord.

Forms of vitamin B$_{12}$ in foods and good food sources

The structure of vitamin B$_{12}$ is shown in Figure 10.7; the various vitamers have different groups chelated to the central cobalt atom: CN$^-$ (cyanocobalamin); OH$^-$ (hydroxocobalamin); H$_2$O (aquocobalamin);

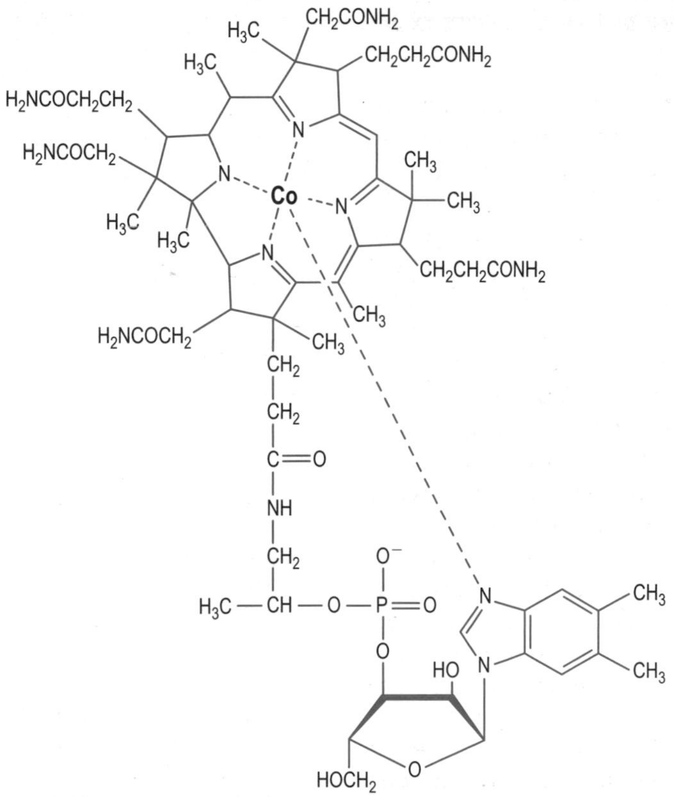

Figure 10.7 Vitamin B$_{12}$.

−CH$_3$ (methylcobalamin); 5'-deoxy-5'adenosine (adenosylcobalamin).

Cyanocobalamin is not an important naturally occurring vitamer; because it is more stable to light than the other vitamers it is used in pharmaceutical preparations.

Vitamin B$_{12}$ is found only in foods of animal origin; there are no plant sources. Rich sources include liver, fish and meat (see Table CD 10.11). A number of reports have suggested that vitamin B$_{12}$ occurs in some algae, but this is probably the result of bacterial contamination of the water in which they were grown.

A number of related compounds in plants do not have vitamin activity (and indeed are antimetabolites of the vitamin), but are growth factors for B$_{12}$-dependent microorganisms, and hence give a misleading result when the vitamin is measured microbiologically.

Absorption and transport of vitamin B$_{12}$

Very small amounts of vitamin B$_{12}$ can be absorbed by diffusion across the intestinal mucosa, but under normal conditions this is insignificant; the major route of vitamin B$_{12}$ absorption is by way of binding to intrinsic factor, a glycoprotein secreted by the gastric parietal cells.

Both gastric acid and pepsin are important in vitamin B$_{12}$ nutrition, serving to release the vitamin from protein binding. Between 10 and 15% of people over 60 show some degree of deficiency as a result of impaired absorption due to atrophic gastritis. In the early stages there is failure of acid secretion, resulting in failure to release the vitamin from dietary proteins, although the absorption of free crystalline vitamin is normal. As the condition progresses, so there is also failure of the secretion of intrinsic factor.

In the stomach, vitamin B$_{12}$ binds to cobalophilin, a binding protein secreted in saliva. In the duodenum cobalophilin is hydrolysed, releasing the vitamin for binding to intrinsic factor. The vitamin B$_{12}$-intrinsic factor complex is absorbed from the distal third of the ileum by receptor-mediated endocytosis. Inside the mucosal cell, the vitamin is released by proteolysis and is bound to transcobalamin II for export from the enterocytes. Tissue uptake is by receptor-mediated endocytosis of holo-transcobalamin II, followed by proteolysis to release hydroxocobalamin, which may either undergo methylation to methylcobalamin in the cytosol, or enter the mitochondria to form adenosylcobalamin.

Although transcobalamin II is the metabolically important pool of plasma vitamin B$_{12}$, it accounts for only 10–15% of the total circulating vitamin. The majority is bound to haptocorrin (also known as transcobalamin I). The function of haptocorrin is not well understood; it does not seem to be involved in tissue uptake or inter-tissue transport of the vitamin. A third plasma vitamin B$_{12}$-binding protein, transcobalamin III, provides a mechanism for returning vitamin B$_{12}$ and its metabolites from peripheral tissues to the liver.

There is considerable enterohepatic circulation of vitamin B$_{12}$; between 1 and 9 μg is secreted in the bile each day, and is mainly reabsorbed bound to intrinsic factor. This seems to be a mechanism for excretion of inactive metabolites of the vitamin; only active vitamin B$_{12}$ binds to intrinsic factor, while transcobalamins and cobalophilins bind a variety of inactive analogues as well.

Metabolic functions of vitamin B$_{12}$

There are three vitamin B$_{12}$-dependent mammalian enzymes:

1. Methionine synthetase, which catalyses the transfer of the methyl group from methyltetrahydrofolate to homocysteine.
2. Methylmalonyl CoA mutase, which catalyses the rearrangement of methylmalonyl CoA, an intermediate in the metabolism of valine, cholesterol and odd-carbon fatty acids, to succinyl CoA.
3. Leucine aminomutase, which catalyses the interconversion of leucine and β-leucine and acts mainly to metabolise β-leucine arising from intestinal bacteria.

Effects of deficiency and excess of vitamin B$_{12}$

Pernicious anaemia is the megaloblastic anaemia due to vitamin B$_{12}$ deficiency, commonly as a result of failure of intrinsic factor secretion, in which there is also spinal cord degeneration and peripheral neuropathy. High intakes of folate prevent the development of megaloblastic anaemia, and in up to one-third of patients the (irreversible) neurological signs develop without megaloblastosis.

Failure of intrinsic factor secretion is often due to autoimmune disease; 90% of patients with pernicious anaemia have antibodies against gastric parietal cells and 70% also have anti-intrinsic factor antibodies. Only about 10% of patients are aged under 40;

by the age of 60 about 1% of the population are affected, rising to 2–5% of people aged over 65, as a result of atrophic gastritis.

The neurological damage is caused by demyelination due to failure of methylation of arginine[107] of myelin basic protein. The nervous system is especially vulnerable to lack of methionine for methylation reactions because, unlike other tissues, it contains only methionine synthetase, which is vitamin B$_{12}$ dependent, and not the vitamin B$_{12}$-independent homocysteine methyltransferase that uses betaine as the methyl donor.

It is difficult to account for megaloblastic anaemia in vitamin B$_{12}$ deficiency; none of the B$_{12}$-dependent enzymes is associated with the synthesis of DNA or nucleotides. The most likely explanation is that vitamin B$_{12}$ deficiency causes functional folate deficiency. Most folate is transported between tissues as methyltetrahydrofolate, and the only reaction that releases free folate is the vitamin B$_{12}$-dependent reaction of methionine synthetase. Hence in vitamin B$_{12}$ deficiency folate is trapped as (unusable) methyltetrahydrofolate.

There is no evidence of any adverse effects of high intakes of vitamin B$_{12}$.

Drug-induced vitamin B$_{12}$ deficiency

Nitrous oxide inhibits methionine synthetase, by oxidising the cobalt of methylcobalamin. Patients with hitherto undiagnosed vitamin B$_{12}$ deficiency can develop neurological signs after surgery when nitrous oxide is used as the anaesthetic agent, and there are a number of reports of neurological damage due to vitamin B$_{12}$ depletion among dental surgeons and others occupationally exposed to nitrous oxide.

The histamine H$_2$ receptor antagonists and proton pump inhibitors used to treat gastric ulcers and gastro-oesophageal reflux act by reducing the secretion of gastric acid, and prolonged use may result in impairment of the absorption of protein-bound vitamin B$_{12}$. However, a number of studies have shown that even prolonged use of these drugs does not lead to significant depletion of vitamin B$_{12}$ reserves.

Assessment of vitamin B$_{12}$ status

Serum vitamin B$_{12}$ is measured by radioligand binding assay. A serum concentration below 110 pmol/l is associated with megaloblastic bone marrow, incipient anaemia and myelin damage. Below 150 pmol/l there are early bone marrow changes, abnormalities

of the dUMP suppression test and methylmalonic aciduria after a valine load; this is considered to be the lower limit of adequacy. Criteria of adequacy are shown in Table CD 10.12.

The Schilling test for vitamin B$_{12}$ absorption

The absorption of vitamin B$_{12}$ is determined by giving an oral dose of [^{57}Co] or [^{58}Co]vitamin B$_{12}$ together with a parenteral dose of 1 mg of non-radioactive vitamin (the Schilling test); urinary excretion of radioactivity shows the absorption of the oral dose. Normal subjects excrete 16–45% of the radioactivity over 24 hours, while patients lacking intrinsic factor or with anti-intrinsic factor antibodies excrete less than 5%.

Atrophic gastritis causes decreased secretion of gastric acid before there is impairment of intrinsic factor secretion. This means that the absorption of crystalline vitamin B$_{12}$, as used in the Schilling test, is normal, but the absorption of protein-bound vitamin B$_{12}$ from foods will be impaired and the test will give a false negative result.

Methylmalonic acid excretion

Moderate vitamin B$_{12}$ deficiency impairs the activity of methylmalonyl CoA mutase, resulting in urinary excretion of methylmalonic acid, especially after a loading dose of valine. This can be used to detect subclinical deficiency. However, up to 25% of patients with confirmed pernicious anaemia excrete normal amounts of methylmalonic acid even after a dose of valine.

The basis for setting dietary requirements of vitamin B$_{12}$

The total body pool of vitamin B$_{12}$ is of the order of 1.8 μmol (2.5 mg), with a minimum desirable body pool of about 0.3 μmol (1 mg). The daily loss is about 0.1% of the body pool in subjects with normal intrinsic factor secretion and enterohepatic circulation of the vitamin. On this basis the requirement is 0.3–1.8 nmol (1–2.5 μg)/day. This is probably a considerable overestimate of requirements, since parenteral administration of less than 0.3 nmol/day is adequate to maintain normal haematology in patients with pernicious anaemia, in whom the enterohepatic recycling of the vitamin is grossly impaired.

Requirements are probably between 0.1 and 1 μg/day; as shown in Appendix Table A14 reference intakes range between 1 and 2.4 μg/day, compared with an average intake of some 5 μg/day by non-vegetarians in most countries.

⊃ Key points

⊃ Dietary deficiency of vitamin B_{12} occurs only in strict vegans; there are no plant sources of the vitamin.

⊃ Functional deficiency, due to failure of absorption, is relatively common among elderly people, as a result of atrophic gastritis.

⊃ Deficiency causes pernicious anaemia – megaloblastic anaemia with spinal cord degeneration. The nerve damage is the result of failure of methylation of myelin basic protein.

⊃ The anaemia is due to functional folate deficiency, as a result of the failure to demethylate methyltetrahydrofolate because of the impaired activity of vitamin B_{12}-dependent methionine synthetase. High intakes of folate can prevent the development of anaemia.

⊃ Vitamin B_{12} status can be assessed by measurement of the serum concentration, the excretion of methylmalonic acid after a test dose of valine, or suppression of the incorporation in vitro of [³H]thymidine into DNA by dUMP.

⊃ The absorption of vitamin B_{12} can be assessed by the Schilling test, using an oral dose of radioactive vitamin and a large parenteral dose of non-radioactive vitamin.

⊃ Current estimates of requirements are almost certainly an overestimate of true requirements, but considerably lower than average intakes by omnivores.

10.7 VITAMIN C (ASCORBIC ACID)

Vitamin C is a vitamin for only a limited number of vertebrate species: human beings and the other primates, the guinea pig, bats, some birds and fishes. It is synthesised as an intermediate in the gulonolactone pathway of glucose metabolism; in those species for which it is a vitamin, one enzyme of the pathway, gulonolactone oxidase, is absent.

Vitamin C is the cofactor for some hydroxylation reactions, and also functions as a non-specific reducing agent and antioxidant.

Forms in foods and good food sources

The physiologically important compound is L-ascorbic acid (Fig. 10.8). It can undergo oxidation to the monodehydroascorbate radical and dehydroascorbate, both of which have vitamin activity because they can be reduced to ascorbate. D-Iso-ascorbic acid (erythorbic acid) has some vitamin activity; it is not a naturally occurring compound, but is widely used, interchangeably with ascorbic acid, in cured meats and as an antioxidant in a variety of foods.

Fruits and vegetables are rich sources; blackcurrants and guava provide about five times the reference intake in a single serving, and potatoes are an important source in many countries (see Table CD 10.13).

Absorption and transport of vitamin C

Some 80–95% of dietary ascorbate is absorbed at intakes up to about 100 mg/day; the absorption of

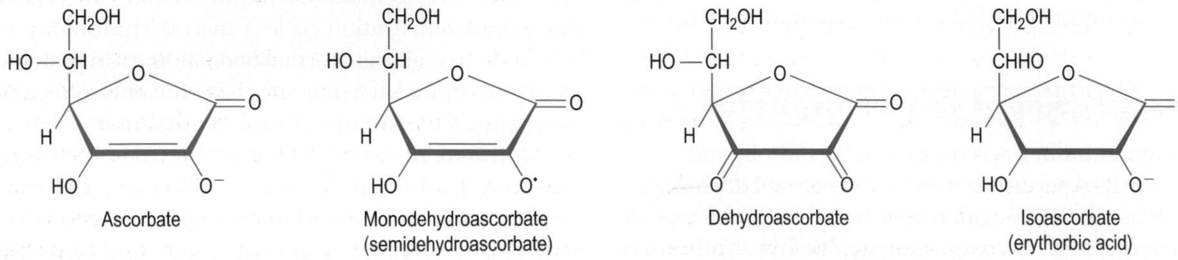

Figure 10.8   Vitamin C.

larger amounts of the vitamin is lower – about 50% of a 1.5 g dose is absorbed. Unabsorbed ascorbate is a substrate for intestinal bacterial metabolism. Ascorbate is absorbed by active transport; dehydroascorbate by a carrier-mediated (equilibrium) transport, followed by reduction to ascorbate inside the intestinal epithelial cell.

Ascorbate enters tissues by way of sodium-dependent transporters, while dehydroascorbate enters by way of the (insulin-dependent) glucose transporter, and is reduced to ascorbate intracellularly. Tissue uptake of dehydroascorbate is impaired in poorly controlled diabetes mellitus, and functional signs of deficiency may develop despite an adequate intake of vitamin C.

About 70% of bloodborne ascorbate is in plasma and erythrocytes (which do not concentrate the vitamin). The remainder is in white cells, which have a marked ability to concentrate ascorbate; mononuclear leukocytes achieve 80-fold, platelets 40-fold and granulocytes 25-fold concentration compared with plasma.

There is no specific storage organ for ascorbate; apart from leukocytes (which account for only 10% of total blood ascorbate), the only tissues showing a significant concentration of the vitamin are the adrenal and pituitary glands. Although the concentration of ascorbate in muscle is relatively low, skeletal muscle contains much of the body's pool of 5–8.5 mmol (900–1500 mg) of ascorbate.

The major fate of ascorbic acid is urinary excretion, either unchanged or as dehydroascorbate and diketogulonate. At plasma concentrations above about 85 μmol/l the renal transport system is saturated, and ascorbate is excreted quantitatively with increasing intake.

Metabolic functions of vitamin C

Ascorbic acid has specific and well-defined roles in two classes of enzymes:

1. Copper-containing hydroxylases, such as dopamine β-hydroxylase and peptidyl glycine hydroxylase. The enzymes contain Cu^+, which is oxidised to Cu^{2+} during the reaction; reduction back to Cu^+ requires ascorbate, which is oxidised to monodehydroascorbate.
2. The 2-oxoglutarate linked iron-containing hydroxylases, of which the best studied are the proline and lysine hydroxylases involved in synthesis of collagen and other connective tissue proteins.

Although ascorbate is consumed in these reactions, it is not stoichiometric with the formation of product. The enzymes contain Fe^{2+}, and the iron is not oxidised during the reaction. However, it is occasionally (accidentally) oxidised to Fe^{3+}, inactivating the enzyme. Ascorbate is required to reduce the enzyme-bound iron back to the active form.

Ascorbate can act as a radical-trapping antioxidant, reacting with superoxide and a proton to yield hydrogen peroxide, or with the hydroxyl radical to yield water. In each case the product is monodehydroascorbate. It is also thought to reduce the α-tocopheroxyl radical formed in cell membranes and plasma lipoproteins during the oxidation of vitamin E, so sparing vitamin E.

Vitamin C deficiency and excess

Although there is no specific site of vitamin C storage in the body, signs of deficiency do not develop until previously adequately nourished subjects have been deprived of the vitamin for 4–6 months, by which time plasma and tissue concentrations have fallen considerably.

The name scurvy for the vitamin C deficiency disease is derived from the Italian *scorbutico*, meaning an irritable person; deficiency is associated with listlessness and general malaise, and sometimes changes in personality and psychomotor performance. The behavioural effects are due to impaired synthesis of catecholamines as a result of reduced activity of dopamine β-hydroxylase.

Most of the other signs of scurvy are due to impaired collagen synthesis. The earliest signs are skin changes, beginning with plugging of hair follicles by horny material, followed by petechial haemorrhage and increased fragility of blood capillaries leading to extravasation of red cells. Later there is haemorrhage of the gums and loss of dental cement. Wounds show only superficial healing in scurvy, with little or no formation of (collagen-rich) scar tissue, so that healing is delayed and wounds can readily be reopened.

Anaemia is common in scurvy, and may be either macrocytic, indicative of folate deficiency, or hypochromic, indicative of iron deficiency. Folate deficiency may be epiphenomenal, since the major sources of folate are the same as those of ascorbate. Iron deficiency in scurvy may well be secondary to reduced absorption of inorganic iron, and impaired mobilisation of tissue iron reserves.

Objectives

By the end of this chapter you should be able to:

- identify the compounds classified as fat-soluble vitamins
- identify good sources of each
- summarise the absorption and transport of each
- summarise the main metabolic functions of each
- describe the main effects of deficiency and excess of each
- be aware of the methods of assessment of status
- discuss the basis for dietary requirements
- appreciate the metabolic interactions between fat-soluble vitamins and other nutrients.

11.1 VITAMIN A: RETINOIDS AND CAROTENOIDS

Vitamin A deficiency is a serious problem of public health nutrition, second only to protein-energy malnutrition worldwide, and is probably the most important cause of preventable blindness among children in developing countries. Marginal deficiency is a factor in childhood susceptibility to infection, and hence morbidity and mortality, in developing countries, and even in developed countries vitamin A (along with iron) is the nutrient most likely to be supplied in marginal amounts.

Preformed vitamin A (retinol) is found only in animals and a small number of bacteria. β-Carotene and some of the other carotenes in plants can be oxidised to retinol. The main physiologically active forms of vitamin A are retinaldehyde (in the visual system) and retinoic acid, which modulates gene expression and tissue differentiation.

Forms in foods and good food sources

The term vitamin A includes both provitamin A carotenoids, and retinol and its active metabolites. The term retinoid is used to include retinol and its derivatives and analogues, either naturally occurring or synthetic, with or without the biological activity of the vitamin. The main biologically active retinoids are shown in Figure 11.1; until the late 1990s only retinol, retinaldehyde, all-*trans*- and 9-*cis*-retinoic acid were known to be biologically active, but a number of other retinoids are now known to have important functions (see Fig. CD 11.1).

Free retinol is chemically unstable, and the main form in foods is the palmitate. Retinoic acid occurs in foods in only small amounts. Liver, full-fat dairy produce, fortified margarine, oily fish and kidneys are good sources of retinol (see Table CD 11.1).

Carotenes that can be oxidised to retinaldehyde are known as provitamin A carotenoids. Relatively few foods are rich sources of retinol, so that carotenes are nutritionally important. In developed countries, with a relatively high intake of animal foods, some 25–30% of vitamin A is derived from carotenoids; in developing countries 80% or more of vitamin A is from carotenoids. The major dietary carotenoids are shown in Figure CD 11.2. Good dietary sources of carotenes are dark green, yellow, red and orange fruits and vegetables (see Table CD 11.2 for information about carotenoid-rich foods and Table CD 11.3 for foods rich in total vitamin A).

International units and retinol equivalents

The obsolete international unit of vitamin A activity was based on biological assay of the ability of the test compound to support growth in animals; 1 iu = 10.47 nmol of retinol = 0.3 μg free retinol or 0.344 μg retinyl acetate.

The total vitamin A content of foods is expressed as μg retinol equivalents – the sum of that provided by retinoids and that from carotenoids; 6 μg β-carotene is 1 μg retinol equivalent. β-Carotene is absorbed very much better from milk than from other foods, and in milk 2 μg β-carotene is 1 μg retinol equivalent. Other provitamin A carotenoids yield at most half the retinol of β-carotene, and 12 μg of these compounds = 1 μg retinol equivalent.

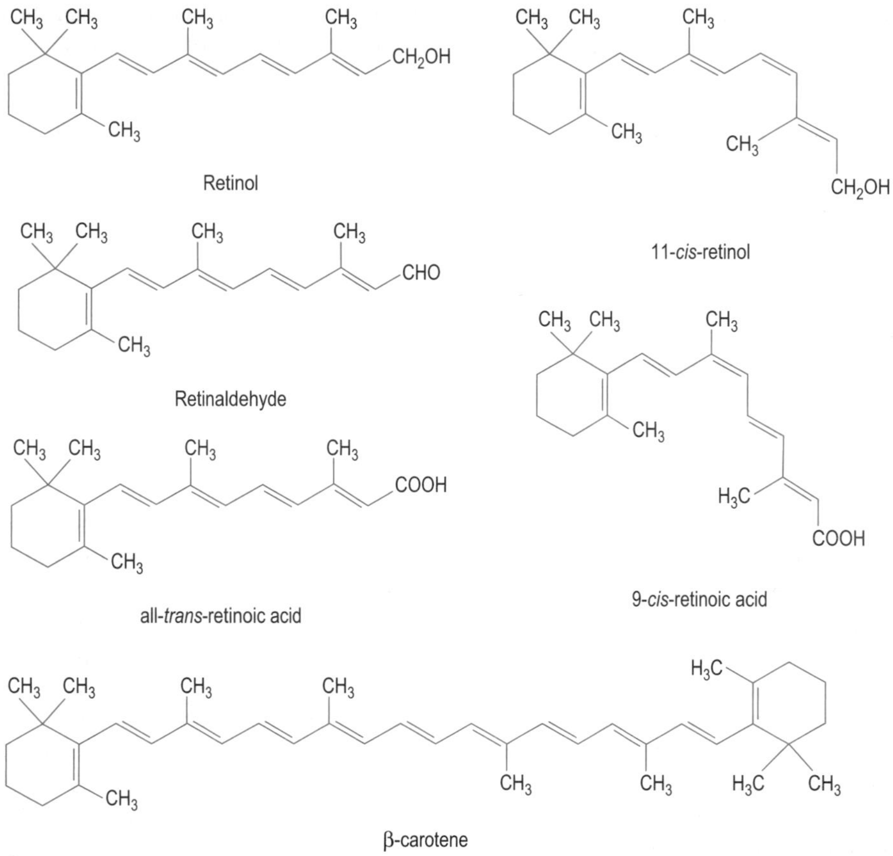

Figure 11.1 Vitamin A vitamers and β-carotene.

On this basis, 1 iu of vitamin A activity = 1.8 μg β-carotene or 3.6 μg of other provitamin A carotenoids.

In 2001 The USA/Canadian Dietary Reference Values report introduced the term *retinol activity equivalent* to take account of the incomplete absorption and metabolism of carotenoids; 1 RAE = 1 μg all-*trans*-retinol, 12 μg β-carotene, 24 μg α-carotene or β-cryptoxanthin. On this basis, 1 iu of vitamin A activity = 3.6 μg β-carotene or 7.2 μg of other provitamin A carotenoids.

Absorption and transport of vitamin A

Dietary retinyl esters are hydrolysed by intestinal lipases, and 70–90% of dietary retinol is absorbed. Uptake into enterocytes is by facilitated diffusion from lipid micelles, followed by esterification to retinyl palmitate, with small amounts of other esters. Retinyl esters enter the lymphatic circulation, and then the bloodstream, in chylomicrons, together with dietary lipid and carotenoids.

Carotenoids are absorbed dissolved in lipid micelles. The absorption of carotene is between 5 and 60%, depending on the nature of the food, whether it is cooked or raw, and the amount of fat in the meal. Provitamin A carotenoids undergo oxidative cleavage to retinaldehyde in the intestinal mucosa, catalysed by carotene dioxygenase. Retinaldehyde is reduced to retinol, then esterified and secreted in chylomicrons.

Only a relatively small proportion of carotene is oxidised in the intestinal mucosa, and a significant amount of carotene enters the circulation in chylomicrons. There is some hepatic cleavage of carotene taken up from chylomicron remnants, again giving rise to retinaldehyde and retinyl esters; the remainder is secreted in very low density lipoproteins, and may be taken up and cleaved by carotene dioxygenase in extrahepatic tissues.

Central oxidative cleavage of β-carotene gives rise to two molecules of retinaldehyde, which can be reduced to retinol. However, the biological activity of β-carotene on a molar basis is considerably lower than that of retinol, not two-fold higher as might be

mobilisation of bone mineral, hypercalcaemia, hypercalciuria, hyperphosphaturia and the development of calcium phosphate renal stones.

Calcitonin is secreted by the C-cells of the thyroid gland in response to hypercalcaemia. Its primary action is to oppose the actions of parathyroid hormone by suppressing osteoclast actions. It also stimulates calcidiol 1-hydroxylation in the kidney.

Metabolic functions of vitamin D

Calcitriol maintains the plasma concentration of calcium by increasing intestinal absorption of calcium, reducing excretion by increasing reabsorption in the distal renal tubule, and mobilising the mineral from bone.

Calcitriol binds to, and activates, nuclear receptors that modulate gene expression. More than 50 genes are known to be regulated by calcitriol, including: calcidiol 1- and 24-hydroxylases; calbindin, a calcium binding protein in the intestinal mucosa and other tissues; the vitamin K dependent protein osteocalcin in bone; osteopontin, which permits the attachment of osteoclasts to bone surfaces; and the osteoclast cell membrane protein integrin. In addition, calcitriol affects the secretion of insulin and the synthesis and secretion of parathyroid and thyroid hormones – these actions may be secondary to changes in intracellular calcium concentrations resulting from induction of calbindin. Calcitriol also has a role in the regulation of cell proliferation and differentiation.

The vitamin D receptor acts as a heterodimer with the RXR retinoid receptor. Binding of calcitriol permits dimerisation with occupied or unoccupied RXR, leading to activation. Abnormally high concentrations of 9-*cis*-retinoic acid result in sequestration of RXR as the homodimers, meaning that it is unavailable to form heterodimers with the vitamin D receptor; excessive vitamin A can therefore antagonise the nuclear actions of vitamin D.

In addition to its nuclear actions, calcitriol has two non-genomic actions:

1. In intestinal mucosal cells it acts to recruit membrane calcium transport proteins from intracellular vesicles to the cell surface, resulting in a rapid increase in calcium absorption, before there has been induction of calbindin.
2. In a variety of cells it acts via cell-surface receptors, leading to opening of intracellular calcium channels and activation of protein kinase C and mitogen-activated protein kinases (MAP kinases). The effect of this is inhibition of cell proliferation, and induction of differentiation.

Calcitriol affects the proliferation, differentiation and immune function of lymphocytes and monocytes. Activated macrophages have calcidiol 1-hydroxylase, and can synthesise calcitriol from calcidiol, suggesting that in addition to its endocrine role calcitriol may have a paracrine role in the immune system.

Calcitriol receptors have been identified in a variety of tumour cells. At low concentrations it is a growth promoter, while at higher concentrations it has both antiproliferative and pro-apoptotic actions in cancer cells in culture. There is an epidemiological association between low vitamin D status and prostate cancer.

Adipocytes have vitamin D receptors, and there is evidence that vitamin D suppresses adipocyte development. It has been suggested that vitamin D inadequacy may be a factor in the development of the metabolic syndrome ('syndrome X', the combination of insulin resistance, hyperlipidaemia and atherosclerosis associated with abdominal obesity). Sunlight exposure, and hence vitamin D status, may be a factor in the difference in incidence of atherosclerosis between northern and southern European countries.

Effects of vitamin D deficiency and excess

Rickets is a disease of young children and adolescents, resulting from a failure of the mineralisation of newly formed bone. In infants, epiphyseal cartilage continues to grow, but is not replaced by bone matrix and mineral. The earliest sign of this is craniotabes – the occurrence of unossified areas in the skull. At a later stage there is enlargement of the epiphyses. When the child begins to walk, the weight of the body deforms the undermineralised long bones, leading to bow legs or knock knees, as well as deformity of the pelvis. Similar problems may develop during the adolescent growth spurt.

Osteomalacia is the defective remineralisation of bone during normal bone turnover in adults, so that there is a progressive demineralisation, but with adequate bone matrix, leading to bone pain and skeletal deformities, with muscle weakness. Women with inadequate vitamin D status are especially at risk of osteomalacia after repeated pregnancies, because of the drain on calcium reserves for fetal bone mineralisation and lactation. The elderly are at risk of osteomalacia, because of both decreased synthesis of 7-dehydrocholesterol in the skin with increasing age and low exposure to sunlight.

Osteoporosis, the loss of bone mineral and matrix that may affect 40% of women and 12% of men as they age, is not due to vitamin D deficiency, but an intake of 10–15 µg/day, together with 1200–1500 mg calcium, is recommended for treatment of osteoporosis, together with hormone replacement therapy or treatment with antiresorptive agents such as bisphosphonates.

Vitamin D toxicity

Intoxication with vitamin D causes weakness, nausea, loss of appetite, headache, abdominal pains, cramp and diarrhoea. More seriously, it also causes hypercalcaemia, with plasma concentrations of calcium between 2.75 and 4.5 mmol/l, compared with the normal range of 2.2–2.5 mmol/l. Above 3.75 mmol/l, vascular smooth muscle may contract abnormally, leading to hypertension. Hypercalciuria may also result in the precipitation of calcium phosphate in the renal tubules and the development of urinary calculi. Hypervitaminosis also results in increased uptake of calcium into tissues, leading to calcinosis – the calcification of soft tissues, including kidney, heart, lungs and blood vessels.

Rickets was more or less eradicated as a nutritional deficiency disease during the 1950s, by widespread enrichment of infant foods with vitamin D. However, some children are sensitive to hypercalcaemia and calcinosis with vitamin D intakes as low as 45 µg/day, and the level of enrichment was reduced because of the development of hypercalcaemia in a small number of susceptible infants. As a result, rickets has re-emerged, especially in northern cities in temperate countries.

The tolerable upper level of intake is 50 µg/day for adults and 25 µg/day for infants. Reports of hypercalcaemia in adults have involved intakes in excess of 1000 µg/day.

Assessment of vitamin D status

Before anatomical deformities are apparent in vitamin D deficient children, bone density is lower than normal – radiological rickets. At an earlier stage of deficiency there is a marked elevation of plasma alkaline phosphatase released by osteoclast activity – biochemical rickets.

The plasma concentration of calcidiol is the most sensitive index of vitamin D status, and is correlated with elevated plasma parathyroid hormone and alkaline phosphatase activity. The reference range of plasma calcidiol is between 20–150 nmol/l, with a two-fold seasonal variation in temperate regions. Concentrations below 20 nmol/l are considered to indicate impending deficiency, and osteomalacia is seen in adults when plasma calcidiol falls below 10 nmol/l. In children, clinical signs of rickets are seen when plasma calcidiol falls below 20 nmol/l (see Table CD 11.8).

The basis for setting dietary requirements

Dietary vitamin D makes little contribution to status, and the major factor is exposure to sunlight. There are no reference intakes for young adults in UK and Europe; for the house-bound elderly, the reference intake is 10 µg/day, based on the intake required to maintain a plasma concentration of calcidiol of 20 nmol/l. This will almost certainly require supplements of the vitamin, since average intakes are less than half this amount. The US/Canadian adequate intake is 5 µg/day up to age 50, increasing to 10 µg between 51 and 70, and to 15 µg over 70 years of age. However, intakes above 5 µg/day are required to prevent osteoporosis and secondary hyperparathyroidism, and normal sunlight exposure may provide the equivalent of 20–50 µg/day.

The vitamin D content of human milk is probably inadequate to meet the requirements of breastfed infants without exposure to sunlight, especially during the winter, when the mother's reserves of the vitamin are low. Infant formulae normally provide 10 µg of cholecalciferol/day, and a similar amount is recommended for breastfed infants and children aged under 3 years – this maintains the plasma concentration of calcidiol above 20 nmol/l.

⮩ Key points

⮩ Vitamin D is really a steroid hormone, and dietary intake is relatively unimportant compared with sunlight exposure for endogenous synthesis, except for infants and the elderly.

⮩ The main body reserve of vitamin D is circulating calcidiol.

because they form stable radicals that persist long enough to undergo reaction to non-radical products. It is therefore to be expected that they are also capable of perpetuating the radical chain reaction deeper into lipoproteins or membranes, and therefore causing increased damage in the absence of co-antioxidants such as ascorbate or ubiquinone.

Non-antioxidant actions of vitamin E

α-Tocopherol (but not other vitamers) inhibits platelet aggregation and vascular smooth muscle proliferation. In monocytes it reduces formation of reactive oxygen species, cell adhesion to the endothelium and release of interleukins and tumour necrosis factor.

α-Tocopherol modulates transcription of a number of genes, including the scavenger receptor for oxidised LDL in macrophages and smooth muscle. As yet no response element for intracellular vitamin E binding protein has been identified on any of the proposed target genes.

In experimental animals, vitamin E deficiency depresses immune system function, with reduced mitogenesis of B- and T-lymphocytes, reduced phagocytosis and chemotaxis and reduced production of antibodies and interleukin-2, suggesting a signalling role in the immune system.

Vitamin E deficiency and excess

Vitamin E deficiency in experimental animals was first described in 1922, when it was discovered to be essential for fertility. It was not until 1983 that vitamin E was demonstrated to be a dietary essential for human beings, when the devastating neurological damage due to lack of vitamin E in patients with hereditary abetalipoproteinaemia was first described.

Vitamin E deficiency in experimental animals results in a number of different conditions, with considerable differences between species. Some of the lesions can be prevented or cured by synthetic antioxidants, and others respond to selenium. Most of these effects of vitamin E deficiency can be attributed to oxidative damage to membranes.

Dietary vitamin E deficiency is not a problem even among people living on relatively poor diets. In depletion studies, very low intakes of vitamin E must be maintained for many months before there is any significant fall in circulating α-tocopherol, because there are relatively large tissue reserves of the vitamin.

Deficiency develops in patients with severe fat malabsorption, cystic fibrosis, chronic cholestatic hepatobiliary disease and in two rare groups of patients with genetic diseases:

Patients with congenital abetalipoproteinaemia, who are unable to synthesise VLDL. They have undetectably low plasma levels of α-tocopherol and develop 'devastating' ataxic neuropathy and pigmentary retinopathy.

Patients who lack the hepatic tocopherol transfer protein and suffer from what has been called AVED (ataxia with vitamin E deficiency), are unable to export α-tocopherol from the liver in VLDL.

In both groups of patients the only source of vitamin E for peripheral tissues will be recently ingested vitamin E in chylomicrons. They develop cerebellar ataxia, axonal degeneration of sensory neurons, skeletal myopathy and pigmented retinopathy similar to those seen in experimental animals.

In premature infants, whose reserves of the vitamin are inadequate, vitamin E deficiency causes haemolytic anaemia. When premature infants are treated with hyperbaric oxygen, there is a risk of damage to the retina (retrolental fibroplasia), and vitamin E supplements may be protective, although this is not firmly established.

Vitamin E has very low toxicity, and habitual intake of supplements of 200–600 mg/day (compared with an average dietary intake of 8–12 mg) seems to be without untoward effect; there are no consistent reports of adverse effects up to 3200 mg/day, suggesting that an acceptable daily intake is in the very wide range between 0.15 and 2 mg/kg body weight.

Very high intakes may antagonise vitamin K and potentiate anticoagulant therapy. On the basis of prolonged prothrombin time in people receiving anticoagulants and consuming vitamin E supplements, the tolerable upper level is set at 1000 mg vitamin E per day.

Assessment of vitamin E status

The most commonly used index of vitamin E nutritional status is the plasma concentration of α-tocopherol; because it is transported in plasma lipoproteins, it is best expressed /mol cholesterol or /mg total plasma lipids. The reference range is 12–37 μmol/l; ranges associated with inadequate and desirable status are shown in Table CD 11.11; an optimum concentration for protection against cardiovascular disease and cancer is >30 μmol/l.

Erythrocytes are incapable of de novo lipid synthesis, so oxidative damage has a serious effect, shortening red cell life and possibly precipitating haemolytic anaemia in vitamin E deficiency. The haemolysis induced in vitro by hydrogen peroxide or dialuric acid provides a means of assessing functional status, albeit one that will be masked by adequate selenium intake and may be affected by other, unrelated, factors.

Overall antioxidant status, rather than specifically vitamin E status, can be assessed by a variety of measures of lipid peroxidation.

The basis for setting dietary requirements

Early reports suggested that vitamin E requirements increase with intake of polyunsaturated fatty acids. Neither the UK nor the EU set reference intakes for vitamin E, but both suggested that an acceptable intake was 0.4 mg α-tocopherol equivalent/g dietary polyunsaturated fatty acid. This should be readily achievable from PUFA-rich oils, which are also rich sources of vitamin E. There is little evidence to support the figure of 0.4 mg α-tocopherol equivalent/g dietary PUFA, and indeed the need for vitamin E (and other antioxidants) depends more on the degree of unsaturation of fatty acids than the total amount.

From the plasma concentration of α-tocopherol required to prevent haemolysis in vitro, the average requirement is 12 mg/day, which was the basis of the 2000 US/Canadian RDA of 15 mg/day. This was a 50% increase on the previous (1989) RDA, partly as a result of considering only the 2R isomers in dietary intake.

Pharmacological uses of vitamin E

Although vitamin E deficiency causes infertility in experimental animals, there is no evidence that deficiency has any similar effects on human fertility, and it is a considerable leap of logic from the effects of gross depletion in experimental animals to the popular, and unfounded, claims for vitamin E in enhancing human fertility and virility.

Animal studies show some protective effects of tocopherol supplements against a variety of radical generating chemical toxicants, and it has been assumed that vitamin E may similarly be protective against degenerative diseases that are associated with radical damage. However, there is little evidence from intervention trials that vitamin E reduces cancer risk, cardiovascular disease, cataract or neurodegenerative diseases and supplements may increase mortality.

⮎ Key points

- ⮎ Vitamin E is the major lipid-soluble antioxidant in cell membranes and plasma lipoproteins.

- ⮎ There are 8 vitamers, with differing biological activity and antioxidant action.

- ⮎ α-Tocopherol has actions in regulating platelet coagulability and vascular smooth muscle proliferation, and gene expression.

- ⮎ The tocotrienols downregulate cholesterol synthesis.

- ⮎ Vitamin E deficiency only occurs in people with severe fat malabsorption, and rare patients with a genetic lack of β-lipoprotein or hepatic tocopherol transfer protein, who suffer devastating nerve damage.

- ⮎ Premature infants have inadequate vitamin E status and are susceptible to haemolytic anaemia.

- ⮎ There is little evidence on which to estimate requirements for vitamin E.

11.4 VITAMIN K

Vitamin K was discovered in 1935 as a result of studies of a haemorrhagic disease of chickens fed on solvent-extracted fat-free diets and cattle fed on silage made from spoiled sweet clover. The problem in the chickens was a lack of the vitamin in the diet, while in the cattle it was due to the presence of dicoumarol, an antimetabolite of the vitamin. It soon became apparent that vitamin K was required for the synthesis of several of the proteins required for blood clotting, but it was not until 1974 that the mechanism of action of the vitamin was elucidated. A new amino acid, γ-carboxyglutamate (Gla), was found to be present in the vitamin K dependent proteins, but absent from the abnormal precursors that circulate in deficiency.

A number of other proteins undergo the same vitamin K-dependent carboxylation of glutamate to γ-carboxyglutamate, including osteocalcin and the matrix Gla protein in bone, nephrocalcin in kidney and the product of the growth arrest specific gene Gas6, which is involved in both the regulation of differentiation and development in the nervous

Preprothrombin is elevated at intakes between 40–60 µg/day, but not at intakes above 80 µg/day.

The US/Canadian Adequate Intake is 120 µg for men and 90 µg for women. This is based on observed intakes, but there is some evidence that average intakes may be inadequate to permit full carboxylation of osteocalcin.

➲ Key points

- ➲ Although intestinal bacteria synthesise vitamin K, it is not known to what extent this contributes to intake and status.

- ➲ The metabolic function of vitamin K is as cofactor for carboxylation of glutamate in precursors of proteins involved in blood clotting and a range of other functions, including the product of the growth arrest specific gene Gas6 that is involved in regulation of growth and development, and osteocalcin in bone.

- ➲ Clinically used anticoagulants for treatment of people at risk of thrombosis act as antimetabolites of vitamin K.

- ➲ Dietary deficiency of vitamin K is rare, and there is little evidence on which to base estimates of requirements.

- ➲ Newborn infants have low vitamin K status and are at risk of severe bleeding unless given prophylactic vitamin K.

- ➲ Vitamin K status is assessed by blood clotting (the prothrombin time) and sometimes measurement of undercarboxylated prothrombin and osteocalcin.

Further reading

Section 11.1 – Vitamin A

Bender D A 2003 Chapter 2, Vitamin A. In: Nutritional biochemistry of the vitamins, 2nd edn. Cambridge University Press, New York

Blomhoff R, Green M H, Green J B et al 1991 Vitamin A metabolism: new perspectives on absorption, transport, and storage. Physiological Reviews 71:951–990

Section 11.2 – Vitamin D

Bender D A 2003 Chapter 3, Vitamin D. In: Nutritional biochemistry of the vitamins, 2nd edn. Cambridge University Press, New York

Chatterjee M 2001 Vitamin D and genomic stability. Mutation Research 475:69–87

Haussler M R, Haussler C A, Jurutka P W et al 1997 The vitamin D hormone and its nuclear receptor: molecular actions and disease states. Journal of Endocrinology 154(suppl):S57–73

Section 11.3 – Vitamin E

Azzi A, Breyer I, Feher M et al 2001 Nonantioxidant functions of alpha-tocopherol in smooth muscle cells. Journal of Nutrition 131:378S–381S

Azzi A, Ricciarelli R, Zingg J M 2002 Non-antioxidant molecular functions of alpha-tocopherol (vitamin E). FEBS Letters 519:8–10

Bender D A 2003 Chapter 4, Vitamin E. In: Nutritional biochemistry of the vitamins, 2nd edn. Cambridge University Press, New York

Packer L, Weber S U, Rimbach G 2001 Molecular aspects of alpha-tocotrienol antioxidant action and cell signalling. Journal of Nutrition 131:369S–373S

Section 11.4 – Vitamin K

Bender D A 2003 Chapter 5, Vitamin K. In: Nutritional biochemistry of the vitamins, 2nd edn. Cambridge University Press, New York

Bolton-Smith C P R, Fenton S T, Harrington D J, Shearer M J 2000 Compilation of a provisional UK database for the phylloquinone (vitamin K1) content of foods. British Journal of Nutrition 83:389–399

Weber P 2001 Vitamin K and bone health. Nutrition 17:880–887

CD-ROM contents

Further reading

Further reading from the book

12

Minerals and trace elements

Paul Sharp

Objectives

By the end of this chapter you should be able to:

- identify the most important food sources of minerals and trace elements
- understand the main features of their absorption, metabolism, and tissue distribution
- describe their important functions in the body
- appreciate the effects of deficiency and excess, and their importance in the UK and elsewhere
- discuss the basis for dietary recommendations.

12.1 INTRODUCTION

This chapter deals with the key minerals and trace elements essential to a number of important biochemical and physiological functions in the body. The focus is placed on dietary sources of the various minerals and their homeostatic regulation in the body (i.e. the balance between bioavailability and absorption versus regulation and excretion). This is followed by discussion of the major metabolic functions of the minerals and trace elements and an appreciation of the consequences of deficiency and excess of individual elements. Each section closes by discussing the current methodologies used to assess the body status of these minerals and trace elements and how all of this knowledge has been processed to provide the current dietary recommendations for adequate intakes of these micronutrients. Five minerals are dealt with in detail. Calcium and phosphorus are discussed together due to their close interrelationship in maintaining bone health. This is followed by a discussion of the essential roles of iron, zinc and iodine in human metabolism. Further information on the essential nature of these micronutrients as well as their interactions with other nutrients will be provided elsewhere in this book: Chapter 11 (Fat-soluble vitamins – the metabolism of vitamin D); Chapter 13 (Inter-micronutrient topics); Chapter 24 (Nutrition and the skeleton); Chapter 25 (Dental disease); Chapter 28 (Deficiency diseases). Additional information is provided on the accompanying CD-ROM.

12.2 CALCIUM AND PHOSPHORUS

Calcium is the most abundant mineral in the body, the majority of which is contained within the adult skeleton in the form of hydroxyapatite, a complex crystalline form of calcium phosphate. Accordingly, phosphorus is also abundant in bone (approximately 85% of total body phosphorus). More details of the roles of calcium and phosphorus in maintaining bone health are provided in Chapter 24.

Food sources

The most important dietary sources of calcium in the Western world are milk and other dairy products including yoghurt, cheese and ice cream (see Table CD 12.1). Phosphorus is also abundant in these products and its concentration is approximately equimolar with calcium. However, while the calcium content of these foods can contribute 50–75% of the daily dietary intake, dairy products only contribute 20–30% of daily phosphorus intake. Cereal and vegetable sources of calcium contribute less to total intake in Western countries (approximately 25%) than in developing countries where grains and cereals are staple foods. Interestingly, the phosphate content of cereals and vegetables is relatively high due to the presence of phytic acid (inositol hexaphosphate) and these foods contribute a further 25–35% of daily phosphorus intake. In addition, carbonated soft drinks, which are often rich in phosphates, may contribute significantly to phosphorus intakes in some diets (e.g. teenagers'). The calcium content of meat and fish is low in comparison to dairy products and cereals. However, sardines (containing bones) are a rich source of both calcium and phosphorus. In addition to its abundance in bone, phosphate is also present at high levels in soft tissues such as muscle and therefore levels of phosphorus in meat and fish are much higher than those of calcium, and contribute a further 25–35% to daily phosphorus intake.

Whilst in most foods calcium is largely present as simple organic and inorganic salts (some of which form larger complexes with other dietary components), dietary phosphorus occurs in several forms including inorganic phosphate, organic phosphoproteins, phosphorylated sugars, sugar alcohols (e.g. phytate) and phospholipids. The relative amounts of organic versus inorganic phosphate varies depending on the food source; for example, organic complexes prevail in meat, whereas 80% of phosphorus in cereals and grains is phytic acid and 33% of phosphorus in milk is present as inorganic salts.

Absorption and metabolism

Bioavailability

Absorption of calcium from a mixed diet is fairly constant (25–35%). Bioavailability of calcium in milk and dairy products is improved by the presence of sugars (lactose) and casein phosphopeptides (Allen & Wood 1994). The absorption from calcium salts used as supplements (such as lactate, carbonate, gluconate and citrate) is similar to that from dairy products (30–40%). However, other dietary acids, especially oxalate and phosphate, inhibit calcium uptake. Oxalate is the most potent inhibitor of calcium absorption and forms a highly insoluble complex, whereas phytate (containing six phosphate groups) is less potent but is present at a much higher concentration in the intestinal lumen and is likely to be the major dietary inhibitor of calcium absorption – a dietary phytate to calcium molar ratio of 0.2 can increase the risk of calcium deficiency.

Phosphorus is absorbed very efficiently from the small intestine (approximately 60–70% of dietary intake) and is always absorbed as inorganic phosphate – phosphate groups are liberated from organic compounds prior to absorption by alkaline phosphatase on the luminal membrane of intestinal enterocytes. This enzyme has little activity towards phytate, which is largely non-bioavailable in its natural form. However, yeast added to leavened bread contains significant levels of the enzyme phytase, which is lacking from the human intestinal secretions. Phytase readily releases phosphate from phytate and about 50% of phytate-derived phosphate in bread is thought to be absorbed.

Absorption

Intestinal calcium absorption occurs via both active transcellular and passive paracellular pathways (see Fig. CD 12.1). The transcellular route is subject to tight homeostatic control by the calcium content of the diet and 1,25-dihydroxycholecalciferol (1,25-$(OH)_2D_3$; vitamin D_3), whereas the passive paracellular route is not regulated and is non-saturable. The trigger for vitamin D_3 synthesis is the release of parathyroid hormone (PTH) in response to decreased plasma calcium. Elevated PTH levels do not regulate intestinal calcium absorption directly, but act indirectly by increasing the production of active vitamin D_3 in the kidney.

The mechanisms involved in phosphate absorption are less well defined than those for calcium (see Fig. CD 12.2). Phosphate absorption is regulated by long-term changes in dietary phosphorus content and body phosphorus status. In addition, there may also be a regulatory role for vitamin D_3 in controlling dietary phosphate absorption.

Tissue distribution

The human body contains approximately 1.2 kg (30 moles) of calcium, 99% of which resides in mineralised tissues such as the bones and teeth. The majority of calcium in these tissues is present as hydroxyapatite, a complex form of calcium phosphate, $Ca_{10}(PO_4)_6(OH)_2$. The remaining 1% is found in blood (where plasma calcium is tightly regulated at 2.5 mmol/l) and extracellular fluid. Intracellular free calcium concentration is extremely low (approximately 100 nmol/l) but can rise dramatically following hormone- or neurotransmitter-induced release of calcium from the intracellular stores (in the endoplasmic/sarcoplasmic reticulum) and influx from the extracellular fluid through plasma membrane calcium channels.

Body phosphorus is also largely associated with the bone; approximately 85% of the 600 g in the body is found in the skeleton. The remaining 15% is found in the soft tissues and blood largely as phospholipids, phosphoproteins, and nucleic acids as well as inorganic phosphate.

Renal excretion and regulation

Plasma calcium levels are tightly regulated at 2.5 mmol/l by the action of parathyroid hormone (PTH) and vitamin D_3, which increase plasma calcium

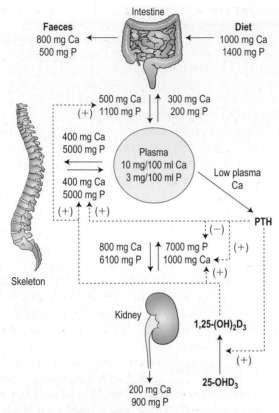

Figure 12.1   Homeostatic regulation of serum calcium and phosphorus. PTH, parathyroid hormone; 1,25-(OH)₂D₃, 1,25-dihydroxycholecalciferol (vitamin D₃).

(Fig. 12.1), and calcitonin, produced in the C-cells of the thyroid gland, which promotes calcium excretion. PTH is released in response to a decrease in plasma calcium levels and has several actions, including promoting the synthesis of 1,25-$(OH)_2D_3$ (the active form of vitamin D_3), which in turn stimulates intestinal calcium absorption. In addition, PTH (and vitamin D_3) promotes bone resorption and increases renal calcium reabsorption. Together, these coordinated actions serve to raise plasma calcium back to normal levels within minutes to hours. Thyroid synthesis of calcitonin is promoted in response to elevated plasma calcium levels and release of this hormone acts to antagonise the effects of PTH, inhibiting bone resorption and renal calcium reabsorption (i.e. promoting excretion of calcium) to lower plasma calcium.

As a consequence of bone resorption induced by PTH and vitamin D_3, plasma phosphate levels also rise. The excess phosphate, which could decrease ionised Ca^{2+} in the plasma, is eliminated via the kidney under the action of PTH, which inhibits its reabsorption in the renal tubules.

Functions

Bone mineralisation

The major function of both calcium and phosphorus is in the formation of the major inorganic bone component, hydroxyapatite (see also Ch. 24). Approximately 60% of the weight of bone is due to the presence of calcium-rich mineral deposits. Calcium is deposited in bone at a rate of 150 mg/day during adolescence as the skeleton develops. In the adult, there is a dynamic equilibrium between calcium and phosphate deposition and resorption (400 mg Ca and 500 mg P are exchanged between the bone and plasma every day) due to the constant remodelling associated with the maintenance of the healthy skeleton.

Blood clotting

Integral to the formation of a blood clot is the presence of a series of irregular fibrils of the protein fibrin, formed by polymerisation of a soluble precursor, fibrinogen. Deposition of fibrin is the end-point of a complicated cascade of enzyme reactions involving at least 10 other factors. This sequence of events can be initiated by blood coming into contact with a foreign surface such as collagen (the intrinsic clotting system) or following tissue damage (the extrinsic clotting system). Ca^{2+} (also known as factor IV) is a key component for the activation of both the intrinsic and extrinsic factor X activator complexes, the point at which the intrinsic and extrinsic coagulations systems converge. Calcium ions are further required at several subsequent stages of this cascade and a decrease in plasma calcium (below 2.5 mmol/l) is associated with a reduced ability to form blood clots (see also Section 11.4, under 'The metabolic functions of vitamin K').

Calcium and cell signalling

In contrast to the requirement to maintain a relatively high extracellular calcium level, intracellular free calcium concentrations are extremely low (less than 100 nmol/l). Low cytosolic calcium is maintained because cell membranes are relatively impermeable to calcium. Any calcium that does enter the cell is rapidly removed from the cytosol through the action of a number of calcium transporters and channels present in the plasma membrane and in the membranes of intracellular organelles, in particular, the smooth endoplasmic/sarcoplasmic reticulum, which sequesters calcium and acts as an intracellular store. However, cytosolic calcium levels can increase dramatically following agonist-induced generation of the second messenger inositol-1,4,5-trisphosphate (IP_3), which binds to specific receptors on the smooth endoplasmic reticulum and leads to an increase in intracellular Ca^{2+} concentration by as much as 10-fold. The release of Ca^{2+} initiates further second messenger activity by binding to various target molecules, for example protein kinase C and calmodulin, which in turn trigger a number of diverse cellular responses including cell division, cell motility, contraction, secretion, endocytosis and fertility.

Phosphorus and energy metabolism

Body phosphorus not involved in bone mineralisation is generally found in the soft tissues. Inside cells phosphorus (as the phosphate ion) participates in a number of processes associated with energy metabolism. Glucose, the primary metabolic fuel for most cellular activities, must first be phosphorylated before it can enter glycolysis. Indeed all of the intermediates between glucose and pyruvate in the glycolytic pathway are phosphorylated. Ultimately, energy produced from metabolism during oxidative phosphorylation in the mitochondria is stored as high-energy phosphate bonds in ATP (plus phosphocreatine in skeletal muscle).

A number of second messenger signalling cascades rely on phosphorylation or dephosphorylation as a mechanism for either activating or deactivating crucial enzymes. One of these second messengers is cyclic AMP, which is generated from ATP by the enzyme adenyl cyclase. Formation of cyclic AMP activates a specific protein kinase (PKA) that modulates the activity of a number of proteins by adding phosphate groups. An example of one such target protein is phosphorylase, the enzyme responsible for the degradation of the carbohydrate storage molecule glycogen to release glucose molecules for utilisation in metabolism.

Effect of deficiency and excess

As we have seen above, every day there are obligatory losses of calcium in the urine and the faeces. If this calcium is not replaced by the dietary supply, plasma calcium is maintained by resorption of bone under the action of PTH. If there is a continual low intake of calcium, or if intestinal absorption is impaired over a prolonged period, bone resorption will cause a severe decrease in bone mass and this dietary imbalance, together with a number of other factors, contributes to an increased risk of osteoporosis (see Ch. 24). It is estimated that more than one-third of women and one-sixth of men will sustain an osteoporotic fracture during their lifetime. Current estimates suggest that the NHS spends over £940 million per year treating more than 200 000 fractures, the majority of which are in the elderly.

Evidence for calcium toxicity is rare and adverse effects are limited to people taking high-level calcium supplements. However, the US Food and Nutrition Board has set a tolerable upper intake level of 2500 mg/day which appears to be safe for most people. There have been some concerns that high intakes of calcium might reduce the absorption of other essential trace elements, especially iron, but whilst calcium can decrease iron absorption from a single meal, there is no evidence to suggest that chronic calcium supplementation alters body iron status in the long term.

Since almost all food contains phosphorus, deficiency syndromes associated with inadequate phosphorus intake are extremely rare. When phosphorus intakes are low the body can adapt accordingly, increasing intestinal absorption and decreasing renal excretion. However, in some circumstances, for example in people with chronic gastrointestinal malabsorption syndromes or uncontrolled diabetes, there can be an imbalance in phosphorus homeostasis, which is regulated by demineralisation of the bone to maintain plasma phosphate levels. In severe situations, this can result in rickets in children or osteomalacia in adults. Similarly, rare genetic defects in the renal reabsorption of phosphate can cause rickets.

Toxicity associated with high phosphorus intakes is rare and is only likely to be a problem when calcium intakes are low. Elevated phosphorus intakes manifest themselves as an increase in plasma phosphate concentration, which is thought to be a risk factor for a decrease in bone mass. When plasma phosphate increases it results in a decrease in the plasma ionised calcium concentration that in turn leads to elevated serum PTH, which promotes bone resorption to re-establish plasma calcium levels. To this end there has been some concern in recent years that increasing dietary phosphorus intakes due to the large consumption of processed foods, which are often rich in phosphates, could have a detrimental effect on bone health.

Status assessment

Presently there are no reliable biochemical indicators to accurately assess calcium status. As we have seen above, plasma calcium is so tightly regulated that it bears little relationship to body calcium status. However, since 99% of body calcium is retained within the skeleton, measures of bone mass such as the bone mineral content (of a specific region such as the femoral neck) and bone mineral density have proved to be useful indicators of body calcium status.

The most common measure of phosphorus status is serum phosphate concentration. However, assessment of phosphorus status has not been considered a major problem due to the rarity of deficiency symptoms. Instead emphasis has been placed on maintaining phosphorus intake on an equimolar basis with calcium.

The basis of dietary recommendations

The dietary reference values (see Table CD 12.2) for the United Kingdom for calcium were determined by factorial analysis of the basal amounts of calcium required for bone growth and the maintenance of bone mineralisation (Department of Health 1991) and are based on published figures for calcium retention by the body for this purpose. In breastfed infants, calcium requirements (reference nutrient intake (RNI): 525 mg/day) are high and are met by the increased bioavailability of calcium from breast milk (about 66% absorption efficiency). Calcium retention in children increases significantly between the ages of 1 and 10 years (from 70 mg/day to 150 mg/day) as the skeleton develops. Absorption efficiency of calcium from a mixed diet in childhood is around 35% (i.e. less than from breast milk) and accordingly, the RNI has been calculated at 350 mg/day at age 2 rising to 550 mg/day at age 10. Assuming retention increases in adolescence to 250 mg/day for girls and 300 mg/day for boys the RNIs increase accordingly to 800 mg/day and 1000 mg/day, respectively. In adults following cessation of growth, there is still a significant calcium requirement based on calcium losses of 150 mg/day in the urine and 10 mg/day in sweat, skin and hair loss. Calcium absorption from an adult mixed diet is assumed to be 30%, giving an RNI of 700 mg/day.

No recommendation has been made for increasing calcium intakes during pregnancy due to higher rates of absorption compared with non-pregnant women. However, in adolescent pregnancies where females are still growing it may be advisable to increase calcium intakes. During lactation, the mother requires increased calcium for milk production, most (if not all) of which is derived from the diet. Initial estimates suggested that an extra 550 mg calcium/day was required for this purpose although this has recently been questioned due to potential adaptations in maternal calcium metabolism during lactation. The UK COMA panel has decided to wait for further evidence before changing the current recommendations (Department of Health 1998). No recommendations for increased intakes were made for postmenopausal women or the elderly.

In the UK and EU, phosphorus requirements are based on an equimolar intake with calcium and current recommendation is that the RNI for phosphorus should be equal to the calcium intake in mmol/day. Recently, the US Food and Nutrition Board set separate RDAs for phosphorus (not based on calcium intakes): for infants (0–6 months) 100 mg/day rising to 275 mg/day by 12 months of age; for children (1–3 years) 460 mg/day rising to 500 mg/day by age 8 years; for adolescents 1250 mg/day; for adults 700 mg/day. No further recommendations were made for pregnant or lactating adult women.

12.3 IRON

Iron is an essential trace metal and plays numerous biochemical roles in the body, including oxygen binding in haemoglobin and acting as an important catalytic centre in many enzymes, for example the cytochromes. However, in excess, iron is extremely toxic to cells and tissues due to its ability to rapidly alter its oxidation state and generate oxygen radicals. Consequently, body iron levels must be tightly regulated to avoid pathologies associated with both iron deficiency and overload. More than 2 billion people worldwide suffer from iron deficiency anaemia, making this the most common nutritional deficiency syndrome. At the same time 1 person in 200 of northern European descent is genetically predisposed to the iron loading disease haemochromatosis. The prevalence of these disorders highlights the importance of maintaining homeostatic control over iron nutriture.

Food sources

Dietary iron is found in two basic forms, either as haem or non-haem iron. Haem is found in meat and meat products that are rich in two major haem-containing proteins, haemoglobin and myoglobin. The most important dietary sources of haem iron are those that are eaten in significant quantities (e.g. mince, steaks, chicken and fish), though these may not necessarily be the richest sources of haem; a lamb chop, for example, contains 1.9 mg iron/100 g whereas calves' liver contains 8.0 mg iron/100 g. Between 25% and 50% of the total iron content of meat is haem; the remainder is non-haem iron largely present in iron storage proteins such as ferritin. Therefore haem iron accounts for approximately 5–10% of the daily iron intake in industrialised countries, whereas in vegetarian diets and in developing countries the haem iron intake is negligible. The main form of iron in all diets is non-haem iron, found in cereals, vegetables, pulses, beans, fruits etc. (see Table CD 12.3). Non-haem iron is present in these foods in a number of compounds ranging from simple iron oxides and salts to more complex organic chelates. In addition to food iron, exogenous iron from the soil can be present in significant quantities on the surface of food. This contaminating iron will enter the dietary pool and may therefore have nutritional importance.

Cereals contribute approximately half of our daily iron intake, yet most of the naturally occurring iron in cereals is in the seed coat. One might expect therefore that the products from processing cereal grains, e.g. flour, would have low iron content. However, since the 1950s in the UK, all wheat flours (other than wholemeal) have been fortified with iron by law so that they contain at least 1.65 mg iron/100 g flour. In addition to flour, breakfast cereals and many infant foods are also fortified with iron. The iron source used to fortify foods is usually small particles of reduced elemental iron, which are partially soluble at gastric pH and therefore readily contribute to the non-haem dietary iron pool.

Absorption and metabolism

The absorption of iron by duodenal enterocytes is influenced by a number of variables, especially dietary factors, e.g. the iron content of foods, the type of iron present, bioavailability, other dietary constituents. Absorption is also regulated in line with metabolic demands that reflect the amount of

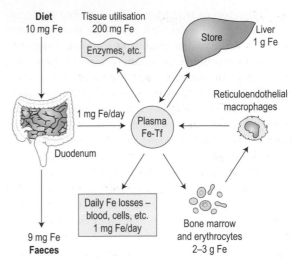

Figure 12.2   Body iron metabolism. Seventy-five per cent of body iron resides at any one time in the bone marrow and circulating erythrocytes; 25% is present in body stores in the liver. Approximately 1 mg Fe/day is absorbed from the diet to replace iron lost through minor bleeding and cell shedding.

iron stored in the body, and the requirements for red blood cell production (Fig. 12.2).

Bioavailability

Haem iron is the most bioavailable form of iron (see Table CD 12.4). Although it only accounts for 5–10% of dietary iron in Western countries, absorption of iron from haem-containing foods is some 20–30%. Compared with non-haem iron, haem absorption is less influenced by the iron status of individuals. The calcium content of the diet is thought to be the only other dietary factor to influence haem iron absorption, though the mechanism for this action is unknown. Food preparation alters haem iron bioavailability; prolonged cooking of meat at high temperatures is thought to degrade the porphyrin ring allowing the iron centre to be removed and join the non-haem iron pool.

Although non-haem iron is the most prevalent form of dietary iron, it is much less bioavailable than haem. Only 1–10% of dietary non-haem iron is absorbed due to the profound influence of other dietary components that can enhance or inhibit non-haem iron bioavailability (see Table CD 12.5). The most potent enhancer is ascorbic acid (vitamin C), which acts by reducing ferric iron to the more soluble and absorbable ferrous form. Other small organic acids, such as citric acid, and alcohol also promote the absorption of non-haem iron, possibly by forming stable soluble complexes with iron, thereby avoiding precipitation in the gut lumen. Meat and fish, as well as being abundant sources of haem and non-haem iron, also significantly promote the absorption of non-haem iron. The nature of the so-called 'meat factor' is still unclear but it might be related to high levels of cysteine- and histidine-containing peptides that could reduce ferric iron to ferrous.

The best-known dietary inhibitors of non-haem iron absorption are phytates, which are salts of inositol hexaphosphates found especially in cereal products. Phenolic compounds found in all plant food sources are also potent inhibitors of non-haem iron absorption. Perhaps the best-known group of compounds are the tannins found in abundance in tea and red wine. Both the phytates and phenolic compounds are thought to form insoluble ferric iron chelates in the intestinal lumen rendering the iron in a non-absorbable form. It is important to note that if the dietary level of ascorbic acid is sufficient it can counteract the inhibitory effect of phytates and phenols.

Intestinal absorption

Both haem and non-haem iron are absorbed in the duodenum (the proximal region of the small intestine), though through completely independent mechanisms (see Fig. CD 12.3). Haem is absorbed intact and inside the enterocyte the iron is removed by the action of haem oxygenase.

Non-haem iron is largely present in the less soluble and non-absorbable ferric form and must first be reduced to ferrous iron before it becomes bioavailable. This is achieved by a combination of dietary reducing agents (e.g. ascorbate) and endogenous enzymic activity of the enterocyte. The fate of the absorbed iron is determined by body iron requirements – it can either be stored in the enterocyte as ferritin when the body stores are replete, or can leave the cell and be loaded onto transferrin for transport in the plasma and delivery to the iron-requiring tissues.

Transport and tissue distribution

Transferrin can bind two ferric iron molecules, delivering the iron to the sites of storage (mainly in the liver) or utilisation (e.g. the bone marrow) (Fig. 12.2). Body iron content is some 3–5 g (approximately 50 mg/kg body weight). Of this, approximately 70% is present in the circulating red blood cells, 20% is stored as ferritin and haemosiderin in

the liver, 5% is incorporated into myoglobin in muscle and 5% bound or utilised by various enzymes. Clearly erythrocyte production and destruction accounts for the majority of metabolic iron turnover in the body. The typical lifespan of a red blood cell is 120 days and after this time senescent erythrocytes are engulfed by cells of the reticuloendothelial system (a combination of splenic macrophages and the Kupffer cells in the liver) and the iron recovered from haemoglobin by the action of haem oxygenase. This liberated iron is transported in the blood bound to transferrin back to the bone marrow for new red blood cell production or to the liver for storage.

Iron homeostasis

There are no defined excretory pathways for excess iron from the body. Iron losses are therefore restricted to that stored in cells shed from the lining of the gastrointestinal and urinary tracts, skin and hair, and losses through bleeding. Basal losses of iron amount to approximately 1.0 mg/day in men and 1.3–1.4 mg/day in premenopausal women (due to menstrual blood loss). These losses must be replaced by dietary intake to maintain body iron levels. Therefore the body has three basic mechanisms for maintaining iron homeostasis: (1) continuous re-utilisation of iron recovered from senescent red blood cells; (2) regulation of intestinal iron absorption to match body iron status; (3) exploitation of an iron storage pool, i.e. ferritin, that acts as an iron reserve, storing and releasing iron in response to excessive metabolic demand.

Functions

Iron-containing enzymes

Iron plays a major role in regulating energy production via oxidative phosphorylation. The cytochromes are haem-containing enzymes consisting of a globin chain plus a haem group containing one iron atom. Whilst the cytochromes do not bind oxygen, they can function as efficient electron carriers and play a crucial role in the mitochondrial oxidation of fuels and formation of ATP. Three cytochromes, *a*, *b* and *c*, are involved in mitochondrial electron transfer leading to oxidative phosphorylation, and other cytochromes are important in the detoxification of foreign compounds.

Iron is also an important component of several other enzymes involved in energy metabolism, e.g. aconitase, succinate dehydrogenase and NADH-dehydrogenase. Iron in these enzymes is present as non-haem iron and forms an iron–sulphur complex that is responsible for the carriage of electrons. Haem iron is an important component of catalase and peroxidase, two key enzymes that act on reactive oxygen metabolites by converting hydrogen peroxide into oxygen and water.

Pro-oxidant activity

Despite its essential role in metabolism, iron is also a prospective pro-oxidant and is therefore potentially harmful (see also Section 13.5). Excess iron promotes lipid peroxidation and tissue damage in vitro, raising the possibility that, via these pro-oxidant effects, disturbances in iron metabolism play a pathogenic role in a number of diseases.

Immune function

The importance of iron as a regulator of immune function is becoming increasingly recognised. Iron is an essential growth factor for most microorganisms and the sequestration of iron in ferritin inside cells and its binding to transferrin in the plasma means that there is a lack of available free iron in the body for microbial growth. When there is an imbalance in body iron homeostasis, as in iron overload, then more iron is available and may predispose an individual to infection. However, iron is an important growth promoter for a number of crucial immune responses including lymphocyte proliferation, and hence cell-mediated immunity may be compromised by iron deficiency.

Effects of iron deficiency and overload

Anaemia

The most common cause of anaemia is nutritional iron deficiency (see Ch. 28). It is estimated that 2 billion of the world's population (largely in developing countries) have marked iron deficiency anaemia (WHO 1997).

Whilst mild anaemia in many individuals is of little health consequence (due to a number of compensatory mechanisms such as increased cardiac output, diversion of blood flow to vital organs and increased release of oxygen from haemoglobin), severe anaemia exceeds the body's ability to adapt, resulting in impaired oxygen delivery to the tissues. This in turn has deleterious effects on a number of important body functions.

Work performance

Work performance, particularly physical work capacity, is severely limited in anaemia. Experimental studies in animals have demonstrated impaired running ability in iron-deficient rats that was accompanied by a reduction in oxidative energy production in skeletal muscle. In human beings also, iron deficiency anaemia limits work performance. In female tea pickers in Sri Lanka and in male Indonesian rubber plantation workers who had hookworm infection, reduced productivity was directly related to the severity of anaemia. Following supplementation therapy, iron-deficient subjects showed improved performance, with the greatest progress seen in those who had the most severe anaemia.

Cognitive function

The relationship between iron deficiency and impaired performance in mental and motor tests in children is well established (Lozoff et al 2000). Brain iron content increases throughout childhood and reaches its maximal levels in young adulthood between the ages of 20 and 30 years. However, experiments with iron-deficient rats suggest that iron accumulation during infancy is especially important in determining both total brain iron content and brain development; an early deficit in brain iron is not compensated for in later years. Compelling evidence demonstrates that infants with iron deficiency anaemia fare less well in an array of psychomotor tests than non-anaemic age-matched counterparts. Even though measurable indices of body iron status can be normalised in these children by giving iron supplements, cognitive function is still impaired some 10 years later in those subjects who were severely iron deficient in childhood.

Haemochromatosis

The majority of cases of primary iron overload are accounted for by the genetic disease haemochromatosis, an autosomal recessive disorder affecting mainly populations of European descent. The disease has a carrier frequency of approximately 1 in 10 and a homozygous frequency for the mutated gene of 1 in 200. Two mutations resulting in the disease have been mapped to the HLA-H (now called HFE) gene region of chromosome 6 and these account for more than 80% of the cases of haemochromatosis in northern Europeans.

Most cases of hereditary haemochromatosis are not diagnosed until patients present with clinical problems associated with organ failure (typically around 40–50 years of age). Simple and effective treatment of these patients can be achieved through the removal of excess body iron by phlebotomy. In the initial stages of treatment, venesection will be performed as often as once per week and continued until the body iron stores are depleted. The patient will remain on venesection therapy (every 3–4 months) for life. It is often stated that haemochromatosis is a clinical and not a nutritional problem of iron metabolism. However, there may be nutritional issues for the 1 in 10 of the population who are heterozygous carriers of the HFE mutations, who may be predisposed to increased intestinal iron absorption resulting in mild iron overloading.

Status assessment

Currently, there is no single test available to determine with complete accuracy perturbations in body iron status. Therefore, a wide variety of biochemical methods are employed to assess a number of key indices of iron metabolism (Table 12.1).

The basis of dietary recommendations

Daily basal iron losses occur as a consequence of desquamation of cells lining the gastrointestinal tract (0.14 mg/day) and urinary tract (0.1 mg/day); blood loss accounts for a further 0.38 mg/day and bile losses amount to 0.24 mg/day (see Table CD 12.6). Minor amounts are lost due to shedding of skin and hair. Thus basal iron losses are estimated at 14 µg/kg body weight/day though these vary on an individual basis. In infants, children and adolescents, in addition to basal losses, iron is also required for growth of the tissues and organs and for the expanding red blood cell mass. Within the first year of life the infant

Table 12.1 Common methods for assessing body iron status		
Status indicator	**Normal range**	**Additional information**
Serum ferritin	30–300 µg/l	1 µg/l serum ferritin = 10 mg tissue stored ferritin 12–15 µg/l indicates empty stores Acute phase protein – false high levels seen in infection and inflammation
Transferrin saturation	25–30%	Values below 16% are indicative of inadequate supply for erythropoiesis Values above 50–60% are generally indicative of haemochromatosis
Erythrocyte protoporphyrin	<80 µmol/mol haem	Protoporphyrin is the final intermediate in haem synthesis – levels rise when iron supply is limited Values >80 µmol/mol haem indicate iron deficiency anaemia Also increased by other diseases, resulting in increased erythroid turnover
Serum transferrin receptor	2.8–8.5 mg/l	A measure of reticulocyte differentiation – shedding of TfR into serum Detectable receptor levels increase in iron deficiency Also increased in all diseases, increasing erythrocyte turnover Not affected by iron overload
Haemoglobin	120–180 g/l	Values below 110 g/l indicative of anaemia Not altered by iron overload Not altered in intermediate phases leading to anaemia
Mean cell volume	80–94 fl	Smaller erythrocyte volume in anaemia Cannot distinguish between iron deficiency anaemia and other anaemias

doubles its iron content and triples its body weight (most of these changes take place between 6 and 12 months of age). Body iron content is again doubled between 1 and 6 years old. The growth spurt in adolescence also increases iron demand, as does the dramatic increase in haemoglobin concentration seen in males during puberty and the onset of menarche in females. In premenopausal women menstrual blood loss must also be taken into account alongside other iron losses (it is estimated that women lose an average of 0.7 mg/day via this route).

Dietary intakes to satisfy the metabolic requirements and iron losses depend largely on the bioavailability of iron in the diet. In most industrialised countries typical diets will be rich in meat, poultry and fish plus food containing high levels of ascorbic acid. Current UK guidelines envisage that iron absorption from typical diets will be 15% and this has been used to calculate the current dietary reference values for iron (Department of Health 1991). Assuming average endogenous iron losses in adults are 1.0 mg/day in men and 1.7 mg/day in women, the estimated average dietary requirements for iron are 6.7 and 11.4 mg/day in men and women, respectively.

The EAR for breast- or formula-fed infants aged 0–3 months is 1.3 mg/day, which trebles (in line with increased growth) over the next 6 months to 3.3 mg/day. There are no recommendations for increasing iron intake during pregnancy as the extra demand should be met by a combination of pre-existing body stores, lack of menstrual blood loss and the increased intestinal absorptive capacity during the second and third trimesters. Likewise, there are no recommendations for increasing iron intake during lactation, where iron losses (i.e. secreted in breast milk) are compensated for by the amenorrhoea associated with lactation.

12.4 ZINC

The essential role of zinc in mammalian nutrition has been known since the 1930s. However, it was believed that human zinc nutrition was not a major public health issue due to the absence of zinc deficiency symptoms in the general population. This continued to be the case until the 1960s when human zinc deficiency was first noted in adolescents living in the Nile delta of Egypt and in rural Iran. Since these observations there has been a huge increase in the understanding of human zinc metabolism. However, there are still significant nutritional questions to be addressed including the assessment of marginal zinc status.

Food sources

Daily zinc intake from an omnivorous diet is typically 10–12 mg/day (see Table CD 12.7). The zinc content of foods varies greatly (see Table CD 12.8), with the highest levels found in meat, whole grains and shellfish (particularly oysters). Animal sources provide the majority of dietary zinc in omnivorous diets (up to 70% of daily intake), mainly due to the high levels of zinc present in muscle (up to 50 mg/kg) where it is bound to proteins and nucleic acids. In contrast, fat has a very low zinc content (5 mg/kg). In general, red meats have higher zinc levels than white meat and fish muscle has a lower zinc content than meat.

In many cultures, cereal products are the major dietary energy sources. The zinc content of these foods is directly related to the degree of refinement. Highest levels are found in whole grains (30–50 mg/kg), with lower amounts present in white flour (8–10 mg/kg). This difference is due to the fact that zinc is contained within the outer layer of the cereal grain, which is removed during processing. In general the zinc content of green leafy vegetables and fruit is low (2–6 mg/kg).

Absorption and metabolism

Bioavailability and absorption

Zinc is variably absorbed from different food groups (see Table CD 12.9). The major inhibitor of absorption is phytic acid, present in large quantities in cereals, legumes and other vegetables. Phytate is negatively charged at food pH and readily forms insoluble complexes with positively charged ions such as zinc, thereby limiting bioavailability. This inhibitory effect on absorption can be partly overcome by food preparation techniques; for example, addition of yeast during bread-making increases phytase activity, reducing phytate levels. On the other hand, diets containing large quantities of unleavened bread are poor providers of zinc and are thought to be associated with the growth defects observed in adolescents living in the Nile delta of Egypt and rural Iran.

Animal protein is thought to act as an 'antiphytic' agent and enhances the bioavailability of zinc. It is thought that small peptides and amino acids released during digestion improve the solubility of zinc and protect against the formation of insoluble phytate complexes. A typical omnivorous diet should provide adequate zinc to maintain body homeostasis, since animal protein intake would be sufficient to outweigh the inhibitory effects of the phytate.

It is also important to note that the diet is not the only source of zinc entering the gastrointestinal tract. Endogenous zinc is also present in the small intestine as a consequence of pancreatic and biliary secretions (zinc is an essential co-factor for the carboxypeptidases involved in protein digestion). This source of zinc is also available for absorption and is taken up by the intestinal epithelial cells by the same route as dietary zinc.

Zinc absorption takes place in the small intestine, with the highest absorption rate in the jejunum. Uptake is transporter mediated (an additional passive component may be evident at high luminal zinc concentrations) though the precise cellular mechanisms involved are still unclear (see Fig. CD 12.4).

Transport and tissue distribution

Zinc entering the blood from the intestinal enterocytes is transported in the portal circulation to the liver bound mainly to albumin (70%) and α_2-macroglobulin (20–30%). Total body zinc amounts to some 2–3 g in a typical adult and is primarily localised intracellularly. Only 0.1% of total body zinc is found in the plasma whereas 60% is found in skeletal muscle and a further 30% is contained within bone (Fig. 12.3).

Homeostatic regulation of body zinc content

There is no recognised storage pool of zinc to act as a reservoir for times when zinc metabolic requirements change. Instead a number of tissues, especially the liver, are highly active in redistributing zinc between body organs. A key feature of this regulation appears to be the intracellular zinc binding protein metallothionein, a cysteine-rich protein that is induced by high dietary zinc levels and is thought to act as an intracellular zinc buffer.

The small intestine ultimately controls body zinc content by regulating both the amount of dietary zinc absorbed and the quantity of endogenous zinc, supplied by the intestinal, biliary and pancreatic secretions, lost in the faeces. Absorption (or

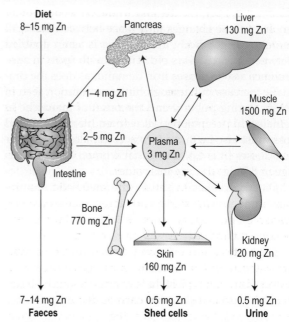

Figure 12.3   Body zinc distribution. Dietary intake (8–15 mg/day) matches endogenous losses in the faeces, urine and shed skin cells. Zinc is mainly an intracellular ion – hence low plasma but high tissue concentrations.

reabsorption) of zinc from both of these sources is directly related to body zinc status. Zinc losses via the intestinal route include not only exogenous and endogenous zinc but also that lost as a consequence of shedding of cells lining the gastrointestinal tract. Total losses via this route normally range from 0.5 to 3 mg/day but can be greater in gastrointestinal disease.

In addition to intestinal losses, excretion of zinc via the kidney usually amounts to 0.5 mg/day in healthy adults. Most of the zinc filtered through the glomerulus is reabsorbed from the renal tubular fluid as it passes along the nephron. Unlike the intestine, zinc reabsorption in the kidney is unaffected by daily fluctuations in dietary zinc intake. However, urinary zinc excretion can be altered significantly in renal disease, insulin-dependent diabetes mellitus, alcoholism and starvation.

Further zinc can be lost from the body via skin, hair and sweat (about 0.5 mg/day). Also zinc accumulates in the prostatic fluids and an ejaculation of semen contains up to 1 mg of zinc.

Functions

The major function of zinc in human metabolism is as a cofactor for over 100 metalloproteins and enzymes.

Zinc can participate directly in the catalytic activity at the active site of many enzymes, catalysing a wide variety of reactions, and in other key proteins the role of zinc is structural, maintaining three-dimensional integrity.

Several key enzymes involved in the synthesis of RNA and DNA are zinc dependent, including the DNA and RNA polymerases. In addition, zinc plays a key role in gene transcription as an essential structural component of the zinc finger motifs found in several nuclear hormone receptors (e.g. those for vitamin D, testosterone and oestrogen) and transcription factors. The ability of zinc finger-containing transcription factors to bind DNA is highly zinc dependent and may be lost in zinc deficiency.

In addition to zinc fingers, structural zinc centres are essential for several enzymes, including superoxide dismutase (SOD), a key antioxidant enzyme. In SOD there are two atoms each of zinc and copper. It is thought that zinc maintains the structural arrangement of the enzyme whilst copper is essential to the catalytic activity required for the removal of the superoxide radical. In addition to its essential role in the antioxidant function of SOD, zinc exhibits further antioxidant actions, including induction of metallothionein synthesis, and the ability to bind to sulphydryl groups on various proteins, protecting them from oxidation.

Zinc has profound effects on carbohydrate metabolism. Zinc-deficient animals have significantly impaired glucose tolerance, due to a reduced ability to secrete insulin from the pancreas in response to an oral glucose load. It has been long recognised that dimerisation of insulin and complexing with zinc are essential for storage and secretion in the pancreatic beta cell. When pancreatic islets are stimulated with glucose or other secretagogues, there is a marked decrease in cellular zinc content that is directly related to the release of insulin. In addition to co-release with insulin from the beta cell, zinc is also thought to increase and stabilise insulin binding to its receptors on target tissues, prolonging its biological actions.

Zinc deficiency and excess

Zinc deficiency

A number of zinc deficiency states of varying severity occur, especially in the developing world. In the UK, zinc intakes are sufficient to replace endogenous daily losses and therefore severe zinc deficiency does not occur. The possibility of people having marginal zinc status in Western countries is more difficult to address and there is a need for the development of better techniques with which to assess zinc status (see below).

The first observations of human zinc deficiency were made in the 1960s in Iran and Egypt (Prasad et al 1961, 1963). It was suggested that zinc deficiency was the major contributing factor to a syndrome in which adolescents presented with dwarfism and hypogonadism. A number of similar cases were subsequently identified, mainly in Middle Eastern countries. The primary causes of zinc deficiency in these patients were two-fold: nutritional deficiency due to poor zinc bioavailability from a diet rich in unleavened bread; and geophagia (the practice of eating clay – up to 0.5 kg/day in some patients), which would further reduce zinc absorption.

Subsequently, severe zinc deficiency has been noted in industrialised countries and is characterised by dermatitis, diarrhoea and impaired immunity leading to greater susceptibility to infections. This syndrome, called acrodermatitis enteropathica, is not thought to have its origins in nutritional deficiency but rather develops due to an autosomal recessive inborn error of zinc metabolism leading to a decrease in the absorption of dietary zinc. Recently, an intestinal zinc transport protein has been shown to be mutated in a number of families affected with acrodermatitis enteropathica, suggesting that this defective protein contributes to the aetiology of the disease.

For many years it has been known that zinc deficiency inhibits growth. The overall effects of zinc deficiency on growth are likely to be multifactorial, with the major inhibitory influences on mitogenic hormones complemented by negative effects of zinc deficiency on food intake, signal transduction pathways, and gene transcription. To date, reduced growth rate is the only clearly demonstrated consequence of mild zinc deficiency in human beings and zinc supplementation studies have shown improved growth in infants and children (Gibson 1994).

Zinc is found in abundant quantities associated with the skeleton where it is thought to play a central role in the turnover and metabolism of the connective tissues. Zinc deficiency has a negative influence on bone formation, which might result from imbalances in DNA synthesis and protein metabolism. Zinc is also an essential cofactor for a number of crucial enzymes including alkaline phosphatase, which plays a major role in bone mineralisation, and collagenase, which is fundamental to the development and remodelling of bone structure.

Zinc excess

Whilst on the whole zinc is considered to have low toxicity, acute excessive intake (of the order of 2 g zinc) can cause symptoms such as nausea, abdominal pain, vomiting, diarrhoea and fever. In addition, there are some concerns that high doses of zinc (75–300 mg/day) over a prolonged period of time might adversely influence the metabolism of other important trace elements, in particular copper and iron.

Status assessment

The intracellular nature of zinc, its tissue distribution (and homeostatic redistribution) and the absence of a defined storage pool make the assessment of zinc status difficult. Several indices of zinc status have been used, including zinc levels in plasma, erythrocytes, leukocytes, neutrophils and hair. In addition, indirect methods associated with zinc-dependent physiological functions have also been studied, including the activity of a number of metalloenzymes, dark adaptation and taste acuity, but with limited success. None of these measures has yet proven successful in determining marginal zinc deficiency. Zinc levels in plasma or serum are the most commonly used measures but are not ideal as they only vary significantly with severe zinc deficiency and do not respond to fluctuations in dietary zinc. In addition serum zinc can be altered dramatically by metabolic variations that are not linked to zinc status. Further research is required therefore to develop more reliable methods for assessing human zinc status and particularly marginal zinc deficiency.

The basis of dietary recommendations

As mentioned above, endogenous losses of zinc are dependent on zinc intake and the homeostatic mechanisms controlling faecal loss. Zinc requirements are based on replenishing basal losses. A number of methods have been used to determine these, including metabolic balance studies, turnover time of radiolabelled endogenous zinc pools and measurement of total endogenous zinc loss. None is an ideal measurement, but they all indicate that in people eating a typical Western diet providing 10–12 mg zinc/day, endogenous losses amount to 2–3 mg/day (recent factorial analysis suggests that basal zinc losses are 2.2 mg/day for men, 1.6 mg/day for women) and this amount needs to be replaced. The dietary reference values for the UK are based on these figures and assume that 30% of dietary zinc is bioavailable for absorption. This translates into RNIs of 9.5 and 7.0 mg/day for men and women, respectively (Department of Health 1991). For infants and children, factorial analysis has suggested that zinc losses are related to body size and that the zinc requirements for growth increase incrementally with age. Consequently, the RNI for infants is 4.0 mg/day, rising to 9.0 mg/day in prepubescent children.

There is evidence that extra zinc is required in pregnancy for the fetus, placenta and amniotic fluid as well as for uterine and mammary tissue development and the increase in the maternal blood volume. However, because additional zinc is accumulated in the last trimester of gestation it is likely that in healthy women this extra zinc plus metabolic adaptation provides adequate transfer of zinc to the fetus and therefore in the UK there is no recommendation for additional zinc in pregnancy. In lactation, additional zinc requirements have been calculated on the basis of a zinc secretion in milk of 2.13 mg/day, giving an increase in the RNI of 6.0 mg/day. Requirements fall after 4 months of lactation, as milk secretion decreases, to an additional 2.5 mg/day over the RNI.

12.5 IODINE

Iodine is an essential micronutrient that forms a vital component of the thyroid hormones thyroxine and triiodothyronine, which are crucial regulators of the metabolic rate and physical and mental development in humans. Iodine deficiency is relatively rare in the UK but is still prevalent in many areas in the world, where it constitutes a major problem of public health nutrition.

Dietary sources

Iodine is usually found in food as inorganic iodide or iodate. The iodine content of plants and cereals varies dramatically (from 10 μg/kg to 1 mg/kg) depending on the iodine content of the soil. Similarly the iodine content of drinking water is also variable (0.1–100 μg/l) and therefore for many population groups does not constitute a major dietary source (see Table CD 12.7). In the UK, cow's milk has become the major iodine-containing food in the diet (0.15 mg/kg) due to the use of supplemented feeds and the provision of iodinated casein as a lactation promoter (Wenlock 1987). The richest sources of iodine in the diet are marine fish (up to 2.5 mg/kg), shellfish (up to 1.6 mg/kg), seaweed (up to 5 mg/kg) and sea salt (up to 1.4 mg/kg). Significant amounts of iodine are also provided by multivitamin and mineral supplements (up to 0.1 mg/day) and in seaweed (kelp) products. In some regions of the world where iodine deficiency is a significant problem, extra iodine is provided in the diet in the form of iodide- or iodate-supplemented salt or bread (see Table CD 12.8).

Absorption and metabolism

Bioavailability

Iodine is rapidly and efficiently absorbed in the proximal small intestine as iodide. In addition, some organic iodine complexes, such as thyroid hormones added to animal feeds, can be absorbed intact (approximately 50% of dietary intake) but to a lesser extent than free iodide. The remaining larger organic complexes are lost in the faeces. Other iodine-containing foods and iodates, which are often used as a salt fortificant or as a food additive (especially in bread as a dough preservative), are readily broken down and reduced to iodide in the intestinal lumen.

Iodine content of foods can be significantly affected by the way that foods are cooked. For example, boiling foods reduces their iodine content by approximately half whereas frying decreases iodine by less than 20%. Bioavailability and absorption is also influenced by other dietary components, especially by brassicas (e.g. cabbage, broccoli etc.) that are rich in sulphur-containing glucosides, which can liberate thiocyanates and isothiocyanates that compete with iodide for absorption and tissue uptake.

Transport and tissue distribution

The mechanisms involved in iodide absorption in the intestine are still unclear; however, following absorption free iodide appears rapidly in the blood. Unlike the majority of trace elements, iodide in the blood does not appear to be bound to plasma proteins and is available for uptake by all the tissues of the body. The majority of the circulating iodide (approximately 80%) is rapidly taken up by the thyroid gland, but significant amounts are also accumulated by the salivary glands, choroid plexus and the lactating mammary gland. Uptake of iodide by all of these tissues employs a similar mechanism utilising a sodium/iodide symporter, which is stimulated by the thyroid-stimulating hormone (TSH) released from the pituitary gland. Total body iodine levels are 15–20 mg in healthy adults. Once the iodine requirements for thyroid hormone production have been met, excess circulating iodide is removed from the blood by the kidney and excreted in the urine (urinary iodide is a good indicator of body iodine status).

Function – the thyroid hormones

Iodide is taken up from the circulation by the follicle cells of the thyroid and passes into the inner colloidal space where it is rapidly oxidised to iodine (I_2), by thyroid peroxidase, and reacts with the tyrosine residues on thyroglobulin, a large glycoprotein, to produce monoiodotyrosine and diiodotyrosine. These two precursors can condense to form the thyroid hormones triiodothyronine (T_3) and thyroxine (T_4). These remain bound to thyroglobulin and are stored within the colloid until the thyroid is stimulated by TSH, whereupon thyroglobulin is taken up by the follicle cells and acted on by lysosomal enzymes to liberate active T_3 and T_4 which are subsequently released into the circulation. T_4 has a relatively low biological activity and serves as a reservoir for the production of the more active T_3 following removal of the 5' iodine by selenium-dependent deiodinases present in the liver, kidney, muscle and pituitary.

The major functions of the thyroid hormones are the maintenance of the metabolic rate, cellular metabolism and growth. Their function is elicited by binding to nuclear receptors that in turn bind to DNA and regulate the transcription of several genes in target tissues, in particular the brain, heart, liver and kidneys.

Effects of iodine deficiency and excess

Iodine deficiency causes a wide range of disorders collectively known as iodine deficiency disorders in which symptoms range from mild, such as goitre, to severe, including mental retardation or cretinism

13

Inter-micronutrient topics

David Thurnham

Objectives

By the end of this chapter you should be able to:

- summarise drug/micronutrient interactions
- describe the role of micronutrients in the immune response
- explain the role of micronutrients in gene expression
- discuss the roles of micronutrients as pro- or antioxidants
- describe the potential protective effects of polyphenols and phytoestrogens.

13.1 INTRODUCTION

Poor diets are rarely just deficient in only one nutrient. The nutrient that is least adequate in the diet may cause the main clinical or subclinical effects but if only that nutrient is replaced, other nutrients may then become limiting, preventing any response to treatment. There is considerable potential for adverse consequences from both single and multi-nutrient supplements through interaction with dietary components. Supplements usually contain a disproportionately large amount of nutrient relative to normal dietary intakes as the objective is to improve nutritional status rapidly (Beaton et al 1993). Giving large amounts of supplements can have surprisingly adverse effects. Nutrients may have toxic effects themselves on the body as in the case of vitamin A. Even non-toxic β-carotene increased mortality from lung cancer in smokers in two large intervention studies. Nutrients can interact with one another and block absorption, as happens with iron and zinc. Supplementary nutrients may exacerbate inflammation and thus worsen the effects of disease on the body. Iron is a good example of this, but there are also reports that supplements of vitamin A can adversely affect respiratory disease and there is one report that vitamin A supplements increased transmission of HIV to infants from the mother.

We adapt to handle nutrients and other substances at the concentrations in our diet and environment. We have in-built safety mechanisms to handle large amounts of nutrients as well as the many thousands of xenobiotics in our diet (Guengerich 1995, Kane & Lipsky 2000). The bio-transformation of such compounds is handled by what are known as phase I and II reactions. Most end-products of such biotransformations can be safely excreted but there are some well-known exceptions. Intermediate compounds formed from dietary nitrosamines and aflatoxins are more active than the original and, in these cases, are carcinogenic. The activity of phase I enzymes can be both depressed and stimulated by substances in our diet and the actual activity of these enzymes may be a product of the habitual dietary environment in which we live. Hence persons regularly consuming diets high in fruit and vegetables may metabolise potential carcinogens differently from those whose diet is low in these foods, and thereby will have a lower risk of developing cancers. A well-balanced diet should contain adequate amounts of nutrients to maintain normal metabolism but also a wide range of non-nutrients to optimise phase I and II metabolic processes.

It is proposed to examine a selection of issues relating to micronutrient interactions. Section 13.2 will address drug–nutrient interactions and this includes lifestyle factors like smoking and alcohol use. Section 13.3 will look at issues relating to the immune response and micronutrients. Section 13.4 will address some issues relating to gene–nutrient interactions. Section 13.5 will address the question of interrelationships between the antioxidant nutrients and their significance in maintaining health. Finally Sections 13.6 and 13.7 deal with two specific groups of antioxidants, namely (1) phenols and polyphenols and (2) phytoestrogens and the possible importance of their antioxidant properties in determining biological activity.

13.2 DRUG–NUTRIENT INTERACTIONS

A drug–nutrient interaction refers to the effect of a medication on nutrients in the food we eat or those already in our bodies or the converse, where food or dietary treatments may have an influence on the effectiveness of a drug. Food ingestion can profoundly affect a drug's pharmacodynamics and can either accelerate or retard drug absorption. Where prolonged medication is prescribed, the potential interaction between food and drugs may be increased and this becomes of greater importance in older people (Thomas & Burns 1998). Risk factors that increase the potential for drug–nutrient interactions are multiple medications, reduced intakes, nutrient loss from poor cooking habits, restrictive diets, anorexia, eating disorders, alcoholism, drug dependency or addiction, renal and hepatic dysfunction.

Drug–nutrient interaction can be categorised as physicochemical, physiological or pathophysiological. An example of a physicochemical interaction is chelation of a nutrient by a drug, causing loss of a nutrient and lower activity of a drug. Physiological interactions include drug-induced changes in appetite, digestion, gastric emptying, metabolism and excretion. Pathophysiological interactions occur when a drug impairs nutrient absorption or metabolism, or a drug causes an inhibition of metabolic processes. For example, female sex hormones alter the metabolism of vitamins A and D, producing higher plasma concentrations of retinol and 25-hydroxycholecalciferol.

Frequently, drug–nutrient interactions are bi-directional. For example, while the bioavailability of minerals is reduced by co-administration with some drugs, drug absorption is also reduced by nutrients, especially minerals. Iron–drug interactions of clinical significance may involve tetracycline derivatives, penicillamine, methyldopa, thyroxine and other drugs. Furthermore, disease itself depresses circulating concentrations of some nutrients and may increase requirements (Thurnham & Northrop-Clewes 2004). Plasma concentrations of iron, retinol, ascorbate and zinc are rapidly and almost universally depressed by the inflammatory response.

Common drugs that influence the handling or turnover of nutrients

Medications may decrease appetite but usually the effects of the drugs are to alter nutrient absorption, metabolism or excretion (Table 13.1). The interactions described in this section are those that may lead to impaired nutritional status.

The short-term use of drugs is less likely to have adverse effects on nutritional status than long-term treatments. The problem is that the long-term use of many drugs is escalating. Over the last forty years, life expectancy has increased by almost 10 years in

industrialised countries and by 20 years in parts of the developing world. As people live longer, the incidence of chronic diseases rises and the use of long-term drug therapy for chronic diseases such as arthritis, hypertension, coronary artery disease and adult onset diabetes will continue to increase. Many classes of drugs including antimicrobials, hypoglycaemic and hypocholesterolaemic agents can be affected by the presence of food, with the elderly patient being particularly at risk.

Aspirin and other non-steroidal anti-inflammatory drugs commonly cause gastric irritation and should be consumed with food. Aspirin is also reported to lower plasma vitamin C concentrations, but the mechanism is not known. Severe irritation to the stomach lining can cause bleeding leading to the loss of blood and the risk of anaemia through iron deficiency. In addition, it is suggested that aspirin alters the transport of folate by competition for binding sites on serum proteins; 70% of patients with rheumatoid arthritis have low plasma folate concentrations.

Antacids neutralise stomach acid and acid blockers reduce its secretion. Antacids may alter a substance's solubility both by modifying gastric pH and by chelation. Aluminium, a constituent of many antacids, can produce a relaxing effect on gastric smooth muscle that leads to a delay in gastric emptying time. Increased gastric pH leads to a reduced absorption of calcium, iron, magnesium and zinc. Regular use of these drugs lowers the absorption of vitamin B_{12} since an acid environment is needed for its release from dietary proteins; as discussed in Section 10.6, the elderly are already at risk of vitamin B_{12} deficiency as a result of atrophic gastritis.

Antibiotics are used to treat bacterial infections. When they are taken by mouth they will reduce the number and range of bacteria found in the large intestine. Although the relative importance of dietary vitamin K (phylloquinone) and intestinal bacterial menaquinones is unclear (see Section 11.4), antibiotics can cause vitamin K deficiency and impair blood clotting. Cephalosporins containing the N-methylthiotetrazole side-chain are inhibitors of hepatic vitamin K epoxide reductase.

Tetracycline antibiotics bind to calcium in dairy products, which is a major food source of calcium in most industrialised countries (Thomas & Burns 1998). The interaction prevents the absorption of both calcium and the antibiotic. Calcium deficiency leads to mobilisation of bone calcium and subsequently to osteoporosis, a common feature of ageing.

Table 13.1 Examples of some drug–nutrient interactions

Altering absorption		Altering nutrient metabolism		Altering nutrient excretion	
Drug	**Nutrient malabsorbed**	**Drug**	**Nutrient**	**Drug**	**Nutrient with increased excretion**
Bisacodyl (laxative)	Potassium	Hydralazine (antihypertensive)	Vitamin B_6 antagonism	Aspirin (anti-inflammatory)	Vitamin C, potassium
Cholestyramine (anti-hyperlipaemic)	Iron, carotene, vitamins A, D and K, folate	Isoniazid (antitubercular)	Vitamin B_6 antagonism	Furosemide (frusemide; diuretic)	Vitamin B_1, potassium, calcium, magnesium, sodium, chloride
Aluminium hydroxide (antacid)	Phosphate, vitamins A and B_1	Methotrexate (antineoplastic, anti-psoriatic)	Folate antagonist, malabsorption of vitamin B_{12} and fat	Spironolactone (diuretic)	Sodium, chloride
Colchicine (anti-gout)	Sodium, potassium, carotene, vitamin B_{12}	Penicillamine (chelating agent)	Inhibits vitamin B_6-dependent enzymes, chelates copper, iron and zinc	Thiazide (diuretic)	Potassium, magnesium and sodium but decrease urinary calcium
Mineral oil (laxative)	Carotene, vitamins A, D, E and K, calcium and phosphorus	Phenobarbital, (anticonvulsant)	Increased turnover of vitamin D due to hepatic enzyme induction	Tetracycline (antibiotic)	Vitamin C
Phenolphthalein (laxative)	Vitamin D, calcium and other minerals	Phenytoin (anticonvulsant)	As above and also decreased folic acid levels		
Sulfasalazine (anti-inflammatory)	Folate	Pyrimethamine (antimalarial)	Inhibits dihydrofolate reductase and lowers folic acid levels		
Captopril (antihypertensive)	Iron and other minerals	Triamterene (diuretic)	Weak folic acid antagonist		
Olestra (anti-obesity)	Small decreases in carotene and vitamins D and E	Aspirin (anti-inflammatory)	Gastric irritation can cause iron deficiency		
Stanols and sterols (anti-obesity)	Small decreases in carotene	Corticosteroids	Anti-vitamin D activity can reduce calcium absorption and cause osteoporosis		
		Oestrogen-containing oral contraceptive	Increase turnover of vitamin C and B_6 Elevate serum retinol concentrations		

Modified from Smith C H, Bidlack W R 1984 Dietary concerns associated with the use of medications. Journal of the American Dietetics Association 84:901–914.

The elderly are also at risk from increasing gastric pH which retards the absorption of calcium and increased use of loop diuretics which enhance urinary loss of calcium.

Anticoagulants such as warfarin slow the process of blood clotting and this can decrease the risk of strokes in persons whose blood shows tendencies to clot too easily. Such drugs function by interfering in the metabolism of vitamin K. Effective therapy is achieved by balancing the amount of anticoagulant against the usual intake of vitamin K. Hence physicians warn against the consumption of foods high in vitamin K in case an elevated dietary intake of the vitamin impairs the effectiveness of the treatment. In addition, haemorrhage caused by the anti-vitamin K action of such drugs can be exaggerated in the elderly by taking antioxidants such as tocopherol or very large doses of vitamin C ($\geq 10\,g$).

Anticonvulsant drugs used to control epilepsy, such as phenytoin, phenobarbital and primidone, can cause diarrhoea and decrease appetite, so reducing the availability of many nutrients. They also increase vitamin D turnover and catabolism by inducing the hepatic microsomal drug metabolising system, so that vitamin D supplements may be needed.

Anticonvulsants also interact with folate; blood levels fall shortly after the onset of therapy. Folate supplements will counter the adverse effects on folate status but they also adversely affect the efficacy of anticonvulsant treatment, so folate supplementation has to be monitored carefully (as discussed in Section 10.5, under 'Upper levels of folate intake', this is one of the problems in considering widespread enrichment of foods with folate). The antiepileptic drug valproic acid is associated with folate deficiency and birth defects; in experimental animals it alters embryonic folate distribution, producing elevated concentrations of tetrahydrofolate and lower concentrations of formylated forms of folate. Such alterations are partially prevented by co-administration of folinic acid and *S*-adenosylmethionine but could cause hypomethylation of DNA and induce teratogenesis.

Antihyperlipaemic drugs are used to reduce blood cholesterol levels. Such drugs work by reducing fat absorption, the side effect of which is a reduction in absorption of the fat-soluble vitamins A, D, E and K and carotenoids. It is also reported that the absorption of vitamin B_{12}, folate and calcium may be affected.

The unabsorbed fat replacer Olestra (a sucrose polyester) and the plant sterols and stanols used to reduce cholesterol absorption cause small variable decreases in plasma carotenoid concentrations but minimal detectable effects on serum concentrations of vitamins A, D, E and K.

Antihypertensive drugs used to control blood pressure can affect body levels of potassium, calcium and zinc. Captopril, a hypotensive drug and an inhibitor of angiotensin-converting enzyme, can bind to iron in the gut if jointly administered with iron-containing mineral preparations, thus reducing absorption of the drug. Food also interferes with the absorption of captopril since food retards gastric emptying and elevates gastric pH.

Antineoplastic drugs used in cancer chemotherapy frequently irritate the lining of the mouth, stomach and intestines and can damage mucosal cells, thus altering digestion. Many cause nausea, vomiting and/or diarrhoea. All of these effects can potentially influence nutrient status.

The antineoplastic drug methotrexate is a folate antagonist that competitively inhibits key enzymes of intracellular folate metabolism and reduces the availability of methyl groups derived from single carbon compounds. Supplies of both folate coenzymes and the tetrahydropteroyl glutamate substrate for the conversion to polyglutamate derivatives (and liver storage) are impaired. Methotrexate also inhibits folate transport across the intestine and into hepatocytes.

The anti-tuberculosis drug isoniazid (isonicotinic acid hydrazide) reacts with pyridoxal phosphate and increases the risk of vitamin B_6 deficiency. Although older treatment regimens using high doses of isoniazid frequently included vitamin B_6, more modern low-dose regimens do not; however, a significant proportion of the population are genetically slow metabolisers of isoniazid, and hence are at risk of vitamin B_6 deficiency even at low doses. Isoniazid-induced vitamin B_6 deficiency frequently presents as the niacin deficiency disease pellagra, as a result of impaired synthesis of niacin from tryptophan (see Section 10.3), although it may also present as seizures due to changes in brain neurotransmitter synthesis. Isoniazid can also inhibit hepatic vitamin D 25-hydroxylation and possibly affect metabolism of the vitamin.

Diuretics stimulate increased excretion of urine and with it the risk of increased excretion of potassium, magnesium and calcium and the water-soluble vitamins. Thiamin status in the elderly is of particular concern in relation to the use of diuretics. Total thiamin body stores are small and thiamin has a high turnover rate with a half-life of 10–18 days, so a regular intake is required in conjunction with diuretics. Furosemide (frusemide), in particular, has been associated with thiamin deficiency in elderly patients; in addition to increased urinary loss, it has been shown to impair the uptake of thiamin by cardiac cells in vitro. However, the clinical importance of this still needs to be confirmed.

Laxatives speed up the movement of material through the digestive tract, so reducing the time for nutrient absorption. They may therefore deplete vitamins and minerals, and there may also be increased fluid losses leading to dehydration.

Influence of nutrients or nutritional status on drug handling

The processing or detoxication of drugs and the many foreign compounds that enter our bodies daily occurs through phase I and phase II reactions. Phase I reactions include oxidation, hydroxylation, reduction or hydrolysis, introducing reactive groups on molecules. They occur predominantly in the liver and comprise the microsomal or mixed function oxidase systems (MFOS), NADPH-dependent enzymes and cytochrome P450, the latter in liver, lung and small intestine (Guengerich 1995). The second phase of the transformation involves conjugation with glucuronate, sulphate or glycine to render the metabolites water-soluble and permit excretion in the urine or bile. In general the intermediate compounds formed by these reactions are safe but there are exceptions, and a number of otherwise inert compounds are rendered carcinogenic by phase I metabolism.

Many nutrients and micronutrients may affect phase I activity; niacin and riboflavin are needed for oxidation, iron and glycine for haem synthesis for cytochrome P450 and minerals like calcium, zinc and magnesium to maintain membranes (Hoyumpa & Schenker 1982). It is difficult to establish to what extent low nutritional status influences MFOS activity but considerable experimental work suggests that the cytochrome P450 system is sensitive to deficiency of vitamins A, B-group, C and E. The pentobarbital sleeping time is prolonged in scorbutic guinea pigs, reflecting slower metabolism of the drug. However, it is uncertain whether human cytochrome P450 enzymes are also sensitive to vitamin C deficiency since the rate of metabolism of ^{13}C-labelled methacetin was not sensitive to vitamin C supplementation. Deficiencies of both protein and carbohydrate, on the other hand, clearly do reduce P450-catalysed oxidations in human beings. For example, children with kwashiorkor have lower rates of drug metabolism.

Some food constituents can reduce human cytochrome P450 activity in amounts that are within the normal dietary intake, including flavonoids, the sulphur compounds in onions and garlic, the isothiocyanates and indoles in cruciferous plants, and capsaicin in capsicum fruits. Experimental studies with compounds that inhibit phase I or activate phase II metabolism show they reduce tumour formation in animals and there is growing evidence of their effectiveness in human beings.

The role of dietary inadequacies and excesses in influencing P450 activity in humans is also of fundamental importance in obtaining a better understanding of the aetiology of several diet-related cancers. For example, alcohol consumption is associated with head and neck cancers, smoking with lung cancers and a diet high in salt is associated with gastric cancers. By contrast, diets high in fruit and vegetables are associated with a general protection against many cancers and as indicated above, there are several classes of compounds now known to inhibit or induce different P450 enzymes with potential anti-cancer properties.

Effects of lifestyle habits on nutrient status

Polyphenol-containing beverages, such as tea, reduce the bioavailability of non-haem iron, raising the possibility that tea consumption might cause anaemia. A review of published studies concluded that tea consumption does not influence iron status in Western populations where most people have adequate iron stores (Temme & van Hoydonck 2002). Among people with marginal iron status there was a weak negative association between ferritin or haemoglobin and tea consumption. Recent experimental work suggests that flesh foods (beef, poultry and seafood), phytic acid and vitamin C are probably the most important dietary factors determining iron bioavailability.

Smoking is associated with lower consumption of many foods including fruit and vegetables and dairy products. Furthermore, smokers frequently have lower plasma concentrations of nutrients (especially vitamin C and carotenoids) than non-smokers even when dietary intake is taken into account. There is some evidence that smoking increases the rate of vitamin C metabolism.

There is an increased risk of bone demineralisation, fractures and osteoporosis in women who smoke and there is some evidence that smokers consume significantly less calcium and vitamin D than non-smokers, never smokers or ex-smokers. Although dietary vitamin D is usually a poor predictor of vitamin D status, since sunlight provides our main supply, one study in the two groups of elderly women reported that plasma 25-hydroxycholecalciferol concentrations were significantly lower in heavy smokers than in non-smokers and this was accompanied by lower calcium absorption, but there was no difference in bone density at any site. In a recent review of the evidence for the effects of smoking and alcohol use on micronutrient requirements in pregnancy, it was suggested that vitamin C requirements increase for pregnant smokers and that plasma β-carotene, vitamin B_{12}, vitamin B_6 and folate concentrations are lower in pregnant than non-pregnant smokers. It is not clear whether the lower concentrations were due to increased requirements, lower dietary or supplement intakes or other factors. There is some evidence that iron supplementation partially ameliorates impaired fetal growth caused by cadmium intake from cigarette smoke.

The consumption of alcohol impairs the absorption of thiamin by inhibiting the active but not the passive process of thiamin absorption and, as discussed in Section 10.1, thiamin deficiency is a significant problem among alcoholics. Reduced absorptive capacity for thiamin persists despite supplementation with thiamin, but the effects of the alcohol are reversible since thiamin absorption, general nutritional status and hepatic morphology return to normal after a 2–3-month period of adequate nutrition and abstinence from alcohol.

Animal studies suggest that chronic alcohol consumption (at levels of 20–50% of energy intake) during pregnancy may mobilise fetal vitamin A from the liver, resulting in increases in vitamin A in various organs and birth defects. These results are of questionable relevance to human beings as the human infant has very little hepatic vitamin A at birth. However, chronic alcohol abuse is known to interfere with the storage of liver vitamin A in adults, and poor control of plasma retinol concentrations could have adverse effects; excess vitamin A is known to be teratogenic (see Section 11.1, under 'Toxicity of vitamin A').

Ethanol is oxidised to acetaldehyde in the liver by two enzyme systems, alcohol dehydrogenase and the microsomal ethanol oxidising system. The predominant enzyme in the latter system is cytochrome P4502E1 (CYP2E1). Isozymes of alcohol and other dehydrogenases convert ethanol and retinol to their corresponding aldehydes in vitro. In addition, new pathways of retinol metabolism have been described in hepatic microsomes that involve, in part, cytochrome P450s, which can metabolise various drugs. In view of these overlapping metabolic pathways, it is not surprising that multiple interactions between retinol, ethanol and other drugs occur. Accordingly prolonged use of alcohol, drugs or both, not only results in decreased dietary intake of retinoids and carotenoids, but also accelerates the breakdown of retinol through cross-induction of degradative enzymes. In addition, acetaldehyde interacts with liver stellate cells, the main storage sites of retinol in the body, stimulating their capacity to produce fibrous tissue and impairing the ability to store retinol.

13.3 MICRONUTRIENTS AND THE IMMUNE RESPONSE

As discussed in Chapter 26, the immune response is part of an orchestrated series of responses by the body known as the acute phase response (APR) that follows infection or trauma. The APR is essentially a protective response of the body against the danger posed by disease and is designed to facilitate both the inflammatory and repair processes, and to protect the organism against the potentially destructive action of inflammatory products. For example, tissue damage can be controlled or reduced by limiting cytokine production, neutralising reactive oxygen intermediates, inhibiting proteinases etc. A reduction occurs in the concentration of several plasma nutrients with the onset of the immune response and these are frequently misinterpreted as nutrient deficiencies (Thurnham & Northrop-Clewes 2004). However, as circulating nutrient concentrations can fall very rapidly, they may be a part of the APR. If such 'apparent-deficient states' are protective, then administering large quantities of micronutrients at such times may upset this homeostasis. This section will attempt to examine some of these issues and suggest explanations for the changes seen. Low plasma nutrient concentrations also occur in nutrient-deficient states when the body maximises mechanisms for nutrient economy and possibly the same mechanisms operate in disease states.

by thymic atrophy and a high frequency of bacterial, viral and fungal infections if not treated.

Zinc influences all immune cell subsets but is especially important in the maturation and function of T-lymphocytes because it is the cofactor for the thymus hormone, thymulin. The control of T-lymphocyte activation is delicately regulated by zinc, and the physiological plasma zinc concentration 12–16 μmol/l is optimally balanced for T-cell function. Th1 lymphocytes are important in cell-mediated immunity and responsible for interleukin-2 (IL-2) and interferon-γ release, while Th2 cells are linked to antibody-mediated immunity and the production of IL-4, IL-6, IL-10 and IL-13. It is suggested that zinc influences Th1 more than Th2 cells.

With the onset of infection, plasma zinc concentrations fall rapidly and in febrile illness the fall can be as much as 70%. The fall in plasma zinc is probably a consequence of monocyte stimulation by bacterial products, because experimental IL-1 infusions decrease plasma zinc concentrations and increase metallothionein transcription in hepatocytes. During this acute phase response, zinc is redistributed from the plasma to the liver and lymphocytes. The advantage to the host of this response may be deprivation of zinc from invading pathogens. It is also important to note that while 12–16 μmol/l is the optimal plasma zinc concentration for T-cell function in healthy subjects, higher concentrations can be inhibitory; thus a reduction in plasma zinc may be anti-inflammatory. The mitogenic properties of zinc, i.e. the direct induction by zinc of cytokine production in polymorphonuclear leukocytes, is enhanced by bacterial LPS and phytohaemagglutinin at concentrations that would not normally be mitogenic. Hence apparent immunological disadvantages of low plasma zinc concentrations at the start of infection may be overcome by synergisms with bacterial antigens.

Low plasma zinc concentrations (<10.7 μmol/l) have been associated with not only reduced growth and development, but also impaired immunity and increased morbidity from infectious diseases. The response to zinc supplements, however, is variable and may be dependent on whether plasma zinc concentrations reflect a true zinc deficiency or an infection-associated depression of plasma zinc. A meta-analysis of supplementation studies in children aged under 13 years showed that overall there was a highly significant positive impact of zinc on change in weight, although a review of eight randomised controlled intervention trials in pregnant women performed in less developed countries found no evidence that maternal zinc supplementation promotes intrauterine growth. There was evidence to suggest beneficial effects on neonatal immune status, early neonatal morbidity and infant infections but evidence was conflicting with respect to labour and delivery complications, gestational age at birth, maternal zinc status and health and fetal neurobehavioural development.

Zinc supplements have been shown to be beneficial against diarrhoea and this is possibly the best evidence of the widespread nature of zinc deficiency in developing countries, since in experimental zinc deficiency, inducible nitric oxide synthase is more readily upregulated in intestinal cells by exposure to infection, with the production of diarrhoea.

Adverse effects of zinc supplementation have also been reported. Fever was greater in patients on home parenteral nutrition with catheter sepsis who were given zinc supplements (30 mg/day) compared with those given 0 or 23 mg/day. Depressed immune responses were observed in another study where patients were given 100–300 mg/day. One study is particularly revealing. Zinc supplements were given to children (6 months to 3 years) 3 days after admission with severe protein-energy malnutrition (PEM) and there was higher morbidity in those who received 6 mg/kg elemental zinc compared with 2 mg/kg. Most of the infants died of sepsis-related conditions and the authors suggested that the higher mortality may have been because many of the children would not have recovered from intercurrent infections present on admission. The study serves to illustrate the importance of the hypozincaemia in the infective process. Hypozincaemia may be important to deprive bacteria of an essential nutrient or reduce the potential pro-oxidant effects of zinc. This is similar to the situation with iron, where early iron supplementation of children with severe PEM also caused high mortality (see 'Transition metals' below).

Selenium

As discussed in Section 12.6, selenium, as selenocysteine, provides the active site of glutathione peroxidase, one of whose main functions is to convert lipid peroxides to hydroxy acids and hydrogen peroxide to water. Thyrodoxin is a specific selenoperoxidase in the thyroid, and selenium deficiency partially blunts the thyroid response to iodine supplements. In addition to this, selenium is required in the deiodinases that form active tri-iodothyronine from thyroxine (see Section 12.5). Selenium deficiency exacerbates the effects of iodine deficiency. When selenium is deficient, a high iodine intake may cause thyroid damage due to a lack of selenium-dependent glutathione peroxidase activity during thyroid stimulation.

Disease and trauma are linked with increases in redox stress within tissues and experimental studies indicate that certain viruses may take advantage of compromised antioxidant status. Keshan disease in China is geographically associated with selenium deficiency but temporal fluctuations in incidence suggested that other factors were involved in its aetiology. Enteroviruses, and particularly coxsackieviruses, are believed to be responsible for the cardiomyopathy of Keshan disease, and experimental studies showed that Se-deficient mice were more susceptible than Se-supplemented mice to the cardiotoxic effects of coxsackievirus B4, which had been isolated from the blood of a patient with Keshan disease. Susceptibility to these viruses was not specifically associated with Se deficiency but could also be increased by vitamin E deficiency or a combination of vitamin E deficiency and polyunsaturated fatty acid (PUFA) excess. A previously avirulent strain of coxsackievirus CVB3/0 was changed to a virulent phenotype when passaged through vitamin E deficient animals. Similar effects have been observed in mice given excess iron and in glutathione peroxidase-'knock-out' mice. Analysis of the genomic structure of the newly developing viruses suggests that increased oxidative stress in disease facilitates the enhanced growth rate of the invading virus, increasing the likelihood of development of more virulent mutations. That is, it was not selenium deficiency specifically that promoted development of more virulent viruses, but impaired antioxidant status in appropriate tissues and cells.

13.4 MICRONUTRIENTS IN GENE EXPRESSION

Vitamins A and D and gene regulation

The process of cell differentiation takes place in all tissues throughout the body. It has been known for a long time that epithelial tissue differentiation is sensitive to vitamin A deficiency as the normal mucus-secreting cells are replaced by keratin-producing cells. This is the basis of the pathological process termed xerosis that leads to drying of the conjunctiva and cornea of the eye in vitamin A deficiency (see Section 11.1, under 'Effects of vitamin A deficiency and excess'). As discussed in Section 11.1, under 'Genomic actions of retinoic acid', it has become clear that vitamin A plays a hormone-like role in controlling differentiation of cells in tissues and organs throughout the body.

As discussed in Section 11.2, under 'Metabolic functions of vitamin D', calcitriol, the active form of vitamin D, also exerts its effects on gene transcription through vitamin D receptors (VDR), and the vitamin D receptor forms a heterodimer with the retinoid X receptor, so that both vitamins A and D are required for many, if not all, of the genomic functions of vitamin D.

It is interesting to speculate whether the possible need for vitamin A to permit vitamin D-induced calcium absorption can explain the effect of oestrogen therapy in the prevention of bone loss in postmenopausal women, apart from the direct effects of oestrogens on bone metabolism (see Ch. 24). Oestradiol has no direct effect on calcium transport, and does not directly increase the effect of calcitriol. However, hormone replacement therapy significantly increases plasma retinol and this might increase tissue retinoic acid concentrations, and so enhance calcitriol actions.

Control of iron metabolism

The regulation of iron metabolism is normally under the control of iron-regulatory proteins (IRP). These are cytoplasmic proteins that coordinate cellular iron traffic by binding to iron-responsive elements on mRNA for a number of proteins responsible for iron uptake, storage and utilisation, protecting them from degradation. In iron deficiency IRP binds to mRNA and promotes the synthesis of transferrin receptor protein while ferritin synthesis is repressed. Hence the utilisation and absorption of iron is increased. When iron is adequate, ferritin synthesis is promoted and iron storage occurs.

In infection, the cytokines tumour necrosis factor-α (TNF-α) and interleukin-1 (IL-1) are increased and these reorganise the normal control of iron metabolism. TNF-α induces the synthesis of ferritin and transferrin receptor and also inhibits the release of iron from macrophages and reduces incorporation of plasma iron into newly synthesised erythrocytes

(Thurnham & Northrop-Clewes 2004). Administration of TNF-α to experimental animals lowers serum Fe concentrations and serum iron falls in the incubation period of most infectious processes. Plasma ferritin levels increase in spite of the hypoferraemia since ferritin mRNA is sensitive to both iron and cytokines.

Nitric oxide (NO) is produced both by macrophages in vivo as a physiological response to infection and by a variety of cell types as an intracellular messenger. It is central to macrophage-mediated cytotoxicity. It is increased in infection and may have a direct role in the post-transcriptional gene regulation mediated by IPR. In a low iron environment, IFN-γ, TNF-α, IL-1 or LPS induces macrophage nitric oxide synthase (NOS). NO activates the mRNA-binding activity of IRP and so mimics iron deficiency. However, NO-induced binding of IRP to iron responsive elements specifically represses the synthesis of the cellular iron-storage protein, ferritin.

Hereditary haemochromatosis is a disease characterised by progressive iron overload which if undetected can lead to cirrhosis, diabetes mellitus, cardiac disease, arthritis or hepatocellular carcinoma or a combination of these. The basic deficit appears to be an increase in iron absorption, decrease in iron excretion and production of preferential deposits of iron in hepatic parenchymal cells rather than Kupffer cells. Recent evidence suggests that TNF-α may be involved in the aetiology of the disease because of its location on chromosome 6 and its effect upon iron transport. The haemochromatosis gene is tightly linked to the HLA complex on the short arm of chromosome 6. Increased production of TNF-α, which is also located on chromosome 6, downregulates iron absorption but decreased production of TNF-α occurs in stimulated monocytes from patients with haemochromatosis.

Polymorphism in the haptoglobin gene, vitamin C and iron

Serum haptoglobin (Hp) comprises two protein chains and there are two forms of the alpha chain, giving rise to three variants of Hp in serum. It seems that Hp 1-1 has the best haemoglobin-binding capacity, while Hp 2-2 is the best at promoting immune function. Caucasians tend to have approximately 10–20% Hp 1-1, blacks 30–50% and Asians <10%. The Hp 2-2 is commonest in Asians (>50%), lowest in blacks and middling in Caucasians.

One phenotype of the haptoglobin gene has been reported to influence vitamin C metabolism. The results indicate a lower stability of vitamin C (a higher rate of oxidation) in haptoglobin Hp 2-2 carriers than in those with Hp 1-1 and Hp 2-1. There is less haptoglobin in the blood of Hp 2-2 individuals, so there will be more haemoglobin iron present in serum, causing the oxidation of ascorbate.

Likewise the Hp 2-2 phenotype has also been reported to influence iron metabolism. People with this phenotype accumulate more iron and have higher serum ferritin concentrations than those of the haptoglobin 1-1 or 2-1 phenotypes. Thus possession of the Hp 2-2 phenotype may make individuals more susceptible to disease by lowering plasma vitamin C concentrations (although this might be viewed as protective – see 'Inflammation and vitamin C' below) and increasing potential inflammatory damage as a result of increased tissue iron concentrations.

Control of plasma homocysteine concentrations

As discussed in Section 10.5, homocysteine is an intermediate in one-carbon metabolism. Intracellular homocysteine is either converted to cysteine via the vitamin B$_6$-dependent *trans*-sulphuration pathway or is re-methylated to methionine by the vitamin B$_{12}$-dependent methionine synthase which requires 5-methyl-tetrahydrofolate as methyl donor. This means that vitamin B$_{12}$ and folic acid are major determinants of plasma homocysteine.

The synthesis of 5-methyl-tetrahydrofolate is catalysed by methylene tetrahydrofolate reductase (MTHFR). A commonly occurring polymorphism of the MTHFR gene reduces the stability and activity of the enzyme and is associated with moderate increases in homocysteine, particularly in subjects with low folate status. Supplementation with folate in doses from 0.2 to 10 mg/day has been shown to reduce both normal and elevated plasma homocysteine concentrations.

As discussed in Section 10.2 under 'Metabolic functions of riboflavin', riboflavin is a precursor of the flavin coenzymes which are cofactors for enzymes involved in the metabolism of folate and vitamins B$_6$ and B$_{12}$. FAD is the cofactor for MTHFR, which catalyses the formation of 5-methyl-tetrahydrofolate, the methyl donor for methionine synthase.

The possibility that riboflavin status might influence homocysteine concentrations was initially demonstrated in blood donors, where plasma homocysteine concentrations were 1.4 μmol/l higher in the quartile with the lowest riboflavin concentrations.

This compared with a 2.8 μmol/l difference between the quartiles for folate and 1.0 μmol/l in the case of vitamin B$_{12}$. The riboflavin–homocysteine relationship was mainly confined to subjects with the unstable variant of the MTHFR gene. Further studies confirm that riboflavin status can be an independent determinant of plasma homocysteine but the modulating effect of genotype is less clear.

13.5 MICRONUTRIENTS AS PRO- AND ANTIOXIDANTS

Antioxidant nutrients

Cellular integrity

Disruption to cellular integrity leads to the rapid release of cytokines by non-specific immune cells of the innate or natural immune system distributed through the body. The cytokines help to mount an inflammatory response and to recruit specialised cells such as mononuclear phagocytes, natural killer cells and neutrophils to the site of damage or infection. It is now known that the rapid induction of the synthesis of these cytokines is coordinated by a common cellular element, a transcription factor known as nuclear factor kappa-B (NF-κB) (Kopp & Ghosh 1995).

NF-κB is critical for the inducible expression of many genes involved in the immune and inflammatory responses including IL-1, -2, -6, -8, TNF-α, TNF-β and serum amyloid A protein. It is reported NF-κB exists in almost all cells but that it remains in the cytoplasm bound to an inhibitory protein, inhibitory kappa-beta (IκB). Exposure of cells to various inducers such as TNF-α leads to the dissociation of the cytoplasmic complex and the translocation of the free NF-κB to the nucleus. Significant activation of NF-κB occurs within minutes, allowing NF-κB to function as an effective signal transducer and rapidly connect events in the cytoplasm to response genes in the nucleus. One such response is the rapid upregulation of IκB-α synthesis, which then helps to shut down the NF-κB response and provide a feedback loop to control a transient inducer of responsive genes. However, a unique feature of signalling through NF-κB is the diversity of both signalling molecules, including viruses, ROIs, mitogens and cytokines and situations that activate NF-κB, and the types of genes responsive to NF-κB. Nevertheless the common feature of the inducers is that they all signal situations of stress, infection or injury to the organism.

NF-κB can be activated by ROI and common inducers can be inhibited by antioxidants. Thus the NF-κB mechanism is of particular interest to those wishing to account for the health advantages associated with antioxidant-rich fruit and vegetable diets. *N*-Acetyl-L-cysteine is a precursor of the antioxidant, reduced glutathione, and a scavenger of ROI, and suppresses the activation of NF-κB by many agents. This supports the idea that the redox state of the cell plays a general role in the activity of NF-κB. However, in vitro studies with micronutrients which influence the redox state have to be interpreted with caution. In neutrophils, deficiency of iron can reduce myeloperoxidase activity and supplements of vitamins C and E suppress production of oxygen free radicals, so potentially both dietary deficiency and dietary excess could impair the killing of bacteria and/or reduce tissue damage. Among the questions that need to be answered are: is there an optimal redox state in vivo to enable efficient bacterial killing with minimal damage to surrounding tissues and are certain antioxidant nutrients more important than others in regulating this state?

Vitamin E

As discussed in Section 11.3 under 'Antioxidant functions of vitamin E', vitamin E is a conventional phenolic antioxidant. The amount of vitamin E in membranes is several thousand-fold less than the amount of potentially oxidisable lipid. Under oxidative stress, vitamin E undergoes a very rapid transfer of phenolic hydrogen to the recipient free radical with the formation of a resonance-stabilised phenoxyl radical from the vitamin E. The phenoxyl radical is relatively unreactive towards lipid or oxygen and therefore does not propagate the chain reaction; however, it is not an antioxidant and to maintain the antioxidant properties of membranes, the vitamin E must be regenerated. Water-soluble vitamin C is believed to be the main reductant of the phenoxyl radical, but thiols and particularly glutathione can also function in vitro.

Vitamin C

As discussed in Section 10.7 under 'Metabolic functions of vitamin C', ascorbic acid is a powerful reducing agent and many if not all of the biological properties of vitamin C are linked to its redox properties. In the eye, vitamin C concentrations are ~50 times higher than those in the plasma and may protect against oxidative damage initiated by light. Spermatogenesis may need ascorbate to protect DNA from oxidative damage. Spermatogenesis needs many more cell divisions than oogenesis, and reports suggest that DNA damage at this site varies inversely with the intake of vitamin C between 5 and 250 mg/day. Vitamin C is superior to other biological antioxidants in protecting plasma lipids exposed ex vivo to a variety of sources of oxidant stress. Lastly, folate, homocysteine and probably many other plasma components, require vitamin C for stability and when blood plasma is separated from erythrocytes, vitamin C is one of the first antioxidants to disappear.

Carotenoids

As discussed in Section 11.1 under 'Vitamin A and carotene in cancer prevention', carotenoids can act as antioxidants because of their extended system of conjugated double bonds and the various functional groups on the terminal ring structures. Although there are many hundreds of carotenoids found in nature, there are relatively few found in human tissues, the five main ones being β-carotene, α-carotene, lycopene, β-cryptoxanthin and lutein. The ROIs scavenged by carotenoids are peroxyl radicals, and carotenoids in general, and especially lycopene, are very efficient at quenching singlet oxygen. Singlet oxygen is generated during photosynthesis; therefore carotenoids are important in protecting plant tissues but there is limited evidence for this role in human beings. However, β-carotene has been used in the treatment of erythropoietic protoporphyria, a light sensitive condition where singlet oxygen might be involved in pathogenesis, with some success. Otherwise results from studies suggesting that β-carotene provides protection against solar radiation are somewhat equivocal. There was no benefit reported when large amounts of β-carotene were used to treat persons with a high risk of non-melanomatous skin cancer. However, lutein and zeaxanthin, which occur specifically associated with the rods and cones in the eye, may protect the retinal pigment epithelium against the oxidative effects of blue light.

The antioxidant properties of carotenoids depend on oxygen tension in the surrounding tissue. At low oxygen tension, β-carotene acts as a chain-breaking antioxidant whereas at high oxygen tension it readily autoxidises and exhibits pro-oxidant behaviour. As discussed in Section 11.1 under 'Vitamin A and carotene in cancer prevention', the widespread distribution of carotenoids in plants and the considerable epidemiological evidence that consumption of fruit and vegetables was protective against heart disease led to three major β-carotene intervention studies. In two of these the subjects were smokers or people who had previously been exposed to asbestos. In both there was excessive mortality from lung cancer in the β-carotene treated groups. In the third study, the subjects were not primarily smokers and the overall conclusion was that β-carotene caused neither benefit nor harm. β-Carotene is essentially non-toxic but one possible explanation is that the large amount of β-carotene induced one or more of the cytochromes that increase carcinogenicity of smoking-associated toxins such as nitroso compounds, and increase the risk of cancer (Paolini et al 1999).

Flavonoids and polyphenols

Polyphenols are compounds which by definition are made up from multiple phenol rings. They can be classified into two groups, flavonoids and non-flavonoids. Flavonoids are the most common and widely distributed group of phenolics; over 4000 individual flavonoids occur in nature. They can be free, polymerised or linked to sugars or other non-flavonoid phenols. Dietary sources of flavonoids are predominantly fruits and vegetables, or products derived from these foods, such as wines and fruit juices. The simpler flavonoids tend to be water-soluble and are usually conjugated with various sugars in the form of glycosides. Cooking usually has little effect on the glycosides but colonic bacterial β-glycosidases will hydrolyse the glycosidic link, releasing the aglycone (Day et al 2000). The aglycones tend to be insoluble and, to be absorbed, must be conjugated to glucuronide or sulphate groups by phase II enzymes (see 'Influence of nutrients or nutritional status on drug handling', above).

Quercetin is a major flavonol (a subclass of the flavonoids) which is found ubiquitously in the diet. There is much evidence to suggest that it is a bioactive constituent of the human diet with powerful antioxidant activity and free-radical scavenging properties. However, most of the experimental work with quercetin has used the aglycone. After feeding sources of quercetin (such as 200 g of onion), only a very small amount is present in plasma as the aglycone; most is present as a variety of metabolites. While some of the metabolites will retain the biological properties of the aglycone, others will not and much work needs to be done to re-evaluate the earlier experimental work with flavonoid aglycones to characterise the important metabolites and their biological activity.

Pro-oxidant nutrients

Most biological antioxidants are potentially pro-oxidants. When an antioxidant molecule accepts an unpaired electron from a free radical, the intermediate formed by the antioxidant becomes itself a free radical. Fortunately, this is mainly a problem of food chemistry rather than physiology. However, in the case of vitamin C, changes in plasma concentrations occur which may be linked to its potential to be a pro-oxidant in inflammatory conditions. Likewise, although iron in healthy subjects is carefully controlled and unlikely to have pro-oxidant effects, in inflammation and disease there is indirect evidence that iron may become pro-oxidant since changes occur in the handling of iron to minimise potential pro-oxidant effects.

Inflammation and vitamin C

Several metabolic changes occur during inflammation which depress the concentration of vitamin C. Within 24 hours of surgery or following an attack of influenza, leukocyte vitamin C concentrations are depressed, due to the mobilisation of new neutrophils from bone marrow, which enter the circulation with low concentrations of ascorbate. The depression continues for 3 to 5 days while the cells gradually acquire vitamin C, probably from the plasma. Granulocytes actively take up ascorbate in vitro and where residual inflammation remains, plasma ascorbate concentration tends also to be low. It has been suggested that granulocytes require the ascorbate to protect them from free radical products that they produce during phagocytosis.

An alternative reason why plasma ascorbate concentrations fall in inflammation may be to prevent oxidation of transition metals. Inflammation is associated with tissue damage which increases the concentration of transition metals in the circulation. Interaction with vitamin C increases the risk of formation of ferrous and cuprous ions from iron and copper. Ferrous iron in particular is a powerful catalyst of the non-enzymic reactions that form hydroxyl radicals, with potentially damaging consequences for any molecule in the vicinity.

Ascorbate frequently catalyses damage in tissues in vitro probably because any tissue preparation is likely to be contaminated with unbound iron. This may be the explanation for the suggestion that ascorbate and many of its derivatives have anti-cancer properties. In vitro experiments with a malignant leukaemia cell line (P388D1) suggested that the concentration of ascorbate that inhibited cell growth by 50% (ED50) was approximately 17 μmol/l, within the range of plasma ascorbate of 11–20 μmol/l seen in populations where there is a risk of chronic disease (e.g. the elderly) or there is increased exposure to disease. Although plasma ascorbate is strongly correlated with dietary intake of vitamin C, healthy populations tend to have higher plasma concentrations than those exposed to sickness/trauma or who are sick.

Other workers have suggested that the cytotoxic properties of the ascorbate derivatives against human tumour cell lines are due to their ability to generate hydrogen peroxide and showed that cytotoxic activity of sodium ascorbate was almost completely inhibited by the addition of catalase to the assay. The generation of hydrogen peroxide by sodium ascorbate is probably an artefact of the experimental conditions, due to reaction of ascorbate with transition metals in the medium. Nevertheless, the treatment of cancer is often aggressive and likely to cause inflammation as indicated by the usefulness of iron chelators to lessen side effects of chemotherapy. However, the use of large amounts (up to 45 g) of vitamin C to treat cancer was not successful, and it was later pointed out that the four patient deaths from haemorrhagic tumour necrosis soon after treatment was started could have been due to the pro-oxidant effects of vitamin C.

Transition metals

In the absence of inflammation, zinc, copper, magnesium and selenium are involved in protecting the body against oxidative stress. Superoxide dismutase (SOD) is found in all aerobic cells and is responsible for the dismutation of the free radical superoxide (to hydrogen peroxide and oxygen). The cytoplasmic enzyme uses zinc and copper as cofactors, while mitochondrial enzyme uses zinc and magnesium. The hydrogen peroxide produced by the reaction is reduced to water by glutathione peroxidase (GPx), a selenium-dependent enzyme, using reduced glutathione as the reductant. Cellular concentrations of

unless destroyed by the leavening process. Likewise, tannic acid in tea has been implicated in interfering with iron absorption, although a recent review of published studies suggested that tea consumption has no significant influence on haemoglobin concentrations in industrialised countries (see 'Effects of lifestyle habits on nutrient status', above).

Much of the work on the assessment of antioxidant properties of polyphenols has used the naturally occurring glycosides or the aglycones. For example, one study compared the effects of feeding red wine extract (equivalent to 375 ml red wine and comprising a mixture of flavonoid glycosides and aglycones) and quercetin aglycone (30 mg) on lipoprotein oxidisability. Following 2 weeks' supplementation to male volunteers, resistance to oxidation was increased by 18% and 16% for the wine extract and quercetin groups, respectively. However, there is no way of comparing the efficiency of absorption of the respective components in these two treatments, since the wine extract contained a mixture of flavonoid glycosides and aglycones while the quercetin was the pure aglycone. Not only do absorption characteristics vary between foods and also between individuals but the type of sugar glycosylating the flavonoid and the position of conjugation will also influence absorption. Furthermore, new metabolites are formed during absorption and structure–activity relationships suggest that they will have different antioxidant properties from those of the pure compounds tested in vitro, with potentially different biological activities. An aspect that should be considered is that the new metabolites may well have less pro-oxidant activity than native flavonoids (see 'Adverse effects of polyphenols', below). Consequently, it is important to determine the exact nature of the metabolites in plasma.

Anti-carcinogenic properties

Quercetin has been shown to be chemopreventative in several animal models and in vitro it inhibits the proliferation of colorectal, breast, gastric, ovarian and lymphoid cancer cell lines. The protective effects of quercetin and other flavonoids have been attributed to inhibition of key signalling enzymes, e.g. protein kinase C, tyrosine kinase and phosphoinositide 3-kinase involved in the regulation of cell proliferation, angiogenesis and apoptosis, as well as antioxidant effects such as radical scavenging.

There is also evidence that polyphenols may inhibit cancer cell growth by effects on P450 enzymes 1A and 2B1 (see 'Influence of nutrients or nutritional status on drug handling', above). Repression of phase I enzymes involved in cancer initiation will guard against cancer development. A number of in vitro and trial cancer models have shown that green tea polyphenols appear to inhibit cancer development by blocking nitrosamine activation. In addition, green tea and citrus fruit polyphenols have been shown to increase the activity of the detoxifying phase II enzymes. However, a review of studies of green tea consumption in relation to various cancers reported mixed results. Only for gastric cancer did most of the evidence suggest that tea consumption might be beneficial, since 6 out of 10 studies found an inverse association. For colon, rectum and bladder cancers, no conclusion could be drawn as tea consumption was associated with both increased and decreased risks. Thus although green tea contains polyphenols with powerful antioxidant effects and one cup of tea usually contains ~400 mg polyphenols, the evidence for a protective effect against cancer in human studies is weak.

Cardiovascular properties

Red wine is an especially rich source of phenolic compounds and the protective effects of moderate wine consumption against heart disease, and in providing a possible explanation for the 'French paradox', are well known. Tea is also a rich source of flavonoids and it has recently been shown that tea consumption can reverse endothelial dysfunction in patients with proven coronary artery disease; both short-term and long-term consumption of tea improved flow-mediated dilatation of the brachial artery.

High flavonoid intake mainly from black tea (61%), onions (13%) and apples (10%) was first associated with a lower mortality from cardiovascular disease and a lower incidence of myocardial infarction in the Zutphen study of older men. Catechin is the main flavonoid in tea but it is also present in wine, fruit juices and chocolate, and later studies suggested that sources of catechin intake from foods other than tea might explain 20% of the reduction in ischaemic heart disease mortality risk. Although not all studies have found similar effects, a recent meta-analysis on 10 cohort and 7 case-control studies suggested that the incidence rate for myocardial infarction in those consuming three cups of tea per day was 11% lower than that in those consuming no tea (Peters et al

2001). Reasons for inconsistencies in the epidemiological data are not clear. The antioxidant properties of black and green teas are similar and although milk is usually added to black tea, the flavonoid–protein complex formed does not appear to inhibit the absorption of flavonoids. For black tea, a cup (235 ml) contains 172 mg flavonoids and dose–response evidence suggests that 150 mg is needed to trigger an antioxidant effect and increase the anti-thrombotic lipid, prostacyclin. However, the strength of tea as drunk varies enormously not only between populations but also within households and this may be the most important factor responsible for inconsistencies in the epidemiological findings.

Adverse effects of polyphenols

In spite of the many potentially health-benefiting effects of polyphenols, adverse effects are known. Many polyphenols are synthesised by plants to protect themselves from predators. For example, resveratrol and catechins are antifungal agents produced by plants grown in conditions that encourage mould growth. Thus possible toxic properties in many of these compounds should be expected.

There are reports that mutagenicity is related to flavonoid-mediated oxidative damage and it appears that some of the same structural attributes that optimise antioxidant capacity may also exacerbate oxidative stress and tissue damage. Pro-oxidant activity is thought to be directly proportional to the total number of hydroxyl groups and in vitro studies show that flavonoids with multiple hydroxyl groups, especially in the B ring, increased the production of hydroxyl radicals in vitro. Various studies have reported cytotoxic and pro-apoptotic effects, induction of DNA strand breakage and even that the unsaturated 2,3-bond and 4-oxo arrangement may promote the induction of ROS in the presence of copper ions and oxygen. However, glycosylation and methylation attenuate the pro-oxidant behaviour of flavonoids, so the production of secondary metabolites of flavonoids following absorption may well be protective.

There are suggestions that hot tea consumption might be one of the factors responsible for the high risk of oesophageal cancer in China, but opinions seem to indicate that it is the hotness rather than the components that is responsible for the risk. Although a cup of green tea may provide 300–400 mg flavonoids, in the author's experience the tea consumed in some parts of China is very weak indeed and little more than ~400 ml scalding hot water containing one or two small leaves. In these circumstances, the hot water hypothesis seems more tenable.

13.7 PHYTOESTROGENS

A number of polyphenols that occur in plant foods as glycosides and other conjugates have weak oestrogenic/anti-oestrogenic actions, and are collectively known as phytoestrogens. As shown in Figure 13.2, they have two hydroxyl groups that are the same distance apart as the hydroxyl groups of oestradiol, and hence can bind to oestrogen receptors. They produce typical oestrogenic responses in animals, with a biological activity 1/500–1/1000 of that of oestradiol.

High consumption of legumes, and especially soya beans, which are particularly rich sources of phytoestrogens, is associated with lower incidence of breast and uterine cancer, as well as lower incidence of osteoporosis. The oestrogenic action is probably responsible for the effects on the development of osteoporosis, while three factors may be involved in the effect on hormone-dependent cancer:

1. The isoflavones are mainly anti-oestrogenic, since they compete with oestradiol for receptor binding, but the phytoestrogen-receptor complex does not undergo normal activation, so has only a weak effect on hormone response elements on DNA. Even those phytoestrogens that have a mainly oestrogenic action will reduce responsiveness to oestradiol because they compete for receptor binding but have lower biological activity.

2. The phytoestrogens increase the synthesis of sex hormone binding globulin in the liver by stabilising mRNA, leading to a lower circulating concentration of free oestradiol.

3. Some of the phytoestrogens inhibit aromatase and therefore reduce the endogenous synthesis of oestradiol, especially the unregulated synthesis that occurs in adipose tissue.

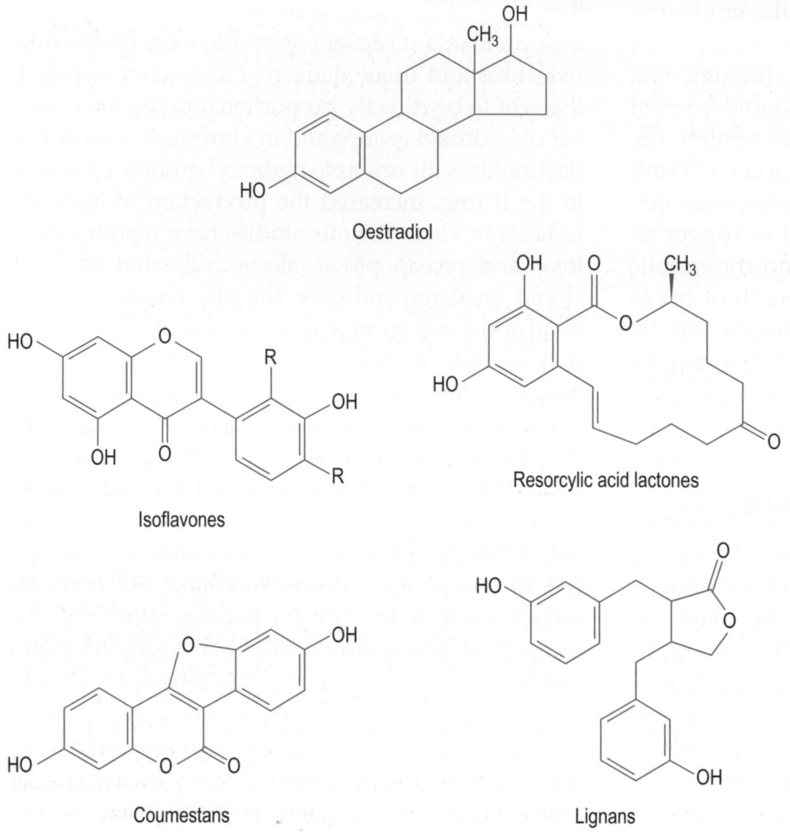

Figure 13.2 The structures of oestradiol and the major phytoestrogens.

Oestradiol

Isoflavones

Resorcylic acid lactones

Coumestans

Lignans

⮑ Key points

- ⮑ A large number of prescribed drugs can interfere with micronutrient metabolism mainly by reducing absorption. The people who are most vulnerable to malnutrition from drug–nutrient interactions are those regularly consuming drugs such as individuals with chronic diseases and the elderly.

- ⮑ Lifestyle factors are well known for their sometimes debilitating effects on nutritional status and for having specific effects on vitamin C and carotenoids (smoking) and thiamin (alcohol). Tea consumption, although suspected of impairing iron absorption, would appear to have little affect on iron status in industrialised countries.

- ⮑ The immune response has a major impact on several nutrients. Plasma retinol, ascorbate, iron and zinc concentrations are depressed as part of the acute phase response, and make important contributions to the body in infection.

- ⮑ Vitamins A and D are important in regulating gene expression.

- ⮑ Many factors control the expression of proteins important in iron regulation especially cytokines, NO and haptoglobin polymorphisms.

- ⮑ Haptoglobin polymorphisms also influence plasma vitamin C concentrations and plasma homocysteine concentrations are influenced by folate, riboflavin and vitamin B_{12} status.

- ⮑ Several micronutrients exhibit antioxidant properties and interact in the maintenance of cellular integrity.

- ⮑ Antioxidant nutrients can potentially become pro-oxidants and depression of plasma vitamin C, iron and zinc at the onset of infection may protect the tissues against excessive free-radical initiated oxidative damage.

- ⮑ Polyphenols from a variety of foods act as radical scavenging antioxidants, and may also be protective against cancer and cardiovascular disease for other reasons as well. Some may also have pro-oxidant actions and may be mutagenic or carcinogenic.

⊃ Some polyphenols (phytoestrogens) have both weak oestrogenic and anti-oestrogenic activity,

and may provide protection against hormone-dependent cancer of the breast, uterus and prostate, as well as protection against post-menopausal development of osteoporosis.

References and further reading

References

Beaton G H, Martorell R, Aronson K J et al 1993 Effectiveness of vitamin A supplementation in the control of young child morbidity and mortality in developing countries. World Health Organization, Geneva

Blomhoff R 1994 Vitamin A in health and disease. Marcel Dekker, New York

Day A J, Canada F J, Diaz J C et al 2000 Dietary flavonoid and isoflavone glycosides are hydrolysed by the lactase site of lactase phlorizin hydrolase. FEBS Letters 468:166–170

Guengerich F P 1995 Influence of nutrients and other dietary materials on cytochrome P450 enzymes. American Journal of Clinical Nutrition 61:651S–658S

Hoyumpa A M, Schenker S 1982 Major drug interactions: effect of liver disease, alcohol and malnutrition. Annual Review of Medicine 33:113–149

Kane G C, Lipsky J J 2000 Drug-grapefruit juice interactions. Mayo Clinic Proceedings 75:933–942

Kopp E B, Ghosh S 1995 NF-κB and rel proteins in innate immunity. Advances in Immunology 58:1–27

Lemire J M 1995 Immunomodulatory actions of 1,25-dihydroxyvitamin D3. Journal of Steroid Biochemistry and Molecular Biology 53:599–602

Paolini M, Cantelli-Forti G, Perocco P et al 1999 Co-carcinogenic effect of β-carotene. Nature 398:760–761

Peters U, Poole C, Arab L 2001 Does tea affect cardiovascular disease? A meta-analysis. American Journal of Epidemiology 154:495–503

Temme E H M, van Hoydonck P G A 2002 Tea consumption and iron status. European Journal of Clinical Nutrition 56:379–386

Thomas J A, Burns R A 1998 Important drug-nutrient interactions in the elderly. Drugs and Aging 13:199–209

Thurnham D I, Northrop-Clewes C A 2004 Effects of infection on nutritional and immune status. In: Hughes D A, Darlington L G, Bendich A (eds) Diet and human immune function. Humana Press, Totowa, NJ, p 35–64

Further reading

Blumberg J, Couris R 1999 Pharmacology, nutrition and the elderly: interactions and implications. In: Chernoff R (ed) Geriatric nutrition: the health professionals handbook. Aspen, Publishers, Gaithersberg, MD, p 342–365

Cooper K A, Chopra M, Thurnham D I 2004 Wine polyphenols and promotion of cardiac health: A review. Nutrition Research Reviews 17:111–129

Goldman P 1997 Olestra: assessing its potential to interact with drugs in the gastrointestinal tract. Journal of Clinical Pharmacology and Therapeutics 61:613–618

Harbourne J B (ed) 1994 The flavonoids: advances in research since 1986. Chapman & Hall, London

Mangelsdorf D J 1994 Vitamin A receptors. Nutrition Reviews 52:S32–S44

Thomas J A 1995 Drug-nutrient interactions. Nutrition Reviews 53:271–282

Thurnham D I 1995 Iron as a pro-oxidant. In: Wharton B A, Ashwell M (eds) Iron, nutritional and physiological significance. Chapman & Hall, London, p 31–41

Thurnham D I 2004 An overview of interactions between micronutrients and of micronutrients with drugs, genes and immune mechanisms. Nutrition Research Reviews 17:211–240

CD-ROM contents

Further reading

Further reading from the book

Part 4

Dietary requirements for specific groups

Edited by Pat Judd

14

Infancy, childhood and adolescence

Elizabeth M. E. Poskitt and Jane B. Morgan

Objectives

By the end of this chapter you should be able to:

- describe the changing characteristics of growth and maturation from birth to adult that alter nutrient requirements
- understand the degree of immaturity of the digestive tract and organs during infancy, including pre-term infants, and the implications for diet
- discuss the composition of maternal milk and compare with alternatives
- explain the weaning process and associated risks
- have an informed opinion about the application of 'healthy eating' beliefs to children, e.g. high fibre, vegetarian/veganism
- be aware of the social and psychological factors that affect food intake during adolescence
- explain the basis of calculation of dietary requirements for infants, children and adolescents.

14.1 INTRODUCTION

Nutrition in childhood must be considered in conjunction with children's age, growth and development. Interactions between individuals' genetic endowments for growth and their nurturing environments determine body size and composition. Growth has specific nutritional needs but is not a steady process, proceeding rapidly in early life, slowing in middle childhood and accelerating at puberty before linear growth ceases. With increasing age also comes physical and psychomotor maturation, which influences activity and body composition and, through feeding skills and food choices, dietary intakes.

14.2 BODY COMPOSITION IN CHILDHOOD

Table 14.1 shows age- and sex-related changes in body composition. After birth total body water falls and the proportion of extracellular fluid also declines. Percentage body weight that is fat (% BF) increases rapidly to a peak between 6 and 12 months. Infancy is followed by a period of natural 'slimming' until around 5 years. Typically this is followed by a second phase of relatively rapid fat deposition (the adiposity rebound) which continues almost unabated in girls until growth ceases. In boys the adiposity rebound reverses with the rapid lean tissue deposition of late puberty.

Each organ has a unique pattern of growth and maturation. At birth, brain weight is 25%, and at 5 years 90%, of expected adult brain weight. Seventy-five per cent of postnatal brain growth takes place in the first 2 years of life. By contrast, about 30% of male adult body mass is acquired during adolescence.

Table 14.1 **Variation in body composition with age in childhood**

Age	Mean weight (kg)	Whole body: water % body weight	Whole body: fat % body weight	FFM: water % LBM	FFM: protein % LBM
Birth	3.5	72	14	84	14
4 months	7	60	26	82	15
12 months	10	59	24	78	19
2 years	12	60	21	78	18
5 years	18	60	21	74	20
10 years	32	60	17	72	20
25-year-old men	70	60	12	72	21
25-year-old women	60	55	25	72	21

FFM, fat-free mass; LBM, lean body mass.
From Poskitt (2003) © John Wiley & Sons Ltd. Reproduced with permission.

14.3 NUTRITIONAL ASSESSMENT IN CHILDHOOD

Body weight for age is frequently used as an indicator of nutritional status but weight-for-age (WFA) is heavily influenced by height-for-age (HFA). Childhood nutritional assessment commonly uses either weight-for-height (WFH) independent of age, or WFA in relation to HFA. The former tends to be used in environments where linear growth retardation is common and age may be uncertain. The latter is more commonly used in situations where children's birthweights are known and reference population means for WFA and HFA are well established and portrayed as centile, or mean with standard deviation (SD), charts or tables. Using SD (or Z) reference tables it is possible to relate individual values to the mean through the SD (Z) score:

$$\text{Standard deviation (Z) score} = \frac{(X - M)}{SD}$$

where: X is the individual value for that parameter (e.g. HFA, WFH), M is the reference population mean for that parameter, and SD is the standard deviation for the reference population for that parameter.

The SD (Z) score (values > mean are positive and < mean are negative) provides a numerical value which represents the individual's position in relation to a population. Centile tables and charts display a population with mean values as the 50th centile. Normally growing individuals follow growth trajectories which usually have similar relationships to population means throughout childhood, although deviating from these temporarily in adolescence.

Reference standards for growth and development (Freeman et al 1990) do not distinguish the abnormal from the extremes of normal. Criteria of 'normality' vary according to the purposes of the nutritional/growth assessment. Scores <−2 or >+2 SD, or <3rd and >97th centiles, are often used as cut-off points for 'normality' but will include overlap between normally and abnormally growing children if only anthropometric criteria are used in assessment. Further, tall parents tend to have tall-for-age children and short parents tend to have relatively short-for-age children. Methods exist for using mid-parental height to judge children's linear growth.

Velocity of growth may be more informative than size attained. Linear growth velocity is influenced by seasonality and, ideally, is recorded over a full year. In practice annual growth velocity may have to be inferred from increments recorded over shorter periods and extended to expected rates/year. Most reference standards are derived from cross-sectional measurements of populations which smooth and flatten curves compared with the individual increments in weight and height at puberty. Longitudinal charts do exist and represent individual growth better over adolescence. Bone age (the relative stage of epiphyseal maturation and development compared with accepted radiological standards) is used to evaluate maturation along with the presence or absence of signs of secondary sexual development.

Undernutrition

Chapter 28 deals with definitions of underweight, wasting and stunting. Stunting, as growth retardation associated with socioeconomic deprivation, is a significant problem in westernised as well as in less affluent societies. Stunting prevalence usually responds better with changes in psychosocial and/or economic environments than with specifically nutritional interventions.

Overnutrition

In adults, body mass index (BMI: weight in kg/(height in m)^2) is used to define overweight and obesity. In children mean BMI varies non-linearly with age. Skinfold thickness, which measures subcutaneous fat only, shows considerable intra- and interobserver error, provides no obvious cut-off points for normality and measurements are not well tolerated by children. Reference charts of waist circumference for age exist but there are no widely recognised 'normal' waist circumference cut-off points.

The International Obesity Task Force (IOTF) defines childhood overweight and obesity as the BMI Z score (BMI SD score) at any age which, if maintained in relation to the reference population throughout childhood, would achieve the adult overweight and obesity BMI cut-off points of 25 and 30 kg/m^2 at 18 years. These definitions need to be used widely to evaluate their specificity and sensitivity, particularly since the use of centiles and Z scores implies the same distribution of obesity/overweight throughout childhood – an implication that is almost certainly incorrect. Lower cut-off points than those quoted here are used to define overweight/obesity in adults from the Indian subcontinent (ISC). Perhaps children from the ISC should also have different cut-off criteria.

eczema in breastfed infants at high risk of atopy in the early months of life. Nevertheless, a follow-up study of combined maternal and infant food allergen avoidance reported no impact on the severity and prevalence of atopic disease at 7 years in a study group when compared with control subjects.

The European Society for Paediatric Allergy and Clinical Immunology (ESPACI) Committee on Hypoallergenic Formulas together with the European Society for Paediatric Gastroenterology, Hepatology and Nutrition (ESPGHAN) Committee on Nutrition have reviewed unresolved issues in the treatment and prevention of food allergy in infants and children (Host et al 1999). Results from trials in both full-term and preterm (PT) infants suggest that the nature and pattern, rather than simply the timing, of solid feeding are important for subsequent development of food allergy.

Development of gastrointestinal function

Digestion and absorption in breastfed infants are promoted by many specific components in breast milk (Table 14.3). Immaturity of gastrointestinal enzymatic function makes digestion and absorption less efficient with infant formula than with breast milk in the first months of life. Fat absorption is particularly likely to be less in formula-fed infants than in breastfed infants. Pancreatic lipase, amylase and bile salt pool size are low in the newborn compared with older infants. Lactase levels in the newborn are quite low, increase as milk feeding begins and may decline later as milk ceases to be the predominant feed. Low lactase levels and lactose intolerance are common in older African and Asian children and adults but less common in Caucasian children and adults.

Development of renal function

Young infants cannot dilute or concentrate their urine as much as older children and adults. This makes them particularly susceptible to fluid overload or to overload from food derived non-metabolisable substances which have to be excreted via the kidney (the potential renal solute load: PRSL). The PRSL is expressed as milliosmoles per litre (mOsm/l) and

Table 14.3 Some specific components of breast milk which facilitate nutrient absorption

Type of nutrient	Specific component of milk	Effects on gastrointestinal absorption
Carbohydrates	Lactose	Digested to glucose and galactose which are readily absorbed. Fermentation of any lactose in colon produces lactic acid and low pH which encourage growth of non-pathogenic colonic bacteria. Facilitates absorption of calcium as soluble calcium lactate
Fats	Presence of bile salt stimulated lipase in breast milk	Helps digestion of fat in milk in young infants in whom pancreatic lipase activity is low
	Relatively small fat droplet size	Small droplets offer larger surface area for volume, encouraging enzymatic digestion
	Saturated fatty acids – palmitic acid	Position of palmitic and other saturated fatty acids in middle of triglyceride molecule facilitates fatty acid absorption as monoacylglycerol which is more readily absorbed than free palmitic acid. Good absorption of palmitic acid discourages precipitation of calcium as calcium palmitate
Nitrogen-containing compounds	Casein:whey ratio	More soluble whey proteins predominate
	Casein composition	Human milk casein micellar structure creates small, easily digested flocculates in stomach
	Urea	May be used as nitrogen source by colonic bacteria to combine with organic acids and form amino acids which can be absorbed
Micronutrients	Lactoferrin and other micronutrient binding compounds	Many specific binding compounds in breast milk facilitate absorption of iron, folic acid, vitamin B_{12}, zinc and other micronutrients

indicates the total number of ionic or molecular particles in the fluid. For infant feeds it is calculated as: PRSL (mOsm/l) = Na + K + P + Cl + (protein (mg)/175) when the dietary intakes of sodium (Na), potassium (K), phosphorus (P) and chloride (Cl) are expressed in mmol/l.

The PRSL for breast milk is 93 mOsm/l; for infant formula ≈ 135 mOsm/l; and for cow's milk ≈ 308 mOsm/l. The unmodified cow's milk formulas used, sometimes with complementary foods, before 1972 gave young infants difficulty excreting sufficiently concentrated urine to expel the necessary solutes. Blood osmolality, plasma sodium and urea were at the upper limits of normal and even mild fluid deficiency precipitated hypernatraemia, uraemia and extracellular hyperosmolality. The ensuing intracellular hyperosmolality, especially in the brain, had disastrous, often fatal, consequences. UK legislation in the early 1970s which lowered the acceptable levels of sodium, phosphate and protein in infant formulas was followed later by similar EC Directives.

The high phosphate content of unmodified cow's milk based formulas also caused problems in young infants who were feeding well. The phosphate ions ingested in large quantities by term infants feeding well on infant formula were not readily excreted. Levels of plasma phosphate rose, precipitating falls in plasma calcium, hypocalcaemic tetany and convulsions in otherwise healthy infants around 7–10 days old. The condition resolved readily with intravenous calcium and change to lower phosphate formula. Changes to low phosphate infant formula have virtually eliminated the problem (Poskitt 1994).

14.5 NUTRITION IN INFANCY

There is now almost universal consensus that breast milk is the best food (Table 14.4) for normal infants with healthy mothers. Despite this consensus, most 1-month-old infants in the UK have received some infant formula and by 10 weeks, 64% of infants are wholly formula fed. It is proving difficult to improve 'breastfeeding statistics' in the UK despite widespread education and publicity promoting breastfeeding.

Table 14.4 **Advantages of human milk for young infants**

Factor	Advantage
Colostrum	High in vitamin A, zinc, sIgA
Convenience	Ready to feed but convenience dependent on local acceptability of breastfeeding
Low cost	Mother may have stores of fat laid down in pregnancy to mobilise for provision of fat in breast milk. Mother does not have to eat expensive food to produce milk
Clean	Breast milk is not sterile but bacteria present are usually non-pathogenic and milk contains antibodies to bacteria in maternal gastrointestinal system
Composition	Appropriate amino acid profile; contains long-chain PUFA; high organic acid residues in infant large bowel may be converted to amino acids by colonic flora
Facilitated absorption of micronutrients	Binding proteins, such as lactoferrin, facilitate absorption of many micronutrients
Enzymes	Breast milk contains enzymes the role of which is not understood in all cases. However, bile salt stimulated lipase may improve efficacy of fat absorption in early infancy
Other non-nutritional factors in breast milk	Breast milk contains hormones, growth promoting factors, cytokines and prostaglandins. The role of many of these is not clear but they may be relevant to the protective effects of breastfeeding against infection and possibly against non-communicable disease of later life
Anti-infective properties	These are varied: see Table 14.7

Proteins

Human milk protein is 30–40% casein to 70–60% whey. Whey proteins include lactalbumin, sIgA, lactoferrin and lysozymes. Casein is a mixture of proteins associated with magnesium, phosphate, and citrate ions, bound with calcium as 'calcium caseinate complex'. Human milk casein forms smaller micelles with looser structure than the casein of cow's milk. The structure facilitates enzymic action. Precipitation of tough, undigested casein curds in the stomach is less likely than with cow's milk or unmodified cow's milk formula. Heat treatment of cow's milk protein in the manufacture of infant formulas affects casein micellar structure and enhances digestibility (Poskitt 1994).

The newborn liver has little cystathionine β-synthase, an enzyme involved in the synthesis of cysteine from methionine. Deficiency is greater in immature infants. However, provided there is sufficient methionine in the diet, cysteine deficiency does not seem to arise. There is cystathionine synthase activity in organs other than the liver which may account for this paradox.

About 25% of total nitrogen in human milk is non-protein nitrogen, of which 50% is urea, with small amounts of glucosamines, nucleotides, free amino acids, polyamines and biologically active peptides. Taurine is present in unusually high amounts amongst the free amino acids (DHSS 1977). Levels of taurine are lower in cow's milk and infant formulas supplemented with taurine. Infants fed low taurine diets conjugate bile acids with glycine rather than taurine and these conjugated bile acids are less stable than taurine-containing bile acids, although evidence of disadvantage for normal full-term infants does not exist. All amino acids are potentially essential in infancy if rapid protein synthesis (e.g. in catch-up growth) outstrips the synthesis of amino acids from precursors.

Fat

Although the quantities of fat in human and cow's milk are not very different, the component fatty acids are very different. Human milk fat is higher in unsaturated fat, particularly the essential fatty acids linoleic (18:2ω6) and α-linolenic (18:3ω3) acids and also contains the long-chain polyunsaturated fatty acids (LCPUFA), arachidonic (20:4γ6), eicosapentaenoic (20:5ω3) and docosahexaenoic (22:6ω3) acids. Interest in the role of these LCPUFAs in neurological development particularly has been huge

since it was shown that the levels of LCPUFAs in the brains of infants who were breastfed were higher than in those fed unsupplemented cow's milk formula. LCPUFAs are seen as conditionally essential for fast growing premature infants who may have difficulty synthesising LCPUFAs from precursors sufficiently rapidly to meet the needs of the rapidly growing premature brain. The real importance of these fatty acids in full-term infants has yet to be determined but LCPUFAs are seen as justifiable fortifying compounds for modern term infant formulas.

The fats in human milk are more readily digested and absorbed than those of cow's milk since saturated fatty acids (especially palmitic) tend to be attached to the middle carbon of the glycerol molecule encouraging absorption bound to micelles as monoglycerides rather than free fatty acids. Fat absorption from breast milk is also facilitated by the presence of bile-salt-stimulated breast milk lipase, although this is probably not of great significance except in immature infants. Most infant formulas now contain fats derived predominantly from vegetable oils with rather different proportions of fatty acids than those found in human milk fat. The relative proportions of fatty acids in plant fats are largely determined by plant genetics. The relative proportions of fatty acids in the milk of mammals (human and otherwise) reflect in part dietary fatty acid content.

Human milk has a surprisingly high level of cholesterol. The explanation for this is not obvious. Human milk also contains relatively high levels of carnitine – an amino acid like substance which is involved in mitochondrial oxidation of fatty acids. Infants can sythesise carnitine, but premature infants and those undergoing very rapid (catch-up) growth may be unable to synthesise carnitine at a sufficiently rapid rate to meet demand. This may limit the rate of fatty acid oxidation.

Enzymes and hormones

The roles of the many enzymes, other than breast milk lipase, and of the hormones in human milk remain largely undetermined. One enzyme – glucuronidase – can cause minor problems in early infancy. Newborn infants are prone to jaundice due to poor hepatic capacity to form bilirubin glucuronide which is excreted via the bile. High levels of glucuronidase in the milk of some mothers deconjugate bilirubin glucuronide excreted in the bile, allowing reabsorption of bilirubin, increased bilirubin load on the liver, and 'breast milk jaundice'. The jaundice, usually developing at 7–10 days, is mild and occurring in otherwise healthy infants who are feeding and gaining weight well. It resolves gradually as liver function matures.

Promoting successful lactation

Lactation is discussed further in Chapter 15. Volumes of milk increase over the first months of lactation as infants develop appetite and grow. Successful lactation is now recognised as promoted by early onset, frequent and night-time suckling especially in the first days of lactation; 'emptying' the breasts; and absence of other foods given to the baby. Maternal nutrition is also important. The stimulus from suckling probably needs to be greater in poorly nourished women than in well-nourished women in order to maintain the prolactin levels needed to promote the same milk output. Once breastfeeding is established, it may be possible to reduce feed frequency to six to eight times a day, although infants vary widely in the nutritional demands they make on their mothers. Night suckling (which particularly stimulates prolactin secretion) is important in maintaining high breast milk output.

Exclusive breastfeeding for 6 months may be ideal but this has to be viewed against the finding that most women in developed societies stop breastfeeding either exclusively or altogether long before that time. The reasons why mothers decide to feed infant formula from birth, or to switch from breast milk to infant formula are complex. Table 14.8 illustrates breastfeeding rates by mothers' ages, educational attainments and location. In the UK the stereotypic description of 'younger, economically disadvantaged mothers living in the North' as less likely to breastfeed is borne out by the findings of the survey by Hamlyn et al (2002). One of the main reasons many women quote for stopping exclusive breastfeeding is that they have 'insufficient' milk. The infants of these mothers are usually growing very satisfactorily so can be presumed to be receiving sufficient milk. Very rarely they are failing to thrive. Commonly breast milk 'failure' results from inappropriate lactation practices, usually at initiation of breastfeeding, leading to lack of confidence by the mother in her ability to produce breast milk to satisfy her infant.

It is widely felt that more women could breastfeed successfully if they were given better advice and

Table 14.8 Estimated incidence of breastfeeding (% who breastfed initially) by mother's age, socioeconomic classification (SEC) and region of the UK in 2000 (adapted from Hamlyn et al 2002)

Variable	Subgroup	Percentage ever breastfeeding
Age (years)	16 or under	54
	17–18	70
	Over 18	88
SEC	Higher occupations	85
	Intermediate occupations	73
	Lower occupations	59
	Never worked	52
	Unclassified	66
Location	England & Wales	62
	Scotland	54
	Northern Ireland	47

support in the perinatal period. UNICEF has developed 'Ten steps to successful lactation' as part of the Baby Friendly Hospital (BFH) Initiative (see Table CD 14.1). These 'Ten steps' are aimed particularly at perinatal hospital practices relating to breastfeeding, with the Initiative giving BFH status to hospitals which have incorporated practices supporting breastfeeding into maternity and paediatric ward.

Mothers should be advised on infant feeding but their choices, once made, should be supported. Many need, or want, to work outside their homes. Some formula feeding, whilst continuing to breastfeed, may enable mothers to avoid abandoning breastfeeding altogether, although the introduction of other formula almost invariably leads to reduction in the volume of breast milk secreted.

Problems which may arise from composition of breast milk

Breastfeeding is not without problems (see Table CD 14.2). As already mentioned, rarely infants present with failure to thrive in association with inappropriate breastfeeding technique or – even more rarely – failure of breast milk production. When this happens the infants present with gross weight loss and sometimes hypernatraemia. Jaundice (already discussed), mother–child transmission of infection and vitamin K deficiency bleeding (VKDB) are other medical concerns.

Table 14.9 **Problems developing in LBW infants which may relate to feeding and nutrition**

Problem	Nutrition-related factors
Hypothermia and hypoglycaemia	Small glycogen content of liver; immature mechanisms for mobilising low fat stores of LBW infants; large surface area to volume encourages heat loss
Bradycardia and apnoea	Gastric overload with feed
Respiratory distress syndrome	Acutely, high fluid intakes and gastric distension can exacerbate cardiorespiratory problems, e.g. respiratory distress syndrome. Chronically, micronutrient deficiencies, especially for antioxidants, may contribute to development of chronic obstructive pulmonary dysplasia
Patent ductus arteriosus	Fluid overload may discourage closure of ductus arteriosus and contribute to cardiac failure
Intestinal obstruction	Inspissated curd syndrome: obstruction with casein flocculates. Less likely in breast milk fed than cow's milk based formula fed infants. Necrotising enterocolitis: intestinal stasis followed by perforation and peritonitis, resulting from intestinal overload with distension of the bowel and ischaemia in the bowel wall
Eye disease of prematurity	Shortage of micronutrients and/or long-chain PUFAs may contribute to eye damage: retrolental fibroplasia
Bone disease of prematurity	Insufficient intake of calcium, phosphorus, vitamin D, sodium, protein
Anaemia of prematurity	Rapid growth rate due to good nutrition outstrips capacity to form haemoglobin. Deficiency of folic acid; riboflavin; copper; or haemolysis due to low vitamin E: essential fatty acid ratio
Reduced cognitive skills in later life	Insufficient intake of long-chain PUFAs to meet needs of rapidly developing brain

infants. Further, expressing breast milk into containers results in cells and fat adhering to the containers with loss of some energy and protective effects. Cells are rapidly lost on storage although immune factors such as sIgA and lactoferrin keep their activity much longer. The benefits of breast milk are thus reduced when it cannot be fed at the breast. However, once enteral feeding is established, commercial or hospital laboratory developed 'breast milk fortifiers' can be used to add extra nutrients to expressed breast milk fed to LBW infants if growth rates are faltering.

Nutritional requirements of LBW infants are estimated as those supporting growth equivalent to the expected growth and nutrient accretion of the post-conception-age-matched fetus. Such nutrient accretion is difficult to achieve in PT infants for minerals such as calcium, phosphorus and zinc. For these reasons LBW infant formulas have increased minerals/unit volume as well as energy and protein (Table 14.6).

Supplements of vitamins A, C and D and folic acid (enterally or parenterally depending on the method of feeding) should be given to LBW infants. Iron supplementation should be avoided before 4 weeks since it may enhance the production of free radicals.

Breast milk banks

These used to be popular as a means of providing breast milk to infants who might benefit but whose mothers were unable or unwilling to provide sufficient milk. Maintenance costs, risks of HIV infection from milk which is not 'own mother's milk', effectiveness of modern intravenous nutrition, and recognition that stored pasteurised breast milk is not nutritionally wholly adequate for PT infants, have led to declining use of stored breast milk that is not 'own mother's milk'. Few UK banks remain.

Kangaroo care

Maternal involvement in PT infant care should be encouraged from birth but parents have few opportunities to feed small, sick, infants in the newborn period. Once a neonate's condition is stable, 'kangaroo care' where the mother carries her infant around next to her skin and between her breasts to encourage warmth, tender loving care and easy breastfeeding can be encouraged. Maternal attachment, growth, time to discharge, and survival rates for PT infants in kangaroo care compare favourably with traditional incubator care.

14.7 THE TRANSITION TO MIXED FEEDING: WEANING OR COMPLEMENTARY FEEDING

Definitions

Weaning, also known as complementary feeding, has been defined as

The process of expanding the diet to include foods and drinks other than breast milk or infant formula. (Department of Health 1994)

For developing countries, WHO (1998) describes weaning as

The period during which other foods or liquids are provided along with breast milk is considered the period of complementary feeding. Any nutrient-containing foods or liquids other than breast milk given to young children during the period of complementary feeding are defined as complementary foods.

Since the term 'weaning' is also used to indicate complete cessation of breastfeeding, WHO recommends that the terms 'weaning' and 'weaning foods' are avoided. We use the term complementary feeding to embrace the use of all foods and liquids other than breast milk or infant formula.

Maternal milk output averages 650 ml/day at 1 month of lactation, 750 ml/day at 3–4 months' lactation and peaks at perhaps 900–1000 ml/day at 4–5 months' lactation. We have already indicated that the energy requirements of infants are currently debated but assuming a need of 80 kcal/kg, average infants would need 850 ml and 1450 ml of breast milk to meet energy requirements at 6 ($\approx$7.5 kg weight) and 12 ($\approx$10 kg weight) months respectively on exclusive breastfeeding. From 6 months, and probably before this for some infants, additional sources of energy and nutrition are needed to complement breast milk. For formula-fed infants, the increasingly large volumes of fluid needed to provide energy requirements become less tolerable to infants.

Physiological and developmental changes (growth, micronutrient status, psychomotor development) all influence the age of introduction of complementary foods. A systematic review found no evidence in support of the modification of the Department of Health (1994) recommendation:

The majority of infants should not be given solid foods before the age of 4 months, and a mixed diet should be offered by the age of 6 months.

However, an expert Consultative Panel, convened by the WHO, commissioned its own systematic review (Kramer & Kakuma 2001) and recommended:

Exclusive breast feeding for 6 months, with introduction of complementary foods and continued breast feeding thereafter.

Relying on this systematic review, WHO formally adopted this policy, and more recently the UK Department of Health did so too:

Breast feeding is the best form of nutrition for infants. Exclusive breast feeding is recommended for the first six months (26 weeks) of an infant's life as it provides all the nutrients a baby needs. (Department of Health website, published Monday 12 May 2003, reference number: 2003/0185)

However, since the 2000 Hamlyn survey (Hamlyn et al 2002) found that 90% of infants are introduced to some non-milk, non-formula, food *before 4 months*, despite education about the age of introduction of complementary foods, this policy seems likely to be an ideal practised by few.

Maternal choice in complementary feeding

Early introduction of complementary feeds is associated with low maternal age, formula feeding, and maternal smoking. Maternal practices seem influenced by infant growth since infant weight at 6 weeks predicts age at introduction of complementary foods better than birthweight or early weight gain, with heavy infants introduced earlier than light infants. Breastfed infants are often 'switched' to infant formula with the introduction of complementary foods.

Digestion is not a problem for full-term infants introduced prematurely to complementary foods. For example, starchy foods (e.g. cereal) fed before pancreatic enzymes reach mature levels (around 4 months of age) can be digested fully. Increased salivary amylase and intestinal glycoamylase activities compensate for low pancreatic amylase. Table 14.10 outlines some advantages and disadvantages of introducing complementary feeds.

What foods

Complementary foods may be home prepared or commercially produced. Initially one small feed is

Table 14.11 Modifications to quality of diet needed for child to progress from infant diet to that of adult

Age	Diet	Nutritional issues
Young infant	Wholly breastfed	Entirely liquid diet Quite low energy food ~0.7 kcal/ml All essential nutrients in one food No fibre in diet >50% total energy from fat
Weaning diet	Milk: formula or breast plus some 'solid' foods as purees and porridges	Diet low energy density ~1 kcal/g Very little or no fibre May be low in fat – some weaning diets even in developed countries may have fat content <30% total energy Often high refined sugar content to diet
Young child	Mixed diet. May be quite limited in variety Little unprocessed meat Children often not keen to chew and whole fruit largely absent Vegetables usually eaten only with reluctance	Varies according to food offered and children's pickiness Fat content may range from 25% to >40% total energy Iron content may be very low Fibre intake largely from breakfast cereals
Schoolchild	Diet may be influenced by school meal. School dinners whether provided from home or canteen often high in total energy, energy from fat and refined sugar and low in vegetable fibre. Micronutrient intake in school dinners commonly low	School dinners may achieve >45% energy from fat Saturated fat may be majority of fat Sugar and sweetened drinks very popular May be high salt intake Fibre predominantly from breakfast cereals
Adolescent	May be a balanced adult diet or a thoroughly irregular diet Diet eaten away from home without supervision. May be excessive soft drink consumption	Important that diet is encouraged to follow recommendations for adults whenever possible Other aspects of 'healthy living' important as well as diet

From Poskitt (2003) © John Wiley & Sons Ltd. Reproduced with permission.

and perhaps two between-meal snacks, the timing of which depends on mealtimes. One snack or meal should be close to bedtime. Small eaters and 'fussy' eaters may have difficulty consuming sufficient energy to meet needs so recommendations for adults to consume <35% dietary energy from fat do not apply to young children. The transition from >50% dietary energy derived from fat provided by exclusive breastfeeding to <35% energy derived from fat should be spread over the first 5 years of life. Similarly, adult recommendations for fibre intake should not apply in early childhood since high fibre content lowers food energy density and phytates reduce absorption of micronutrients. Diets with <30% energy derived from fat are quite common amongst preschool children who consume

large quantities of 'juice' and sweets instead of meals of varied content. They are likely to lead to FTT if prolonged.

Persuading children to eat family meals is not always easy. All over the world children seem reluctant to eat green leafy vegetables. Inexperience with chewing may be a contributing factor. UK government recommendations for supplementary vitamins A and D to children under 5 years recognise the difficulties of achieving varied diets in young children. However, relatively few children receive supplementary vitamins after infancy.

As children grow up they become more independent in their eating habits. Meals should be spread over the day and snacks regulated to facilitate recognition of hunger and satiety.

Nutritional problems in children and adolescents

Failure to thrive (FTT)

Failure to thrive (FTT) is failure to gain in weight and height at the expected rate, the expected rate being that indicated by the child's weight and/or height velocity compared with reference standards for age (see Table CD 14.5 for further details). Resolution of FTT through catch-up growth (CUG) can be very rapid with treatable cause and the provision of extra nutrients to support catch-up. Where resolution of the precipitating cause is impossible, as with cystic fibrosis and with some congenital heart disease with high cardiac output, increasing the energy and nutrient density of the diet so children ingest more energy and nutrients without increasing food volume can lead to improved growth rates.

FTT: psychosocial deprivation syndrome

Psychosocial deprivation (PSD) may be the commonest form of FTT in the UK today although often unrecognised. Overt cases come from homes where the nurturing environment is in some way deficient in the love, warmth, enjoyment and stimulus which enable normal growth. The explanation for the poor growth must be multifactorial with inadequate food offered or ingested as the most reasonable explanation for some cases. Some children steal food, eat food off others' plates at school, and show other attention-seeking behaviours. Children with PSD may have low levels of growth hormone and ACTH secretion when in their deprived environments. Changing the adverse environments so as to provide more positive nurture rapidly normalises hormone levels and results in catch-up growth.

Obesity

The definition of childhood obesity has been discussed earlier. In the UK the proportion of obese children has doubled in the past 10 years and is still increasing. Other westernised countries show similar disturbing prevalences of childhood obesity. Childhood obesity is a matter of major public health concern. Psychological distress and the physical handicap of gross size contribute to underachievement at school. More childhood overweight/obesity and more prevalent adult obesity inevitably means more overweight/obese children continue into adult overweight and associated complications. Type 2 diabetes mellitus (previously considered only an adult disease) is increasing in prevalence among children and adolescents in western Europe (including the UK) and North America.

The vast majority of obese children have no recognisable underlying medical cause for their obesity. Around 80% of obese children have one obese parent and 20–40% have both parents obese. Presumably a genetic predisposition and an obesogenic environment combine in many children to produce obesity. Very rare, single gene defect, obesity syndromes associated with abnormalities of leptin metabolism are described. Such children usually show unrelenting increase in fatness from birth but dramatic and sustained fat loss with leptin therapy.

A few uncommon medical conditions are also associated with increased risk of obesity in children (see Table CD 14.6). Most childhood obesity 'secondary' to other recognised conditions includes short stature as a feature, often with other clinical findings and/or psycho-developmental problems. Prader–Willi syndrome is the most likely condition to present with obesity as the prime concern, although short stature and low IQ usually alert clinicians to the possibility of 'secondary' obesity.

Explanations for the rise in childhood obesity must be multifactorial (see Table CD 14.7). Surprisingly, recorded energy intakes have been falling in the UK for several decades. For example, the National Diet and Nutrition Survey (Gregory & Lowe 2000) showed mean energy intakes lower than previous surveys. Total energy intakes for 10–11-year-old UK children decreased on average by 1.6 MJ/day between 1983 and 1997. For the same period and age group, the percentage of energy derived from fat decreased from a mean of 37.4% energy from fat in 1983 to 35.7% in 1997. These dietary patterns are replicated in all age groups in the National Diet and Nutrition Survey (NDNS) studies and in other countries as well. Some of this decline may reflect failure of previous studies to account adequately for food eaten outside the home.

Energy expenditures must have declined more than energy intakes to explain the increased prevalence of obesity. For the same movement the obese expend more energy than their lean lighter peers, making it difficult to judge energy needs. Studies in the USA and Mexico show that obesity in teenage boys increases in proportion to time spent watching television – a pastime associated with very low energy expenditure. Increased sedentary behaviour could be the most significant societal change leading to increased prevalence of childhood overweight/obesity. In westernised countries, obesity is more common amongst the socially deprived.

lower respiratory tract infections. The soft lower rib cage is pulled in by diaphragmatic contraction during respiration, causing the typical indrawing of the lower chest or 'Harrison's sulcus'. This, with the swelling at the costochondral junctions which cause the 'rickety rosary', gives the characteristic appearances of the chest.

Secondary hyperparathyroidism in response to the fall in plasma calcium with vitamin D deficiency leads to bone demineralisation and loss of phosphate through the kidney. Thus the biochemical findings in rickets are usually those of borderline low plasma calcium, low plasma phosphate and very high alkaline phosphatase. Alkaline phosphatase, a manifestation of osteoclastic activity, may remain high throughout the healing period. Oral vitamin D (cholecalciferol) is very effective in restoring bone architecture to normal after time. However, with adolescent girls there may be insufficient growth time left for resolution of pelvic deformity and the risk of cephalopelvic disproportion during childbirth.

Metabolic bone disease ('rickets of prematurity') is common in PT infants but is more complex in aetiology than simple vitamin D deficiency. Mineral needs are high in rapidly growing PT infants and bone disease can result from calcium or phosphate deficiency. Use of the diuretic furosemide (frusemide) for fluid overload can worsen the situation by increasing urinary excretion of phosphate. Modern PT infant formulas and intravenous nutrition solutions aim to meet PT infants' needs for bone growth and mineralisation. However, nutritional requirements cannot always be met when infants are sick and not tolerating large fluid volumes either enterally or parenterally. Vitamin D supplementation of all LBW infants is advisable to maximise calcium absorption. The parathyroid hormone response to low plasma calcium is poorly developed in PT and newborn infants. Symptomatic hypocalcaemia (tetany and convulsions) in neonatal vitamin D deficiency is common whilst plasma phosphate levels are often more or less normal.

Bone health and later life

The likelihood of the loss of bone mineral in middle and old age leading to clinical osteoporosis is partly determined by peak bone mass (PBM). Weight-bearing activity in adult life and old age appears to reduce the loss of bone mineral with age but in childhood weight-bearing activity contributes positively to developing PBM. Although calcium intakes should have some influence on bone mineralisation, work from The Gambia suggests that normal bone mineralisation can take place on diets that are very low in calcium compared with recommended requirements. Calcium supplementation (1000 g/day) to pre-adolescent children on very low calcium traditional diets improves bone mineralisation but has no effect on growth.

Macronutrient undernutrition may also have negative impact on bone mineralisation. Anorexic individuals, as well as ballet dancers and gymnasts who deliberately undereat so as to remain light and small, have low PBM. The importance of energy and protein for developing the collagen matrix on which bone mineral is deposited may explain the apparently better response to calcium supplementation in trials where calcium is supplied as extra milk – with all its extra nutrients – rather than as calcium salts.

14.9 CONCLUSIONS

Growth, dependency and development make infants and children susceptible to nutritional imbalance and deficiencies. It may seem that broad knowledge of nutrition is necessary in order to feed children appropriately. Clearly this is not so since the nutritional knowledge of most families is slight yet the majority of children survive with good nutrition even in environments less advantageous than in western Europe. Nevertheless, it is wise to promote meals varied in content, texture and taste for children. Variety leads, almost certainly, to nutritionally adequate combinations of macro- and micronutrients, even when there is no specific nutritional knowledge.

Meals should be made enjoyable social affairs offered without excessive pressure to eat. Snacks should be planned rather than opportunistic (or continuous). Wholemeal cereals, fruits and vegetables should be seen as enjoyable components of the diet. In this way children can eat to requirement whilst allowing opportunity to develop and recognise satiety and hunger. Linking family nutrition with a caring, stimulating environment encourages both normal growth and development, and the prospect of sustainable healthy lifestyles continuing into adulthood. Table CD 14.14 suggests how this may be achieved.

⊃ Key points

- ⊃ There are sound and varied physiological reasons why breast milk is most suitable for the young infant.

- ⊃ The adaptations in modified formula milks accommodate the needs of young infants, even those with very low birthweight or with inborn errors of metabolism, where breast milk may have limitations.

- ⊃ The transition from breast milk/formula milk to a solid diet is a time when young children are vulnerable to nutritional problems.

- ⊃ Vitamin and mineral deficiencies present problems in child nutrition even in affluent developed countries.

- ⊃ Overnutrition as overweight and obesity is a problem of increasing concern to public health and child nutrition. It presents challenges which involve not only diet but lifestyle change for prevention or cure.

- ⊃ Adolescence is an age of both nutritional vulnerability and opportunity for nutritional education for a healthy adult lifestyle.

- ⊃ Healthy nutrition encompasses not only what is eaten but when and how it is consumed and includes many aspects of lifestyle such as activity.

References and further reading

References

Barker D J P 1998 Mothers, babies and health in later life, 2nd edn. Churchill Livingstone, Edinburgh

Department of Health 1994 Weaning and the weaning diet. Report on health and social subjects no 45. HMSO, London

DHSS 1974 Present day practice in infant feeding. Report on health and social subjects no 9. HMSO, London

DHSS 1977 Composition of human milk. Report on health and social subjects no 12. HMSO, London

DHSS 1980 Present day practice in infant feeding. Report on health and social subjects no 20. HMSO, London

Freeman J V, Cole T J, Chinn S et al 1995 Cross sectional stature and weight reference curves for the UK 1990. Archives of Disease in Childhood 73:17–24

Gregory J R, Collins D L, Davies P S W et al 1995 National diet and nutrition survey: children aged 1½–4½ years, Volume 1. Report of the diet and nutrition survey. HMSO, London

Gregory J R Lowe S 2000 National diet and nutrition survey – young people aged 4 to 18 years, Volume 1: Report of the diet and nutrition survey. The Stationery Office, London

Hamlyn B, Brooker S, Lleinikova K, Wands S 2002 Infant feeding 2000. The Stationery Office, London

Host A, Koletzko B, Dreborg S et al 1999 Dietary products used in infants for treatment and prevention of food allergy. Archives of Disease in Childhood 81:80–84

Kramer M S, Kakuma R 2001 The optimal duration of exclusive breast feeding. A systematic review. Department of Nutrition for Health and Development. World Health Organization, Geneva

Li R, Ogden C, Ballew C et al 2002 Prevalence of exclusive breastfeeding among US infants: the Third National Health and Nutrition Examination Survey (Phase II, 1991–1994). American Journal of Public Health 92:1107–1110

Poskitt E M E 1994 Use of cows' milk in infant feeding with emphasis on the compositional differences between human and cows' milk. In: Walker A F Rolls B A (eds) Infant nutrition: issues in nutrition and toxicology 2. Chapman & Hall, London, p 162–185

Poskitt E M E 2003 Nutrition in Childhood. In: Morgan J B, Dickerson J W T (eds) Nutrition in Early Life. John Wiley, Chichester, p 291–323

Stordy B J, Redfern A M, Morgan J B 1995 Healthy eating for infants – mothers' actions. Acta Paediatrica 84:733–741

WHO 1972 Nutritional anemia. WHO Technical Report Series number 3. WHO, Geneva

WHO 1998 Complementary feeding of young children in developing countries: a review of current scientific knowledge. WHO/NUT/98.1. WHO, Geneva

Further reading

Burniat W, Cole T J, Lissau I, Poskitt E M E 2002 Child and adolescent obesity. Cambridge University Press, Cambridge

Fomon S J 1993 Nutrition of normal infants. Mosby, St Louis

Morgan J B, Dickerson J W T 2003 Nutrition in early life. Wiley, Chichester

Websites

World Health Organization

http://www.who.dk/nutrition/Infant/20020808

http://www.who.dk/nutrition/Infant/20020730

(Both refer to baby-friendly hospital initiatives.)

Objectives

By the end of this chapter you should be able to:

- discuss the risks for healthy conception
- describe the changes in body composition during pregnancy and lactation and determining factors such as metabolic changes, activity, control of intake
- explain the impact of nutrition in pregnancy on birthweight and long-term health
- discuss the effects of lactation on birth spacing and mother's nutritional status
- describe the effects of inadequate nutrition on milk volume and composition
- explain the basis of calculating requirements for pregnancy and lactation.

15.1 INTRODUCTION

It is self-evident from worldwide demographic change that human reproduction is a highly successful process. High rates of infant survival to adulthood have enabled humans to populate many parts of the world. Optimal nutrition prior to pregnancy, during pregnancy and in lactation will make a significant contribution to that success. It is appropriate to look at the outcomes of these processes in terms of a continuum and the idea of a continuum of reproductive casualty has been suggested (Table 15.1). Of couples across the globe attempting to achieve a pregnancy 90% will have been successful after approximately 18 months of regular sexual intercourse. The remaining 10% are subfertile but many of these couples can now be helped to have a successful pregnancy as a result of medical management, in particular assisted reproductive techniques such as in vitro fertilisation (IVF). Once pregnancy has been achieved and in the absence of any medical interference the maternal death rate is approximately 1 in 200 pregnancies and 1 in 20 babies will die before birth, or in the first week of life. Intervention by health professionals, including nutritional advice, results in a change to these figures to 1/10 000 pregnancies resulting in a maternal death and 1 in 200 pregnancies resulting in the loss of the infant. Of course, both these figures may be higher than this in the developing world where deficiency of specific nutrients, poor provision of medical services and/or intercurrent infectious disease may each play a part (Rush 2000).

The concept of the continuum of reproductive casualty is, however, quite useful because when recommending an intervention such as a nutritional supplement perhaps to achieve a beneficial outcome in one aspect of the continuum, e.g. to reduce miscarriage, one must be careful that the result of the intervention does not lead to an increase in unwanted effects elsewhere in the continuum such as the birth of more infants with congenital malformations. A recent suggestion for instance has been that the periconceptional supplementation with folic acid of a woman planning a pregnancy, which will reduce her risk of producing an infant with a neural tube defect (spina bifida), may have the unwanted effect of increasing the spontaneous twinning rate. As twinning increases infant deaths and handicaps, principally because of an excess of premature births, the overall burden of disease and disability achieved by this intervention in the continuum of reproductive casualty may be greater than before. This important concept must be understood by all those who would wish to advise or prescribe for the would-be pregnant or pregnant woman. It is also prominent in the minds of such women – the constant query to the health professional offering advice on nutrition or pharmaceutical drug use in pregnancy is – 'will it harm my baby?'

Table 15.1 Continuum of reproductive casualty

- Fecundability/fertility
- Maternal morbidity
- Maternal mortality
- Miscarriage
- Late fetal death
- Aneuploidy
- Structural congenital anomaly
- Neonatal death
- Cerebral palsy/psychomotor impairment
- Susceptibility to disease in adult life

15.2 PREPREGNANCY

Nutritional requirements for healthy conception

The opinions of Frisch and her colleagues regarding the relevance of body composition in achieving pregnancy, particularly with respect to the percentage of fat in the body of the adult female, are now generally accepted (Frisch 1994). Her principal observation was that an improved plane of nutrition in adolescent girls was associated with an increasingly early date of menarche signalling the onset of fertility. The mean body weight at which menarche occurred in US girls was 48 kilograms (SE ± 0.5 kg) with a mean height of 1.59 m (SE ± 0.005 m) at 12.9 years (SE ± 0.1 years). Of the mean body weight at the completion of growth (16–18 years) 16 kg was fat representing an energy reserve for reproduction of 144 000 kcal (602 MJ). Such an energy reserve would provide the theoretical energy requirement of both pregnancy and 3 months of lactation. Of course in athletes in training or those involved in hard physical work this body weight can be achieved with a relatively low proportion of fat. Frisch's observation was that body fat proportion of less than 22% of body weight was associated with the absence of ovulation and that healthy fertile women who were ovulating on a monthly basis had an average body fat proportion of 28%. Menarche and the onset of fertility can be delayed by athletic training or eating disorders and accelerated by excess nutrient consumption. Interestingly early menarche may be a particular problem in girls exposed to famine in childhood who are then re-fed with a high energy diet. If they live in a society where the onset of menarche is a trigger for marriage and reproduction they may get into serious difficulties in trying to give birth before they have achieved full adult stature and their bony birth canal has reached full adult dimensions. Natural labour may become obstructed if the baby's head is too large to pass easily through the mother's pelvis.

The basic mechanism involved in body fat as a determinant of a healthy conception appears to be a requirement for a certain energy store to permit reproduction to take place. In natural experiments when severe famine has affected populations of women who are *already* established in pregnancy there is no significant change in mean birthweight if this occurs during the first 6 months of pregnancy. There is a modest reduction in birthweight of approximately 5–10% if famine affects women during the last

3 months of pregnancy. Most surprisingly perhaps, successful lactation can continue for up to 3 months in the face of severe energy deprivation of the mother. These physiological adaptations in extreme conditions are clearly factors in successful human reproduction. What is seen in the non-pregnant female population exposed to acute famine is a failure of ovulation in at least 50% of females even before the fat store has been catabolised.

In summary, a population exposed to a low plane of nutrition during childhood will have a relative delay in reaching full adult stature and reproductive maturity. Refeeding of the chronically undernourished child may lead to accelerated development and onset of puberty, which may lead to pregnancy before full adult stature has been obtained. In the absence of adequate medical and midwifery resources such pregnant young women may die as the result of neglected obstructed labour. When energy deficits affect women after the achievement of natural puberty and full adult stature there is an acute reduction in fertility and with chronic undernutrition ovulation will cease. In acute undernutrition during an established pregnancy utilisation of stored energy from the maternal adipose tissue is capable of protecting the baby's nutrient supply to a large extent during pregnancy and indeed through the early months of lactation.

Influence of obesity on conception

In the situation of excess nutrient consumption evidence suggests that obesity with or without the problem of the polycystic ovarian syndrome (PCOS) is associated with a doubling in the rate of ovulatory infertility (Rich-Edwards et al 1994) (see Fig. CD 15.1). What is important from the nutritional point of view however is that in both polycystic ovarian syndrome and simple obesity weight reduction is associated with a return of ovulation, menstruation and fertility, in many cases.

It is therefore appropriate to assess body mass index (BMI) and general nutritional status in women who wish to get pregnant but are anovulatory. Therapies designed to raise or lower the BMI into the normal weight range represent a simple non-pharmacological and often successful approach to anovular infertility. Anti-obesity drugs such as orlistat (Xenical) and sibutramine may be prescribed to achieve weight targets that will return a

from about 10 to 16 weeks of gestation, possibly related to the high levels of human chorionic gonadotrophin (HCG) when levels of this hormone peak. Observational studies have, however, found no association between absolute HCG levels in serum and symptoms in the individual woman. In about 1% of cases the vomiting is severe enough to require hospital admission and parenteral nutritional support (hyperemesis gravidarum). Although it is a major concern for many women that their nutrient intake is severely compromised by the duration of nausea and vomiting there is no evidence, except in the most severe cases, of fetal harm resulting from a temporary acute fall in nutrient intakes. In fact the evidence is that those women who suffer more from nausea and vomiting have relatively higher birthweight infants.

A further common symptom is ptyalism, the sensation of producing excessive saliva, which may be spat out rather than swallowed when the woman is nauseated. Objective testing has not shown any measured increase in saliva production.

Relaxation of the cardiac sphincter in the stomach is thought to be at the root of the common symptom of acid reflux which results in heartburn. Delayed gastric emptying can lead to a feeling of fullness after meals. Motor sluggishness in the small intestine increases transit time from stomach to caecum from a mean of 52 hours in the non-pregnant, to 58 hours in pregnant subjects. Animal studies report an increase in villous density and absorptive area in the small bowel in pregnancy. Assuming such changes appear in the human the combined effect would be to increase nutrient uptakes. Evidence for this is scanty but calcium absorption is greater in early pregnancy up to 24 weeks, with no subsequent increase. Iron absorption in contrast increases throughout pregnancy and may be 40% higher towards the later stages. In contrast again experiments with oral folate uptake demonstrated no increased absorption in pregnancy.

The reduced peristalsis in the large bowel is associated with increased water reabsorption and production of hard stools leading to the common symptom of constipation.

Placental transfer

The placenta is responsible for maternal fetal exchange and grows with the fetus. Obviously the placenta is a fetal organ perfused on the fetal side by fetal blood and on the maternal side by maternal blood, exchange taking place across the cellular interface which is the syncytiotrophoblast. Major physiological changes take place in the terminal branches of the uterine artery at the placental site to allow expansion of the placental blood flow with advancing pregnancy. At term the placental blood flow reaches 800 ml/min.

The structural modifications of these terminal arteries follow invasion of the trophoblast into the uterine wall and the arterial walls in the first half of pregnancy. A failure of adequate trophoblast invasion is a feature of disorders such as pre-eclampsia. Despite this abnormal vascularisation placental perfusion is adequate in early pregnancy whilst the demands are small but fails to increase progressively in later gestation leading to retardation of fetal growth. Other barriers to adequate placental perfusion and therefore normal late fetal growth include factors operating on the maternal side of the placental such as the effect of maternal cigarette smoking. Placental transfer of nutrients takes place through four mechanisms, which are highlighted in relation to specific nutrients below; these are simple diffusion, facilitated diffusion, active transport and pinocytosis. In addition to its transport functions, the placenta is the source of several placental proteins with endocrine functions including HCG (the hormone detected in the maternal blood or urine in pregnancy testing), human placental lactogen and human placental growth hormone. The latter two have insulin counter-regulatory effects and therefore may modify the nutrient substrate mixture presented to the placenta by the mother. A number of other pregnancy-specific placental proteins have been identified, most of which appear to have a role in early pregnancy to facilitate uterine implantation.

Transfer of the principal fetal substrates is discussed below.

Maternal homeostasis of fetal nutrient substrates

A general observation is that plasma levels of water-soluble and fat-soluble nutrients adopt different homeostatic relationships in the maternal plasma in pregnancy. These changes, which can be characterised as a fall in maternal plasma levels of the water-soluble nutrients and a relative rise in the plasma levels of lipid soluble nutrients, are established at two stages in pregnancy. The majority of changes have taken place by about 10 to 12 weeks following fertilisation, long before fetal demands could cause maternal depletion. The implication is that these are homeostatic resettings which in various ways are potentially beneficial to the fetus but the relationships have not as yet been well characterised. A second wave of apparently physiological changes in substrate availability occurs at the end of the mid trimester, approximately 24 to 28 weeks into the pregnancy, when women in the developed world almost universally show a picture of relative insulin resistance. Insulin resistance is associated with an increased availability of all potential fetal substrates, particularly in the postprandial period when glucose, amino acid and lipid levels are raised. Insulin resistance is also a factor in enhanced lipolysis which is seen during overnight fasting in pregnancy and generates glycerol and free fatty acids as potential fetal or maternal energetic substrates.

It is of interest in making a judgement about these physiological relationships that women on typical diets of the developing world, particularly those that are rich in unrefined carbohydrate sources, do not show the picture of insulin resistance in the second half of pregnancy and therefore are presenting a different substrate mix to the placental circulation. The implication of these observations for normal fetal growth and proportions of fetal body composition remains the subject of continuing research.

Carbohydrates

Glucose provides at least 75% of fetal energy requirements. There is a physiological resetting of glucose homeostasis which results in approximately 15 to 20% lower plasma levels during overnight fasting and during the post-absorptive phase throughout gestation. Postprandially, however, the glucose peaks are relatively higher and there is increased glucose flux across the placenta during the postprandial period, particularly in the second half of pregnancy when insulin resistance has been established.

Glucose transport is by transcellular carrier-mediated facilitated diffusion up to a saturable maximum of 17 mmol/l. Experiments with large animals suggest an eight-fold rise in fetal glucose requirements between mid and late gestation. This is facilitated by the presence of increased amounts of the GLUT1 transporter in syncytiotrophoblast and endothelial cells and an increase in the density of GLUT1 in fetal endothelial cells.

It is of interest that the human fetoplacental unit appears to have no mechanism to prevent excess glucose transfer across the placenta below the saturable maximum, and in the pathological model of pregnancy complicated by maternal diabetes the excess glucose transfer has serious harmful effects on fetal growth and development (see Section CD 15A).

Protein and amino acids

Although small IgG class immunoglobulins may cross the placenta by the process of pinocytosis the placenta is effectively a barrier to the transport of larger protein molecules. Amino acids are actively transported across the placenta by both sodium-dependent and sodium-independent mechanisms. Amino acids appear in higher concentrations in the fetal than maternal circulation. In the studies of Phelps and colleagues (1981) measurements of eight neutral amino acids showed a similar profile (leucine, isoleucine, valine, tyrosine, phenylalanine, serine and proline) to that of glucose in that fasting and preprandial levels were lower in pregnancy but post-meal increments were greater and more sustained than in non-pregnant women. Throughout the diurnal cycle these amino acids appear in higher concentrations in the fetal circulation than the maternal circulation as a result of active transport across the placenta. There are at least 15 transport systems in the placenta for amino acids, some of which are sodium dependent, others not. Transferred amino acids are required for new tissue formation in the fetus, placental metabolism and consumption and placental interconversion. Basic amino acids are transferred to the fetus in adequate amounts for new tissue formation. Neutral amino acids are transferred in excess of requirement for new tissue formation and may be utilised as an energy source.

Lipids

Fat accumulates in the fetus at a rapid rate in the last third of pregnancy when fetal synthesis makes a significant contribution. Triglycerides do not appear to cross the placenta but fatty acids will cross the placenta by concentration-dependent diffusion. The pattern of fatty acids seen in fetal triglycerides after re-esterification mimics the triglyceride pattern in the mother's adipose tissue.

Placental transfer of lipoprotein complexes is slow but significant in that up to half of fetal cholesterol is of maternal origin. This transfer follows proteolysis in placental lysosomes. Phospholipids are hydrolysed by the placenta and resynthesised by the fetus. Research suggests that selective transport mechanisms for n-3 and n-6 essential fatty acids (EFAs) are present for the requirements of placental metabolism and fetal central nervous system (CNS) development during the second half of pregnancy. Concerns

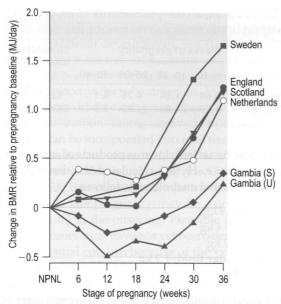

Figure 15.1 Changes in basal metabolic rate (BMR) from the non-pregnant state and at 6-weekly intervals in pregnancy in women studied by indirect calorimetry in four European countries and one African country. Gambian women were on their normal diet (U) or randomised to receive a high calorie supplement (S). (Adapted from Prentice et al 1989, with permission.)

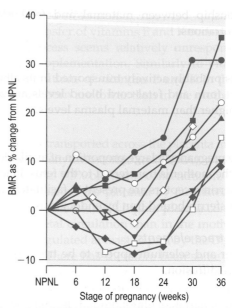

Figure 15.2 Changes in basal metabolic rate in eight individual European subjects studied by direct calorimetry. Baseline is the non-pregnant non-lactating (NPNL) state. (Adapted from Prentice et al 1989, with permission.)

tissue approximately 8000 kcal (33 MJ). This represents a cumulative increased calorie requirement over the whole of pregnancy of 80 to 85 000 kcal (356 MJ), or a daily calorie increase of approximately 320 kcal (1.3 MJ). This gave rise to the widespread advice that women, in order to have a successful pregnancy, must increase their energy intakes by 250 to 300 calories per day (1–1.5 MJ) – the widespread layperson's idea that the mother should 'eat for two'. The fat store in the mother comprises 3.8 kg of new adipose tissue. This major change in fat deposition is not seen in comparable studies from the developing world and the reasons for these differences in energetic costs of pregnancy are the subject of speculation (see below). Dietary surveys have been performed to assess women's responses to pregnancy in terms of the nutrient intake and to see whether their consumption matches the theoretical calculations. By and large they do not; an excellent example is the longitudinal study of energy balance performed in healthy pregnant women in Glasgow by Durnin et al (1987). This study showed a gradual rise in intakes during the duration of pregnancy, but the calculated total extra energy intake in pregnancy was less than 20 000 kcal (84 MJ). Basal metabolic rate

(BMR) calculated by indirect calorimetry showed a fall in early pregnancy followed by a rise during the last 10 weeks. There was no excess requirement for energy in the first 30 weeks of pregnancy and the increase in the last trimester could have been met by either a small increase in energy intake or a reduction in physical activity. Durnin's study was expanded by further recruitment to become part of a collaborative international project where longitudinal studies of BMR in pregnancy were performed by indirect calorimetry in selected developing and developed countries.

These studies using basal metabolic rates (BMR) assessed by indirect calorimetery show very wide geographical variations in the increase in BMR in pregnancy. Whereas women in the developed world have increases in BMR compatible with increased total energy expenditure (TEE) similar to the hypothetical calculation above (Fig. 15.1), women in the developing world may go through pregnancy with an apparent *reduction* in energy expenditure. This would be a very powerful adaptation to guarantee reproductive success against a background of an unreliable food supply. Most interestingly, however, the individual studies using whole body calorimetry on eight healthy women studied in Cambridge by Prentice et al (1989) show a very variable individual pattern in total energy expenditure. Approximately 50% of

Table 15.3 EAR energy for women in the UK

	Energy MJ/day (kcal/day)
Women (19–50)	8.1 (1940)
Pregnancy	+0.8 (200)[a]
Lactation (1 month)	+1.9 (450)
Lactation (2 months)	+2.2 (530)
Lactation (3 months)	+2.4 (570)
Lactation (4–6 months)[b]	+2.0 (480)
Lactation (4–6 months)[c]	+2.4 (570)
Lactation (>6 months)[b]	+1.0 (240)
Lactation (>6 months)[c]	+2.3 (550)

[a]Third trimester only.
[b]Non-exclusive breastfeeding – weaning commenced.
[c]Exclusive breastfeeding – weaning not commenced.

healthy European women were energy profligate during pregnancy whilst the other 50% were energy sparing (Fig. 15.2). Against this background, and with no easy way to assess the plane of energy expenditure adopted by any individual woman during her pregnancy, it is impossible to recommend an ideal energy intake. Current estimated average requirements (EARs) for energy intake in pregnancy and lactation are shown in Table 15.3.

Effects of activity on pregnancy and of pregnancy on activity

Whilst there is now much interest in the developed world in the relationship of activity and exercise to pregnancy outcomes it must be borne in mind that for many women in the developing world manual labour throughout pregnancy is not something they have a choice about. In addition, both in the developed and developing world the mother who has the day-to-day care of younger children at the time of the pregnancy may find that she does not have the opportunity to significantly reduce her physical activity.

For those who are able to reduce activity or give up demanding physical work during the last few weeks of pregnancy, the altered pattern of energy expenditure is bound to have an effect on substrate availability to the fetus. Studies such as that of Clapp & Dickstein (1984) suggested that women who maintained a high level of recreational exercise throughout pregnancy gained less weight, delivered their children earlier, and produced infants of lower birthweight. A study from the developing world, of women who were involved in hard physical work despite lower than recommended caloric intakes, again found there was a lowering of birthweight.

In summary, women who exercised before pregnancy and continued to do so during pregnancy tended to weigh less initially, to gain less weight, and to deliver smaller babies than (non-randomised) control subjects. There is insufficient evidence in the literature to make a judgement whether active women have better pregnancy outcomes than women who are predominantly sedentary in the second half of pregnancy, although one observational study from France reported that premature delivery rates more than doubled in women working more than 40 hours a week during pregnancy compared to those working for less than 40 hours per week. Apart from this there is little information from good quality studies to suggest whether active women have better pregnancy outcomes than less active women. The American College of Obstetricians and Gynecologists have issued some guidance to women about exercise patterns during pregnancy. Whilst these are empirical they may be useful as a practical guide (see Section CD 15B for details).

An important consideration when advising women about exercise in pregnancy is to consider diet as well. Diets high in carbohydrate, particularly from low glycaemic index sources, will alter the availability of fetal substrates, and thus a relatively unrefined diet associated with hard physical work or programmed exercise in pregnancy can lead to a reduction in birthweight. It is an interesting argument as to whether the non-exercising woman on the usual Western diet or her exercising sister on a high carbohydrate traditional type of diet should be recognised as the physiological norm in studies of pregnancy outcome.

Nutrient requirements of pregnancy

The current UK recommendations for nutrient intakes in pregnancy are summarised in Table 15.4. The reference nutrient intake (RNI) represents a nutritional intake at which about 97% of the population will obtain their daily requirements. Increased requirements are recommended during pregnancy for a small number of nutrients discussed below.

Protein
The recommendation for increased dietary protein content is based on the protein requirement of the new tissue formation outlined above. It is likely, however, that maternal resources would be made available to the fetus on a short-term basis in the face of any acute deficiency of protein intake.

Iodine

Iodine deficiency remains a major problem on a geographical basis in some areas of the developing world. It is particularly important in relation to pregnancy because of the risk of mental impairment in the offspring of iodine-deficient mothers. Where iodine deficiency is known to exist, iodised table salt or iodised cooking oil should be available to all the population and pregnant women in particular.

Nutrition and adverse pregnancy outcomes

Foodborne disease in pregnancy

Listeriosis is a disease more common in the immunocompromised. Pregnancy represents a state of relative immune compromise and in the rare case of primary infection during pregnancy transplacental infection of the fetus has been responsible for fetal death. Because of the behaviour of the organism and its proliferation in common foodstuffs such as mould ripened cheese, liver pate and cook-chill foods, major anxiety has been provoked amongst pregnant women in recent years. Sensible advice is that women should avoid mould-ripened cheese whilst pregnant and only eat pate from manufacturing processes where pasteurisation has taken place. As far as cook-chill food is concerned it should be consumed within the recommended shelf life and properly heated through before serving.

Toxoplasma gondii is a parasitic protozoal infection which non-immune women may be at increased risk of during pregnancy. It is caught from the ingestion of parasites from undercooked meat or from contact with cat faeces as a result of gardening or cleaning cat litter trays. In the fetus it can be responsible for brain infection and particularly defects of vision. Sensible advice to women in pregnancy who may be at risk is to cook all meat thoroughly before consumption and to either avoid gardening or cat litter trays or only to undertake these tasks with strong rubber gloves.

Maternal mortality

Maternal mortality rates are extremely low in the developed world, in the order of 1 in 10 000 births, but in the developing world rates may be as high as 6 per 1000 pregnancies. Nutrition may contribute to this increased mortality in two respects. Firstly protein calorie malnutrition, or rickets in childhood may lead to a failure to reach full genetic potential of adult height. This in turn may be associated with inadequate pelvic dimensions and obstructed labour in adulthood. Obstructed labour is a major cause of maternal death where facilities for safe caesarean section are not available.

Severe anaemia is also a contributor to maternal death, often in association with intercurrent illness such as malaria and the absence of safe blood transfusion to deal with antepartum or postpartum haemorrhage. Evidence, reviewed by Rush (2000), would suggest that moderate anaemia is not a major risk factor but severe anaemia (Hb < 8.0 g/dl) has been associated with a doubling of death rates in urban dwelling women and a quadrupling of death rates in rural dwelling women. For example, when the relationship between haematocrit and maternal death in northern Nigeria was examined there were 36 maternal deaths amongst 760 anaemic women (4.7%) but only 142 deaths in 11 699 non-anaemic women (1.2%), a relative risk of death of 3.9.

Low birthweight

Poor weight gain in pregnancy has been associated with poor fetal growth but of course to some extent this is self-fulfilling as the normal growth of the products of conception must be a factor in the maternal weight gain. Although advice to increase energy intakes will result in enhanced maternal weight gain there is no published evidence that this enhanced weight gain acts in the fetal interest.

In any obstetric population the prevalence of low birthweight is a good surrogate marker for risk of perinatal death (this is a combination of deaths before birth plus those in the first week of life). There are two principal causes of low birthweight – preterm delivery in which the infant may be normally grown but born in an immature state, and intrauterine growth retardation (IUGR) where inefficient placental transfer of oxygen and/or nutrients has led to a reduced rate of growth. The WHO definition simply is a 'birthweight of less than 2.5 kg'. This must include a mixture of the two diagnostic groups, although the proportions may vary depending on factors such as maternal stature, smoking and alcohol consumption, altitude above sea level, etc. Evidence is that low calorie intakes do not significantly contribute to low birthweight above a threshold value of an average energy intake somewhere between 1400 and 1700 kcal (5.8–7 MJ). Below this threshold there is good evidence that carbohydrate supplementation can significantly reduce the number of low birthweight babies. Above the threshold there is no clear evidence of such a benefit from supplementation.

Energy supplementation experiments both in the developed and developing world in women with calorie intakes above the threshold have negligible effects on birthweight and indeed experiments with protein dense supplements have been associated with a relative *reduction* in birthweight. Rush reviewed the published studies in 1989 and reported a reduction in birthweight when the percentage of calories as protein in supplements exceeded 20% (Rush 1989). Nutrient supplementation of healthy pregnant women at a time of enhanced energetic efficiency may simply result in increased rates of maternal obesity postpartum.

The effect of individual nutrient supplements in the prevention of low birthweight has been studied. Calcium supplementation appears be effective in the reduction of both preterm birth and the incidence of low birthweight (Atallah et al 2001). It may be that calcium supplementation has a role in the prevention of pregnancy-induced hypertension (see below) and that the increased mean birthweight is simply a reflection of prolongation of pregnancy. Although several experiments have been performed there is no evidence to support the use of magnesium supplementation during pregnancy to prevent low birthweight. There is similarly no evidence that routine iron supplementation prevents low birthweight. There is some suggestion from trials that folate supplementation may be effective in reducing the incidence of low birthweight in infants born at full term but folate supplementation has no preventative effect on preterm labour. In contrast, trials of zinc supplementation have suggested that lower rates of preterm delivery may be seen, although this evidence is not considered strong enough to influence practice at present. Meta-analyses of zinc supplementation studies suggest a non-significant reduction in low birthweight at term which again does not justify zinc supplementation in practice. Some studies suggest that vitamin D supplementation in pregnancy may have a beneficial effect on fetal growth but these are not of sufficient quality to influence practice and further research is indicated in this particular area.

No other specific nutrient supplement has been shown to be beneficial in properly designed trials in either reducing preterm birth rates or reducing term intrauterine growth retardation.

Obesity and pregnancy outcome

Obesity creates problems throughout the continuum of reproductive casualty. A BMI above 30 is associated with a doubling of the rate of ovulatory infertility and an even greater increase when the obesity is associated with the polycystic ovarian syndrome (see Fig. CD 15.1). During pregnancy obese women are at increased risk of developing gestational diabetes, venous thromboembolism and pregnancy-induced hypertension. There is also evidence that labour in the obese is more likely to be prolonged and unsuccessful, and should delivery by caesarean section be necessary, the procedure can be technically fraught because of difficulties with surgical access to the uterus through the obese abdomen. Offspring of obese mothers are heavier than those of height- and age-matched non-obese women when obese diabetic women are excluded from the analysis.

Nutrition and the hypertensive disorders of pregnancy

Pregnancy is complicated by the development of hypertension in about 8% of cases worldwide, with a predominance of first pregnancies. When hypertension is established and accompanied by proteinuria the condition is referred to as pre-eclampsia and is associated with increased maternal and perinatal mortality and morbidity. There have been many attempts to identify the causes of pre-eclampsia and several nutritional hypotheses have been tested. Early observational studies for instance suggested that the conditions were more common in omnivores than in strict vegetarians. Generalised nutritional deprivation in wartime has also been associated with a reduction in the frequency of pregnancy-associated hypertension. More recently attempts to prevent the condition have been made by dietary interventions including high protein diets, or establishing a high plane of general nutrition by eating a well-balanced diet. In contrast, some workers have suggested that voluntary dieting leading to weight gain restriction in pregnancy was beneficial in preventing hypertensive disease.

The evidence for dietary prevention of hypertension in pregnancy is of limited quality – and there is no suggestion that manipulating the diet can alter the incidence of these conditions. It may be able to prevent or moderate the secondary effects of disease in some circumstances.

As stated earlier, maternal obesity is associated with increased rates of pregnancy-associated hypertension and high weight gains during pregnancy have been reported in association with this disease. Once again this is probably self-fulfilling as these hypertensive conditions are often accompanied by fluid retention in the form of oedema.

In the past women have been recommended to reduce their salt intake but the only comparative study

Once again there is some evidence that lactation is associated with physiological shifts towards energy conservation and most women are probably in an energy-efficient mode during lactation (Fig. 15.3).

Nutrient requirements of lactation

Although essential fatty acid concentrations are low in human milk and low in breast milk substitutes, there is no evidence that maternal supplementation with essential fatty acids is beneficial. In lactation there is a recommendation for increased calcium intake to match losses in the milk. In prolonged lactation bone mineral density reduces in relation to the volume of breast milk produced. The bone mineral density is restored rapidly on cessation of lactation and there is no evidence that lactation contributes to an increased risk of osteoporosis in postmenopausal life. Phosphorus requirements are judged to be equimolar to calcium requirements and phosphate deficiency is unrecognised in normal diets.

The recommended increases in nutrients for lactation are calculated based on the assumption that the energy costs of lactation are added to the typical energy expenditure of the non-pregnant, non-lactating state. The comments above with regard to alterations in diet-induced thermogenesis and possible metabolism of maternal stored fat obviously influence the validity of these calculations in the individual.

Essential fatty acid contents of breast milk range from 0.1 g/100 g total fat to 1.4 g/100 g total fat in different population groups. The predominant n-6 long-chain polyunsaturated fatty acid (LCP-UFA) is arachidonic acid and docosahexaenoic acid (DHA) is the most common and most important n-3 LCPUFA in breast milk. The ratio of n-6 to n-3 fatty acids depends almost entirely on the intakes in the maternal habitual diet.

Dietary reference values

See Table 15.4.

Unwanted components of maternal diet which pass into milk

General concerns about the effect of components of the maternal diet on infants' tolerance of breast milk are probably overstated. Essential oils in foods such as garlic and some spices produce characteristic odours in milk which the infant may object to, although in one study maternal garlic consumption was associated with increased length of suckling and the rate of suckling at subsequent feeds. Foods which can produce problems of tolerance for the infant are cabbage, turnips, broccoli and beans, which seem capable of producing colic in some infants. The same effect has been ascribed to rhubarb, apricots and prunes. It might be sensible to exclude such food items when a breastfed infant appears to be distressed by colic after feeds.

Undernutrition in lactation

As suggested before, there are significant adaptive mechanisms to protect the newborn baby despite acute or chronic maternal undernutrition. The classic Bacon Chow studies performed in Taiwan women who were given a nutrient-dense supplement or placebo during pregnancy and lactation revealed marginally improved weight retention through lactation in the supplemented women (Adair et al 1984). Some placebo-treated women, however, maintained their weight or even increased it during a period of 12 months of lactation following birth. Skinfold thicknesses in undernourished women were greater at the end of lactation after the second studied pregnancy whether given supplements or not. The conclusion drawn was that most mothers maintain an appropriate energy balance, compromising neither their own health status nor that of their developing infants despite the apparent marginal nutritional status of the whole population. Mothers on low energy intakes in lactation maintain their weight well and lactate successfully, suggesting that important adaptive mechanisms are operating.

Lactational amenorrhoea, birth spacing and effects of maternal nutritional status

Fertile couples reproducing in the developing world without access to contraception typically show birth intervals of 3 to 4 years. This includes the duration of the pregnancy and approximately 18 to 24 months of lactational amenorrhoea during which there is no ovulation. In the developed world, freely available high calorie intakes are associated with periods of lactational amenorrhoea which may be as short as 6 to 8 weeks after the delivery. Thus paradoxically a high nutritional plane may be associated with a shorter inter-pregnancy interval and possibly physiological derangements associated with frequent childbearing in the developed world, compared with the developing world. Studies performed in Bangladesh in poorly nourished women reported average durations of amenorrhoea of 17.9 months compared to 16.8 months in well-nourished women from the same population. Similar studies performed in Guatemala found periods of amenorrhoea of 14.8 months in the undernourished compared to 13.2 months in the better nourished. This is a different pattern of response in developed compared to developing countries and once again there may be a trigger related to body mass index for the resumption of ovulation and menstruation.

⊃ Key points

- ⊃ Nutritional status throughout the human reproductive cycle can affect outcomes.

- ⊃ Anovulatory infertility is seen in under-nourished and overnourished women.

- ⊃ Periconceptional nutritional deficiencies may be associated with congenital malformations.

- ⊃ There is extensive maternal homeostatic change to produce a milieu favouring fetal growth and development.

- ⊃ Energy costs of pregnancy are variable and unpredictable.

- ⊃ Foodborne diseases such as listeriosis may be fatal for the fetus.

- ⊃ Maternal nutrient deficiencies such as iron predict increased maternal mortality in the developing world.

- ⊃ Reduced diet-induced thermogenesis is an energy-sparing mechanism in lactation.

References and further reading

References

Adair L S, Pollitt E, Mueller W H 1984 The Bacon Chow study: effect of nutritional supplementation on maternal weight and skinfold thicknesses during pregnancy and lactation. British Journal of Nutrition 51:357–369

Atallah A N, Hofmeyr G J, Duley L 2001 Calcium supplementation during pregnancy for preventing hypertensive disorders and related problems (Cochrane Review). In: The Cochrane Library, Issue 3. Oxford: Update Software

Campbell-Brown M, Hytten F 1998 Nutrition. In: Chamberlain G, Broughton-Pipkin F (eds) Clinical physiology in obstetrics, 3rd edn. Blackwell Science, Oxford, p 165–191

Clapp J F, Dickstein S 1984 Endurance exercise and pregnancy outcome. Medicine and Science in Sports and Exercise 16:556–562

Czeizel A E, Dudas I 1992 Prevention of the first occurrence of neural-tube defects by periconceptional vitamin supplementation. New England Journal of Medicine 327:1832–1835

Doyle W, Srivostova A, Crawford M A et al 2001 Interpregnancy folate and iron status of women in an inner city population. British Journal of Nutrition 86:81–87

Durnin J V, McKillop F M, Grant S, Fitzgerald G 1987 Energy requirements of pregnancy in Scotland. Lancet ii:897–900

Frisch R 1994 The right weight: body fat, menarche and fertility. Proceedings of the Nutrition Society 53:113–129

Illingworth P J, Jung R T, Howie P W et al 1986 Diminution in energy expenditure during lactation. British Medical Journal 292:437–441

Naylor K E, Iqbal P, Fledelius C et al 2000; The effect of pregnancy on bone density and bone turnover. Journal of Bone and Mineral Research 15:129–137

Phelps R I., Metzger B E, Freinkel N 1981 Carbohydrate metabolism in pregnancy. XVII Diurnal profiles of plasma glucose insulin free fatty acids, triglycerides, cholesterol and individual amino acids in late normal pregnancy. American Journal of Obstetrics and Gynecology 140:730–736

Prentice A M, Goldberg G R, Davies H L et al 1989 Energy sparing adaptations in human pregnancy assessed by whole body calorimetry. British Journal of Nutrition 62:5–22

Prentice A M, Spaaij C J, Goldberg G R et al 1996 Energy requirements of pregnant and lactating women. European Journal of Clinical Nutrition 50(suppl 1):S82–S118

Rich-Edwards J W, Goldman M B, Willet W C et al 1994 Adolescent body mass index and infertility caused by ovulatory disorder. American Journal of Obstetrics and Gynecology 171:171–177.

Rush D 1989 Effects of changes in maternal energy and protein intake during pregnancy, with special reference to fetal growth. In: Sharp F, Milner R D G,

Objectives

By the end of this chapter you should be able to:

- describe the physiological and pathological changes of ageing relevant to nutrition

- discuss important aspects of macro- and micronutrient intakes in older people

- understand the interactions of current measures of nutritional status with ageing, disability and disease and the consequent limitations for use in elderly people

- discuss the role of nutrition in the development, susceptibility to and outcome of common chronic disabling diseases in the elderly

- understand current important public health messages to maintain and improve nutritional status in elderly people.

16.1 INTRODUCTION

The number of older people is growing rapidly worldwide and looks set to continue increasing in the future. This has created a need for a more complete understanding of age-related changes relevant to nutrition and the role of nutrition in the prevention and treatment of chronic disabling diseases in the elderly. It is well recognised that with advancing age there is an increased incidence of chronic diseases, and evidence points to the importance of nutrition in the development, susceptibility to and outcome of these diseases. Undernutrition is recognised as a potential problem among the elderly, especially in the oldest age groups. There are, however, difficulties in diagnosing undernutrition in the elderly because of physical and biochemical changes which may take place as part of normal ageing. In addition, the neglect of nutritional assessment in the setting of acute clinical medicine is well known. For example, in Britain, undernutrition is prevalent but largely unrecognised in elderly patients on admission to hospital and tends to deteriorate further during their hospital stay. There is no doubt that good nutrition contributes to the health and well-being of elderly people and to their ability to recover from illness.

16.2 DEMOGRAPHIC TRENDS IN THE UK

Since the early 1930s the number of people aged over 65 in England has more than doubled (**Fig. 16.1**) and today a fifth of the population is over 60. Between 1995 and 2025 the number of people over the age of 80 is set to increase by almost a half and the number of people over 90 will double. The 2000 national statistics on the health of older people in England revealed that 4% of those aged 65 and over were resident in care homes and just over three-quarters of these residents were women, compared with a figure of 57% women among those aged 65 and over in private households. Two-thirds of permanent admissions to care homes were from private households and 14% were from hospital. Women were more likely than men to have been living alone before admission. Chronic illness and disability are both important determinants of the need for elderly people to enter residential care. Although no national register of disability or disabled older persons in Britain exists, nearly two-thirds of disabled people are aged 65 or older. The National Health Service (NHS), for example, spent around 40% of its budget – £10 billion – on people over the age of 65 in 1998/99. In the same year social services spent nearly 50% of their budget on the over 65s, some £5.2 billion.

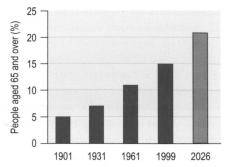

Figure 16.1   The percentage of people aged 65 and over amongst the UK population (Adapted from ONS 2001).

16.3 AGE-RELATED PHYSIOLOGICAL AND PATHOLOGICAL CHANGES RELEVANT TO NUTRITION

Ageing in humans may be accompanied by changes that impair the search for food and its subsequent intake, but such changes are complex and difficult to document. Anorexia and weight loss are common and important clinical problems in the oldest age groups and the causes are multifactorial. There is a growing recognition that age-related physiological anorexia may predispose to protein-energy undernutrition (PEU) in the elderly, particularly in the presence of other 'pathological' factors associated with ageing, such as social, psychological, physical and medical factors, some of which are responsive to treatment.

Physiological changes

Hormonal changes

The mechanisms of physiological anorexia of ageing are poorly understood but they have been the focus of recent research. Current evidence suggests that a combination of reduced sensory perception within the gastrointestinal tract, a decline in opioid modulation of feeding, particularly in older women, and an increase in the satiating effects of cholecystokinin (CCK) contribute to this anorexia. CCK, the best characterised of the gastrointestinal hormones, is known to play a role in the control of food intake (see Section 5.6). There is evidence that sensitivity to the satiating effects of CCK increases with age. The combination of increased circulating CCK concentrations and enhanced sensitivity to the satiating effects of CCK in older people suggests that CCK may be a significant contributor to the anorexia of ageing. With age the time taken for the emptying of the stomach after large volumes of food is increased, and this affects satiation. This may explain why older adults feel a greater satiating effect of an average meal compared to younger adults. Other hormones (e.g. leptin), neurotransmitters (e.g. opioids and nitric oxide) and cell signalling molecules (e.g. cytokines) may also have a role to play in anorexia and weight loss of ageing (MacIntosh et al 2000).

Gastrointestinal tract

Objective changes in smell and taste have been observed which may directly decrease food intake or alter the type of foods selected. In addition, the ability to identify foods while blindfolded decreases with advancing age. This is a common perceived problem among elderly individuals who complain of loss of both taste and smell (Exton-Smith 1980). A reduction in taste and smell, which may occur in up to 50% of elderly people, is often associated with impaired appetite. Taste thresholds are higher in institutionalised than in healthy elderly men and the use of drugs, particularly antihypertensive medication, appears to be a contributing factor. Dental health is important in old age and 45% of the free-living elderly in the most recent National Diet and Nutrition Survey in the UK were found to be edentulous (Finch et al 1998). Although there is evidence linking nutritional status to dentition, a causal relationship is yet to be established in randomised controlled intervention trials (see Section 25.2, under Geographic and social class differences and Section CD 16A).

Other gastrointestinal changes in the elderly have been documented which could affect their food intake. For example, changes in peristaltic activity of the oesophagus occur which may result in delay of oesophageal emptying. Absorption of some nutrients, in particular vitamin B_{12}, may be impaired because of mild ageing-related achlorhydria. Some researchers have reported widespread nutritional deficiencies associated with bacterial contamination of the small bowel, whilst others found no association between bacterial contamination of the small bowel and nutritional status. The most likely interpretation of these apparently conflicting reports is that bacterial contamination of an anatomically normal small bowel in the elderly is the result rather than the cause of undernutrition. The mechanisms through which undernutrition might cause bacterial growth are not fully understood but there is evidence that the activity of several enzyme systems involved in bactericidal processes may be reduced in undernutrition.

Body composition

Changes in body composition seen with ageing include a decrease in lean body mass, which occurs faster after the eighth decade, and an increase in body fat. The decline in lean body mass is predominantly that of muscle, and the loss of muscle mass with ageing contributes to a loss of mobility and an increased frequency of falls in elderly people. A decrease in lean body mass is associated with a

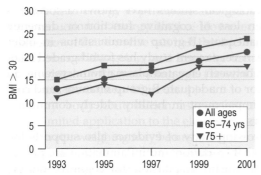

Figure 16.2 Prevalence of obesity amongst men in England (Adapted from ONS 2001).

suggested for the delivery of such services:

- BMI 25–30: Primary care can help individuals in the population to take responsibility for their own management of weight maintenance/reduction.

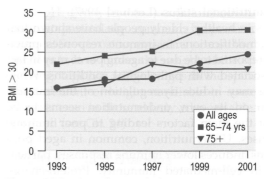

Figure 16.3 Prevalence of obesity amongst women in England (Adapted from ONS 2001).

- BMI 30–40: Secondary and primary care (provision to be agreed locally in GP surgeries and local general hospitals).
- BMI 40+: Specialist services.

16.4 AGE-RELATED CHANGES IN ENERGY AND PROTEIN REQUIREMENTS

Energy requirements

To date, the scientific evidence regarding energy requirements in the elderly has been incomplete and highly variable. The reasons for this include paucity and variability of data on energy intake and requirements, and most important of all, diversity of physical activity patterns in the elderly population. In a series of studies, elderly subjects from the USA consumed on average more energy than subjects in European studies. However, the US trials included fewer people than the European studies. The Department of Health and Social Security (DHSS) longitudinal study in the UK, which examined energy intake in 365 elderly people in 1967/8 and 5 years later, found that the average energy intake fell from 2235 to 2151 kcal per day for men and from 1711 to 1636 kcal per day for women. The most recent National Diet and Nutrition Survey of British people aged 65 years and over (Finch et al 1998) found that the mean energy intake appears to be even lower; for free-living men it was 1909 kcal and for women it was 1422 kcal. A similar trend for energy intakes to fall with age over 5 years was observed in a study of 269 elderly people in Gothenburg, Sweden.

Energy expenditure

Basal metabolic rate (BMR)

BMR reflects the energy requirements for maintenance of the intracellular environment and the

mechanical processes, such as respiration and cardiac function, which sustain the body at rest. It usually accounts for between 60% and 75% of total energy expenditure. The FAO/WHO/UNU Expert Consultation (WHO 1985) used equations to predict BMR. These equations may be less appropriate for elderly populations, especially older men, because of small numbers in the study. BMR increases with body size, particularly with lean body mass. This explains why it is higher in men than women, and 10–20% lower in old people compared with younger adults because of reduced muscle mass and increased fat mass with ageing.

Physical activity

In most working populations physical activity accounts for 10–35% of total energy expenditure. The energy expenditure of different activities depends on the amount of work being carried out, the weight of the individual and the efficiency with which that work is carried out. In general, ageing is associated with a reduction in efficiency, which may make standard tasks like walking up to 20% more energy-expensive in older people. This reduced efficiency may be one reason why older individuals slow down. For example, the energy cost of normal activities has been reported to increase with age for men. In Nottingham, healthy women aged 70 years had a 20% higher energy cost for walking at a standard speed than either men of the same age or younger women.

In a questionnaire survey based on a sample of the general population resident in private (non-institutional) households in Britain, information was collected from 3691 people aged 65 or over about participation in physical activities in the previous 4 weeks. In the 60–69-year age group about 70% recorded no outdoor activity in the previous 4 weeks and this proportion was even higher in the over 70-year age group. A survey in Nottingham of customary activity of elderly people found that the average reported daily time in active pursuits was less than one hour and lower still in those aged 75 years or more. Four years later a significant decline in activity levels was found in the 620 survivors. Another feature of ageing which may restrict physical activity is the liability to a variety of degenerative and chronic diseases such as chronic obstructive airway disease, angina and arthritis.

Thermogenesis

The term thermogenesis encompasses a wide variety of phenomena which include energy expenditure and heat generation associated with feeding, body temperature maintenance and thermogenic response to various specific stimuli such as smoking, caffeine and drugs. Thermogenesis has also been postulated to play a part in the regulation of body weight (see Ch. 5). This field of research is complex in humans, and the underlying theory is derived mainly from animal models. In the elderly, resting circulating catecholamine concentrations are elevated, and the responsiveness to catecholamines may decline with age, as is the case in experimental animals. The thermic response to meal ingestion appears to be influenced by age, physical activity and body composition. It is possible that the fall in the capacity for thermogenesis with age may explain the increased risk of hypothermia in the elderly. However, in most cases of hypothermia there is a precipitating physical cause such as stroke, which may or may not have a direct effect on thermogenesis.

Protein requirements

Determination of protein requirements in humans is a complex subject posing difficult questions for nutritionists. (For a detailed discussion see Ch. 8, Section 8.5.) Lean body mass protein falls with age and protein synthesis, turnover, and breakdown all decrease with advancing age. The progressive loss of protein appears to be a major feature of ageing throughout adult life. This appears to affect some tissues, notably skeletal muscle, more than others. There is no direct evidence to suggest that this erosion of tissue protein is due to lack of adequate amounts of protein in the average diet.

Ill health, trauma, sepsis and immobilisation may upset the equilibrium between protein synthesis and degradation. A group of researchers studied the dietary protein requirements of 12 elderly men and women aged 56–80 years using short-term nitrogen balance techniques and calculations recommended by the 1985 Joint FAO/WHO/UNU Expert consultation. They also recalculated nitrogen balance data from three previous protein requirement studies in elderly people. From the current and retrospective data they reported that a safe protein intake for elderly adults would be 1.0–1.25 g/kg per day.

16.5 AGE-RELATED CHANGES IN MICRONUTRIENT INTAKE AND REQUIREMENTS

Vitamins

Because of a reduced energy requirement and the associated lower food intake and the increased incidence of physical diseases, which may interfere with absorption, metabolism and utilisation, deficiency of certain vitamins is more likely in the elderly than in younger adults. The most recent diet and nutrition survey of the elderly carried out in the UK revealed average vitamin intakes of most vitamins to be above current RNIs. However, older people comprise a very heterogeneous group within which there are subgroups at more risk of vitamin inadequacies than others. Vitamin D status is more likely to be poor among institutionalised elderly, particularly during the winter months. Evidence of lower vitamin intakes among lower socioeconomic groups, reported in younger people, appears to track into old age, and this seems to be true for folate and vitamin C. Poor folate status in some old people has been linked with poor cognitive function and poor vitamin C status has been associated with evidence of impaired collagen metabolism, likely to contribute to poor wound healing in elderly people.

Table 16.2 Some drugs that may interfere with nutritional status in elderly people (Durnin & Lean 1992)

	Increase	Decrease
Energy intake (appetite/absorption)	Phenothiazines Tricyclic antidepressants Corticosteroids	Metformin Digoxin Many antibiotics Anticancer drugs Most analgesics Theophylline
Vitamins		Isoniazid (pyridoxine) Metformin (folate, B_{12}) Phenothiazines (folate) Tricyclics (folate) Methotrexate (folate) Colchicine (B_{12}) Cholestyramine (A, B_{12}, D, E, K) Tetracycline (C) Aspirin (C) Corticosteroids (C) Anticoagulants (D, folate)
Minerals and electrolytes	Amiloride (K) Spironolactone (K) Corticosteroids (Na) Phenylbutazone (Na) Carbenoxolone (Na) Ethanol (Fe)	Diuretics (Na, K, Ca, Mg, Zn) Phosphates (Fe) Tetracycline (Fe) Antacids (Fe) NSAIDs (Fe) Iron supplements (Zn)

possible effects of illness on nutritional status, many drugs which are commonly used in the elderly may interact with nutritional factors such as energy and nutrient intake, appetite, and mineral and electrolyte homeostasis (Table 16.2).

16.9 NUTRITIONAL SUPPORT OF ELDERLY PEOPLE

Why elderly patients need nutritional support and when

Prior to coming into hospital elderly people in the community are likely to have premorbid decreases in energy or calorie intake, low lean body mass and impaired immune response, all of which may be associated with poor nutritional status. Their nutritional status is likely to deteriorate further as the result of the catabolism associated with the acute illness. This is compounded further by the demands of the sometimes prolonged period of rehabilitation. Nutritional depletion during rehabilitation, however, may be more serious than during acute illness, since rehabilitation periods may extend over weeks and months, and weight loss, although less marked than in the early catabolic phase, may be greater overall.

Recent work has shown that baseline nutritional status of elderly stroke patients was worse among those who later died or remained in hospital compared with those discharged, and most patients who remained in hospital showed marked and significant deterioration in all measures of nutritional status during the hospital stay (Gariballa et al 1998). Nutritional status was a strong and independent predictor of morbidity and mortality at 6 months following acute stroke (FOOD Trial Collaboration 2003). Studies on the nutritional status and energy intake of 350 randomly selected admissions to a geriatric rehabilitation unit found that protein-energy malnutrition was a strong predictor of in-hospital and post-discharge mortality. A recent study of predictors of early non-elective hospital readmission in elderly patients found that individuals with any amount of weight loss and no improvement in albumin concentrations during the first month after hospitalisation were at a much higher risk of readmission than those who maintained or increased their post-discharge weight and had repleted their serum albumin concentrations.

A recent meta-analysis reported that aggressive nutritional support in surgical and critically ill patients, who are known to be hypermetabolic (with a loss of 20–40 g of nitrogen/day) and have increased nutrient requirements, did not influence the overall mortality. However, it may reduce complication rates in already malnourished patients. A larger, systematic Cochrane Library review on protein and energy supplementation in elderly people at risk from malnutrition included 31 trials with 2464 randomised participants. The authors concluded that supplementation produces a small but consistent weight gain. There was a statistically significant beneficial effect on mortality and a shorter length of hospital stay. Additional data from large-scale multicentre trials are still required to provide clear evidence of benefit from protein and energy supplements on

mortality and length of hospital stay. Too few data were reported and the time scale of most studies was too short to have a realistic chance of detecting differences in morbidity, functional status and quality of life. Furthermore, most trials do not address the organisational and practical challenges faced by practitioners trying to meet the individual needs and preferences of those at risk from malnutrition (Milne et al 2002). Based on present evidence it is possible that the poor outcome in elderly patients following acute illness may at least be partly due to undernutrition and that aggressive nutritional support during the convalescent period is more likely to improve nutritional status and lead to better rehabilitation outcome, decreased readmission rate, improved quality of life and contribute to reducing Health Service cost.

See Section CD 16A for a summary of the latest UK National Diet and Nutrition Survey of people aged 65 and over (1998), Section CD 16B for discussion of nutritional support studies in elderly patients, Appendix Tables A1–A27 for recommended energy and nutrient intakes including older people, and the CD Additional references and Further reading sections for additional reading.

⊃ Key points

⊃ Healthy elderly people's dietary patterns and the foods eaten are not likely to be that much different from what is known about those of younger people.

⊃ The majority of 'pathological' factors associated with ageing, which may predispose to malnutrition, are responsive to treatment.

⊃ Older people should be advised to eat a balanced diet containing a variety of nutrient-dense foods.

⊃ Elderly people should be encouraged to lead an active life, especially after episodes of inter-current illness.

⊃ Future research should focus on understanding complex factors determining intake of food and the role of adequate nutrition in prevention and treatment of disease in the ageing population.

References and further reading

References

Dawson D, Hendershot G, Fulton J 1987 Ageing in the eighties: functional limitations of individuals 65 and over. NCHS Advance Data from Vital Health Statistics no. 133

Department of Health and Social Security 1979 Nutrition and health in old age (Report on health and social subjects no 16). HMSO, London

Durnin J V G A, Lean M E J 1992 Nutrition – consideration for the elderly. In: Brocklehurst J C, Tallis R C, Fillit H M (eds) Textbook of geriatric medicine and gerontology. Churchill Livingstone, London

Exton-Smith A N 1980 Nutritional status: diagnosis and prevention of malnutrition. In: Exton-Smith A N, Caird F I (eds) Metabolic and nutritional disorders in the elderly. John Wright, Bristol

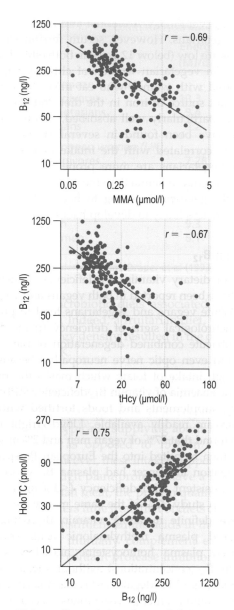

Figure 17.1 Indices of vitamin B_{12} deficiency in British vegan men. Plasma concentrations of methyl-malonic acid (MMA) $> 0.75 \, \mu$mol/l, homocysteine (tHcy) $> 15 \, \mu$mol/l and holotranscobalamin (HoloTC) < 25 pmol/l indicate vitamin B_{12} deficiency. Source: Lloyd-Wright et al (2003).

Table 17.2 Polyunsaturated fatty acids (wt %) in the breast milk of vegans, vegetarians and omnivores

Fatty acids	Vegans	Vegetarians	Omnivores
18:2 n-6	23.8	19.5	10.9
18:3 n-3	1.36	1.25	0.49
20:3 n-6	0.44	0.42	0.4
20:4 n-6	0.32	0.38	0.35
22:6 n-3	0.14	0.3	0.37

Source: Sanders & Reddy (1992).

contain significant amounts of linolenic acid (Sanders 1999a). However, the levels of DHA in blood, arterial and breast milk lipids are approximately only one-third of those found in omnivores (Table 17.2). Supplementation with linolenic acid does not lead to an increase in DHA in these lipids but relatively small amounts (~200 mg) of preformed DHA lead to a substantial increase. Products acceptable to vegans, fortified with an algal source of DHA, are now available. While there are cogent reasons for believing that a supply of DHA is important for normal visual and neurological development in the neonate, as yet there is no clear indication that the consumption of DHA by vegans has any clear health benefits.

Vitamin D and calcium

Vegetarians who consume milk and cheese regularly have relatively high intakes of calcium but vegans tend to have low intakes of calcium, usually well below the reference nutrient intake. Vegetarian diets may contain significant quantities of modifiers of the absorption of calcium such as phytic acid contributed by legumes and unrefined cereals (especially unleavened breads and brown rice). A high prevalence of rickets has been noted in children reared on macrobiotic diets who are predominantly vegetarians. However, rickets and osteomalacia do not appear to be significant problems among the white vegetarian population. To be acceptable to vegetarians, vitamin D needs to be provided as ergocalciferol in fortified foods and supplements. Rickets among vegans and vegetarians appears to be more related to the bioavailability of calcium from the diet than any other factor. High intakes of phytate from cereals such as brown rice or unleavened bread appear to be the main precipitating factor even in climates where exposure to sunlight may be high.

n-3 Fatty acids

Docosahexaenoic acid (22:6 n-3; DHA) is believed to play an important role in the development of the retina and the central nervous system. It can be synthesised from linolenic acid (18:3 n-3) or obtained preformed in the diet from food of animal origin, especially fish. Vegan diets are devoid of DHA but

17.4 PREGNANCY

The duration of pregnancy was found to be approximately 4–5 days shorter in Hindu vegetarians and earlier onset of labour and caesarean section are more common than in the white population in the UK. Babies born to Hindus are lighter than those born to Muslims or white omnivores even when adjustments are made for gestational age and maternal frame size. Birthweights appear normal in white vegetarian women but a shorter duration of pregnancy has been observed in vegans. The pathophysiological significance of a slightly lower birthweight is uncertain. However, according to Barker's nutritional programming hypothesis, a lower birthweight and smaller head circumference may increase the risk of developing diabetes and cardiovascular disease in later life.

17.5 CHILD GROWTH AND DEVELOPMENT

Widdowson & McCance (1954) in their classic experiment carried out at the end of World War II clearly demonstrated that children will grow and develop quite normally on a diet consisting of plenty of bread and vegetables with minimal amounts of milk and meat. The growth rate of the white Seventh-Day Adventists vegetarian population appears to be virtually indistinguishable from that of white omnivores except for a later age of menarche. Lower rates of growth, particularly in the first 5 years of life, have been reported in children reared on vegan and macrobiotic diets. Despite these lower rates of growth in the first few years of life, catch-up growth occurs by the age of about 10 years. Height is normal but there is still a tendency for these children to be lighter in weight for height than children on mixed diets. The slower rates of growth observed in some of these children under the age of 5 can be attributed to low energy intakes. The significance of slightly slower rates of growth is debatable, but a small fraction of vegan children do show evidence of impaired growth.

It needs to be more widely recognised that severe nutritional deficiencies do occur in children reared on inappropriate vegetarian and vegan diets. With the increasing popularity of vegetarian diets and the trend for a small majority to ignore conventional nutritional wisdom, it seems inevitable that more children will fall victims to their parental folly.

17.6 THE HEALTH OF VEGETARIANS AND VEGANS

The health of Western vegetarian groups has been extensively studied and generally appears to be good, providing the known dietary pitfalls – low energy density, inadequate intakes of iron, vitamin B_{12} and D – are avoided. Assessing the health impact of vegetarianism is often compounded by other lifestyle factors such as socioeconomic status, non-smoking status and health consciousness. One approach has been to compare biomarkers of disease (such as plasma cholesterol and blood pressure) in vegan, vegetarian and omnivore groups. These studies show that on average serum cholesterol is 20% (~1mmol/l) lower in vegans than in omnivores with intermediate values in vegetarians. Blood pressure has also been found to be lower in vegetarians and this appears to be an effect independent of salt intake or body mass index and appears to be due to a higher consumption of potassium from fruit and vegetables. Recent research has reported elevated homocysteine in vegetarians and vegans. This was particularly marked in subjects recruited in the report by Lloyd-Wright et al (2003) and was attributable to a low vitamin B_{12} intake rather than a low folate intake. This would be regarded as an adverse finding as elevated plasma homocysteine is associated with endothelial dysfunction and increased risk of cardiovascular disease (ischaemic heart disease, stroke and deep-vein thrombosis). Epidemiological studies suggest that a $3\,\mu mol/l$ increase in plasma homocysteine is associated with a 15% increase in risk of cardiovascular disease (Wald et al 2002). The mean plasma homocysteine concentration in B_{12}-deficient vegans was $22\,\mu mol/l$ compared with $10\,\mu mol/l$ in healthy controls. Despite the findings of Lloyd-Wright et al (2003) elevated plasma homocysteine is often indicative of poor folate status, which is thought to have implications for risk of cancers at various sites.

An almost universal finding has been that vegetarians and vegans are lighter in weight than their meat-eating counterparts. The Oxford cohort of the EPIC Study found a difference of 1 unit of BMI

exhaustion and heat stroke. In the case of maximal performance, the availability of carbohydrate together with fluid may limit performance. In this respect both carbohydrate and sodium have beneficial characteristics stimulating water absorption. On the other hand, from a number of observational as well as experimental studies, it has become clear that a higher frequency of gastrointestinal distress symptoms occur when athletes are dehydrated, especially when fluid loss exceeds 4% of body weight.

Restoration of fluid balance after exercise is an important part of recovery. Rehydration after exercise can be achieved effectively only if both electrolyte as well as water losses are replaced. The sodium content of most sports drinks lies within a range of 200 to 600 mg/l. These values are already at the lower level for an effective rehydration solution. An ideal post-exercise rehydration drink should contain around 1100 mg/l sodium to optimise water retention. In comparison, regular soft drinks contain virtually no sodium and are therefore less suitable as a rapid rehydration solution.

Micronutrients

Vitamins have attracted much attention in the world of sport because of their supposed capacity to enhance performance. Vitamin supplements are widely used by both professional and recreational athletes, often with extreme levels of intake exceeding 10 to 100 times the RDA. It is fair to assume that vitamin requirements are increased in the athlete involved in rigorous exercise training, due to the increased energy expenditure, sweat loss, core temperature etc. However, as the increased energy expenditure in the athlete is compensated for by an increase in energy intake and assuming a healthy diet, increased vitamin intake fully compensates for any increase in vitamin requirements. As such, there are no indications that long-term vitamin intake among athletes is in any way insufficient. The only exception may be athletes involved in regular intense exercise training who consume either a (very) extreme low (<4.2 MJ/day) or high (>21 MJ/day) energetic diet for a prolonged period. The latter is explained by the fact that athletes requiring such an extreme high energy intake tend to consume energy-dense food and beverages (often during prolonged endurance exercise trials) which from a dietary viewpoint often tend to be of a lesser quality. These athletes (such as cyclists during the Tour de France)

as well as those consuming extremely low energetic diets (like female endurance runners, gymnasts and ballet dancers) are prone to a marginal vitamin intake and can be at risk of developing vitamin deficiencies. Therefore, vitamin supplementation at moderate levels can contribute to adequate daily intake in these athletes. A vitamin deficiency will result in decreased performance and/or increased susceptibility to illness. However, vitamin supplementation with quantities exceeding those needed for optimal blood levels has never been shown to improve performance.

In addition, vitamin E, C and β-carotene are important antioxidants. The growing interest in the health-related aspects of antioxidants has also raised the interest of sport nutritionists. Exercise has been associated with increases in free radical production in skeletal muscle, with potential for tissue damage. It is suggested that especially in a state of overtraining the balance between oxidative stress and repair has been interrupted, leading to dysfunction of membranes and increased lipid peroxidation. However, it has also been shown that athletes have increased levels of cellular antioxidant enzymes, such as superoxide dismutase (SOD), catalase and glutathione peroxidase compared to untrained individuals. Most probably this is the result of a physiological adaptation to the higher oxidative stress and therefore it is questionable whether additional supplementation of antioxidants above the normal adequate intake levels are of any benefit. So far, in this respect the available literature does not allow any claims.

With respect to the minerals, iron has probably attracted most attention regarding the advice on additional supplementation in athletes. Although other minerals, such as calcium, chromium, magnesium, zinc, copper and selenium, are just as important, the status of these minerals is generally adequate in most athletes. Iron loss is increased in athletes, partly due to some iron loss in sweat, increased gastrointestinal and/or urinary blood loss and foot strike haemolysis, as a consequence of the intensity and duration of the exercise. However, as mentioned before regarding other (micro)nutrients, increased iron loss is usually well compensated for by the increased dietary intake associated with the higher energy expenditure. Though many athletes, in particular females, tend to be iron depleted, true iron deficiencies are rarely seen. Iron deficiency may be suspected in athletes who have a slightly lower than average haemoglobin (Hb) from the so called athletes' anaemia (Hb <14% in male and <12% in female endurance athletes). This is usually a training-induced physiological condition, caused by an increase in plasma volume. Despite a slightly reduced haemoglobin, the total red cell mass is normal or greater than usual. Although athletes' anaemia may be associated with low serum ferritin, this physiological condition does not respond to iron supplementation. Therefore, iron supplement use is generally considered unnecessary and supplementation without medical indication is not advised. The latter, because excessive iron supplementation can cause gastrointestinal disturbances and/or even haemosiderosis. Iron supplements have not been shown to enhance performance capacity, except where iron deficiency anaemia exists.

18.5 ERGOGENIC AIDS

Following the recognition of glycogen loading and carbohydrate supplementation as means to improve exercise performance, much attention has been directed towards the use of nutritional supplements to optimise sports performance. In response, various nutrition companies started to develop specific sports nutrition products. Since then, sports nutrition has become a thriving branch of the food industry, and a wide variety of (sports) supplements is now available. These supplements range from the well-known sports drinks, high-energy bars and protein-shakes to a multitude of supplements containing vitamins, minerals, free amino acids etc. These supplements are, in some cases, useful to compensate (temporarily) for a less than adequate diet, to meet the special nutrient demands induced by intense exercise training and/or to optimise exercise performance. An increasing interest has been directed towards novel ergogenic supplements, often referred to as functional foods or nutraceuticals. From the term nutraceuticals it is already clear that these supplements should be categorised somewhere between nutritional supplements and pharmaceuticals. In most cases these nutraceuticals contain compounds that do occur in a normal diet but are supplemented in amounts far above nutrient RDA levels, or the amounts typically provided by food. Most of these supplements are proposed to increase performance capacity, often through a more pharmacological rather than a physiological effect. However, most of these claims rely on theoretical or anecdotal support rather than on documented results from scientific trials. It must be noted that such products are not registered like regular pharmaceuticals and, as such, are not under appropriate legislation or obligatory safety requirements. In short, at this moment no clinical trials need to be performed before these products are allowed to be advertised and marketed. Though the majority of the advertised nutraceuticals have not been clinically tested on their ergogenic potential nor on their safety, some nutraceuticals (e.g. caffeine, creatine, carnitine and sodium bicarbonate) have received much attention from scientists because of their proposed potential to affect muscle metabolism. Here, we will discuss the efficacy of a few currently popular ergogenic aids.

Caffeine

Caffeine is a well-known ergogenic aid, and was until January 2004 included on the banned substances list used by the IOC (International Olympic Committee), with an acceptance limit of $12\,\mu g/ml$ in the urine. Several studies have provided evidence for the ergogenic properties of caffeine ingestion during prolonged endurance exercise tasks. These ergogenic effects have been observed even when caffeine was ingested in doses leading to urine concentrations well below IOC limits. An effective ingestion dose lies between 2 and $5\,mg/kg$ body weight, comparable to the amount of caffeine in 2–6 cups of coffee. The performance-enhancing effect of caffeine is often attributed to its proposed stimulating effect on adipose tissue lipolysis and subsequent increase in fat oxidation rate. However, no direct in vivo evidence for this mechanism has yet been provided. A more plausible explanation would be the stimulating effect of caffeine on the central nervous system, the release and/or activity of adrenaline. As such caffeine stimulates motivational aspects which probably explains the improved performance observed mainly during long-term endurance exercise tasks. Caffeine supplementation could be detrimental to performance capacity when an athlete is particularly sensitive to its diuretic effect. Other negative side effects associated with caffeine use include gastrointestinal distress, decreased motor control, shivering, headache, dizziness, and minor elevations in blood pressure and resting heart rate.

Objectives

At the end of this chapter you should:

- know the prevalence of cardiovascular disease in different parts of the world and be aware of the changing mortality rates in different countries
- know the risk factors for cardiovascular disease and their nutritional determinants
- be aware of the clinical trials in which diet has been modified to reduce cardiovascular risk
- have an understanding of how information from epidemiological studies may be translated into practical dietary advice for individuals and populations.

19.1 INTRODUCTION

Cardiovascular diseases account for an appreciable proportion of total morbidity and mortality in adults throughout the world. The different conditions assume varying degrees of importance in different countries. For example, in developing countries rheumatic heart disease (which affects the heart valves) and cardiomyopathy (which affects the heart muscle) are common, but these conditions are relatively infrequent in most affluent societies, where coronary heart disease (CHD) has assumed epidemic proportions. This chapter describes cardiovascular diseases in which nutritional factors play an important role in aetiology and management. Thus, the emphasis is on CHD rather than cerebrovascular disease (stroke) or peripheral vascular disease (claudication) since there is considerably less evidence concerning the importance of nutritional factors in these conditions. Most of these cardiovascular diseases primarily affect the arteries with symptoms and signs resulting from the consequent reduction in blood supply. It is important to appreciate the terminology used to describe the pathological process and clinical entities.

Atherosclerosis is the basic pathological lesion which tends to occlude the arteries to a varying extent. A superimposed *thrombus*, or clot, may produce further narrowing to the extent that the artery is totally blocked. A variety of cells and lipids are involved in the pathogenesis of the atherosclerotic plaque and the arterial thrombus, including lipoproteins, cholesterol, triglycerides, platelets, monocytes, endothelial cells, fibroblasts and smooth muscle cells. Nutrition may influence the development of atherosclerosis by modifying one or more of these factors. Two major clinical conditions may occur when atherosclerosis, with or without a superimposed thrombus, affects the coronary arteries (arteries supplying the heart muscle itself). *Angina pectoris* is characterised by pain or discomfort in the chest which is brought on by exertion

Table 19.1 Risk factors for coronary heart disease

Irreversible
- Masculine gender
- Increasing age
- Genetic traits, including monogenic and polygenic disorders of lipid metabolism
- Body build

Potentially reversible
- Cigarette smoking
- Dyslipidaemia: increased levels of: cholesterol, triglyceride, low-density and very low-density lipoprotein and low levels of high-density lipoprotein
- Oxidisability of low density lipoprotein
- Obesity, especially when associated with high waist circumference or waist/hip ratio
- Hypertension
- Physical inactivity
- Hyperglycaemia and diabetes
- Increased thrombosis: increased haemostatic factors and enhanced platelet aggregation
- High levels of homocysteine
- High levels of C-reactive protein

Psychosocial
- Low socioeconomic class
- Stressful situations
- Coronary-prone behaviour patterns: type A behaviour

Geographic
- Climate and season: cold weather
- Soft drinking water

or stress, and which may also radiate down the left arm and to the neck. It results from a reduction or temporary block to the blood flow through the coronary artery to the myocardium. The pain usually passes with rest and seldom lasts for more than

15 minutes. A *coronary thrombosis* or *myocardial infarction* results from prolonged total occlusion of the artery, which causes infarction or death of some of the heart muscle and is associated with prolonged and usually excruciating central chest pain. The terms coronary thrombosis and myocardial infarction are used to describe the same clinical condition, although they really describe the two pathological processes which underlie the disease. Together these two conditions are referred to as *coronary heart disease* or *ischaemic heart disease*. The terms are regarded as synonymous and relate to the two different pathological processes, the former to the disease of the coronary arteries which provide the heart with its blood supply whereas the latter describes the effects of reduced blood supply on the myocardium or heart muscle. When a similar disease process influences the blood supply to the brain a *cerebral thrombosis* or *stroke* occurs. A typical consequence of the effect on brain tissue is weakness or paralysis of one side of the body though the precise nature of the abnormality will depend upon where the block has occurred in the arterial system. This condition is comparable with a coronary thrombosis or myocardial infarction. A less than total block may produce short-term consequences (less than 24 hours) involving weakness on one side and difficulty with speech, known as a *transient ischaemic attack*. Such a clinical event is akin to angina. These conditions are referred to as *cerebrovascular diseases*. Reduced blood supply to the muscles of the legs resulting from atherosclerosis to the arteries most distant to the heart (iliac and femoral arteries) causes pain on exercise in the muscle group(s) supplied by the affected arteries. This is known as intermittent claudication.

This chapter describes the epidemiology of cardiovascular disease, the risk factors (Table 19.1), nutritional determinants and the potential for dietary modification to reduce cardiovascular risk.

19.2 PREVALENCE OF CARDIOVASCULAR DISEASE

In most industrialised countries CHD is the commonest single cause of death. Overall rates are higher in men than women, though as women age CHD contributes a greater proportion of total mortality. In England and Wales about one-third of all deaths are the result of CHD. In recent years, in addition to the approximately 156 000 deaths every year in England and Wales, there have been more than 100 000 hospital discharges. This is still an appreciable underestimate of the total morbidity resulting from CHD. Many cases of myocardial infarction, especially in older people, are not admitted to hospital and there are no statistics regarding the far greater number of people who are debilitated by angina pectoris even though they may not have suffered an acute myocardial infarction. It should be noted that in more than half of all fatal myocardial infarctions, death occurs in the first hour after the attack. Most CHD deaths, therefore, occur too rapidly for treatment to influence the prognosis. In Britain more than £500 million per annum is spent on patients suffering from CHD, which accounts for 10% of all working days lost due to illness, and sickness benefits amount to more than £250 million.

There are marked international differences in the rate of occurrence of CHD (Fig. 19.1). Mortality rates are more than five times higher in countries comprising the previous Soviet Union than they are in Japan. In Europe there is almost an approximately four-fold difference between France, Italy and Spain on the one hand and such countries as Finland, Scotland and Northern Ireland on the other, but now, eastern European countries such as Hungary, former Czechoslovakia and the former USSR are in the worst position (Bobak & Marmot 1995). Some of the variation between countries is undoubtedly due to differences in diagnostic practice and coding of death certificates, but numerous studies using comparable methods have confirmed that real differences do exist in the frequency of the disease.

These international comparisons have played an important part in the search for causes. The experience of migrants suggests that these variations between countries are likely to be the result chiefly of environmental and behavioural differences. People who have migrated from a low-risk country (e.g. Japan) to a high-risk country (e.g. the USA) tend to have rates of CHD approaching that of the host country. There is also some evidence for the reverse: Finns living in Sweden have appreciably lower rates than those in their country of origin. In the UK, where CHD rates are appreciably higher in Scotland and Northern Ireland than in England, CHD risk depends upon country of residence at the time of death rather than country of birth.

Despite this body of evidence suggesting a link between high intakes of saturated fatty acids and CHD, predominantly via an LDL-elevating mechanism, some inconsistencies have emerged. In particular, it was noted that the French had relatively high intakes of saturated fatty acids and lower than expected rates of CHD. This has been attributed to the mitigating effects of protective factors (see below) and has sometimes been referred to as the 'French Paradox'. A similar phenomenon has been observed in other countries. It is also noteworthy that some within-population prospective studies have not demonstrated an increased cardiovascular risk associated with high intakes of saturated fatty acids nor a protective effect of n-6 polyunsaturated fatty acids. This is probably due to the range of intakes in a single population being too narrow to demonstrate an association.

Other cardiovascular risk factors

Risk factors for CHD have principally been identified in prospective epidemiological studies. Like The Seven Country Study, the Framingham Study (Stykowski et al 1990), one of the earliest such cohort studies, confirmed increasing levels of cholesterol, blood pressure and cigarette smoking as important determinants of cardiovascular risk. The presence of diabetes and impaired glucose tolerance, obesity and lack of physical activity were also identified as cardiovascular risk factors at a relatively early stage of the research in this field. All these factors are associated with a graded increase in risk and in the case of cholesterol and blood pressure there is convincing evidence from randomised controlled intervention trials that lowering the risk factor reduces risk, thus providing robust evidence that the association is a causal one and that benefit is likely to accrue in populations as well as in individuals if the risk factor is modified. More recent analyses from the Framingham Study as well as very many more recent prospective studies have identified a host of physico-chemical as well as psychosocial risk factors some of which are potentially modifiable and some not (Table 19.1). Several are potentially amenable to modification by lifestyle changes. The role of individual dietary factors has been directly studied in only relatively few prospective studies since reliable dietary data are difficult to gather in studies of this type, usually involving tens of thousands of subjects. Most of the recent data regarding food and nutrients are derived from the

various studies of health professionals studied by Willett and colleagues from Harvard. The section which follows describes the key results of these studies and the dietary determinants of some of the individual risk factors.

Nutritional and dietary determinants of cardiovascular risk

Most of the early attempts to study dietary determinants of CHD rates were based on food or nutrient data derived from national food consumption data, the balance sheets of the Food and Agriculture Organization or, in the UK, more reliably, on household food surveys and on the national mortality statistics before 1970, during which time CHD was increasing (at least in men) in most affluent societies. The studies have either been cross-cultural comparisons at a single point in time, or an examination of increasing trends in relation to changing food consumption data in one or more countries. Positive associations with saturated fat, sucrose, animal protein and coffee, and negative correlations with flour (and other complex carbohydrates) and vegetables are some of the best described.

Perhaps more interesting are relatively recent studies from the USA, the UK, Australia, New Zealand and Iceland, which have examined the downward trend of CHD rates in relation to dietary change (Tuomilehto et al 1986, Pietinen et al 1996). There are certainly associations between falling CHD rates apparent in these countries and changes in some foods and nutrients, but in view of the strong correlations (positive and negative) among different dietary constituents it is difficult to be sure which dietary factor is principally involved, or indeed whether dietary change is simply occurring in parallel with some other more important environmental factor, e.g. increasing physical activity and reduction in cigarette smoking (Stykowski et al 1990). Furthermore, population food consumption data are notoriously unreliable (they are usually derived from local production figures, imports and exports, often with an incomplete account of quantities not utilised as food), and the accuracy with which mortality is recorded varies from country to country. Consequently, such data do not provide direct evidence concerning aetiology, only clues for further research. The sections that follow describe associations which have been demonstrated as a result of direct measurements and corroborated in experimental situations.

Fish and n-3 polyunsaturated fatty acids

The Eskimo people (Inuits) of Greenland appear to have low rates of CHD despite a high intake of fat. The fat in the diet of the Greenland Eskimo is derived almost exclusively from marine foods, which contain large quantities of the n-3 fatty acids eicosopentaenoate (EPA, C20:5) and docosahexaenoate (DHA, C22:6). This observation was largely responsible for a considerable body of experimental and epidemiological research which suggested that regular consumption of fish, especially oily fish and fish oil, is protective against CHD. Reduced platelet aggregation appears to explain the reduced cardiovascular risk. The n-3 fatty acids (C20:5 and C22:6) form the anti-aggregatory prostanoid, PGI_3. Platelet aggregation is largely controlled by a balance between the pro-aggregatory compound thromboxane A_2 (synthesised from arachidonic acid released from the platelet membrane after injury to the blood vessel wall) and the anti-aggregatory substance prostacyclin PGI_2 (also synthesised from arachidonic acid in the endothelial cells of the arterial wall). C20:5 and C22:6 inhibit conversion of arachidonic acid to thromboxane A_2 as well as facilitating the production of the additional anti-aggregatory substance PGI_3 (Fig. 19.2). The n-3 fatty acids may also reduce cardiovascular risk via effects on cardiac electrophysiology, arterial compliance, endothelial function, blood pressure, vascular reactivity and inflammation.

n-6 Unsaturated fatty acids

In addition to their potential to reduce LDL, polyunsaturated fatty acids of the n-6 series may also reduce CHD risk by reducing platelet aggregation by providing the series 1 prostanoid PGE_1, which is anti-aggregatory. Oleic acid may also act as an inhibitor of platelet aggregation, though the effect is less than for polyunsaturated fatty acids.

Trans-unsaturated fatty acids

Trans-unsaturated fatty acids are geometrical isomers of *cis*-unsaturated fatty acids that adopt a saturated fatty acid-like configuration. Partial hydrogenation, the process used to increase shelf-life of polyunsaturated fatty acids (PUFAs), creates *trans* fatty acids and also removes the critical double bonds in essential fatty acids. Metabolic studies have demonstrated that *trans* fatty acids render the plasma lipid profile even more atherogenic than saturated fatty acids, by not only elevating LDL cholesterol to similar levels but also by decreasing HDL cholesterol and increasing lipoprotein (a). Several large cohort studies have found an increased risk of CHD associated with an increased intake of *trans* fatty acids. Most *trans* fatty acids in the diet are derived from industrially hardened oils. Even though *trans* fatty acids have been reduced or eliminated from retail fats and spreads in many parts of the world, deep-fried fast foods and baked goods are a major and increasing source.

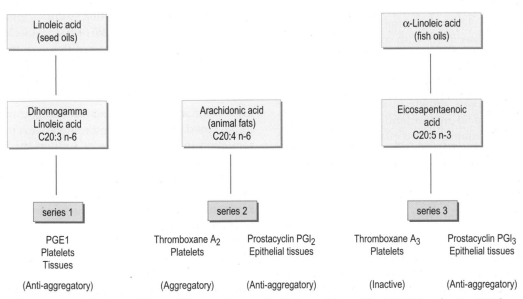

Figure 19.2   Prostanoids formed from different fatty acids (Adapted from Ulbricht & Southgate 1991).

Antioxidant nutrients, flavonoids

Low-density lipoproteins appear to be atherogenic primarily when the constituent lipid is oxidised. Many experimental studies have shown that several dietary antioxidants, notably β-carotene, vitamin E and vitamin C, reduce LDL oxidation in vitro. Prospective epidemiological studies confirm these observations, the findings being particularly consistent for vitamin E as well as a group of biologically active substances known as flavonoids in berries, fruits and some vegetables (see Section 13.5 in Ch. 13). It is of interest to note that more recent cross-country comparisons similar to those undertaken in the original Seven Country Study have suggested that CHD risk may be predicted more accurately when antioxidant nutrient status is considered in addition to the conventional major risk factors. A high intake of nutrients and other substances with antioxidant activity may be at least a partial explanation for the 'French Paradox', the term used to describe the apparently paradoxical observation that the French have a remarkably low rate of CHD despite cholesterol levels that do not differ markedly from those in other European countries with much higher rates of CHD. Reduced susceptibility of LDL to oxidation may offset the detrimental effects of this potentially atherogenic lipoprotein. However, intervention trials using antioxidant nutrients have not generally been shown to be effective at reducing CHD risk (see 'Heart Outcomes Prevention Evaluation (HOPE) Study' and 'Overall perspective of the trials', below).

B vitamins

Case-control and prospective cohort studies have shown that an elevated plasma homocysteine concentration is associated with an increased risk of cardiovascular disease (Mangoni & Jackson 2002). Folic acid, vitamins B_2, B_6 and B_{12} all act as coenzymes for the metabolism of homocysteine and many studies have shown an inverse relationship between folic acid intake (and to a lesser extent, these other B vitamins) and plasma homocysteine concentration. The consumption of folate-fortified foods has also been shown to lower plasma homocysteine, even in apparently healthy people (Venn et al 2002), but the consumption of large quantities of naturally folate-enriched foods seems to be necessary to be effective at homocysteine-lowering.

Wholegrain cereals and dietary fibre (non-starch polysaccharides)

The suggestion that unprocessed or lightly processed carbohydrate-containing foods might be protective against coronary heart disease as well as diabetes first received prominence in the 1970s when Trowell drew attention to the low rates of both conditions in Uganda where such foods provided a very high proportion of total energy. Of course there were many potentially confounding variables but high intakes of wholegrain cereals have now been repeatedly shown to be associated with cardioprotection in prospective studies (Truswell 1995). There are many possible explanations. High intakes of carbohydrates may be associated with reduced intakes of total and saturated fat. Wholegrain cereals are rich in dietary fibre (non-starch polysaccharide; NSP), which has been shown to be protective against CHD and diabetes in some prospective studies. Soluble rather than insoluble forms of NSP reduce total and LDL cholesterol, and these carbohydrates occur to a greater extent in legumes, pulses and certain vegetables and fruits than in wholegrain cereals. Wholegrain cereals are also rich in unsaturated oils and some antioxidant nutrients, notably vitamin E.

Sodium and potassium

High blood pressure is a major risk factor for CHD and both forms of stroke (ischaemic and haemorrhagic). Of the many risk factors associated with high blood pressure, the dietary exposure that has been most investigated is daily sodium intake. It has been studied extensively in animal experimental models, in epidemiological studies and in controlled clinical trials. Data from these studies show convincingly that sodium intake is directly associated with blood pressure. An overview of observational data obtained from population studies suggests that a difference in sodium intake of 100 mmol (2.3 g) per day is associated with average differences in systolic blood pressure of 5 mmHg at age 15–19 years and 10 mmHg at age 60–69 years). Diastolic blood pressures are reduced by about half as much, but the association increases with age and magnitude of the initial blood pressure. It is estimated that a universal reduction in dietary intake of sodium by 50 mmol (1.5 g) per day would lead to a 50% reduction in the number of people requiring antihypertensive therapy, a 22% reduction in the number of deaths resulting from strokes and a 16% reduction in the number of deaths from CHD.

Cutler et al (1997) carried out a systematic review of the effects of dietary salt reduction on blood pressure levels. Based on an overview of 32 methodologically adequate trials, Cutler et al concluded that a daily reduction of sodium intake by 70–80 mmol was associated with a lowering of blood pressure in both hypertensive and normotensive individuals, with systolic and diastolic blood pressure reductions of 4.8/1.9 mmHg in the former and 2.5/1.1 mmHg in the latter. Clinical trials have also demonstrated the sustainable blood pressure lowering effects of sodium restriction in infancy as well as in the elderly in whom it provides a useful non-pharmacological therapy. One low sodium diet trial showed that low sodium diets, with 24-hour sodium excretion levels around 70 mmol, are effective and safe. Some individuals appear to be more sensitive to the blood pressure raising effects of sodium, but there is no clearly defined method of identifying such individuals.

A meta-analysis of randomised controlled trials reported that potassium supplements, typically 60–100 mmol/day (median 75 mmol/day) reduced mean blood pressures (systolic/diastolic) by 1.8/1.0 mmHg in normotensive subjects and 4.4/2.5 mmHg in hypertensive subjects (Whelton et al 1997). Several large cohort studies have also found an inverse association between potassium intake and risk of stroke. While potassium supplements have been shown to have protective effects on blood pressure and cardiovascular disease (CVD), there is no strong argument for their long-term use to reduce the risk for CVD. The levels of fruit and vegetable intake recommended by the World Health Organization and many national bodies should ensure an adequate intake of potassium. The DASH trials, which have examined dietary approaches to reduce blood pressure, found the maximum effect to be achieved by a high intake of vegetables, fruit and low fat dairy products in conjunction with a low sodium intake.

Nuts

Several large epidemiological studies have demonstrated that frequent consumption of nuts is associated with decreased risk of CHD. Most of these studies considered nuts as a group, combining many different types of nuts. Nuts are high in unsaturated fatty acids and low in saturated fats, and may contribute to cholesterol lowering by altering the fatty acid profile of the diet as a whole. However, because of the high energy content of nuts, advice to include them in the diet must be tempered in accordance with the desired energy balance.

Alcohol

There is convincing evidence that low to moderate alcohol consumption lowers the risk of CHD. In a systematic review of ecological, case-control and cohort studies in which specific associations were available between consumption of beer, wine and spirits, and risk of CHD it was found that all alcoholic drinks were linked with lower risk. The beneficial effect may result from an HDL-raising effect of alcohol or the antioxidant content of some alcoholic beverages. However, other cardiovascular and health risks associated with alcohol do not favour a general recommendation for its use as a preventive measure against cardiovascular disease.

Boiled, unfiltered coffee

Boiled, unfiltered coffee raises total and LDL cholesterol because coffee beans contain a terpenoid lipid called cafestol. The amount of cafestol in the cup depends on the brewing method: it is zero for paper-filtered drip coffee, and high in the unfiltered coffee still widely drunk, for example, in Greece, the Middle East and Turkey. Intake of large amounts of unfiltered coffee markedly raises serum cholesterol and has been associated with CHD in Norway. A shift from unfiltered, boiled coffee to filtered coffee has contributed significantly to the decline in serum cholesterol in Finland.

Soya protein

Soya protein has been shown to inhibit atherosclerosis in animals. While there is no conclusive evidence of such an effect in humans, soya protein undoubtedly has a favourable effect on several cardiovascular risk factors. The beneficial effect on plasma lipoproteins (LDL cholesterol, triglyceride and possibly HDL cholesterol) has been the basis of the US Food and Drug Administration's approval of a health claim that '25 g of soya protein a day, as part of a diet low in saturated fat and cholesterol, may reduce the risk of heart disease'. Soya isoflavones have been shown to lower blood pressure. There is also some evidence of beneficial effects on vascular and endothelial function, platelet activation and aggregation, LDL oxidation and smooth muscle cell proliferation and migration. Several trials indicate that soya has a beneficial effect on plasma lipids (see Additional references section on the CD-ROM).

Cardioprotective dietary patterns

It should be clear from the above that a range of dietary patterns may be protective against CHD. The Mediterranean diet has probably received the most attention, with populations consuming the traditional diets of countries surrounding the Mediterranean Sea having low rates of CHD. Several attributes of such diets (e.g. high intakes of fruit and vegetables, and unsaturated vegetable oils) are associated with reduced levels of cardiovascular risk factors. However, it is important to emphasise that there are other equally cardioprotective dietary patterns including traditional Asian diets and indeed a modified typical Western diet. Attributes of cardioprotective dietary patterns are listed in Table 19.2. In a recent study, a 'portfolio' of such dietary changes, together with the use of plant sterol enriched margarine, was shown to be associated with a reduction in LDL cholesterol equivalent to that observed on a statin drug, known to have powerful cholesterol-lowering effects (Jenkins et al 2003). Furthermore, the experimental diet was associated with a reduction in C-reactive protein, an inflammatory marker now known to be associated with increased cardiovascular risk.

While the concept of potentially beneficial eating patterns may be useful as a preventive strategy against cardiovascular disease, it is important to bear in mind that adopting individual attributes of such patterns may not confer benefit. For example, consuming substantial quantities of olive oil in the context of an otherwise inappropriate diet may confer little or no advantage. Further it should be noted that traditional cardioprotective patterns have been altered by many of the people consuming them, so that modern Mediterranean or Asian diets may for instance be high in saturated fatty acids and thus have, at least to some extent, lost their health benefits.

Table 19.2 Attributes of cardioprotective diets

- Low intakes of saturated fatty acids
- High intakes of raw or appropriately prepared fruit and vegetables
- Lightly processed cereal foods and wholegrains are preferred
- Fat intakes are derived predominantly from unmodified vegetable oils[a]
- Fish, nuts, seeds and vegetable protein sources are important dietary components
- Meat, when consumed, is lean and eaten in small quantities
- Energy balance reduces rates of obesity

[a]Coconut oil and palm oil are not encouraged because they tend to elevate LDL.

19.4 CLINICAL TRIALS OF DIETARY MODIFICATION

While prospective epidemiological studies provide strong evidence of risk or protection associated with individual nutrients or foods, proof of causality and the ultimate level of evidence for dietary recommendations can only be derived from randomised controlled trials. The early trials all attempted to lower cholesterol levels, usually by increasing the dietary polyunsaturated:saturated ratio (P:S), i.e. they were single factor intervention trials. More recent trials have involved multifactorial interventions, including dietary change intended to improve all nutrition-related risk indicators as well as attempts to modify risk factors that are not diet related (e.g. cigarette smoking). Dietary intervention trials have been undertaken in people with and without evidence of CHD at the time the study was started (i.e. secondary and primary prevention trials). This review describes briefly a few landmark trials (Table 19.3) and presents an overview of all the important investigations of this kind. For full references to the clinical trials see Additional references (Section 19.4), on the CD-ROM.

Los Angeles Veterans Administration Study

This was the first of the major intervention trials, in which 846 male volunteers (aged 55–89 years) were randomly allocated to 'experimental' and 'control' diets taken in different dining rooms. The control diet was intended to be typical North American (40% energy from fat, mostly saturated). The experimental diet contained half as much cholesterol, and predominantly polyunsaturated vegetable oils (n-6 PUFA) replaced approximately two-thirds of the animal fat, achieving a P:S ratio of 2. The trial was conducted under double-blind conditions. During the 8 years of the trial, plasma cholesterol in the experimental group was 13% lower, and coronary events, as well as deaths due to cardiovascular disease, were appreciably reduced, compared with the controls (Table 19.3). The beneficial effect of the cholesterol-lowering diet was most evident in those with high cholesterol levels at the start of the study. Deaths due to other and uncertain causes occurred

Table 19.3 **Results of selected intervention trials (confidence intervals are given in parentheses)**

Trial	No. of subjects	% reduction in cholesterol	Odds ratios (experimental vs control)	
			Total mortality	Fatal and non-fatal CHD
Veterans Administration	846	13	0.98 (0.83–1.15)	0.77
Oslo	1232	13	0.64 (0.37–1.12)	0.56
DART				
Fat advice	2033	3.5	0.98 (0.77–1.26)	0.92
Fish advice	2033	Negligible	0.74 (0.57–0.93)	0.85
Lyons Heart	605	Negligible	0.30 (0.11–0.82)	0.24
CHAOS	2002	NA	1.30	0.60
GISSI-Prevenzione				
n-3 fatty acids	2836	NA	0.80 (0.67–0.94)	0.80
Vitamin E	2830	NA	0.86 (0.72–1.02)	0.88
HOPE	1511	NA	1.00 (0.89–1.13)	1.05

NA, not available.

more frequently in the experimental group, though no single other cause predominated. This increase in non-cardiovascular mortality in the experimental group raised for the first time the possibility that cholesterol lowering might be harmful in some respects, despite the reduction in CHD. However, this has not been substantiated in subsequent studies.

Oslo Trial

Middle-aged men at high risk of CHD (smokers or those having a cholesterol in the range 7.5–9.8 mmol/l) were divided into two groups; half received intensive dietary education and advice to stop smoking, the other half served as a control group. An impressive reduction in total coronary events was observed (Table 19.3) in association with a 13% fall in serum cholesterol and a 65% reduction in tobacco consumption. There was also an improvement in total mortality and there were no significant differences between the two groups with regard to non-cardiac causes of death. Detailed statistical analysis suggested that approximately 60% of the CHD reduction could be attributed to serum cholesterol change and 25% to smoking reduction. The composition of the experimental diet was quite different from that used in the Veterans Administration trial: total and saturated fat were markedly reduced without any appreciable increase in n-6 PUFA, and fibre-rich carbohydrate was increased. These differences could have accounted for the different results with regard to non-cardiovascular diseases.

Diet and Reinfarction Trial (DART)

This was the first trial to examine the effects of diets high in n-3 PUFA. Burr et al randomised 2033 men who had survived myocardial infarction to receive or not to receive advice on each of three dietary factors: (i) a reduction of fat intake and an increase in the ratio of polyunsaturated to saturated fat, (ii) an increase in fatty fish intake, and (iii) an increase in cereal fibre. For those unable to eat fatty fish, a fish oil supplement was recommended. Within the short (2 years) follow-up period, the subjects advised to eat fatty fish or a fish oil supplement had a 26% reduction in all causes of mortality compared with those not so advised. The other two diets were not associated with significant differences in mortality, but in view of the fact that fat modification only achieved a 3–4% reduction in serum cholesterol, compliance with the fat-modified and high fibre diets may have been less than that on the fish diet. Furthermore, diets aimed to reduce atherogenicity (n-6 PUFA) are likely to take longer to show a beneficial effect than those aimed to reduce thrombogenicity (n-3 PUFA). These results are the first to find that very simple advice aimed to reduce thrombogenicity (at least two weekly portions, 200–400 g of fatty fish) appears to reduce mortality appreciably.

Lyons Heart Study

This study is the most recent in the series of multifactorial dietary intervention studies in the secondary prevention of cardiovascular disease. Six hundred and five individuals with clinical ischaemic heart disease received conventional dietary advice or advice to follow a traditional Mediterranean diet ('experimental diet'). The experimental diet was lower in total and saturated fat (30% and 8% total energy) than the control diet (33% and 12% total energy) and contained more oleic (13% versus 10% total energy) and α-linolenic acid (0.80% versus 0.27%). Dietary linoleic acid was higher in the control group (5.3% versus 3.6%). The Mediterranean diet included more bread, legumes, vegetables and fruit and less meat and dairy products. Those in the experimental group were also provided with a margarine rich in α-linolenate (C18:3 n-3). The marked reductions in risk ratios for cardiovascular events as well as total mortality associated with the experimental diet are difficult to interpret. The confidence intervals are wide and it is difficult to understand why cholesterol levels did not fall despite the reduced intake of saturated fatty acids. The latter observation has led to the suggestion that the beneficial effect must have resulted from an antithrombogenic effect of the diet or a reduction in the risk of dysrhythmias as a result of the increase in n-3 fatty acids. The study has been widely quoted as providing strong evidence for the health benefits associated with the Mediterranean diet.

Cambridge Heart Antioxidant Study (CHAOS)

Several early clinical trials involving supplementation with antioxidant nutrients (vitamins C and E and β-carotene) without concomitant dietary change suggested no benefit in terms of cardiovascular risk reduction despite strong evidence of a cardioprotective effect in epidemiological studies. This study from Cambridge involved the randomisation of over 2000 participants with pre-existing cardiovascular disease to receive either placebo or α-tocopherol 400 iu or 800 iu daily (268 or 537 mg, respectively). After 1.4 years non-fatal myocardial infarction was substantially reduced in those receiving α-tocopherol at either dose (14 out of 1035) as compared with the control group (41 out of 967). However, there were marginally more total deaths in the α-tocopherol than in the control group (36 out of 1035 compared with 26 out of 967).

GISSI-Prevenzione Study

This large study examined the effect of supplementation with very long-chain n-3 fatty acids (eicosapentaenoic and docosahexaenoic acids) or vitamin E (300 mg) or both in 2830 subjects who had had a myocardial infarction. The trial was not conducted in a double-blind manner, but was nevertheless interesting in view of its size. Supplementation with n-3 fatty acids was associated with a statistically significant 15–20% reduction in all the important end-points (non-fatal myocardial infarction, cardiovascular deaths and total mortality). A smaller reduction in event rate in association with vitamin E supplementation did not achieve statistical significance.

Heart Outcomes Prevention Evaluation (HOPE) Study

Patients at high risk of cardiovascular events because they had cardiovascular disease or diabetes and one other risk factor were randomised to receive placebo, 400 iu vitamin E (268 mg) or drug treatment (an angiotensin-converting-enzyme inhibitor, ramipril) and followed for 4.5 years. A primary outcome event (myocardial infarction, stroke or death from a cardiovascular cause) occurred in 16.2% (772 of the 4761) patients assigned to the vitamin E group and 15.5% (739 of the 4780) assigned to placebo. Furthermore, there were no differences between the two groups when considering total mortality or indeed any other cardiovascular end-points.

The 2003 WHO/FAO Report 'Diet Nutrition and the Prevention of Chronic Diseases' has classified each of the nutritional factors which have been related to cardiovascular disease according to level of evidence. Table 19.4 summarises the findings of this report (Joint WHO/FAO Expert Consultation 2003).

Overall perspective of the trials

It is inappropriate to aggregate the results of the dietary intervention trials in a meta-analysis in view of the wide range of interventions that have been employed. Nevertheless certain conclusions may be drawn from the results of the various studies. There is convincing evidence that cholesterol lowering by dietary means reduces coronary events in the context of both primary and secondary prevention. Indeed there is confirmation of the rule derived from observational epidemiology that a 2–3% reduction in coronary events results from each 1% of cholesterol lowering achieved. There would seem to be reasonably strong evidence that lowering of total cholesterol (reflecting principally a reduction in LDL cholesterol) should primarily be achieved by reducing total and

Table 19.4 **Summary of the findings of the WHO/FAO Report, 'Diet, Nutrition and the Prevention of Chronic Diseases' relating to lifestyle factors and risk of developing cardiovascular disease**

Evidence	Decreased risk	No relationship	Increased risk

Convincing	Regular physical activity
	Linoleic acid
	Fish and fish oils (EHA, DHA)
	Vegetables and fruits
	  (including berries)
	Potassium
	Low-moderate alcohol intake
	  (for CHD)
		Vitamin E supplements	Myristic and palmitic acids
			Trans unsaturated fatty acids
			High sodium intake
			Overweight
			High alcohol intake
			  (for stroke)

Probable	α-Linolenic acid Oleic acid Non-starch polysaccharide Wholegrain cereals Nuts (unsalted) Plant sterols/stanols Folate	Stearic acid	Dietary cholesterol Unfiltered boiled coffee
Possible	Flavonoids Soya products		Fats rich in lauric acid Impaired fetal nutrition β-carotene supplements
Insufficient	Calcium Magnesium Vitamin C		Carbohydrates Iron

EPA, eicosapentaenoic acid; DHA, docosahexaenoic acid.

saturated fatty acids. While increasing n-6 polyunsaturated fatty acids (chiefly linoleic acid C18:2 n-6) might further decrease LDL, the clinical trials do not suggest that replacement energy be derived entirely from this source. Rather they suggest that when substitution is required oleic acid (C18:1 n-9), carbohydrate from lightly processed cereals (wholegrains), vegetables and fruit as well as linoleic acid might all contribute replacement energy. Two trials provide some support for the suggestion that dietary modification has the potential to reduce cardiovascular risk by means other than cholesterol lowering. The DART trial achieved appreciable reduction in cardiovascular mortality with minimal change in cholesterol, presumably because the increase in C20:5 n-3 and C22:6 n-3 in the fish or fish oil supplements resulted in reduced tendency to thrombosis or perhaps reduced the risk of dysrythmias. Similarly the experimental diet in the Lyons Heart Study was not associated with appreciable cholesterol lowering. It is impossible to identify which of the many nutritional changes might have been responsible for the beneficial effects. There was undoubtedly an increase in a range of antioxidant nutrients which may have reduced oxidisability of LDL despite minimal change in cholesterol. Non-starch polysaccharide (dietary fibre) as well as starch increased because of the increase in cereals, vegetables and fruit. Total saturated fatty acids decreased while oleic and α-linolenic acids increased. The authors of the study regarded the last mentioned change to be of particular importance. However, it would seem more plausible that a combination of all these factors contributed to the overall risk reduction resulting from favourable modification of several of the risk factors listed in Table 19.1.

When attempting to extrapolate the findings of the various trials into practical recommendations it is important not to be seduced by the many 'experts' (who are presently advocating the Mediterranean diet as the most appropriate means of cardiovascular risk reduction). On the basis of existing evidence it seems more appropriate to conclude that there are probably several dietary patterns which are associated with a low risk of cardiovascular disease. These include the Mediterranean diet, a traditional Asian or African diet or indeed a more conventional Western diet which has been modified to reduce levels of cardiovascular risk factors. A low intake of saturated fatty acids appears to be the most consistent feature of the various dietary patterns associated with low CHD risk. While a Mediterranean diet does offer one means by which this dietary modification can be achieved, it can also be achieved by other eating patterns (e.g. Asian, modified Western).

The trials of nutrient supplements have generally been disappointing apart perhaps from the GISSI-Prevenzione Study, which suggests potential benefit of supplementation with modest amounts of fish oils. There is no clear explanation as to why antioxidant nutrient supplementation trials have been largely negative despite strong suggestions of benefit from epidemiological data. The most likely explanation would seem to be either that a longer time frame might be necessary in order to demonstrate benefit or that a blend of these nutrients in proportions similar to those found in foods might be required to produce benefit, rather than a pharmacological dose of a single antioxidant nutrient. It is also possible that the antioxidant nutrients may be acting as a marker for some other protective factor present in the foods that contain these vitamins or flavonoids. Trials are presently under way to determine whether supplementation with folic acid and other dietary determinants of homocysteine levels have the potential to reduce cardiovascular risk.

19.5 IMPLEMENTATION OF DIETARY ADVICE

Cardioprotective dietary patterns are appropriate for patients with established cardiovascular disease, those with cardiovascular risk factors, and entire populations in order to reduce population risk or to maintain rates amongst groups which currently have low rates. While people at high risk of a first or subsequent cardiovascular event will clearly reap the greatest individual benefit, a population approach is essential to reduce the epidemic proportions of cardiovascular diseases in many countries, or to prevent escalating rates in other countries. The level of intensity of required dietary modification depends upon level of risk and nature of individual risk factors. For example, those with markedly raised levels of total and LDL cholesterol should reduce saturated fatty acids to 8% or less of total energy. For those with high blood pressure emphasis may be on salt reduction and an increase in fruit, vegetables and low fat dairy products. Details of nutritional targets and sample eating plans are provided in Tables CD 19.1, CD 19.2 and CD 19.3. The greatest challenge for the future will be to develop approaches that will facilitate compliance amongst individuals and populations with nutritional recommendations.

⊃ Key points

- ⊃ Geographic variation and time trends indicate the importance of environmental determinants of cardiovascular disease.

- ⊃ Nature of dietary fat is an important determinant of CHD in populations, influencing lipoprotein-mediated risk and other risk factors.

- ⊃ Saturated and *trans*-unsaturated fatty acids increase CHD risk; n-6 and n-3 polyunsaturated fatty acids are protective.

- ⊃ Antioxidant nutrients, flavonoids, folate and other B vitamins, non-starch polysaccharides, wholegrain cereals, nuts, soya protein and alcohol appear to protect against CHD via an influence on several important risk factors for CVD.

- ⊃ Randomised controlled clinical trials demonstrate the potential for dietary change to reduce CHD rates.

- ⊃ A range of different dietary patterns are cardioprotective.

- ⊃ There is adequate evidence to recommend dietary change in high risk populations and individuals.

References and further reading

References

Bobak M, Marmot M 1995 The East-West health divide and potential explanations. In: Harrington P, Ritsatakis A (eds) Health challenges for countries of central and eastern Europe and the newly independent states. WHO, Copenhagen, p 8–43

Cutler J A, Follmann D, Allender P S 1997 Randomized trials of sodium reduction: an overview. American Journal of Clinical Nutrition 65:643–651

Jenkins D J A, Kendall C W C, Marchie A et al 2003 Effects of a dietary portfolio of cholesterol-lowering foods vs lovastatin on serum lipids and c-reactive protein. Journal of the American Medical Association 290:502–510

Joint WHO/FAO Expert Consultation 2003 Diet, nutrition and the prevention of chronic diseases. WHO Technical Report Series 916, Geneva

Keys A 1980 Seven Countries: a multivariate analysis of death and coronary heart disease. Harvard University Press, Cambridge, MA

Keys A, Anderson J T, Grande F 1965 Serum cholesterol response to changes in diet. IV. Particular saturated fatty acids in the diet. Metabolism 14:776–778

Kris-Etherton P, Daniels S R, Eckel R H et al 2001 Summary of the scientific conference on dietary fatty acids and cardiovascular health: conference summary from the nutrition committee of the American Heart Association. Circulation 103(7):1034–1039

Mangoni A A, Jackson S H 2002 Homocysteine and cardiovascular disease: current evidence and future prospects. American Journal of Medicine 112:582–565

Pietinen P, Vartiainen E, Seppanen R et al 1996 Changes in diet in Finland from 1972–1992: impact on coronary heart disease risk. Preventive Medicine 25:243–250

Stykowski P A, Kannel W B, D'Agostino R B 1990 Changes in risk factors and the decline in mortality from cardiovascular disease. The Framingham Heart Study. New England Journal of Medicine 322:1635–1641

Tuomilehto J, Geboers J, Salonen T et al 1986 Decline in cardiovascular mortality in North Karelia and other parts of Finland. British Medical Journal 293:1068–1071

Truswell A S 1995 Dietary fibre and plasma lipids. European Journal of Clinical Nutrition 49(Suppl 3): S105–109

Ulbricht T V L, Southgate D A T 1991 Coronary heart disease: seven dietary factors. Lancet 338:985–992

Venn B J, Mann J I, Williams S M et al 2002 Dietary counseling to increase natural folate intake: a randomized, placebo-controlled trial in free-living subjects to assess effects on serum folate and plasma total homocysteine. American Journal of Clinical Nutrition 76:758–765

Further reading

Armstrong B K, Mann J I, Adelstein A M, Eskin F 1975 Commodity consumption and ischaemic heart disease mortality with special reference to dietary practices. Journal of Chronic Diseases 28:455–469

Kris-Etherton P M, Zhao G, Binkoski A E et al 2001 The effects of nuts on coronary heart disease risk. Nutrition Reviews 59:103–111

Law M R, Frost C D, Wald N J 1991 By how much does salt reduction lower blood pressure? III, Analysis of data from trials of salt reduction. British Medical Journal 302:819–824

Sacks F M, Svetkey L P, Vollmer W M et al 2001 Effects on blood pressure of reduced dietary sodium and the Dietary Approaches to Stop Hypertension (DASH) diet. New England Journal of Medicine 344:3–10

Vessby B, Uusitupa M, Hermansen K et al 2001 Substituting dietary saturated for monounsaturated fat impairs insulin sensitivity in healthy men and women: the KANWU Study. Diabetologia 44:312–319

Whelton P K, He J, Cutler J A et al 1997 Effects of oral potassium on blood pressure. Meta-analysis of randomized controlled clinical trials. Journal of the American Medical Association 277:1624–1632

Whelton P K, Appel L J, Espeland M A et al 1998 Sodium reduction and weight loss in the treatment of hypertension in older persons. Journal of the American Medical Association 279: 839–846 (erratum appears in JAMA 1998; 279:1954)

CD-ROM contents

Tables
Table CD 19.1 Guidelines for optimal food choices
Table CD 19.2 Ranges of population nutrient intake goals (global)
Table CD 19.3 Recommendations for dietary nutrients (UK)

Figures
Figure CD 19.1 Rates of coronary heart disease over time in men aged 45–64 in Canada, England, New Zealand, Australia, Finland and Poland

Figure CD 19.2 Data from the original Seven Country Study showing the association between CHD and the dietary saturated fat content
Figure CD 19.3 The different risks of smoking for CHD in countries with different diets

Additional references related to specific chapter sections

Further reading from the book

Objectives

By the end of this chapter you should be able to:

- know the definitions and their rationale of overweight and obesity in adults and children
- describe their prevalence in Western countries
- compare with other countries and describe time trends
- summarise the health risks of obesity and their mechanisms
- discuss the relative importance of causal factors
- compare critically different approaches to prevention and treatment.

20.1 INTRODUCTION

Obesity has become the major nutrition-related disease of this decade, and is defined as a condition of excessive body fat accumulation to an extent that increases the risk of complicating diseases. Overweight and obesity cause the development of diabetes, and contribute to high blood pressure, adverse blood lipid profile, infertility, birth complications and arthritis, and amplify asthma and a poor health status. Obesity is largely preventable through changes in lifestyle, especially diet.

20.2 EPIDEMIOLOGY OF OBESITY

Definition of obesity

Obesity is not a single entity, but it is most commonly classified by a single measure, the body mass index (BMI), a ratio of weight and height (BMI = weight (kg)/height^2 (m^2)). The World Health Organization (WHO) classifies underweight, normal weight, overweight and obesity according to categories of BMI (Table 20.1). This height independent measure of weight allows comparisons to be made more readily within and between populations of the same ethnic origin. The definition of the 'normal' range of BMI was based primarily on North American mortality data, and the cut-offs are different for Asian populations. The suggested categories are: <18.5 kg/m^2 underweight; 18.5–23 kg/m^2 increasing but acceptable risk; 23–27.5 kg/m^2 increased risk, and 27.5 kg/m^2 or higher, high risk. BMI does not, however, distinguish fat from lean tissue or water nor identify whether the fat is accumulated in particular sites such as the abdomen where it has more serious metabolic consequences. Techniques such as bioelectric impedance to estimate body fat and DEXA scans to separate body mass into fat-free mass and fat mass are increasingly used. DEXA (dual energy X-ray absorptiometry), MR (magnetic resonance), and CT (computer tomography) scans are used for an accurate assessment of intra-abdominal adipose tissue, although simple waist circumference is increasingly recognised as an easy and valid measure of abdominal obesity. Waist–hip ratio and skinfold thickness may also be used to verify fatness in individuals.

Table 20.1 The classification of underweight, normal weight and classes of overweight White individuals according to WHO

Classification	BMI (kg/m^2)	Risk of co-morbidities
Underweight	<18.5	Low (but risk of other clinical problems increased)
Normal range	18.5–24.9	Average
Overweight[a]	≥25	
Pre-obese	25.0–29.9	Mildly increased
Obese	**>30.0**	
Class I	30.0–34.9	Moderate
Class II	35.0–39.9	Severe
Class III	>40.0	Very severe

[a] The term overweight refers to a BMI ≥ 25, but is frequently adapted to refer to BMI 25–29.9, differentiating the pre-obese from the obese categories.

Prevalence and time trends of overweight and obesity

The prevalence of obesity is increasing worldwide in almost every country and in all age groups. The steep increase has prompted this development to be called an epidemic, and because it is worldwide, a pandemic. In 2001 14% of adult men and 17% of women in Denmark were obese, and in the UK 21% of men and 24% of women were obese and a further 47% of men and 33% of women were overweight (BMI 25–30 kg/m^2). In the USA the situation is even worse. In the USA in 2000 the prevalence of obesity was 31% compared to 23% in 1988–94. Southern European countries like Greece have similar levels to the USA. The rates of increase in obesity prevalence in these countries are very similar. Europe is following the track of the USA, but is about 10 years behind, so in 10 years can expect to reach the same level of obesity that exists in the USA today.

Obesity is now apparent in even some of the poorest countries of the world. Normally the obesity problem first appears in a country in the more affluent parts of the population, but in recent decades obesity is characteristically higher among groups with low levels of education, low income and low social class.

The proportion of obese people increases with age until around the age of retirement. Beyond this age the impact of obesity-related premature death and disease-related weight loss leads to a modest decline in the proportion of obese adults. People who today are in their 60s or older were born at a time of austerity and limited food supplies. Younger people have largely grown up in a world where a greater variety of food than ever before has become available and at relatively low cost and so are more prone to develop obesity at a younger age.

Attention is increasingly focused on young people where the problem of overweight and obesity has become more pronounced. Among young Danish males attending draft boards there has been a dramatic increase in the prevalence of obesity from 0.1% in 1955 to about 8% in 2000, corresponding to an 80-fold increase. In UK in 1997 among 4–18 year olds, 4% were obese and a further 15% were overweight, with a higher rate of obesity among young people in Scotland and Wales, relative to England. Rates of overweight and obesity range from 10% to 20% in northern Europe and are higher still in southern Europe – from 20% to as high as 36% in parts of southern Italy.

There is a higher than expected level of obesity among certain ethnic groups living in Europe, probably due to increased genetic susceptibility to the European lifestyle. Obesity rates are highest among people of Indian, Pakistani and black Caribbean origin, and the prevalence of obesity in young people of Asian origin is 3–4 times higher than among whites.

⊃ Key points

- ⊃ Body weight classes are defined based on body mass index (BMI): weight (kg)/height^2 (m^2).

- ⊃ Overweight is defined as BMI >25 kg/m^2, and obesity as BMI >30 kg/m^2.

- ⊃ Overweight and obesity have become highly prevalent and obesity affects 15–35% of the adult population in the developing countries, and the majority have a BMI of more than 25 kg/m^2.

- ⊃ The obesity prevalence is increasing in all countries, in both genders and in all age groups.

- ⊃ Even the developing countries experience a major increase in obesity.

20.3 RISKS OF OBESITY

Health and social risks

The risks and complications of obesity and abdominal overweight are poorly recognised, but can account for more than 5% of all health costs. Even a normal BMI, but with abdominal fat accumulation, can be responsible for hypertension, hyperlipidaemia, type 2 diabetes, and cardiovascular disease, which makes it important to identify increased fatness as the underlying cause of the condition or disease. The increase in obesity rates has an important impact on

the global incidence of cardiovascular disease, type 2 diabetes mellitus, cancer, osteoarthritis, infertility, birth complications, work disability and sleep apnoea. Obesity has a more pronounced impact on morbidity than on mortality, but a BMI of 40 kg/m^2 is associated with a decreased life expectancy of around 10 years. Increases in the prevalence of obesity will potentially lead to an increase in the number of years that subjects suffer from obesity-related morbidity and disability.

Symptoms and consequences

Most overweight subjects suffer from low self-esteem and self-loathing, and also commonly phobias. They are discriminated against, even in the health sector, and can experience heat intolerance, intertrigo (inflammation of skin folds due to heat, moisture, friction, and lack of air circulation), difficulties with physical activity, and sexual problems of a psychological and physical nature. These social and psychological problems often tend to be more pronounced than the somatic complications associated with obesity.

Type 2 diabetes (see Ch. 21)

Definition

Type 2 Diabetes mellitus is a chronic condition that arises when the pancreas does not produce enough insulin to overcome the insulin resistance in the peripheral tissues. Failure of insulin secretion, insulin action, or both, leads to hyperglycaemia. This hyperglycaemia is associated with long-term damage, dysfunction and failure of various organs and tissues, particularly small vessel complications affecting the eyes (retinopathy), kidneys (nephropathy) and nerves (neuropathy), and large vessel complications affecting the heart and blood vessels (cardiovascular disease). Previously known as insulin-dependent diabetes mellitus (IDDM) and non-insulin-dependent diabetes mellitus (NIDDM) respectively, the terms type 1 and type 2 are used to avoid individuals being classified based on their treatment, rather than the cause of the disease.

Role of overweight and obesity

Overweight and obesity are the major causes of the development of type 2 diabetes in individuals with a high genetic susceptibility to the disease. Type 2 diabetes occurs 50–100-fold more frequently in obese subjects than in lean subjects. In observational studies overweight, obesity, physical inactivity, smoking, and diet composition can account for almost all cases of type 2 diabetes (Hu et al 2001). The genetic make-up determines if an obese individual develops type 2 diabetes or not, and many morbidly obese subjects without the genetic predisposition maintain a normal glucose tolerance throughout life. Diabetes is the most important medical consequence of obesity because it is common, has serious complications, is difficult to treat, reduces life expectancy by 8–10 years and is expensive to manage.

Obesity-related mortality caused by diabetes

Although diabetes is not directly the cause of most of the excess mortality among obese subjects, the metabolic abnormalities underlying type 2 diabetes (see 'Metabolic syndrome', below) are clearly the result of obesity, which in itself predisposes to hypertension and cardiovascular disease (see Ch. 21).

Prevention of type 2 diabetes by weight loss

Some of the metabolic defects accompanying impaired glucose tolerance (IGT) and type 2 diabetes are reversible with weight loss, unless the diabetes has persisted for too long a time with irreversible damage to insulin secretion (Harder et al 2004). In high risk subjects, such as obese subjects with IGT, weight loss can prevent and almost eliminate type 2 diabetes. In a Swedish surgical weight loss intervention study on obesity, the 2-year incidence of diabetes was 6.3% in the control group and only 0.2% in the weight loss group (Astrup 2004). This intervention study shows that >95% of new cases of type 2 diabetes among obese individuals can be prevented by a major (20–25 kg) sustained weight loss. Most of the benefit was maintained at 10 years when the incidence of diabetes was still five-fold lower than in controls, which corresponds to an 80% protection against developing diabetes. More recent intervention studies have very clearly demonstrated that even a modest weight loss of 3–5% achieved by diet and slightly increased daily physical activity is sufficient to prevent nearly 60% of all new cases over a 4–5-year period. Further analyses have shown that it is the weight loss per se, not a specific diet or the physical activity, that is important.

Increased blood pressure (hypertension)

The risk of developing hypertension is 5–6 times greater with obesity. Blood pressure is positively correlated with both abdominal circumference and with the degree of obesity. Insulin resistance and hyperinsulinaemia appear to be responsible for the hypertension. Insulin has an anti-natriuretic effect that causes increased extracellular and intravascular volume. It is also possible that the hyperinsulinaemia has a direct trophic effect on the smooth muscle cells of the arterioles, which can lead to a chronically hyperactive sympathetic nervous system.

The hypertension associated with obesity is just as harmful as hypertension from other causes, and should be controlled and treated with the same vigour as in the normal weight patient. Even a small weight loss can result in a marked drop in blood pressure, and weight loss is a much more effective treatment than salt restriction.

Atherosclerosis, ischaemic heart disease and stroke

Obesity, and abdominal obesity in particular, are associated with a significant increased risk of atherosclerotic manifestations. The risk of developing ischaemic heart disease or stroke is 2.5 and 6 times greater, respectively, with a pronounced abdominal fat distribution than with a low waist measurement, i.e. even distribution. The cause of the increased risk is related to the unfavourable blood lipid profile associated with obesity and abdominal distribution, and to increased plasma fibrinogen and reduced fibrinolytic activity.

Arthritis urica (gout)

Gout is a frequent complication of obesity. Plasma urate is increased in the majority of patients, but clinical symptoms are observed in only a minority.

Metabolic syndrome (see Sections 19.3 and 21.2)

A number of studies point to the existence of a particular metabolic syndrome encompassing insulin resistance, hypertension, increased plasma VLDL and reduced HDL cholesterol and abdominal obesity. This syndrome is also known as insulin resistance syndrome, since the main consequence is reduced sensitivity to the action of insulin. A variety of risk factors for the development of cardiovascular disease appear to be associated with this syndrome, which links obesity with the most significant health complications (type 2 diabetes, hypertension and atherosclerosis). In addition to the level of obesity,

other factors are significantly associated with the metabolic syndrome – fat distribution, level of physical activity and genetic disposition. A suggested definition of the syndrome is given by WHO and shown below:

- Insulin resistance (hyperinsulinaemia: fasting plasma insulin $\geqslant$25% quartile)
- And at least two of the following components:
  1. Abdominal obesity: waist width – for men >94 cm; for women >80 cm; or BMI >30 kg/m^2
  2. Glucose intolerance: fasting plasma glucose >6.0 mmol/l
  3. Arterial blood pressure: $\geqslant$149/90 mmHg (or antihypertensive medical treatment)
  4. Dyslipidaemia: fasting triglyceride: >2.0 mmol/l and/or fasting HDL cholesterol <1.0 mmol/l (or cholesterol lowering medical treatment).

The way in which overweight and obesity contribute to the metabolic syndrome is not entirely clear, but hormones and substrates secreted by the adipose tissue are thought to be the main cause. An increased metabolism of free fatty acids and reduced secretion of the fat tissue hormone adiponectin, as well as increased secretion of cytokines, appear to play an important role in the development of insulin resistance in the muscle tissue. Treatment of the metabolic syndrome is weight loss and physical activity.

Other complications

Obesity is also associated with hypoventilation syndrome and sleep apnoea, liver and gallstone diseases, osteoarthritis and numerous cancers. People who are more than 40% overweight have a risk of cancer 50% higher than in normal weight individuals. In men colorectal cancers are common, but women are more typically affected by endometrial and gall bladder cancer, and by cancer of the cervix, breast and ovary. In addition, obesity is a risk factor for osteoarthritis in the weight-bearing joints, infertility and numerous endocrinological conditions.

The nature of obesity makes many clinical and paraclinical studies difficult to perform and surgical measures are associated with an increased risk of complications. The length of hospital admission time is also generally prolonged when obese patients are treated for other complaints.

⊃ Key points

- ⊃ The risks and complications of obesity and abdominal overweight can account for more than 5% of all health costs.

- ⊃ Even a quite normal BMI with abdominal fat accumulation can be responsible for hypertension, hyperlipidaemia, type 2 diabetes, and cardiovascular disease.

- ⊃ The increase in obesity has an important impact on the global incidence of cardiovascular disease, type 2 diabetes mellitus, cancer, osteoarthritis, infertility, birth complications, work disability and sleep apnoea.

- ⊃ Obesity has a more pronounced impact on morbidity than on mortality, but a BMI of 40 kg/m² is associated with a decreased life expectancy of around 10 years.

- ⊃ Increases in the prevalence of obesity will potentially lead to an increase in the number of years that subjects suffer from obesity-related morbidity and disability.

20.4 CAUSAL FACTORS

Genetics

In only a minority of cases is obesity caused by a chromosome abnormality, a mutation in a single gene or classic endocrine disorder. Most cases of obesity are due to an inadequately functioning appetite regulation and energy metabolism, where the energy density and fat content of food and drink are too high, mealtimes are irregular, daily physical activity is limited and inactivity has become a characteristic of everyday life. An unlimited supply of cheap, tasty foodstuffs and larger food portions also help to promote overweight and risk of obesity. The disposition towards obesity is not necessarily genetic, since other influences, for example chemicals or hormones transferred from mother to fetus during pregnancy may programme the offspring to be susceptible to an obesity-promoting lifestyle. It is possible that a number of environmental factors, currently unknown, play an important role in the development of obesity. For example, recent studies suggest that severe overweight or excessive weight gain during pregnancy increases the offspring's predisposition to obesity within an obesity-inducing lifestyle. Further evidence shows that an adenovirus infection in the central nervous system (CNS) can induce obesity in animals, although human studies are not conclusive.

Chromosome and gene abnormalities

Prader–Willi syndrome is the most common genetic obesity disorder. It is caused by absence of a paternally derived region on chromosome 15, manifested as either a deletion or a double maternally derived region. The syndrome is characterised by cognitive impairment, low stature, genital hypoplasia and infertility, neonatal and infantile hypotonia, distinctive facial features and small hands and feet. Because of severe hunger, low energy metabolism and reduced intellect, dietary treatment is often impossible and surgical treatment may instead be indicated. Other less frequent congenital obesity disorders include Bardet–Biedl, Alström and Cohen's syndromes.

Single-gene mutations that cause obesity in humans are extremely rare, though they have led to an important understanding of the physiological mechanisms for appetite regulation (Hebebrand et al 2003). A deficit of the satiety hormone leptin, produced by adipose tissue, can be found in children in a few families with mutations in the leptin gene. These children are characterised by a severe hyperphagia and respond with considerable weight loss when treated with leptin injections. Obesity caused by mutations in the gene coding for the leptin receptor is also found in a few individuals. The most common form of obesity due to a single gene mutation involves mutations in the melanocortin-4 receptor, which occur in 3–4% of children with severe obesity. Other mutations, such as in the genes for proopiomelanocortin and the prohormone convertase 1, are similarly associated with obesity. Mutations in the systems involved in appetite regulation are extremely rare and account for only a very small percentage of the total cases of obesity. Many of the genes on a number of chromosomes are currently being screened in connection with obesity, but no definite association with the most usual form of obesity has so far been found.

Genetic disposition

It is commonly observed that obesity 'runs' in families, but it has been difficult to determine the difference between genuine genetic inheritance and inheritance of environmental/lifestyle factors; for example, hormonal transfer from an overweight mother to the fetus or inheritance or influence of the parents' dietary and exercise habits. Many Nordic studies of twins and adopted children have suggested that adult body weight and particularly obesity appear to have a significant genetic component. About half of the phenotypic variation of weight and fat mass in a given fat-inducing environment is thought to have a genetic basis, but it is difficult to determine the source of the inheritance even in these types of studies, since an early influence, for example in the womb or during infancy, can be critical and be mistakenly interpreted as being genetic inheritance.

The supposed genetic component is generally not perceived in such a way that the development of obesity is fixed in the genes from the outset and can therefore only be changed with difficulty. The genetic component is rather perceived as a predisposition, which is expressed only when certain environmental factors are favourable. The most important obesity-triggering environmental factors that are generally acknowledged are a high dietary fat content, energy-rich drinks, a low level of physical activity and irregular mealtimes, though stopping smoking and pregnancy also play a role. It is still not precisely known how the genetic component is expressed physiologically, although a number of studies suggest that an abnormal lipid metabolism, which promotes fat deposition and inhibits oxidation, a poorly regulated appetite at a low level of physical activity, increased preference for fatty tastes, and a reduced ability to spontaneously increase physical activity during periods of overeating are the most important candidates.

Changes in environment and lifestyle

Diet composition and drinks

The prevalence of obesity rose slowly from about 1920, with a dramatic increase in the years after World War II. During this period the diet has changed from consisting mainly of carbohydrate-rich foods (potatoes and other root vegetables, legumes, vegetables, grains, wholemeal bread) with a modest amount of fat, to the recent diet, where the consumption of meat, cheese, butter and other rich milk products and of alcohol has increased at the cost of more energy-poor, carbohydrate-rich foods. The fat content of the diet has risen considerably. Obesity is seldom seen among people who traditionally live on a diet with moderate fat content and a high content of energy-poor vegetables and wholemeal products. A rich, energy-dense diet with plentiful supply of sugary drinks tends to increase energy intake. In people with no special disposition towards obesity such a fat-promoting diet can result in a marked weight gain and overweight. When the predisposed individual is exposed to this type of diet, the weight increase can be considerable and eventually lead to obesity (Astrup 2001).

The weak satiating effect of a fat-rich diet is linked to the high energy density, whereas the stronger satiating effect of carbohydrate and protein is less dependent on energy density. Typical carbohydrate-rich foods with a low content of fibre are less satisfying than similar products with a high fibre content, but the quantitative significance for weight regulation is poorly defined. The same applies to the glycaemic index of the carbohydrate-rich foods (see Ch. 6). While there is no basis to suggest that sugar in solid form satiates less than starch, there is growing evidence that sugar in drinks satiates less than sugar in solid form and studies have suggested that a high consumption of sugary drinks leads to a marked weight increase (Raben et al 2002).

Alcohol

It is normally assumed that the energy content of alcohol is added to the energy from the diet, such that alcohol increases the total energy intake. However the Health Survey of England indicated that non-drinkers are more likely to be obese than those who consume alcohol. Among alcohol consumers there is a gender difference in the effect on body weight. Somewhat surprisingly, alcohol intake does not increase weight among men, whereas women seem to lose weight with increasing alcohol intake. In women the energy intake from food is suppressed by alcohol; women who drink a couple of units per day appear to eat less. The problem, however, is that most of the current knowledge is based on observational population studies, where confounding effects are possible. Thus other factors cannot be ruled out, for example smoking tobacco at the same time as drinking alcohol could instead be responsible for the attributed 'slimming' effect.

through a direct effect on the brain via blood glucose and insulin and partly through a satiating effect mediated by oxidation in the liver when glycogen depots in the liver have become fully loaded. The extent to which the satiating effect of simple carbohydrates like sucrose can be differentiated from that of more complex sugars is not entirely clear. There is also no evidence that replacement of sugar with artificial sweeteners leads to weight loss, unless it occurs as part of a strict calorie-controlled programme.

Triggering factors

Obesity can present itself from earliest childhood to senility, slowly or suddenly, with or without triggering factors. Several factors can potentially disturb the energy balance to such an extent that a large weight increase is involved.

Pregnancy

Fifty per cent of overweight women cite pregnancy as the main cause of their obesity (Linne et al 2002). First-time pregnant, non-smoking, hypertensive and already overweight women are a special risk group for excessive weight gain. The normal weight increase from conception to birth is 10–14 kg (about 20%), and the average gain from conception to a year after birth is 2 kg. This average figure, however, hides the fact that 30% have lost weight whilst the majority have gained – 15% more than 5 kg and 2% more than 10 kg. For underweight women a greater gestational weight gain is accompanied by increased birthweight and reduced perinatal mortality, while for normal and overweight women a gestational weight increase of >12 kg simply indicates a greater risk of caesarean section and lasting increased fat mass. The energy expenditure during pregnancy is about 330 MJ, of which the cost of fat storage accounts for only 10%, and increased energy intake accounts for the rest. In cases of severe overweight (>60%), weight gain during pregnancy should be limited to 5 kg, and with lesser degrees of obesity, energy restriction during pregnancy is not contraindicated, although greater attention should be placed on the quality of the diet.

Immobility

Acute weight gain is often seen with a sudden cessation of a habitually high level of physical activity,

due to a specific occupation or sport. Obesity frequently occurs in taxi and bus drivers, as well as in chronically immobilised patients.

Stress

Stress can increase the risk of weight gain and obesity, particularly among individuals with increased genetic risk as a result of polymorphisms in the glucocorticoid receptor. Glucocorticoid excess has a powerful stimulating effect on appetite and fat deposition is typically of the android pattern.

Psychological trauma

Serious psychological trauma is often accompanied by voracious hyperphagia and weight increase in some individuals, whilst others react with anorexia and weight loss. Both manifestations can occur with grieving due to the loss of a close family member or after divorce. The incidence of the phenomenon is overestimated, since weight increase has sometimes been brought about by the use of psychotropic drugs, the weight-stimulating effects of which have only been acknowledged in recent years.

Stopping smoking

Tobacco smoking suppresses appetite and nicotine stimulates the sympathetic nervous system, so that 15–20 cigarettes a day can increase the daily energy metabolism by 10%. Smokers tend to be slimmer than non-smokers, but have more abdominal fat distribution, which is a risk factor for cardiovascular disease and diabetes. The average weight gain after stopping smoking is 3 kg for men and 4 kg for women over a 10-year period. For some the weight gain is merely normalising, but for most it is excessive. Risk groups are heavy smokers, and younger slim women with sedentary employment. Even though the health consequences of weight gain are secondary compared to the benefits of giving up smoking, the phenomenon is nevertheless important, since weight increase is the most frequent reason for taking up smoking again.

Endocrine obesity

Many endocrine disorders can be linked to weight gain and result in obesity. In patients with obesity, however, they represent a minority of causes.

Myxoedema (hypothyroidism) is often accompanied by weight gain, which can be attributed to the fact that energy expenditure can fall by up to 40%. Despite effective treatment the weight seldom normalises. With thyrotoxicosis weight loss is most commonly seen, but increase in weight can also occur in younger overweight women treated with anti-thyroid drugs. Treatment results in a weight gain of 5–7 kg within a year. Abdominal obesity is a frequent clinical trait of Cushing's syndrome (due to excess cortisol production), and with the concomitant presence of hypertension, oedema, hirsutism and non-insulin-dependent diabetes, diagnosis of the condition is significantly distinct from simple abdominal obesity. Obesity is only occasionally seen with the insulin-secreting tumour insulinoma, whereas an acute development of severe treatment-resistant obesity often accompanies hypothalamic damage.

Drug-induced obesity

A number of prescription drugs are associated with weight gain, a phenomenon that is all too often neglected by doctors (Tardieu et al 2003). Lithium, neuroleptics, cyclic antidepressants, and the epilepsy drugs valproate and carbamazepine are among the most potent. Oestrogen, glucocorticoids and insulin can also cause weight gain, as can the anti-cancer drugs tamoxifen and megestrol acetate. During the treatment of AIDS patients with antiviral agents, a condition called lipodystrophy is sometimes induced, which is associated with an increased risk of type 2 diabetes and cardiovascular disease.

> ### ⊃ Key points
>
> ⊃ In only a minority of cases is obesity caused by a chromosome abnormality, a mutation in a single gene or classic endocrine disorder.
>
> ⊃ Most cases of obesity are due to a disposition towards an inadequately functioning appetite regulation and energy metabolism.
>
> ⊃ Weight gain and obesity may be triggered in susceptible individuals when the energy density and fat content of the diet's food and drink is too high, mealtimes are irregular, and daily physical activity is limited.
>
> ⊃ An unlimited supply of cheap, tasty foodstuffs and larger food portions also help to promote overweight and risk of obesity.
>
> ⊃ The disposition towards obesity is not necessarily genetic, since other influences, for example chemicals or hormones transferred from mother to fetus during pregnancy, may programme the offspring to be susceptible to an obesity-promoting lifestyle. Obesity can be triggered by pregnancy, immobility, stress, drugs, psychological trauma, stopping smoking or rarely endocrine disorders.

20.5 PREVENTION AND TREATMENT

Principles to achieve diet-induced weight loss

In almost every overweight and obese patient the diet must be adjusted to reduce energy intake. Dietary therapy consists of instructing patients as to how to modify their dietary intake to achieve a decrease in energy intake while maintaining a nutritionally adequate diet. Due to their enlarged body size, obese subjects have higher energy requirements for a given level of physical activity than their normal weight counterparts (Fig. 20.1). Obese diabetics have slightly higher energy requirements than obese subjects without diabetes for a given body size and composition, due to increased hepatic glucose production. Reducing the total energy intake of the obese patient to that of a normal weight individual will inevitably cause weight loss, consisting of about 75% fat and 25% lean tissue, until weight normalisation occurs at a new energy equilibrium. For patients with class I obesity this requires an energy deficit of 300 to 500 kcal/day, and for patients with class III obesity 500 to 1000 kcal/day. The desirable rate of weight loss for most people is 0.5–1 kg per week after the first month of dieting, with younger, taller and more overweight subjects aiming for the upper limit and older, shorter and less overweight subjects for the lower rate. With higher rates of loss there may be excessive loss of lean tissue. During the first month weight loss will be more rapid because of the loss of water associated with glycogen.

There is evidence to support the idea that differences in diet composition exert some effects on energy absorption and energy expenditure, but these differences have less clinical importance compared with

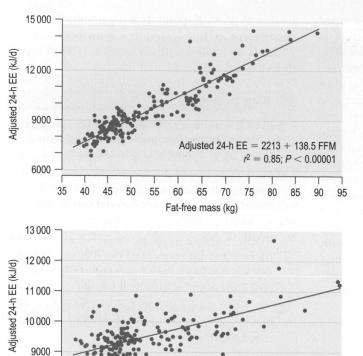

Figure 20.1 Energy expenditure (energy requirements) of normal weight, overweight and obese subjects. Relationship between body weight and energy requirements assessed by measurement of energy expenditure or by apparent energy intake during weight stability. The growing under-reporting with increasing body fatness makes the self-reported energy intake invalid for estimation of energy requirements in obese patients. Klausen et al (1997). Adapted with permission by the *American Journal of Clinical Nutrition.* © Am J Clin Nutr. American Society for Clinical Nutrition.

the major goal to reduce total energy intake. This can be achieved by setting an upper limit for energy intake. The larger the daily deficit in energy balance the more rapid the weight loss. A deficit of 300 to 500 kcal/day will produce a weight loss of 300 to 500 grams/week, and a deficit of 500 to 1000 kcal/day will produce a weight loss of 500 to 1000 grams/week. Greater initial energy deficits may produce even larger weight loss rates. Total energy expenditure declines and normalises along with weight loss, and total energy intake should therefore gradually be further reduced to maintain the energy deficit. Alternatively, advantage can be taken of the differences in the satiating power of the various dietary components in order to cause a spontaneous reduction in energy intake. This is the principle of the ad libitum low fat diet.

Choosing the dietary energy deficit

Initially the target of a weight loss programme should be to decrease body weight by 5–10%. Once this is achieved a new target can be set. Patients will generally want to lose more weight, but it should

be remembered that even a 5% weight reduction improves risk factors and risk of co-morbidities. Several factors should be taken into consideration, e.g. the patient's degree of obesity, previous weight loss attempts, risk factors, co-morbidities, and personal and social capacity to undertake the necessary lifestyle changes.

To prescribe a diet with a defined energy deficit it is necessary to estimate the actual energy requirements of the patient. It would seem natural to estimate the patient's habitual energy intake from self-reported diet record over 3 to 7 days of weight stability. However, these estimates are invalid due to systematic under-reporting of energy intake by obese individuals amounting to 30–40% (Fig. 20.1). Energy requirements should therefore be assessed indirectly by estimation of total energy expenditure. Resting metabolic rate (RMR) can be measured by indirect calorimetry, or be estimated with great accuracy using equations based on body weight, gender and age (Table 20.2) or, even better, estimated from information on the size of fat-free mass and fat mass. Total energy expenditure (= energy requirement) is estimated by multiplication of RMR (kcal/day) by an activity factor (PAL; physical activity

Table 20.2 **Estimating energy needs: revised WHO equations for estimating basal metabolic rate (BMR)**

Men	
18 to 30 years	=(0.0630 × actual weight in kg + 2.8957) × 240 kcal/day
31 to 60 years	=(0.0484 × actual weight in kg + 3.6534) × 240 kcal/day
Women	
18 to 30 years	=(0.0621 × actual weight in kg + 2.0357) × 240 kcal/day
31 to 60 years	=(0.342 × actual weight in kg + 3.5377) × 240 kcal/day

Estimated total energy expenditure = BMR × activity factor

Activity level	*Activity factor*
Low (sedentary)	1.3
Intermediate (some regular exercise)	1.5
High (regular activity or demanding job)	1.7

Reproduced with permission from: Astrup A (2004) Treatment of obesity. In: Ferrannini E, Zimmet P, De Fronzo R A, Keen H (eds) International textbook of diabetes mellitus. Copyright John Wiley & Sons Limited.

level) (Table 20.2). The energy level of the prescribed diet is defined as the patient's energy requirement minus the prescribed daily energy deficit.

Theoretical versus clinical outcome

Translating the physiologically based considerations regarding energy balance and weight loss into clinical practice requires a high degree of compliance, which can be difficult to obtain. Weight loss results tend to be much better in clinical trials conducted in specialised clinics than in trials conducted by non-specialists without sufficient resources and access to auxiliary therapists (dietitians, psychologists etc.). Compliance and adherence to the diet are the cornerstones of successful weight loss, and are the most complicated part of the dietary treatment of obesity. To improve adherence consideration should be given to the patient's food preferences, as well as to personal, educational and social factors. Great efforts should be made to see the patient frequently and regularly. Furthermore, long-term weight reduction is unlikely to succeed unless the patient acquires new eating and physical activity

habits. These behavioural changes should be an integral part of the treatment programme.

Options for weight loss diets

Therapeutic obesity diets distinguish between several recognised weight reduction regimens. Low-energy diets (LED) usually provide 800–1500 kcal/day and use fat-reduced foods, though weight loss occurs independent of the diet composition. Diets providing 1200 kcal/day or more have been classified as balanced-deficits diets, but this definition will not be used in this chapter. Very low energy diets (VLED) are modified fasts providing 200–800 kcal/day that replace normal foods. Ad libitum low fat diets do not restrict energy intake directly, but target a restriction of ad libitum fat intake to 20–30% of total energy intake. Energy intake is spontaneously reduced because of the higher satiating effect of this diet and a modest weight loss occurs.

Very low energy diets (VLED)

Starvation (less than 200 kcal/day) is the ultimate dietary treatment of obesity, but it is no longer used because of the numerous and serious medical complications associated with prolonged starvation. Starvation has been replaced by VLED (200–800 kcal/day), which aims to supply very little energy but all essential nutrients. Reducing the energy content of a diet requires an increased nutrient density. This can be difficult to obtain with natural foods if the diet is to be acceptable once the energy content of the diet becomes lower than 800 kcal/day. This has led to the commercial production of VLEDs, supplemented with all nutrients in RDA amounts. For decades 250–400 kcal/day formula diets were extremely popular. The first VLEDs were clearly nutritionally insufficient, but reports of adverse effects and results from research have brought about a gradual increase in energy level Some concern has been raised about the cardiac safety of the use of VLEDs with less than 800 kcal/day, and patients using VLEDs have an increased risk of developing gallstones (Table 20.3). Their use without medical supervision has generally been abandoned and should not be recommended.

A number of studies have shown that VLEDs with energy levels of less than 800 kcal/day do not produce a greater weight loss and are less well accepted than those comprising 800 kcal/day. Today the

Dietary weight maintenance programmes

In professional weight loss programmes LEDs induce a 5% weight loss in almost all patients, and frequent clinical attendance during the initial 6 months of weight reduction appears to facilitate achievement of the therapy goals. Larger success criteria (>10% weight loss) can be met by the majority of patients if the treatment programme also includes group therapy and behaviour modification. The real challenge is to maintain the reduced body weight and prevent subsequent relapse (Fig. 20.3). In a systematic review of long-term (>3 years' follow-up) efficacy of dietary treatment of obesity success was defined as maintenance of all weight initially lost or maintenance of at least 9 kg of initial weight loss. Initial weight loss was 4–28 kg, and 15% of the followed up patients fulfilled one of the criteria for success, and the success rate was stable for up to 14 years of observation. Diet combined with group therapy leads to better long-term success rates (27%) than diet alone (15%), or diet combined with behaviour modification and active follow-up, though active follow-up produces better weight maintenance than passive follow-up (19% versus 10%).

Whereas the principle of energy restriction (LED) is successful for weight loss induction independent of dietary composition, the low fat, high protein/carbohydrate diet seems to be more effective for long-term weight maintenance and preventing weight regain. In a study by Toubro and Astrup, patients were randomly assigned to two different weight maintenance groups, receiving either a low fat diet ad libitum or a fixed-energy diet (LED) for one year after having lost a mean of 13.6 kg on energy-restricted diets. There was only a small weight regain during the weight maintenance programme over one year. However, 2 years after the weight loss the LED group had regained 11.3 kg whereas the low fat group had regained only 5.4 kg. Forty per cent of the patients in the LED group and 65% of the patients in the low fat group had maintained a weight loss of >5 kg.

Does diet composition matter?

Numerous popular diet books promote changing diet composition in accordance with principles that are claimed to have a particularly favourable impact on weight loss and maintenance. Generally these claims are unsubstantiated and scientifically

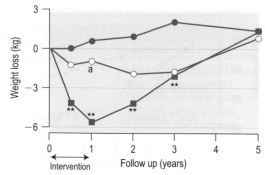

Figure 20.3 A 5-year follow-up of a 1-year randomised controlled trial of a reduced-fat ad libitum diet versus a usual diet (Swinburn et al 2001). Obese IGT patients were randomised to a reduced-fat diet (solid squares) or control (solid circles), and participated in monthly small-group education sessions on reduced-fat eating for 1 year. Weight decreased significantly in the reduced-fat diet group; the greatest difference was noted at 1 year (−3.3 kg), best in the most compliant group, but diminished at subsequent follow-up. Glucose tolerance also improved in patients on the reduced-fat diet; a lower proportion had type 2 diabetes or impaired glucose tolerance at 1 year (47% versus 67%). This difference disappeared in subsequent years, but the more compliant 50% of the intervention group maintained lower fasting and 2-hour glucose at 5 years compared to control subjects. The line with open circles (a) stands for a subgroup of the reduced-fat intervention group with poor compliance. The asterisks denote statistically significant difference between the reduced-fat and the control group. Copyright © 2001 American Diabetes Association. From Diabetes Care, Vol. 24, 2001; 619–624. Adapted with permission from *The American Diabetes Association*.

improbable, and some may even promote nutritionally insufficient diets. With LEDs, slightly more patients will be successful and fewer will drop out if the diet has a low (25% energy) rather than a high (45% energy) fat content (Petersen et al 2004). With ad libitum diets, and weight maintenance diets particularly, differences in the satiating effects of different macronutrients may have some importance.

Carbohydrate types

The high carbohydrate content of low fat diets stems mainly from the complex carbohydrates of different vegetables, fruits and whole grains, which are more satiating for fewer calories than fatty foods and are a good source of vitamins, minerals, trace elements and fibre. A high fibre content may further improve the satiating effect of the diet and a diet rich in soluble fibre, including oat bran, legumes, barley, and most fruits and vegetables, may be effective in reducing blood cholesterol and blood pressure levels. The recommended intake is 20 to 30 grams of fibre daily.

The role of simple carbohydrates in low fat diets remains controversial, mainly due to the lack of proper RCTs. Low fat diets, high in either complex or simple carbohydrates, induce similar fat loss in overweight and obese subjects, and a diet high in simple carbohydrates has no detrimental effects on blood lipids. However, recent evidence suggests that a high intake of sugar from soft drinks may have a special fattening property.

Glycaemic index (GI)

Some scientists have warned against the fattening properties of high GI foods such as potatoes, white bread, bagels and rice – foods that people are otherwise advised to eat more of as part of the currently recommended low fat diet. Instead they advise people to eat more wholegrain products, and types of rice and potatoes characterised by a low GI. Low GI foods are beneficial for glycaemic control in diabetics and have a modest beneficial effect on cardiovascular risk factors but their effect on body weight regulation is controversial (see Ch. 21).

The proponents of the GI hypothesis suggest that high GI foods produce rapid and transient surges in blood glucose and insulin which are in turn followed by rapidly returning hunger sensations and excessive caloric intake, but the scientific evidence is not conclusive. The effect of GI on weight loss is similarly undocumented. The lack of robust evidence prohibits issuing general dietary advice that low GI foods are preferable to high GI foods in preventing weight gain, although it appears likely that this dietary change will have beneficial effects on risk factors of cardiovascular disease and diabetes, and unlikely that it will exert any adverse effects. However, the GI concept is complicated for patients and comprehensive tables are required in order to calculate the diet. Newer research shows that the GI of meals cannot be accurately calculated from the carbohydrate source alone, but requires information about the energy, fat and protein content as well. There is a need for well-powered, randomised, long-term trials to show the potential for low versus high GI diets to produce weight loss or maintenance, and for a more patient-friendly classification of carbohydrate foods.

Protein content

A large body of experimental human data suggests that protein possesses a higher satiating power per calorie than carbohydrate and fat. The impact on weight loss of replacing carbohydrate with protein in ad libitum low fat diets has been addressed in only one RCT. The protein-rich diet produced a larger weight loss than a high carbohydrate diet, had no adverse effect on blood lipids, renal function or bone mineral density, and seemed to have a positive influence on the atherogenic risk factor profile in abdominally obese men. Replacement of some dietary carbohydrate by protein in ad libitum low fat diets may improve weight loss. More freedom to choose between protein-rich and complex carbohydrate-rich foods may encourage obese subjects to choose more lean meat and dairy products and hence improve adherence to low fat diets in weight reduction programmes. Increased protein allowances in weight reduction diets should await confirmation of these results by other studies. The dietary principles promoted in recent popular diet books advocating high protein, low carbohydrate diets are not supported by the existing evidence.

Fat quality and high MUFA diets

Although similar amounts of different fats contain nearly the same amount of energy, differences may exist in their satiating effects, which could influence total energy intake of ad libitum low fat diets and weight maintenance diets. From a biochemical and physiological view saturated fatty acids behave very differently from monounsaturated fats (MUFA), which seem to be more neutral than saturated or polyunsaturated fats in relation to cardiovascular disease, insulin resistance and cancer. However, animal studies suggest that MUFAs increase body weight more than polyunsaturated fatty acids (PUFA). In a cross-sectional, observational study in 128 males the highest positive correlation was found between the intake of MUFAs and body fat mass, whereas no significant association was found between PUFAs and body fat, and only a weak association with saturated fat was seen. Two experimental appetite studies have concordantly shown that meals/infusions with MUFAs produce lower satiety, and that they suppress energy intake for the remainder of the day less than PUFAs. These preliminary reports suggest that a high MUFA content in the diet may promote passive overconsumption and obesity.

(For further information see Section CD 20.5(b).)

of weight loss, and so corrects high serum trigly-ceride levels and low HDL cholesterol levels in obese patients. Sibutramine also increases weight loss and improves maintenance of reduced weight in obese patients who have previously lost weight on a very low calorie diet. For more information on relevant clinical trials see Section CD 20.5(c).

Sibutramine is generally well tolerated and has few side effects. These include symptoms such as dry mouth, headache, insomnia and constipation. The adverse effects of sibutramine include increases in blood pressure and heart rate. Although these increases are generally mild and without clinical relevance, blood pressure should be monitored on a regular basis. Increases in blood pressure may lead to discontinuation of treatment in about 5% of patients.

Obese patients with well-controlled hypertension (calcium channel blockers, beta-blocking agents, ACE inhibitors, thiazide diuretics) do not experience any rise in blood pressure with sibutramine therapy, and their overall risk factor profile will benefit from the induced weight loss.

Surgical treatment of obesity

See Section CD 20.5(d).

⟲ Key points

- ⟲ Prevention and treatment of obesity requires a reduced energy intake and increased expenditure through physical activity.

- ⟲ Energy intake should be reduced by a reduction in energy density and portion sizes of meals, and by avoiding drinks containing calories.

- ⟲ To achieve a weight loss a reduced energy intake is pertinent, while both a changed diet composition and 30–60 minutes of daily physical activity is required for subsequent weight maintenance.

- ⟲ Low energy diets, either consisting of normal foods or meal replacements, are effective to induce a weight loss of 5–10% in most patients.

- ⟲ The optimal diet is reduced in fat, with increased content of fibre-rich carbohydrates and protein from meat and dairy products. Many popular fad diets might produce transient weight loss mainly by a high protein content, and/or ketosis.

- ⟲ Currently approved weight loss drugs improve the mean weight loss and increase the proportion of subjects who achieve more than 5–10% weight loss.

References and further reading

References

Astrup A 2001 Healthy lifestyles in Europe: prevention of obesity and type II diabetes by diet and physical activity. Public Health Nutrition 4(2B):499–515

Astrup A 2004 The effect of exercise and diet on glucose intolerance and substrate utilization? In: Allison S P, Go V L W (eds) Metabolic issues of clinical nutrition. Karger, Basel, p 93–109

Astrup A, Grunwald G K, Melanson E L et al 2000 The role of low-fat diets in body weight control: a meta-analysis of *ad libitum* intervention studies. International Journal of Obesity 24:1545–1552

Harder H, Dinesen B, Astrup A 2004 The effect of a rapid weight loss on lipid profile and glycemic control in obese type 2 diabetic patients. International Journal of Obesity 28:180–182

Harper A, Astrup A 2004 Can we advise our obese patients to follow the Atkins diet? Obesity Reviews 5:93–94

Hebebrand J, Friedel S, Schauble N et al 2003 Perspectives: molecular genetic research in human obesity. Obesity Reviews 4(3):139–146

Hu F B, Manson J E, Stampfer M J et al 2001 Diet, lifestyle, and the risk of type 2 diabetes mellitus in women. New England Journal of Medicine 345(11):790–797

Klausen B, Toubro S, Astrup A 1997 Age and sex effects on energy expenditure. American Journal of Clinical Nutrition 65:895–907

Linne Y, Barkeling B, Rossner S 2002 Long-term weight development after pregnancy. Obesity Reviews 3(2):75–83

Petersen M, Taylor M, Saris W et al 2004 A 10 weeks randomised trial of hypocaloric low-fat versus medium-fat diet – the NUGENOB study. International Journal of Obesity (in press)

Raben A, Vasilaras T H, Møller AC, Astrup A 2002 Sucrose compared with artificial sweeteners: different effects on ad libitum food intake and body weight after 10 wk of supplementation in overweight subjects. American Journal of Clinical Nutrition 76:721–729

Saris W H M, Blair S N, van Baak M A et al 2003 How much physical activity is enough to prevent unhealthy weight gain? Outcome of the IASO 1st Stock Conference and consensus statement. Obesity Reviews 4(2):91–100

Swinburn B A, Metcalf P A, Ley S J 2001 Long-term (5-year) effects of a reduced-fat diet intervention in individuals with glucose intolerance. Diabetes Care 24:619–624

Tardieu S, Micallef J, Gentile S, Blin O 2003 Weight gain profiles of new anti-psychotics: public health consequences. Obesity Reviews 4(3):129–138

Toubro S, Astrup A 1997 Randomised comparison of diets for maintaining obese subjects' weight after major weight loss: ad lib, low fat, high carbohydrate diet v fixed energy intake. British Medical Journal 314:29–34

Further reading

Astrup A 2004 Treatment of obesity. In: Ferrannini E, Zimmet P, De Fronzo R A, Keen H (eds) International textbook of diabetes mellitus, 3rd edn. John Wiley, Chichester

Astrup A, Toubro S 2004 Drugs with thermogenic properties. In: Bray G A, Bouchard C, James W P T (eds) Handbook of obesity, 2nd edn. Marcel Dekker, New York, p 315–328

Astrup A, Larsen T M, Harper A 2004 Atkins and other low-carbohydrate diets: hoax or an effective tool for weight loss? Lancet 364:897–899

Ayyad C, Andersen T 2000 Long-term efficacy of dietary treatment for obesity: a systematic review of studies published between 1931 and 1999. Obesity Reviews 1(2):113–120

British Nutrition Foundation 1999 Obesity. The Report of the British Nutrition Foundation Task Force. Blackwell Science, Oxford

Goran M I, Astrup A 2002 Energy metabolism. In: Gibney M J, Vorser H H, Kok F J (eds) Introduction to human nutrition. The Nutrition Society, Blackwell Science, Oxford, p 30–45

WHO Consultation on Obesity 2000 Obesity: Preventing and managing the global epidemic. WHO Technical Report 894, Geneva

---

CD-ROM contents

Expanded material

Section CD 20.4 Central regulation of energy balance

Section CD 20.5(a) Ad libitum low fat diets – effect on cardiovascular risk factors

Section CD 20.5(b) Fat quality and high MUFA diets

Section CD 20.5(c) Sibutramine

Section CD 20.5(d) Surgical treatment of obesity

Further reading from the book

Useful websites

Objectives

By the end of this chapter you should be able to:

- understand the aetiology and pathophysiology of diabetes mellitus
- be able to distinguish between type 1 and type 2 diabetes mellitus
- have an insight into the link between diabetes and obesity
- understand insulin resistance and how to reduce it essentially through lifestyle modifications
- have a basic knowledge of how to prevent long-term complications of diabetes.

21.1 INTRODUCTION

Diabetes mellitus is a metabolic disorder of multiple aetiology characterised by chronic hyperglycaemia associated with impaired carbohydrate, fat and protein metabolism. These abnormalities are the consequence of either inadequate insulin secretion or impaired insulin action, or both. Diabetes has been recently reclassified by the World Health Organization into four distinct types (Table 21.1): type 1, type 2, gestational diabetes mellitus, other specific types (WHO 1999). Type 1 diabetes is characterised by a cell-mediated autoimmune destruction of pancreatic beta-cells that results in a partial or total inability to secrete insulin, and life-long need for insulin administration. Type 2 diabetes, until recently referred to as non-insulin-dependent diabetes, is characterised by disorders of insulin action and secretion, either feature being the predominant impairment. These individuals may not require insulin treatment either initially or ever, although it may be undertaken in some cases as the most appropriate blood glucose-lowering treatment. The specific aetiologies of this form of diabetes are yet to be found, but it is known that most of these patients are obese or have increased body fat, predominantly in the abdominal region. Other specific types of diabetes include less common causes – where the underlying defect may be genetic, secondary to pancreatic disease, endocrine disorders, infections, drug or chemical toxins. Gestational diabetes is defined as any degree of glucose intolerance with onset or first recognition during pregnancy.

Table 21.1 Aetiological classification of diabetes mellitus

1. Type 1 diabetes
   A. Immune-mediated
   B. Idiopathic
2. Type 2 diabetes
3. Gestational diabetes
4. Other specific types
   A. Genetic defects in beta-cell function (MODY)
   B. Genetic defects in insulin action
   C. Disease of the endocrine pancreas
   D. Endocrinopathies
   E. Drug or chemical induced
   F. Infections
   G. Uncommon forms of immune-mediated diabetes
   H. Other genetic syndromes associated with diabetes

21.2 EPIDEMIOLOGY AND DIAGNOSIS OF DIABETES MELLITUS

The diagnostic criteria for diabetes mellitus have also been modified based on the new classification. Diabetes can be diagnosed in three ways, and – in the absence of specific symptoms of the disease – each must be confirmed on a subsequent occasion: casual plasma glucose concentration $\geqslant 11.1$ mmol/l (200 mg/dl), or fasting plasma glucose $\geqslant 7.0$ mmol/l (126 mg/dl), or 2-hour plasma glucose $\geqslant 11.1$ mmol/l (200 mg/dl) during an oral glucose tolerance test (OGTT) with 75 g of glucose.

Two other categories of impaired glucose metabolism are impaired glucose tolerance (IGT) and impaired fasting glucose (IFG), which can be considered a metabolic state halfway between normal glucose homeostasis and diabetes. IGT is diagnosed by the 2-hour plasma glucose after OGTT >140 and <200 mg/dl with fasting value <126 mg/dl, while IFG is defined by fasting plasma glucose >110 and <126 mg/dl. These two categories are strong risk factors for future diabetes and/or cardiovascular disease. If untreated, approximately one-third of people with IGT develop type 2 diabetes within 5–10 years, one-third remain stable and one-third revert to normoglycaemia (Vaccaro et al 1999). In individuals with IGT, the mortality due to cardio-vascular and cerebrovascular disease is approxi-mately twice that of people with normal glucose tolerance.

IGT and type 2 diabetes are often associated with other metabolic disturbances and cardiovascular risk factors; this condition has been defined as the insulin resistance syndrome or metabolic syndrome. There is no internationally agreed definition of the metabolic syndrome, which is generally considered as an association of impaired glucose regulation (IGT or IFG) or type 2 diabetes, raised arterial pres-sure, raised plasma triglycerides, low HDL and central obesity (see Ch. 20). A recent statement from the US National Cholesterol Education Program (NCEP) attempts to define diagnostic criteria for the metabolic syndrome based exclusively on these clinical parameters (Expert Panel on Detection, Evaluation, and Treatment of High Blood Cholesterol in Adults 2001). Other abnormalities often associ-ated with the metabolic syndrome are micro-albuminuria, hyperuricaemia, non-alcoholic liver steatosis and coagulation disorders. There is grow-ing evidence pointing to insulin resistance as the common aetiological factor of this condition, con-sidered to be associated with increased risk for car-diovascular disease (Reaven 1988).

Type 2 diabetes mellitus accounts for almost 85–95% of all cases of diabetes. Its estimated preva-lence is 2–6% of the population: half of these are diagnosed, while a similar number remain unrecog-nised. The prevalence is known to be much higher in older people and in some ethnic communities (up to 40% of Pima Indians). WHO has predicted that the global prevalence of type 2 diabetes will more than double, from 135 million in 1995 to 300 million in the following years. Long-term complications of type 2 diabetes include retinopathy with potential loss of vision, nephropathy leading to renal failure, peripheral neuropathy with risk of foot ulcers, and autonomic neuropathy which contributes to erectile dysfunction and cardiac arrhythmia. However, most of the morbidity and mortality associated with dia-betes is attributable to macrovascular complications such as myocardial infarction, heart failure and acute stroke. Diabetes is associated with an age-adjusted cardiovascular mortality that is between two and four times that of the non-diabetic population, while life expectancy is reduced by 5 to 10 years in middle-aged patients with type 2 diabetes. Several observa-tional studies suggest that diabetes is primarily a lifestyle disorder; the highest prevalence rates occur in developing countries and in populations under-going 'Westernisation' or modernisation. Under such circumstances, it seems that genetic sus-ceptibility interacts with environmental changes, such as sedentary lifestyle and overnutrition, lead-ing to type 2 diabetes. Populations with the highest recorded prevalence of diabetes, such as Nauru or Pima Indians, share the common experience of change from a hunter-gatherer or agriculture-based lifestyle to one of sedentary living and a diet of energy-dense processed foods. A better under-standing of the impact that lifestyle may have, not only on the risk of diabetes, but also on its key mechanisms, should help implement more effective preventive measures focused on more specific targets.

21.3 AETIOLOGY AND PATHOPHYSIOLOGY OF DIABETES MELLITUS

Type 1 diabetes mellitus

Type 1 diabetes is characterised by absolute insulin deficiency caused in most cases by immune-mediated destruction of the beta-cells (autoimmune type 1A). A minority of patients with type 1 dia-betes, generally of African or Asian origin, have no evidence of autoimmunity although they are insulinopenic and ketosis-prone. This form of dia-betes has been referred as type 1B. The pathogenesis of type 1 diabetes involves genetic, immunological and environmental factors.

Genetic factors

Evidence for the involvement of genetic factors in the aetiology of type 1 diabetes comes from studies on animals, families and human twins. Studies on animal models of type 1 diabetes (NOD mouse, BB rat) have demonstrated that the susceptibility to dis-ease is mostly linked to the major histocompatibility system (HLA), although some non-HLA loci have also been found to be associated with the disease. A link between type 1 diabetes and the HLA system has been confirmed by population studies showing that genetic susceptibility to disease is related to

HLA-DR and HLA-DQ genes located on chromosome 6. Studies on families with multiple members affected by type 1 diabetes have demonstrated that the risk of a sibling developing the disease is increased by up to 27 times by the age of 16. However, between monozygotic twins, the concordance rate for the disease is 35–70% (depending on the length of follow-up), indicating that genetic factors, although important, cannot completely explain the occurrence of the disease, which seems to be multifactorial in nature.

Immunological factors

The evidence that type 1 diabetes is an autoimmune disease rests on the evidence of lymphocytic infiltration of pancreatic islets, abnormalities of cell-mediated immune response and circulating autoantibodies (Bottazzo & Bonifacio 1991). Histological studies of pancreatic tissues from type 1 diabetic patients who died shortly after diagnosis revealed the presence of macrophages, T- and B-lymphocytes and other inflammatory cells that combine to give an inflammatory picture known as 'insulitis'. Abnormalities of circulating cell-mediated immunity consist of an increased number of activated lymphocytes CD4+, which are known to play a major role in beta-cell destruction. Autoantibodies against a variety of pancreatic islet components are commonly observed in patients with type 1 diabetes. These include antibodies to islet cells (ICA), insulin (IAA), glutamic acid decarboxylase (GAD), carboxypeptidase H, and several other minor antigens. Most of these antibodies appear shortly after diagnosis or even prior to the clinical onset of diabetes and tend to fall progressively thereafter. The early detection of these immunological markers paved the way to the possibility of predicting the disease in high-risk subjects, such as first-degree relatives of patients with type 1 diabetes. In these subjects the presence of multiple markers indicates a high risk (above 80%) of developing the disease within the subsequent two years. Based on this rationale, a number of clinical trials have been performed in an attempt to prevent the disease in high-risk subjects using different strategies, e.g. nicotinamide (Deutsche Nicotinamide Intervention Study (DENIS) and European Nicotinamide Intervention Trial (ENDIT studies)) and subcutaneous insulin (Diabetes Prevention Trial 1). Unfortunately, none of these approaches has been shown to effectively reduce the risk of developing the disease.

Environmental factors

Environmental factors could contribute to the pathogenesis of type 1 diabetes mellitus through several mechanisms: (1) exerting a direct toxic effect on the beta-cells, (2) triggering an autoimmune reaction against the beta-cell, (3) damaging beta-cells so as to increase their susceptibility to auto-immune destruction. Environmental factors include drugs or chemicals (e.g. alloxan, streptozotocin, pentamidine), viruses and dietary factors. Among viruses potentially involved in human type 1 diabetes, clinical evidence points to mumps, coxsackie B, cytomegalovirus and rubella viruses as the most likely candidates. The viral aetiology is supported by seasonal variability in the incidence of the disease, with a peak in spring and autumn. In addition, clinical and epidemiological studies have shown a close relation between appearance of diabetes and preceding episodes of viral infections. However, despite its attractiveness, the viral hypothesis requires caution since clinical evidence is far from conclusive. Recently, growing attention has been focused on the potential role of dietary factors. In particular, there is evidence of a close relationship between cow's milk consumption and incidence of type 1 diabetes in childhood. The hypothesis is that antibodies produced against bovine seroalbumin may cross-react with antigens of beta-cells, triggering an autoimmune response. A multicentre trial is in progress to evaluate whether an early elimination of cow's milk from diet may prevent type 1 diabetes in infants with genetic risk for the disease.

Clinical manifestations

Because subjects who develop type 1 diabetes often have a rather abrupt onset of symptoms (polyuria, polydipsia (thirst), or even ketoacidosis), it was long assumed that beta-cell damage occurs rapidly. It is now accepted that type 1 diabetes gradually develops over many years. Some authors have proposed dividing the natural history of the disease into five stages: (1) genetic susceptibility, (2) triggering events (environmental), (3) active autoimmunity, (4) gradual loss of glucose-induced insulin secretion, (5) appearance of overt diabetes. Thus, the presence of islet cell autoantibodies occurs long before the clinical appearance of the disease at a time when there is no elevation in blood glucose and glucose tolerance is near normal. When fasting hyperglycaemia develops, at least 80–90% of the functional capacity of beta-cells is irreversibly lost. Thus, the basic pathophysiological mechanism responsible for type 1 diabetes is the total and irreversible loss of beta-cell function. Insulin deficiency leads to multiple abnormalities of intermediary metabolism that culminate in hyperglycaemia and increased levels of ketone bodies with proneness to ketoacidosis (Fig. 21.1). Hyperglycaemia results from both increased glucose production by the liver and reduced glucose utilisation by peripheral tissue, mainly the skeletal muscle. Hepatic glucose production increases as a consequence of high rates of both glycogenolysis and gluconeogenesis. Under conditions of insulin deficiency, an accelerated flux of gluconeogenic substrates (alanine, lactate, glycerol) takes place from peripheral tissues to the liver, which fuels gluconeogenesis. Glucose utilisation decreases as a result of the lack of insulin stimulatory effect on glucose transport and the increased availability of free fatty acids, which are known to inhibit glucose transport across the muscle membrane through operation of the glucose–fatty acid (Randle) cycle. In uncontrolled type 1 diabetes, fatty acid mobilisation from adipose tissue is markedly increased. Normally, in the liver fatty acids undergo beta-oxidation to acetyl CoA, which is totally oxidised in the Krebs cycle to water and carbon dioxide. When there is an excessive breakdown of fatty acids, as occurs in an insulin-deficient state, the capacity of the liver to oxidise all acetyl CoA is exceeded and two carbon fragments combine to form acetoacetate. Hepatic ketone body synthesis is further enhanced by the low insulin to glucagon ratio that critically regulates the activity of key enzymes of ketogenesis. All these metabolic abnormalities account for the classic symptoms and signs of the disease, such as glycosuria, polyuria, polydipsia and weight loss. However, there is wide variability in clinical manifestations, with some individuals presenting acute signs of decompensation and others being asymptomatic thanks to good control with insulin therapy.

Type 2 diabetes mellitus

Although type 2 diabetes has strong genetic components, modes of inheritance are largely unknown. One exception is the variant represented by MODY (maturity onset diabetes of the young) that conforms to autosomal dominant inheritance with high penetrance. The role of heredity in type 2 diabetes is supported by familial aggregation, a concordance of 60–90% for the disease in identical twins, and marked differences in its prevalence in different ethnic groups.

For the more common forms of type 2 diabetes, it is believed that both genetic and acquired factors contribute to the disease. Genetic factors somehow confer susceptibility to develop glucose intolerance; the occurrence of diabetes will depend on the presence of non-genetic, environmental factors that disrupt the fine balance between insulin secretion and insulin action. Among environmental factors, obesity and sedentary lifestyle are the major factors known to impair glucose tolerance. Also of great interest is the recent evidence that dietary factors, especially a high intake of saturated fats, are associated with an increased risk of developing diabetes. Patients with type 2 diabetes have two major metabolic defects: (1) impaired insulin secretion, and (2) resistance to insulin action on target tissues, namely the liver, skeletal muscle, and adipose tissue.

Defect of insulin secretion

In type 2 diabetic patients fasting insulin levels have been reported as low, normal or even elevated. This does not imply that insulin secretion is normal because, although fasting insulin is normal in absolute terms, it is inappropriately low for the ambient glucose level. At matched plasma glucose concentration, normal subjects would have a much higher insulin concentration. The main abnormality of beta-cell function in type 2 diabetes is the loss of glucose-induced insulin secretion. In normal subjects a rapid rise in plasma glucose elicits a biphasic insulin release: a first (early) phase lasting 5–10 minutes and a second (late) phase persisting for the duration of hyperglycaemia (Fig. 21.2). Although most of the insulin is secreted during the second phase insulin response, the first-phase is recognised as serving an important physiological function, i.e. to stimulate glucose utilisation by peripheral tissues

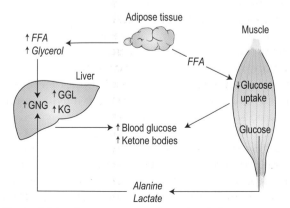

Figure 21.1 Consequences of insulin deficiency in type 1 diabetes mellitus. GNG, gluconeogenesis; GGL, glycogenolysis; KG, ketogenesis.

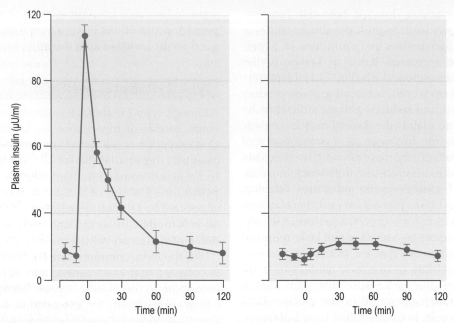

Figure 21.2 Insulin release elicited by an intravenous glucose load in normal subjects (left) and in patients with type 2 diabetes mellitus (right).

and to inhibit glucose production by the liver in order to prevent an exaggerated increase in plasma glucose in the postprandial state. In type 2 diabetic patients, the first phase insulin response is characteristically lost while the late phase is preserved or only attenuated (Fig. 21.2). The main characteristics of this secretory defect have been extensively investigated over the last decades (Kahn 1996). They can be outlined as follows: (1) the defective insulin release is specific for glucose whereas insulin response to other secretagogues (arginine, isoproterenol, secretin) is substantially unaltered; (2) the potentiating effect of glucose on insulin response to secretagogues is reduced, confirming that in type 2 diabetes the beta-cell is selectively unresponsive to glucose; and (3) beta-cell glucose unresponsiveness may be partially restored by correction of hyperglycaemia, suggesting that it may be, at least in part, an acquired defect caused by the toxic effect of high blood glucose on the beta-cells (glucose toxicity hypothesis).

Other abnormalities of insulin secretion have been documented in type 2 diabetes and include disruption of the pulsatile insulin secretory pattern. In normal subjects, plasma insulin displays 5–10 minute oscillations, which disappear in diabetic patients. In addition, diabetic patients are characterised by increased levels of proinsulin and proinsulin/insulin ratio, indicating an abnormal processing of insulin precursors within the beta-cells.

Although beta-cell dysfunction is clearly evident in patients with type 2 diabetes, it is not clear whether the defect in insulin secretion is the result of a reduction of the beta-cell mass or a dysfunction of a normal number of beta-cells. Autopsy studies of pancreases of diabetic patients have shown the presence of both qualitative and quantitative alterations. Beta-cell mass appears to be reduced by about 50% of the normal value while the proportion of alpha-cells (secreting glucagon) is increased. The most characteristic morphological change is represented by amyloid deposition in the islets. These deposits consist of insoluble fibrils formed from a peptide designated 'islet amyloid polypeptide' (IAPP or amylin) that is co-secreted with insulin. The function of this peptide is unknown at present but its presence in secretory granules of the beta-cells suggests a regulatory role. Recently, some animal studies have demonstrated a relation between dietary fat intake and production and/or secretion of amylin in the beta-cells.

Insulin resistance

Insulin resistance is a major pathogenic component of type 2 diabetes. Insulin resistance is a state in which a given concentration of insulin produces a less than normal biological response. As known, insulin exerts its biological effects by initially binding to its specific cell-surface receptors. After this, a number of signals are generated that interact with a variety of effector units (enzymatic systems) leading to multiple metabolic effects. Insulin promotes the storage of nutrients by stimulating glycogen synthesis, protein synthesis and lipogenesis and by inhibiting lipolysis, and glycogen and protein breakdown. In addition, insulin regulates water and electrolyte balance and stimulates cell growth and differentiation. This complex hormonal activity involves different intracellular pathways and mediators, which explains why some effects of insulin may be impaired (e.g. glucose metabolism) whereas others may not be (e.g. cellular growth). The cellular mechanisms underlying insulin resistance have been extensively investigated and all the receptor and post-receptor events that mediate insulin action have been carefully analysed. Defects in insulin signalling, glucose transport and metabolic pathways of intracellular glucose utilisation have been documented in type 2 diabetic patients (De Fronzo 1997). However, it is still unclear what the primary defect is, which defect is genetically determined and which is secondary to acquired factors, such as hyperglycaemia itself.

With regard to glucose metabolism, it is known that insulin lowers blood glucose through two mechanisms: (1) by suppressing glucose production from the liver, and (2) by promoting the uptake of glucose by peripheral tissues, especially the skeletal muscle. Under conditions of insulin resistance, as occurs in type 2 diabetes, the effect of insulin on the liver and peripheral tissues is impaired, thus producing the two major metabolic abnormalities observed in diabetic patients; i.e. fasting and postprandial hyperglycaemia.

Liver

As a result of impaired insulin action on the liver, type 2 diabetic patients tend to have abnormally increased glucose production in the post-absorptive state, which contributes to fasting hyperglycaemia. A strong positive correlation has been found between hepatic glucose production, measured by isotopic techniques, and fasting blood glucose level. The excess of hepatic glucose production is almost entirely accounted for by an increased rate of gluconeogenesis, which is ~40% higher in diabetic patients than in normal subjects. Such an increase is due to an increased supply of 3-carbon compounds (lactate, alanine, glycerol) from peripheral tissues to the liver as well as to a more efficient hepatic conversion of these substrates into glucose. Not only is hepatic glucose production increased in the basal state but it

is less suppressed after glucose ingestion. This failure of the liver to adequately suppress its glucose production in response to insulin contributes to the impairment of postprandial glucose homeostasis. In addition, the ability of the liver to take up and dispose of dietary glucose also seems to be reduced.

Skeletal muscle

Skeletal muscle is another important site of insulin resistance in patients with type 2 diabetes. By means of a number of different techniques, it has been demonstrated that the ability of insulin to stimulate glucose uptake by the skeletal muscle is reduced by 40–50% in diabetic patients as compared with normal subjects. Subsequent studies employing ^{13}C magnetic resonance spectroscopy have established that the defect responsible for impaired muscle glucose uptake involves the glucose transport step. In vitro studies have demonstrated a defect in the translocation and/or activity of GLUT-4, the glucose transporters located in skeletal muscle. In addition, the activity of two of the key enzymes that regulate non oxidative (glycogen synthase) and oxidative (pyruvate dehydrogenase) glucose metabolism is reduced in diabetic patients. However, this defect is likely to be secondary to the reduced glucose transport.

Adipose tissue

Insulin profoundly influences adipocyte metabolism by stimulating glucose transport and triglyceride synthesis (lipogenesis), as well as inhibiting lipolysis. In type 2 diabetes, particularly when associated with obesity, the ability of insulin to suppress lipolysis is markedly impaired. In addition, because glucose transport in the adipocyte is reduced, less glycerophosphate is formed through glycolysis and made available for triglyceride synthesis. The consequence is an increased flux of free fatty acids (FFA) from adipose tissue and a rise in their plasma concentration. It is important to consider that not only are FFA concentrations elevated in the fasting state, but they fail to be appropriately suppressed after meals. The result is a chronic elevation of FFA and triglyceride levels together with excessive deposition of fat in various tissues (including the skeletal muscle) in patients with type 2 diabetes, particularly when associated with obesity. In addition, there is evidence that a chronic elevation in FFAs has detrimental effects on insulin secretion and on the action of insulin in peripheral tissues (lipotoxicity).

What are the defects causing beta-cell dysfunction and insulin resistance?

It is widely accepted that beta-cell dysfunction and insulin resistance in type 2 diabetes are due to both genetic and acquired factors. An inherited defect in any part of the complex cascade that leads from glucose elevation to insulin processing and release could be a potential cause of beta-cell dysfunction. Mutations in the glucokinase gene, in the beta-cell glucose transporter (GLUT 2) gene, in mitochondrial DNA and in the insulin gene itself have been identified in some diabetic patients. However, the importance of these alterations in the common form of type 2 diabetes is questionable as these mutations have not been detected in populations with high prevalence of diabetes (e.g. Pima Indians). Other emerging factors associated with insulin secretory dysfunction include low birthweight (attributed to poor fetal development of the pancreas because of malnutrition) and deficiencies of some amino acids that seem to exert trophic effects on the beta-cells.

With regard to genetic factors responsible for insulin resistance, a number of candidate genes have been identified. Some mutations of the insulin receptor gene lead to altered insulin receptor biosynthesis, others impair the binding of insulin to its own receptor or insulin signalling. However, these mutations produce rare syndromes of severe insulin resistance but do not explain the insulin resistance associated with the common form of type 2 diabetes. The current view is that insulin resistance is not due to a few 'major' genes but to a large number of 'polygenes', each with a relatively minor effect.

The role of acquired factors in deteriorating insulin secretion and insulin action is well expressed by the concept of 'glucose toxicity' and 'lipotoxicity'. According to the glucose toxicity hypothesis, a chronic increment in plasma glucose concentration leads to progressive impairment in insulin secretion and insulin sensitivity. This hypothesis is mainly based on animal studies showing that rats made diabetic by partial pancreatectomy develop hyperglycaemia and, concomitantly, a progressive impairment in insulin secretion and insulin action. Interestingly, when chronic hyperglycaemia is corrected by phlorizin, a substance that increases glucose urinary loss without any effect on the beta-cell, both the first and second phase insulin secretion are restored to normal. In parallel, peripheral insulin sensitivity substantially improves with correction of hyperglycaemia. In addition, clinical studies in diabetic patients have shown that a tight glycaemic control, independent of the method by which it is achieved (diet, insulin or hypoglycaemic agents), ameliorates considerably insulin secretion and insulin action.

Like hyperglycaemia, the chronic elevation of FFAs may impair beta-cell function and contribute to the decreased uptake of glucose into peripheral tissues. This phenomenon has been referred to as 'lipotoxicity'. Studies in diabetic patients have shown that FFAs exert adverse effects on insulin sensitivity by interfering with the activity of GLUT-4, the glucose transporter located in skeletal muscle. This mechanism is likely to play a role in the impaired glucose tolerance associated with a high fat diet.

Natural history of type 2 diabetes

A major question, and one that continues to be the subject of considerable debate, is which of the two defects, insulin resistance or insulin secretory dysfunction, comes first. An important advance in understanding the natural history of diabetes comes from longitudinal studies that have followed for several years people who progressed from the stage of normal glucose tolerance to impaired glucose tolerance to frank diabetes. Collectively, these studies show that defects in both insulin secretion and insulin action occur at an early stage during the development of diabetes and progressively worsen over time. These defects are likely to be genetically determined. The progressive deterioration is caused by the detrimental effects of some environmental factors, mainly obesity (particularly visceral fat accumulation), sedentary lifestyle, high fat intake, glucose toxicity and lipotoxicity. To compensate for reduced peripheral insulin sensitivity, the beta-cell usually increases its insulin secretion so as to prevent persistent hyperglycaemia. In this way, a near-normal blood glucose is maintained at the expense of increased insulin levels. However, when pancreatic beta-cells are no longer able to compensate with an appropriate increase in insulin secretion (because of a genetic defect or a progressive functional exhaustion), frank diabetes will develop (Weyer et al 1999). Understanding the temporal sequence of changes in insulin secretion and insulin action as well as their interaction in the progression of diabetes may have important implications for prevention of diabetes and suggests that lifestyle modifications should preserve both insulin secretion and insulin sensitivity.

21.4 VASCULAR COMPLICATIONS

Microangiopathy

Microangiopathy or microvascular complications of diabetes mellitus include retinopathy, nephropathy and neuropathy, although the contribution of microangiopathy to neuropathy is still not completely understood. The incidence of retinopathy increases with duration of diabetes in type 1 diabetic patients: after 20 years of diabetes, over 95% of patients have background retinopathy, although mostly without visual impairment. The risk of proliferative retinopathy, the main cause of blindness in type 1 diabetic patients, increases rapidly between 10 and 15 years after the onset of diabetes, then remains remarkably constant, reaching a cumulative risk of about 60% after 40 years of diabetes. In type 2 diabetic patients retinopathy can be present at the onset of the disease (from 7% to as many as 38%) perhaps due to the fact that this condition sometimes remains unrecognised for years. It then increases, reaching, after 20 years, a prevalence of about 60% for any kind of retinopathy and 20% for proliferative retinopathy.

Diabetic nephropathy affects 20–40% of patients with type 1 diabetes, while it is rarer in those with type 2. Diabetic microvascular complications result from the interaction of multiple genetic and metabolic factors, among which hyperglycaemia is almost certainly the most important one (Walker and Viberti 1991). In fact, all these complications are specific to diabetes and do not occur in the absence of long-lasting hyperglycaemia. The importance of hyperglycaemia in the determination and progression of microvascular complications has been proven beyond any doubt by the results of some intervention trials performed in the last few years in both type 1 and type 2 diabetic patients. These studies have clearly shown that improving blood glucose control significantly reduces the onset and progression of retinopathy, nephropathy and neuropathy. Besides hyperglycaemia and genetic factors, which determine a variable degree of susceptibility and which have not been fully identified, other factors are important in determining microvascular complications, such as hypertension, smoking and hyperlipidaemia. Hypertension has been shown to play a very important role, especially in the genesis of diabetic nephropathy. Intervention trials in type 2 diabetic patients have clearly shown that improving blood pressure control significantly reduces the onset and progression of both nephropathy and retinopathy.

How all these factors may lead to diabetic microangiopathy is still a matter of debate. Many hypotheses have been put forward and only partly proven. One possible pathway is illustrated in Figure CD 21.1. Hyperglycaemia, together with other factors, may lead, through different mechanisms, to abnormal endothelium function, haemodynamic effects and changes in blood rheological characteristics. All these abnormalities may induce a thickening of basement membrane and an increased permeability with subsequent occlusive angiopathy, tissue hypoxia and organ damage.

Macroangiopathy

Atherosclerotic arterial disease may manifest clinically as coronary heart disease, cerebrovascular disease or peripheral vascular disease. In diabetic patients these lesions are qualitatively similar to those present in the non-diabetic population, except that their progression appears to be accelerated. Both mortality and morbidity for all cardiovascular diseases are significantly increased in diabetic patients. In particular, both coronary heart disease and cerebrovascular disease mortality is increased from two- to four-fold in diabetic patients compared to the non-diabetic population. Moreover, about half of all lower limb amputations occur in diabetic patients.

The high prevalence of arterial disease in diabetes is explained partly by the increased frequency of the most important cardiovascular risk factors, and partly by other factors closely associated with diabetes (Table 21.2). Serum cholesterol remains one

Table 21.2 **Main risk factors for cardiovascular disease in diabetic patients**

General risk factors	Diabetes-related risk factors
Smoking	Hyperglycaemia
Hyperlipidaemia	Hyperinsulinaemia/insulin
Hypertension	resistance
Hypercoagulability	Microalbuminuria/proteinuria
Obesity	Both sexes affected almost
Physical inactivity	equally
Family history	

of the most important cardiovascular risk factors in diabetic patients. Recent intervention studies performed in diabetic patients with hypolipidaemic drugs, particularly statins, have clearly shown that LDL cholesterol reduction significantly decreases cardiovascular events. Beside LDL cholesterol, other lipid abnormalities, more typical of type 2 diabetes, such as increased triglycerides, VLDL and IDL particles, and decreased HDL cholesterol, may have an important role in determining the high cardiovascular risk of diabetic patients.

With regard to the role of high blood pressure, the data are very consistent and similar to those on LDL cholesterol. There is strong evidence that reducing blood pressure significantly decreases cardiovascular events in diabetic patients. The data concerning the role of hyperglycaemia in explaining, at least in part, the excess cardiovascular risk of diabetic patients, are somewhat more controversial. Epidemiological data, as a whole, support the relationship between hyperglycaemia and cardiovascular disease, even if the association is not as strong as for microvascular complications. Moreover, intervention studies show that improvement in blood glucose control reduces the incidence of cardiovascular events in type 2 diabetic patients, if the improvement is part of a multi-factorial intervention that also includes targets for optimal plasma lipid and blood pressure levels (Gaede et al 2003).

Insulin resistance and/or hyperinsulinaemia, typical features of type 2 diabetic patients, are associated with an increased cardiovascular risk. It is not completely clear if this association is fully explained by the clustering of other cardiovascular risk factors with insulin resistance, such as lipid abnormalities, high blood pressure, coagulation abnormalities, high uric acid levels and so on, or whether there is also a

Table 21.3 Optimal goals for cardiovascular disease prevention in patients with diabetes
BMI <25 kg/m^2 HDL cholesterol >45 mg/dl Physical activity: 1/2 hour of brisk walking every day *or* at least 3–4 days/week Abstinence from smoking Optimal blood glucose control

direct link between insulin resistance and/or hyperinsulinaemia and the atherosclerotic process. In any case, all these risk factors, together with others less well identified, may induce, through different mechanisms, endothelial injury. Different and repeated injuries increase the permeability of the endothelium to lipids as well as its adhesion to monocytes and platelets. This in turn increases the procoagulant activities of the endothelium and increases the expression of vasoactive molecules, cytokines and growth factors, which promote the migration of monocytes and proliferation of smooth muscle cells. In this way the atherosclerotic process starts and will continue until the formation of the atherosclerotic plaque, with progressive narrowing of the arterial lumen and arterial stenosis or plaque rupture, thrombus formation and acute ischaemia.

In conclusion, many factors may contribute to the excess cardiovascular risk typical of both type 1 and type 2 diabetic patients. Therefore, in order to reduce this risk, it is necessary to act not only on blood glucose control, but also on plasma lipids, blood pressure, hypercoagulable state, obesity, physical activity, smoking habits, to try to reach the goals indicated in Table 21.3.

21.5 MANAGEMENT OF DIABETES MELLITUS

Diet

Nutritional management is the cornerstone of therapy for diabetes mellitus. In many patients with type 2 diabetes it may be the only therapy required, in the others (type 1 and 2) it allows a more accurate blood glucose control with lower doses of oral hypoglycaemic drugs or insulin. In any case, the aims of nutritional management must be not only the optimisation of blood glucose control but also

and, perhaps more importantly, the reduction of risk factors for cardiovascular diseases. Dietary recommendations for people with diabetes are very similar to those given to the general population for the promotion of good health. Of course, since diabetes mellitus is a chronic disease, diet therapy has to be considered as a lifelong practice and therefore it is essential that all nutritional programmes be adapted to the specific needs of the individual.

Total dietary energy

Most patients (60–70%) with type 2 diabetes are over-weight or obese, and the frequency of moderate over-weight has increased over the last years also in type 1 diabetic patients, especially those following intensive insulin therapy. All these patients should be encouraged to reduce their calorie intake and increase their energy expenditure. There is a very large body of evidence showing that body weight reduction, even if modest (5–10% of basal body weight), is able to improve blood glucose control, reduce insulin resistance and favourably affect the other cardiovascular risk factors, such as blood pressure and lipid abnormalities, often present in diabetic patients.

Two intervention trials performed recently, one in the USA (Diabetes Prevention Program Research Group 2002) and the other in Finland (Tuomilehto et al 2001), have clearly shown that a moderate weight reduction (about 5% of initial body weight), together with increased physical activity and changes in the dietary composition (reduction in saturated fat, increased consumption of dietary fibre), is able to prevent type 2 diabetes, reducing its incidence in high risk individuals by 60%. From a practical point of view, weight reduction may be achieved by reducing the consumption of energy-dense foods, especially those rich in fat, to achieve a caloric deficit of 300–500 kcal/day. To be effective also in the long run this advice should be incorporated into structured, intensive lifestyle education programmes. The prescription of a very low energy diet should be restricted to special cases (BMI >35 kg/m^2) and administered only in specialised centres.

Composition of the diet

According to the recommendations for the nutritional management of patients with diabetes mellitus (Riccardi & Rivellese 1999), the most important aspect in relation to the composition of the diet is the consumption of saturated fat <10% of total energy or, even, <8% for patients at higher cardiovascular risk. This strong recommendation is supported by the high rates of cardiovascular diseases in people with diabetes and by the fact that saturated fat intake has very unfavourable effects on lipid metabolism (increase in LDL cholesterol), insulin resistance and blood pressure. Together with saturated fat, cholesterol intake should also be reduced to less than 300 mg/day for all people with diabetes and less than 250 mg/day for those with raised LDL cholesterol. Taking into account that protein intake should range between 10 and 20% of total energy (0.8 g/kg body

weight/day for those with incipient or established nephropathy) the remaining 80–90% of the total energy should be provided by a combination of carbohydrates and unsaturated fat (especially monounsaturated fatty acids) according to clinical circumstances and local or individual preferences. As to carbohydrates, foods rich in dietary fibre (legumes, vegetables) and/or with low glycaemic index are recommended, while high glycaemic index foods must be restricted and replaced with unsaturated fat (Table 21.4). Fibre-rich foods (legumes, vegetables, fruit, cereal-derived foods) have been shown to improve blood glucose control and lipid profile in both type 1 and type 2 diabetic patients. Therefore, an intake of dietary fibre of 15–20 g/1000 kcal, which can be achieved following the suggestions given in Table 21.4, are recommended for diabetic patients as well as for the general population.

Dietary fibre is only one of the factors able to modulate the glycaemic response to carbohydrate-rich foods, which can be influenced also by other factors (physical state of foods, type of starch, presence of antinutrients). Due to the variety of factors that influence the impact of a meal on blood glucose, it is not possible to predict the postprandial glycaemic response of each food on the basis of its chemical characteristics. Therefore, it is necessary to examine the glycaemic response of foods in vivo and calculate their so-called glycaemic index. This index is based on the increase in blood glucose concentrations (the incremental area under the curve of blood glucose concentrations) after the ingestion of a portion of a test food containing 50 g of carbohydrates, divided by the incremental blood glucose area achieved with the same amount (50 g) of carbohydrates present in an equivalent portion of a reference food (glucose or white bread). According to this index, carbohydrate foods can be divided into broad categories characterised by a high or low glycaemic index. Fibre-rich foods have a low glycaemic index, although some foods with low fibre content (pasta, parboiled rice) may also have a low glycaemic index.

It is now well documented that a diet containing mainly low glycaemic index foods improves metabolic control in diabetic patients and may have favourable effects on other cardiovascular risk factors. Therefore foods with a low glycaemic index (e.g. legumes, oats, pasta, parboiled rice, certain raw fruits) should replace, whenever possible, those with a high glycaemic index. Moreover, the diet for diabetic patients, in accordance with general guidelines for the promotion of good health, should be

Table 21.4 'Optimal diet' for the treatment of diabetes. Provided that saturated fat is reduced and most carbohydrate-rich foods have either a high fibre content or a low GI, some flexibility is allowed in the amount of fat and carbohydrate, e.g. exchanging about 10% energy between monounsaturated fat and carbohydrate-rich foods with high GI

100%		100%
PROTEINS 15%	More fish and vegetable proteins	**PROTEINS 15%**
CARBOHYDRATE 55%	Vegetables, fruit, legumes, low GI starchy foods	**CARBOHYDRATE 45%**
	High GI starchy foods	
FAT 30%	Monounsaturated	**FAT 40%**
	Polyunsaturated	
	Saturated	
0%		0%

Alcohol <30 g/day.
Salt <6 g/day.

moderately restricted in salt intake (<6 g/day) and alcohol intake (20–30 g per day, 250 ml red wine, perhaps less for those who are overweight, hypertriglyceridaemic or have high blood pressure).

Physical exercise

Aerobic physical exercise of moderate intensity but performed on a regular basis (daily or at least not less than four times/week) has been shown to improve blood glucose control, reduce insulin resistance, induce favourable effects on other cardiovascular risk factors, prevent the incidence of type 2 diabetes and, finally, reduce cardiovascular and total mortality (see Section CD 21.5(a); Table CD 21.1). Therefore, half an hour of brisk walking every day or, at least, four times/week is strongly recommended not only for diabetic patients but for all people. This kind of exercise may be carried out by any diabetic patient without particular precautions. Of course diabetic patients may wish to perform heavier exercises (necessarily aerobic); in these cases some precautions must be taken and some advice should be given (see Table CD 21.2). In type 2 diabetic patients, exercise increases peripheral glucose uptake but decreases insulin secretion; therefore, hypoglycaemia is rare and extra carbohydrate is generally not required. In type 1 diabetic patients, glycaemic changes during exercise depend largely on blood insulin levels and, therefore, on insulin administration. Hyperinsulinaemia may cause

hypoglycaemia, while hypoinsulinaemia, combined with counter-regulatory hormone excess, may lead to hyperglycaemia. The risk of hypoglycaemia may be reduced by consuming 20–40 g extra carbohydrate before and hourly during exercise and/or by reducing pre-exercise insulin dosages (see Table CD 21.3).

Oral hypoglycaemic agents

When optimal blood glucose control (glycated haemoglobin, HbA_{1c} <7.0%, fasting and pre-meal blood glucose 80–120 mg/dl; 2-hour postprandial blood glucose 100–140 mg/dl) is not achieved in type 2 diabetic patients by non-pharmacological approaches (nutritional management + physical exercise), oral hypoglycaemic drugs should be added, if specific contraindications are not present (see Section CD 21.5(b)). Drugs commonly used in the treatment of diabetes are listed in Table CD 21.4. Following the results of the UK Prospective Diabetes Study (UKPDS), showing that metformin significantly reduces cardiovascular risk in overweight type 2 diabetic patients, metformin is considered the first choice drug in the treatment of overweight diabetic patients. Therapy with metformin is also useful in these patients because of the weight loss that is generally associated with use of this drug (2–3 kg). Indications for the use of other drugs are based more on a pathophysiological basis than on their effects on cardiovascular end-points. A possible flow-chart for the pharmacological treatment of type 2 diabetic patients is shown in Figure CD 21.2: metformin as first choice in overweight patients, sulphonylureas in normal weight patients; if optimal blood glucose control is not achieved with only one drug, the other (sulphonylureas or metformin) should be added; if the target values for blood glucose control are still not reached, bedtime insulin can be added or insulin therapy (3–4 administrations/day) can replace oral drugs. For each of these points α-glucosidase inhibitors, which slow down carbohydrate absorption, may be added.

New hypoglycaemic oral drugs have been introduced in the last few years for the treatment of type 2 diabetic patients. These are: (1) thiazolinediones, which act especially on peripheral insulin action and are therefore useful instead of metformin or in addition to metformin and/or sulphonylureas, in the attempt to further reduce insulin resistance and its associated metabolic abnormalities; (2) glinides (GND) (regaglinide, nateglinide), which increase insulin secretion, especially the first phase, with a very short time of action. These drugs may be useful in place of sulphonylureas when it is necessary to reduce postprandial blood glucose. In the use and choice of oral hypoglycaemic drugs it is important to consider the possibility of side effects, specific for each drug (see Table CD 21.4) and the absolute contraindications (hepatic, renal and heart failure), which are valid for all drugs with some exceptions for α-glucosidase inhibitors and glinides.

Insulin therapy

Insulin therapy is an essential lifesaving drug for type 1 diabetic patients, and can be used also in the treatment of type 2 diabetic patients when non-pharmacological therapy plus oral hypoglycaemic drugs are no longer able to achieve optimal blood glucose control (see Section CD 21.5(c)). The types of insulin available today are generally based on human insulin, produced by DNA recombinant techniques, and, according to their time of action, may be divided into short-, intermediate- and long-acting insulin (see Table CD 21.5). In the last few years other types of modified insulin molecules have been introduced in clinical practice. These are the so-called insulin analogues, one with a very short time of action (lispro, aspart) and the other type with a very long time of action (glargine) (see Table CD 21.5). The first are very rapidly absorbed subcutaneously and therefore are particularly useful in reducing postprandial blood glucose. The second seems able to produce quite stable basal insulin concentrations for up to 24 hours. Insulin therapy must be tailored to the individual patient and adjusted on the basis of blood glucose control. Therefore, there are no strict rules for its dosage and type of administration. However, some schemes of insulin therapy are more commonly utilised than others, the most common being that based on three injections of short-acting insulin before breakfast, lunch and dinner plus an injection of intermediate insulin at bedtime. In place of short-acting insulin, rapid-acting analogues may be used, adding, if necessary, a few units of intermediate insulin before breakfast and lunch. Moreover, long-acting insulin analogues may be used instead of intermediate insulin at bedtime or before dinner. Whatever the type and the scheme of insulin therapy utilised, doctors and patients must always try to reach and maintain optimal blood glucose control (HbA$_{1c}$ < 7%; fasting and pre-meal blood glucose 80–120 mg/dl; postprandial blood glucose 100–140 mg/dl). To achieve this, frequent blood glucose self-monitoring by patients is essential.

⊃ Key points

- ⊃ Diabetes mellitus is a major cause of morbidity and mortality. Its prevalence is increasing all over the world due to increased prevalence of obesity and low levels of physical exercise.

- ⊃ Type 1 diabetes is characterised by severe insulinopenia and absolute need of exogenous insulin to prevent ketoacidosis and death.

- ⊃ Type 2 diabetes is frequently associated with obesity. Pathogenic mechanisms are: a defect in beta-cell function and a decrease in insulin action at the level of peripheral tissues (insulin resistance).

- ⊃ The incidence of diabetes can be reduced by about 60% through lifestyle modifications, such as weight reduction, increased physical activity, and reduced saturated fat consumption.

- ⊃ Microangiopathic complications can be prevented or delayed by good glycaemic control.

- ⊃ Cardiovascular complications can be reduced by about 50% through multifactorial treatment of the major cardiovascular risk factors.

References and further reading

References

Bottazzo G F, Bonifacio E 1991 Immune factors in the pathogenesis of insulin-dependent diabetes mellitus. In: Pickup J, Williams G (eds) Textbook of diabetes. Blackwell Scientific Publications, Oxford

De Fronzo R A 1997 Pathogenesis of type 2 diabetes: metabolic and molecular implications for identifying diabetes genes. Diabetes Reviews 5(3):177–269

Diabetes Prevention Program Research Group 2002 Reduction in the incidence of type 2 diabetes with lifestyle intervention or metformin. New England Journal of Medicine 346:393–403

Expert Panel on Detection, Evaluation, and Treatment of High Blood Cholesterol in Adults 2001 Executive Summary of the Third Report on the National Cholesterol Education Program (NCEP). JAMA 285:2486–497

Gaede P, Vedel P, Larsen N et al 2003 Multifactorial intervention and cardiovascular disease in patients with type 2 diabetes. New England Journal of Medicine 348:383–393

Kahn S E 1996 Regulation of beta-cell function in vivo: from health to disease. Diabetes Reviews 4(4):372–389

Reaven G M 1988 Role of insulin resistance in human disease. Diabetes 37:1595–1607

Riccardi G, Rivellese A A 1999 Diabetes nutrition in pre-vention and management. Nutrition, Metabolism and Cardiovascular Diseases: NMCD 9(4; suppl):33–36

Tuomilehto J, Lindstrom J, Eriksson J G et al 2001 Prevention of type 2 diabetes by changes in lifestyle among subjects with impaired glucose tolerance. New England Journal of Medicine 344:1343–1350

Walker J D, Viberti G C 1991 Pathophysiology of microvascular disease: an overview. In: Pickup J, Williams G (eds) Textbook of diabetes. Blackwell Scientific Publications, Oxford

Weyer C, Bogardus C. Mott D M, Pratley R E 1999 The natural history of insulin secretory dysfunction and insulin resistance in the pathogenesis of type 2 diabetes mellitus. Journal of Clinical Investigation 104:787–794

WHO 1999 Definition, diagnosis and classification of diabetes mellitus and its complications: report of a WHO consultation. World Health Organization, Geneva

Vaccaro O, Ruffa G, Imperatore G et al 1999 Risk of diabetes in the new diagnostic category of impaired fasting glucose. Diabetes Care 22:1490–1493

Further reading

Flechter G F, Balady G, Amsterdam E A et al 2001 Exercise standards for testing and training: a statement for health care professionals from the American Heart Association. Circulation 104:1694–1740

Riccardi G, Rivellese A, Williams C 2003 The cardiovas-cular system in nutrition and metabolism. In: Gibney M J, Macdonald I A, Roche H M (eds) Nutrition and metabolism. The Nutrition Society Textbook Series, Blackwell Publishing, Oxford

Tanasescu M, Leitzmann M F, Rimm E B et al 2003 Physical activity in relation to cardiovascular disease and total mortality among men with type 2 diabetes. Circulation 107:2435–2439

CD-ROM contents

Expanded material
Section CD 21.5(a) Physical exercise
Section CD 21.5(b) Oral hypoglycaemic agents
Section CD 21.5(c) Insulin therapy

Tables
Table CD 21.1 Exercise and diabetes
Table CD 21.2 Recommendations for physical exercise in diabetic patients

Table CD 21.3 Guidelines for exercise in type 1 diabetes
Table CD 21.4 Main oral hypoglycaemic drugs
Table CD 21.5 Different types of insulin

Figures
Figure CD 21.1 A possible pathogenic pathway of diabetic microangiopathy
Figure CD 21.2 Treatment of type 2 diabetic patients

Further reading from the book

22

Cancers

Timothy J. Key

22.3 PATHOPHYSIOLOGY OF CANCER

Most cancers develop from a single cell that grows and divides more than it should, resulting in the formation of a tumour (growth) or cancer. Cancers growing in most tissues take the form of a lump that grows, invades local non-cancerous tissues, and may spread to other parts of the body through the bloodstream. Cancers arising in the cells of the blood, such as leukaemia, do not form a lump because the cells are floating freely throughout the bloodstream.

The change from a normal cell into a cancer, termed carcinogenesis, is a multistage process. Cancers represent a form of dedifferentiation that is associated with the loss of growth control and disturbances in the regulation of the cell cycle. The fundamental changes that determine carcinogenesis are mostly alterations (mutations) in the DNA; therefore cancer can be viewed as a genetic disease at the level of somatic cells. Typically the change from a normal cell to a cancer requires mutations in a few different genes, perhaps five to ten (Stewart & Kleihues 2003). Mutations in many different genes can result in cancer, but certain genes are especially important and are very frequently involved; in particular, cancer usually results from changes in the function of genes that control cell division (mitosis) and cell death (apoptosis). The key genes in carcinogenesis can be considered in two classes: oncogenes, genes that when over-activated lead to over-stimulation of cell growth and cell division; and tumour suppressor genes, which normally control (i.e. limit) the rate of cell division but, if inactivated by a mutation, allow uncontrolled cell division.

The genetic mutations that result in an originally normal cell giving rise to a cancer can result from various causes. Some mutations are inherited, while others are caused during the lifetime of an individual by factors such as replication errors, ionising radiation, chemical carcinogens, viruses, and endogenous damage due for example to intracellular oxidants. The development of cells containing mutations into a new cancer is strongly influenced by various growth-promoting agents, especially hormones.

Chance plays an important role in determining the occurrence of cancer. In very simplified terms, if mutations in several important genes occur in several different cells then the behaviour of all these cells could well remain normal, but if the same mutations all occur together within one cell, then this individual cell could give rise to a cancer. The reality is certainly much more complex than this theoretical illustration, but the principle holds that chance is an important factor in carcinogenesis. Chance, however, plays no role in determining the cancer rates of populations (Doll and Peto 2003).

The process of carcinogenesis in humans usually extends over many years or even decades. Individuals who inherit a mutation in a key gene could be regarded as being born with the first step of carcinogenesis already present in all their cells. Mutations in cells accumulate throughout life, from in utero life to old age.

Most deaths due to cancer are caused by the spread of the cancer from its site of origin into adjacent areas and to other parts of the body. The transfer of the cancer from one site to another site not directly connected with it is called metastasis.

22.4 INHERITED GENETIC FACTORS IN CARCINOGENESIS

At the cellular level, cancer is a genetic disease, as discussed in the previous section. Genetic factors are also involved in the determination of whether or not individuals develop cancer, but the importance of this role of genetic factors has sometimes been exaggerated. For the common types of cancer, current estimates are that inherited genetic factors contribute to around 5% or less of the cases of cancer arising in a population (Stewart & Kleihues 2003). Inherited genetic factors (as opposed to mutations in genes that can occur during a person's lifetime) can be considered in two classes: high risk mutations, and low risk genetic polymorphisms.

High risk mutations

Inherited high risk mutations confer a high risk for developing cancer, perhaps 10 to 50 times higher than the risk in individuals who do not have the mutation. The prevalence of these mutations, however, is low, generally around 1 in 1000 or less (Stewart & Kleihues 2003). As a consequence of the high risk conferred, these mutations cause clusters of cancers within families of closely related individuals that can be readily recognised by the medical profession and then studied by genetic epidemiologists. Well-known examples of genes which when mutated confer a high risk for common cancers are HNPCC (hereditary non-polyposis colon cancer gene) that gives a high risk for colon cancer, and BRCA1 and BRCA2 that give high risks for both breast and ovarian cancer. At present, there is no strong evidence that dietary factors can modulate the effects of genes such as these on cancer risk.

Low risk polymorphisms

Low risk genetic polymorphisms are variations in genes that are termed polymorphisms (rather than mutations) because they occur at a prevalence of more than 1% in a population. Such polymorphisms appear to confer a risk of cancer only moderately higher (around 20% to 50%) than the risk in individuals with the 'wild type' allele. Since the increase in risk is small to moderate, this class of genetic factor does not cause obvious clustering of disease in families, and can only be identified by analytical epidemiological studies that compare the prevalence of a particular allele in individuals affected by cancer with the prevalence in unaffected controls. In fact, despite considerable interest and research activity in this area in the last decade, establishing relationships between genetic polymorphisms and cancer risk has proved difficult, with many false-positive reports from small studies, and few definite findings. However, polymorphisms remain of great interest and potential importance, because, although they may only cause a moderate increase in the risk for an individual, their high frequency in populations means that they could contribute to an important proportion of cancer cases. Furthermore, the proposed mechanism of effect for many putative low risk polymorphisms is that they may modify the impact of environmental factors such as diet on cancer risk, for example by affecting the rate of detoxification or activation of mutagenic chemicals present in some foods.

22.5 NON-DIETARY CAUSES OF CANCER

The proportions of cancer due to avoidable causes have been estimated by Doll and Peto (Doll & Peto 2003; see Table CD 22.2). These estimates apply to Western countries such as the USA or the UK; in developing countries the overall ranking of factors would be broadly similar, but the proportion of cancer due to infective factors would be higher and therefore some of the other factors correspondingly lower, due particularly to much higher rates of cancers of the liver (caused by hepatitis B virus and hepatitis C virus) and cervix (caused by human papillomavirus).

countries. The most important numerically are cancer of the liver (hepatitis B virus and hepatitis C virus), cancer of the cervix (human papillomavirus), and stomach cancer (*Helicobacter pylori*). In some parts of the world parasites are important causes of cancer; for example, major causes of liver cancer (cholangiosarcoma) in China, Thailand and other parts of Asia are the liver flukes *Clonorchis sinensis* and *Opisthorchis viverrini*, and a major cause of bladder cancer in Egypt and Tanzania is the trematode worm *Schistosoma haematobium*.

Tobacco

Worldwide, the most important preventable cause of cancer is tobacco, which causes approximately 30% of cancers in Western countries. Tobacco causes cancers of the mouth, pharynx, oesophagus, larynx, lung, pancreas, kidney (pelvis) and bladder.

Infections

Infectious agents are responsible for about 9% of cancers worldwide, with the proportion being higher in developing countries and lower in developed

Hormonal and reproductive factors

Hormonal and reproductive factors are important determinants of three types of cancer in women, cancers of the breast, ovary and endometrium (lining of the womb). Childbirth reduces the risk for all three of these cancers; the mechanism of this protective effect varies by cancer site, and is probably due to inducing terminal differentiation of the epithelial cells in the breasts, by stopping ovulation in the ovaries, and by stopping cell division in the susceptible cells in the endometrium. Hormonal factors may also be important in the aetiology of cancers of the

diet-related factors may account for up to 80% of the between-country differences in rates. The best established dietary-related risk factor is overweight/obesity. Alcohol probably causes a small increase in risk. Adult height, which is partly determined by the adequacy of nutrition in childhood and adolescence, is weakly positively associated with increased risk, and physical activity has been consistently associated with a reduced risk. These factors together, however, do not explain the large variation between populations, and there is almost universal agreement that some aspects of a Western diet are a major determinant of risk. These include the following:

Meat

International correlation studies show a strong association between per capita consumption of meat and colorectal cancer mortality, and several mechanisms have been proposed through which meat may increase cancer risk. Mutagenic heterocyclic amines and polycyclic aromatic hydrocarbons can be formed during the cooking of meat at high temperatures, and nitrites and related compounds found in smoked, salted and some processed meat products may be converted to carcinogenic N-nitroso compounds in the colon. In addition, high iron levels in the colon may increase the formation of mutagenic free radicals. The results of observational studies of meat and colorectal cancer have varied; a recent systematic review concluded that preserved meat is associated with an increased risk for colorectal cancer but that fresh meat is not, and most studies have not observed positive associations with poultry or fish. However, mortality rates for colorectal cancer are similar in Western vegetarians and comparable non-vegetarians. Overall, the evidence is not conclusive but suggests that high consumption of preserved and red meat probably increases the risk for colorectal cancer (Department of Health 1998).

Fat

As with meat, international correlation studies show a strong association between per capita consumption of fat and colorectal cancer mortality. Possible mechanisms proposed to explain such an association are that a high fat intake may increase the level of potentially mutagenic secondary bile acids in the lumen of the large intestine. However, the results of observational studies of fat and colorectal cancer have, overall, not been supportive of an association

with fat intake, especially after adjusting for total energy intake.

Fruit, vegetables and fibre

Burkitt suggested in the 1970s that the low rates of colorectal cancer in Africa were due to the high consumption of dietary fibre, and there are several plausible mechanisms for a protective effect, as described above in 'Dietary fibre and bowel function'. Many case-control studies of colorectal cancer have observed moderately lower risk in association with high consumption of dietary fibre, and/or fruits and vegetables, but the results of recent large prospective studies have been inconsistent. Furthermore, results from randomised controlled trials have not shown that intervention over a 3- to 4-year period with supplemental fibre or a diet low in fat and high in fibre and fruit and vegetables can reduce the recurrence of colorectal adenomas. It is possible that some of the inconsistencies are due to differences between studies in the types of fibre eaten and in the methods for classifying fibre in food tables. Other possibilities are that the association with fruits and vegetables is principally due to an increase in risk at very low levels of consumption, or that high intakes of refined flour or sugar (rather than low intakes of fibre) increase risk through chronic hyperinsulinaemia or other mechanisms. At present, the hypothesis that fruit, vegetables and fibre may reduce the risk for colorectal cancer has not been firmly established.

Folate

Some recent prospective studies have suggested that a diet low in folate is associated with an increased risk of colon cancer; there is also some evidence that this increased risk associated with low folate intake is exacerbated by a high alcohol intake. Also, use of folic acid-containing multiple vitamin supplements has been associated with lower risk of colon cancer. A diminished folate status may contribute to carcinogenesis by alteration of gene expression and increased DNA damage and chromosome breakage. The finding that a common polymorphism in a key gene involved in folic acid metabolism (methylene tetrahydrofolate reductase) may also be associated with colorectal cancer strengthens the hypothesis that dietary folate may be an important factor in colorectal carcinogenesis, but the details of these associations are complex and not yet well understood (see Section CD 22.6(c)).

Calcium and vitamin D

Another promising hypothesis is that relatively high intakes of calcium may reduce the risk for colorectal cancer, perhaps by forming complexes with secondary bile acids and haem in the intestinal lumen and thus inhibiting their damaging effects on the epithelium. Several observational studies have supported this hypothesis, and two trials have suggested that supplemental calcium may have a modest protective effect on the recurrence of colorectal adenomas. There is also some evidence that relatively high blood levels of vitamin D may reduce the risk for colorectal cancer, and may perhaps augment a protective role of calcium. More data are needed to evaluate this hypothesis.

Cancer of the liver

Liver cancer was estimated to account for 564 000 cases and 549 000 deaths in 2000, worldwide. Approximately 75% of cases of liver cancer occur in developing countries, and liver cancer rates vary over 20-fold between countries, being much higher in sub-Saharan Africa and Southeast Asia than in Europe and North America. The major risk factor for hepatocellular carcinoma, the main type of liver cancer, is chronic infection with hepatitis B, and to a lesser extent, hepatitis C virus. Ingestion of foods contaminated with the mycotoxin aflatoxin is an important risk factor among people in developing countries with active hepatitis virus infection. Excessive alcohol consumption is the main diet-related risk factor for liver cancer in Western countries, probably via the development of cirrhosis and alcoholic hepatitis (Tomatis et al 1990, Doll & Peto 2003). Little is known about possible nutritional cofactors for viral carcinogenesis, but this may be an important area for research.

Cancer of the pancreas

Cancer of the pancreas was estimated to account for 216 000 cases and 214 000 deaths in 2000 and is more common in Western countries than in developing countries. Time trends suggest that both incidence and mortality for cancer of the pancreas are increasing in most parts of the world, although some of this apparent increase may be due to improvements in diagnostic methods. Overweight/obesity possibly increases the risk. Some studies have suggested that risk is increased by high intakes of meat, and reduced by high intakes of vegetables, but these data are not consistent and come mostly from case-control studies. Over the next few years there will be substantially more prospective data on diet and cancer of the pancreas from studies such as EPIC (see Section CD 22.6(a)), and it is possible that more clear-cut associations with dietary factors will emerge.

Lung cancer

Lung cancer is the most common cancer in the world and was estimated to account for 1 239 000 cases and 1 103 000 deaths in 2000. Heavy smoking increases the risk by around 30-fold, and smoking causes over 80% of lung cancers in Western countries. The possibility that diet might also have an effect on lung cancer risk was raised in the 1970s following the observation that, after allowing for smoking, increased lung cancer risk was associated with a low dietary intake of vitamin A. Since then, numerous observational studies have found that lung cancer patients generally report a lower intake of fruits, vegetables and related nutrients (such as β-carotene) than controls. The only one of these factors to have been tested in controlled trials, namely β-carotene, has, however, failed to produce any benefit when given as a supplement for up to 12 years.

The possible effect of diet on lung cancer risk remains controversial. Several recent observational studies have continued to observe an association of fruits and vegetables with reduced risk, but this association has been weak in prospective studies. This apparent relationship may be partly due to residual confounding by smoking, since smokers generally consume less fruit and vegetables than non-smokers, but there might also be some protective effect of these foods. In public health terms, however, the overriding priority is to reduce the prevalence of smoking.

Breast cancer

Breast cancer is the second most common cancer in the world and the most common cancer among women. Breast cancer was estimated to account for 1 105 000 cases and 373 000 deaths in women in 2000. Incidence rates are about five times higher in Western countries than in less developed countries and Japan. Much of this international variation is due to differences in established reproductive risk factors such as age at menarche, parity and age at birth, and breastfeeding, but differences in dietary habits and physical activity may also contribute. In fact, age at menarche is partly determined by dietary factors, in that restricted dietary intake during childhood and adolescence leads to delayed menarche. Adult height, also, is weakly positively associated with risk, and is partly determined by dietary factors

accompanied by abdominal pain, steatorrhoea, blood loss and dehydration. Adult disease may also present with more subtle and variable symptoms such as anaemia, bone disease, neurological abnormalities and abnormal liver function. As stated previously, latent and silent cases of coeliac disease show no symptoms whatsoever. A suspicion of coeliac disease may be confirmed by the presence of serum antibodies to gliadin, endomysium or transglutaminase. However, definitive diagnosis demands a jejunal biopsy confirming total or partial villous atrophy. The biopsy should be repeated after 6 months on a gluten-free diet to confirm histological improvement.

Aetiology

The cause of coeliac disease was unknown until 1950 when the Dutch paediatrician Dicke reported significant improvement of symptoms in patients with the condition during war time famine in the Netherlands, when supplies of wheat were scarce. He identified the toxic fraction in wheat as gluten. Gluten is the insoluble mass that remains when wheat dough is washed to remove starch granules and other soluble constituents. The major protein fractions of gluten are gliadin and glutenin and all forms of gliadin have been shown to be toxic to coeliac patients. It is believed that a small bowel mucosal enzyme, tissue transglutaminase (tTG), is important in modifying peptides derived from gliadin so that they become capable of forming autoantibodies.

Genetic factors are important in the pathogenesis of coeliac disease and it has now been shown that subjects who have human leukocyte antigen (HLA) DQ2 or DQ8 are at much greater risk of developing the disease. More than 95% of patients with coeliac disease share one or other haplotype. The physical role of the HLA system is to present peptide fragments of antigens to T-cells. A 33 amino acid peptide derived from gliadin has been shown to be remarkably stable and found in foods toxic to coeliac patients, including wheat, barley and rye, but not in oats, rice and maize. It is an excellent substrate for tTG and the deamidated peptide had a much higher affinity for DQ2. When incubated with T-cells from coeliac patients it caused a marked increase in lymphocyte proliferation. This might lead to release of cytokines from leukocytes and mucosal damage. Thus an autoantibody is formed by the action of tTG on gliadin and coeliac disease is associated with other autoimmune disorders including type 1 diabetes, thyroid disease, rheumatoid arthritis and dermatitis herpetiformis. This is important because certain cases of coeliac disease may only be diagnosed by the appearance of the other autoimmune conditions; in addition, many believe that a gluten-free diet improves the control of the associated disease.

Nutrition

As a result of damage to the gastrointestinal mucosa there is reduced production of digestive enzymes and subsequent reduction in digestive capability. Secondary to intestinal villous atrophy there may be significant reduction of mucosal surface area, causing malabsorption of macro- and micronutrients. Nutritional deficiencies will depend on the length and severity of small intestine affected. Iron deficiency anaemia is common. The duodenum is the primary absorption site for iron and the region in which lesions occur. Albumin concentrations may be reduced secondary to leakage into the gastrointestinal lumen. In cases where there is prolonged severe diarrhoea, levels of serum sodium and potassium may be decreased. Malabsorption severe enough to cause steatorrhoea may impair calcium and fat-soluble vitamin absorption by binding unabsorbed fats to form insoluble soap complexes. Calcium absorption may also be reduced by defective calcium transport mechanisms. Low bone mineral density and osteoporosis are subsequently common chronic features of the disease. Low serum folate concentrations are frequent in untreated disease, but are not usually severe enough to cause a megaloblastic anaemia, although this may be associated with elevated plasma homocysteine, which is itself a risk factor for cardiovascular disease. B_{12} deficiency is not as common, but may develop secondary to folate deficiency or if the disease affects the distal ileal mucosa. Increased loss of endogenous zinc may occur irrespective of disease severity. Serum copper concentrations may also be affected. Improvement of nutritional status may require adjunctive therapy in severe cases. In less severe presentations significant improvement may be achieved following introduction of a gluten-free diet and may not require replacement therapies.

The treatment of coeliac disease is the exclusion of gluten from the diet. The avoidance of gluten in the diet has traditionally required the strict exclusion of the prolamins in wheat (gliadin), barley (hordein), rye (secalin) and oats (avenin). The toxicity of avenin is now considered controversial.

Recent research suggests that it may not be as toxic as previously thought, as it occurs in much lower concentrations than the other prolamins present in wheat, barley and rye. Sources of gluten may be obvious or hidden in manufactured products, making the diet difficult to follow (see Table CD 23.1). Ingredients listed on manufactured products cannot guarantee that a food is gluten-free and therefore safe to eat. The charity Coeliac UK (see Useful web links on the CD-ROM for links to international societies) produces a regularly updated list of manufactured foods that are guaranteed gluten-free. Their medical advisory council has produced guidelines for professionals on inclusion of oats in the gluten-free diet, advising that up to 50 g of oats, uncontaminated by wheat, rye or barley, may be consumed daily by coeliac patients without risk, although not in severe cases.

In addition to following a gluten-free diet, the British Society of Gastroenterology and Coeliac UK suggest that all patients with coeliac disease should be advised to take 1500 mg of calcium per day, using supplements if required.

Some patients may fail to respond to the gluten-free diet. This may be due to poor compliance or inadvertent inclusion of gluten in the diet. In patients who are successfully avoiding gluten, transglutaminase antibodies become negative. Dietary education with regular input from a dietician is essential in order for the individual to establish and maintain a diet that is gluten-free and nutritionally complete. Complications of undiagnosed coeliac disease or failure to comply with dietary exclusion of gluten increases risk of intestinal lymphoma, carcinoma of the oesophagus or colon, osteoporosis and general malnutrition.

23.4 CROHN'S DISEASE

Pathology

Crohn's disease is a chronic inflammatory disorder of the alimentary tract, characterised by episodes of relapse and remission. It most commonly affects the terminal ileum and colon. Segments of intestine that are affected with inflammation are often separated by apparently normal areas; known as 'skip' lesions, they may occur throughout the length of the bowel. Inflammation may extend through the layers of the gastrointestinal wall (transmural). Ulceration of the mucosal wall with oedema and inflammation of the bowel in between give the mucosal surface the 'cobblestone' appearance that is typical of this disease (Fig. 23.3). Fistulas, abnormal communications between two internal organs, or any part of the gastrointestinal tract and the skin, may arise in areas of the bowel that are severely affected. If the condition is given opportunity to become well established, the bowel wall may thicken and the lumen narrow, predisposing the individual to strictures and intestinal obstruction.

Clinical features

Presentation varies according to the site and the extent of the disease. Symptoms associated with Crohn's disease are abdominal pain, diarrhoea (defined as an increase in the number of stools with a loose or watery consistency which may contain blood), weight loss or in children failure to thrive, fever and lethargy. Other organ systems may also be affected, especially the eyes (iritis), the skin where painful nodules develop on the front of the legs (erythema nodosum) and joints, especially sacroiliac joints, knees and ankles.

Biochemical characteristics include raised inflammatory markers such as C-reactive protein (CRP) or other acute phase proteins and a raised platelet count. Patients become anaemic and albumin concentrations in the blood are reduced. Increased migration of white cells through the bowel wall into the intestinal lumen occurs at sites of active disease where they accumulate in large numbers. If white cells are

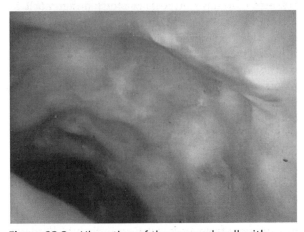

Figure 23.3 Ulceration of the mucosal wall with oedema and inflammation of the bowel in between give the mucosal surface the 'cobblestone' appearance that is typical of this disease.

labelled with radio-isotopes, areas of active disease are clearly identified on scans taken with a gamma camera. This is known as white cell scanning, and the diagnosis may be confirmed by characteristic changes on radiographs with contrast media such as barium or by endoscopy and biopsy.

Aetiology

The aetiology of Crohn's disease is unknown. Both genetic and environmental factors are believed to contribute to the development of the disease. Individuals who have a first degree relative with Crohn's disease have a risk of developing the disease two to three times greater than the rest of the population. Recent research has suggested that genes conferring susceptibility to CD exist on chromosomes 5, 6, 12, 14 and 19. A specific gene, nod 2, has been identified on chromosome 16 and is present in 20% of cases of CD. Intensive research continues in this field.

Environmental factors linked to Crohn's disease include smoking, diet and the oral contraceptive pill (OCP). Smoking increases the risk of CD two- to five-fold, in contrast to ulcerative colitis where it appears to be protective. One study has linked the OCP with the disease, but subsequent studies have not confirmed this.

Prompted by epidemiological evidence, the role of diet in the aetiology of Crohn's disease has been examined carefully. Refined sugar consumption, fat, dietary fibre, fruit and vegetable intake, cereals (cornflakes), 'fast food', margarine and baker's yeast have been investigated. The data are difficult to interpret because of the inconsistency of results and limitations of the methodologies. Aspects of study design such as dietary recall of foods eaten years previously, effect of disease state on appetite and food choice (important in cross-sectional studies), and trial design affect the validity of the research. A number of studies have reported that patients with Crohn's disease consume greater quantities of refined sugar foods than controls, but attempts to link this to the onset of CD is hampered by limitations in study design. In addition, intervention trials have demonstrated that disease activity is not influenced by low sugar diets (Riorden et al 1998).

Fats have also been implicated in the pathogenesis and clinical course of CD. Epidemiological data from Japan show the incidence of CD has increased, displaying a strong correlation with increased fat consumption, and increase in the ratio of n-6 to n-3 fatty acids in the national diet, implicating altered lipid metabolism as a factor (Shoda et al 1996).

Replacement of n-6 arachidonic acid by other polyunsaturated fatty acids derived from the n-3 pathway may reduce prostaglandin and thromboxane production, suppressing inflammation and maintaining immunocompetence.

The role of nutritional factors in the pathogenesis of CD is supported by studies on the importance of the faecal stream. This is composed of gastrointestinal secretions, but also food residues and bacteria. It has been known for many years that diversion of the faecal stream away from the colon by performing an ileostomy allows CD in the lower bowel to heal. Rutgeers and his colleagues in Belgium performed endoscopic examinations of the colon in patients who had been given temporary ileostomies after gastrointestinal resections for CD to allow the anastomosis to heal. No evidence of CD was found in any patient. The ileostomies were then reversed so that the faecal stream returned to the lower bowel. After 6 months, all the patients had endoscopic evidence of Crohn's recurrence.

The beneficial effects which antibiotics frequently produce suggest that the bacteria of the faecal stream are important in CD. Furthermore, there is an immune response to the gastrointestinal bacteria, as in active CD over 80% are coated with immunoglobulin. The equal importance of food residues is suggested by the finding that this coating of bacteria falls back to normal (20%) when patients with CD are fed an enteral feed, containing virtually no fermentable residue, for 2 weeks. Enteral feeds where nitrogen may be presented as either amino acids, oligopeptides or single proteins, are all effective in producing remission in CD, with reduction of pro-inflammatory cytokine mRNA and healing of mucosal ulcers.

Nutrition

Dietary therapy in CD may be used to correct nutritional deficiencies or as primary treatment for the condition.

Nutritional deficiency is a common complication of Crohn's disease, affecting both macro- and micronutrients (see Table CD 23.2). Because of its relapsing and remitting nature, deficiency states may develop insidiously over a number of years, remaining undetected until they are multiple and severe. Although assessment of nutritional status is often made by measuring circulating concentrations of nutrients such values may not reflect long-term dietary intake and therefore data should be interpreted with caution.

Serum concentrations of the fat-soluble vitamins A (retinol), D (calciferol) and K (phylloquinone) are affected by Crohn's disease itself. Serum retinol may be decreased secondary to reduced concentrations of circulating retinol binding protein, a negative acute phase protein. Plasma levels of circulating retinol binding protein fall as part of the acute phase response and therefore low serum retinol concentrations may not be reflective of a deficiency state. Vitamin K produced endogenously by bacteria fermenting non-starch polysaccharides (NSP) in the colon may be reduced because of altered concentrations of gastrointestinal flora arising from antibiotic therapy or extensive large bowel resection. Low serum levels of 25-hydroxycholecalciferol have been reported in 23–75% of inpatients, probably due to malabsorption in Crohn's disease. Vitamin D metabolism and calcium homeostasis are closely linked (see Ch. 24) and many patients with Crohn's disease develop osteoporosis. Various mechanisms are thought to be involved, including reduced dietary intake of calcium, malabsorption and the direct effect of pro-inflammatory cytokines on bone metabolism. However, long-term corticosteroid treatment appears to be the most important. Bone mineral density measurements in patients whose Crohn's disease was treated by diet are reportedly similar to control values and significantly higher than patients who had been treated predominantly with corticosteroids. Thus bone density appears to be affected predominantly by steroid usage and not disease activity. Vitamin C (ascorbic acid) status may fall because of reduced dietary intake or possibly as a direct response to disease activity. Iron deficiency anaemia is a frequent complication in Crohn's disease and may develop secondary to gastrointestinal blood loss, reduced dietary intake and small bowel malabsorption or resection. Serum magnesium levels are kept constant at the expense of body stores, whereas serum zinc may be reduced in the presence of inflammation, reflecting albumin concentrations, despite normal tissue concentrations. Deficiencies of either may arise as a result of persistent diarrhoea, small bowel malabsorption or resection and reduced intakes. Selenium deficiency in CD has been reported in the literature and various potential mechanisms have been proposed including use of corticosteroids and bowel resection. Thus, although some conventional measures of nutrient status would suggest specific deficiencies in patients with CD, there is limited evidence that deficiencies arise through inadequate dietary intake. On the other hand, the pathology of the disease and the associated medication do appear to limit absorption and handling of some nutrients.

Nutrient deficiency may arise by a number of different mechanisms.

Reduced dietary intake

Many patients eat inadequately because they develop anorexia or sitophobia (fear that eating may produce symptoms). Changes in taste may be caused by deficiency of trace elements such as zinc, copper and nickel or as a result of drug therapy. Strictures may cause abdominal pain and vomiting.

Malabsorption

The absorptive area of the small intestine may be considerably reduced as a result of inflammation or following surgery. A fistula may cause a short circuit, reducing the length of gastrointestinal tract available for digestion and absorption. Damage to the ileum frequently reduces absorption of vitamin B_{12}. Loss of the terminal ileum prevents reabsorption of bile salts, whose deficiency may cause malabsorption of fat-soluble vitamins. The small intestine is normally sterile but Crohn's disease may allow colonisation by bacteria, which compete for nutrients.

Intestinal losses

Extensive intestinal ulceration leads to loss of albumin and iron as a result of leakage of blood and plasma from inflamed mucosa. Rapid intestinal transit may lead to loss of fluid and electrolytes and may hamper absorption. Fistulas from the upper intestine to the skin in particular may lead to significant deficiencies of nutrients, fluid and electrolytes.

Increased metabolic requirements

Protein requirements in patients with IBD are usually increased. Inflammation leads to increased production of cytokines, eicosanoids, catecholamines and glucocorticoids which gives rise to a catabolic response producing protein breakdown and negative nitrogen balance. Protein requirement will depend on disease severity; 1–2 g/kg body weight per day may be required to achieve a positive nitrogen balance in comparison with current UK RNI of about 0.8 g/kg/day (see Ch. 8). Current evidence suggests that caloric requirements may only be increased, relative to recommendations for a healthy population, in patients who are less than 90% of ideal body weight.

Drug–nutrient interactions

Corticosteroids are commonly used in the treatment of active Crohn's disease. Steroids reduce calcium absorption and increase its urinary excretion.

Sulfasalazine causes competitive inhibition of folate absorption and cholestyramine binds many nutrients in the gastrointestinal tract, especially fat-soluble vitamins.

Protein energy malnutrition

Reduced intake, increased metabolism and intestinal losses may cause protein energy malnutrition (PEM) in the acute phase of the disease. A reduced serum level of the protein albumin (hypoalbuminaemia) is common but should be used as a marker of disease activity rather than a measure of nutritional status, for which determination of pre-albumin is more suitable. Low albumin may be a result of the inflammatory response on the acute phase plasma proteins as well as increased intestinal losses.

The role of diet as a primary treatment

The role of diet in CD is not only to correct nutritional deficiencies. Dietary therapy may also be used as a primary treatment although its use remains controversial. However, comparisons show that the remission rate with elemental diet in compliant patients is equal to that achieved with corticosteroids (Kelly et al 1989). Up to 20% of patients are unable to comply with enteral feeds. This is unfortunate because the side effects of dietary therapy are much less serious than those for steroid use.

The first stage of diet therapy involves the use of enteral feeding to achieve remission, which may be successful in up to 85% of compliant patients. The second stage involves the maintenance of remission. There is still disagreement as to whether a second stage involving dietary manipulation to detect food intolerances is necessary.

Elemental diet (ED) is a liquid containing a mixture of essential and non-essential amino acids, glucose, lipid, vitamins, minerals and trace elements. Other liquid diets shown to induce remission in Crohn's disease are semi-elemental (peptide based) and polymeric diets (PD). Polymeric diets are whole protein feeds. Trial results of these feeds indicate varying degrees of success. Several advantages of PD over ED include palatability, cost, lower osmolarity, which reduces the incidence of diarrhoea, and greater concentration of energy per millilitre; however, these may be outweighed by the effectiveness of ED in achieving remission.

The efficacy of enteral diets may be influenced by duration of treatment and formula concentration. The mode of action of enteral feeds as a primary therapy remains unclear. Hypotheses include reduced antigenicity of the diet, immunomodulatory effects, improvement of nutritional status and alteration of intestinal microbial flora. As yet no consensus has been reached and this remains a focal point for ongoing clinical trials.

Once remission is achieved there are a number of methods used in clinical practice to insure against further relapse. Although this remains a controversial area, there is a general consensus that remission durations are disappointingly short if normal diet is resumed as soon as symptoms have cleared. Many paediatricians use enteral feeds for extended duration of up to 3 months and claim patients may subsequently return to a normal diet. Other authorities advise a search for food intolerance once remission is achieved. A low fibre, fat-limited exclusion diet (LOFFLEX) has been developed for use in Crohn's patients by the gastroenterology research unit at Addenbrooke's Hospital, Cambridge. The LOFFLEX diet is used as an alternative to elimination diets, which are time-consuming, complicated and require considerable patient motivation. Developed from data gathered from patients completing the elimination diet, the core diet excludes foods that are most likely to cause symptoms. During the food reintroduction phase patients are able to identify and exclude foods that may trigger symptoms, ensuring remission is maintained. A comparison of the elimination diet with the LOFFLEX diet showed no significant difference in length of remission at 2 years in compliant, non-strictured patients with CD. The percentage of patients still in remission at 2 years was 59.4% and 55.6%, respectively. Two-year remission rates following steroid treatment only were 31–35%. Other maintenance diets have been suggested by various centres but these have not yet been scientifically validated.

23.5 ULCERATIVE COLITIS

Pathology

Ulcerative colitis (UC) is an inflammatory disease that affects the mucosa of the colon starting from the anus and extending proximally. Mild cases may affect merely the rectum (proctitis) but commonly inflammation extends as far as the splenic flexure of the large intestine (left sided colitis) and severe disease may affect the whole colon (pancolitis). Unlike Crohn's disease, UC does not affect the small intestine.

The biochemical characteristics are similar to those of CD. However, if inflammation is limited to the rectum, a rise in C-reactive protein is unusual, unless particularly severe.

Clinical features

The characteristic symptoms of UC are diarrhoea and rectal bleeding with the passage of mucus. Blood loss may lead to anaemia and hypoalbuminaemia, which may be severe enough to cause peripheral oedema. Abdominal pain is common and is usually worse after meals. Anorexia leads to weight loss. Severe diarrhoea may cause loss of water and electrolytes, leading to dehydration, hypomagnesaemia and hypocalcaemia. The development of megacolon, dilatation of the large intestine with thinning of the gastrointestinal wall and a high risk of perforation, is a medical emergency requiring surgery. As in Crohn's disease drugs used in the treatment of UC may also contribute to nutritional deficiency.

Aetiology

The cause of UC is not known. Although its onset often appears to follow gastroenteritis, no specific pathogen has yet been discovered. In contrast to normal individuals, the bacterial flora of the colon in patients with UC is highly unstable and may vary considerably over short periods of time. It has been reported that in UC a higher percentage of bacteria in the colon are coated with immunoglobulin than in normal controls and it has been suggested that mucosal inflammation may arise from an immune reaction to the resident colonic microflora. As in Crohn's disease, there is a strong familial tendency but so far no specific gene has been identified that increases susceptibility to UC.

Butyrate is a short-chain fatty acid which is the main fuel of the colonocyte and is obtained primarily as a result of fermentation in the colonic lumen. It has been suggested that in UC butyrate uptake may be impaired by hydrogen sulphide and mercaptides, compounds produced by bacterial fermentation, which may be found in the bowel in higher concentration in patients with UC. This effect is more marked in colonocytes taken from the distal colon where colitis is more common. Sulphide is produced by sulphate-reducing bacteria, which are present more frequently in UC than in controls. However, there is as yet no evidence that giving supplementary butyrate by enemas helps in UC and the therapeutic value of reducing colonic sulphide by low sulphate diets remains unproven.

The colonic mucosa in UC is inflamed and swollen with an increased blood flow. In more severe cases ulceration arises. Ulcers are initially small and discrete but may coalesce and enlarge, extending more deeply in to the lamina propria. The colonic wall may become completely denuded, increasing the risk of perforation or leading to the dilated bowel known as a megacolon. Healing may result in scarring and stricture formation or the development of inflammatory pseudo-polyps from isolated islands of mucosa. Although long-term UC carries a markedly increased risk of the development of colon cancer, these pseudo-polyps are not premalignant. It is believed that the development of colonic cancer in UC is a consequence of chronic inflammation, rather than the development of adenomatous polyps which may arise in uninflamed bowel.

The pharmacological treatment of UC is similar to that of CD with prednisolone and other corticosteroids being the cornerstone of the management of many cases. In proctitis and left-sided disease these may be given by enema, but systemic administration is necessary in severe cases. Drugs releasing 5-aminosalicylic acid are very helpful and patients who become steroid dependent or resistant may require immunosuppressive agents such as azathioprine.

Nutrition

There is little place for diet as primary therapy. Truelove reported relapse in patients when cow's milk was reintroduced into the diets of patients with UC but a subsequent trial concluded only 20% of patients with UC improve on a milk-free diet and that many of these suffer from unrelated hypolactasia. Enteral feeds may be used to improve nutritional status but unlike Crohn's disease they do not reduce colonic inflammation. Supplementation with omega-3 or omega-6 fatty acids in the hope of reducing inflammation has not proved successful.

23.6 IRRITABLE BOWEL SYNDROME

Pathology and clinical features

The Rome criteria have been established to ensure that the clinical presentation of IBS patients included in research studies is reasonably homogeneous. They include a 3-month history of abdominal pain accompanied by a change in bowel habit, which may be diarrhoea or constipation. Other symptoms include flatulence, bloating, a feeling of incomplete evacuation, urgency, straining and mucus. No abnormality, however, can be found to account for these symptoms after radiology and endoscopy of the gastrointestinal tract and standard haematological and biochemical screening. Stool culture reveals no pathogens. The diagnosis therefore is by negative exclusion of other pathology.

Aetiology

Irritable bowel syndrome (IBS) is the single most common condition referred to gastroenterologists in the Western world. It has been estimated that as many as 15% of Westernised populations suffer from the condition at some time in their lives. This figure also includes fast developing eastern European countries such as Russia. Prevalence in China, including Hong Kong, remains lower and is estimated at 3.6%. The high level of incidence makes it all the more frustrating that it is the least well understood of all gastrointestinal (GI) conditions. Treatment is often ineffective and symptoms may continue for years. Many patients seek treatment from homeopaths and alternative practitioners.

Confusion about IBS is compounded because it is not a single discrete entity but a syndrome made up of several quite separate conditions that may produce abdominal pain with or without a change in bowel habit. The lack of pathological findings has led many authorities to believe IBS is primarily a psychological condition. Approximately 20–25% of IBS patients suffer from an anxiety state. Anxiety in this group of patients may lead to hyperventilation and air swallowing; patients commonly present with pain, bloating and flatulence, which may be accompanied by other anxiety symptoms such as breathlessness, palpitations and dizziness. The Nijmegen questionnaire (see Table CD 23.3) is invaluable in detecting those IBS patients whose symptoms are predominantly caused by anxiety. Depression may also cause

GI symptoms. Abdominal pain may arise from musculoskeletal causes or menstrual disturbances, which need to be distinguished from cases presenting with food intolerant IBS.

Burkitt and Painter proposed that IBS might be the result of insufficient intake of dietary fibre. They demonstrated whole gastrointestinal transit times in native Africans, who rarely suffer IBS, considerably shorter than those encountered in the British population. Fibre can be classified according to its ability to absorb water. Soluble fibre (e.g. pectin, guar, ispaghula) forms a viscous solution accessible to bacterial enzymes which rapidly ferment it with production of gases such as hydrogen and methane and other compounds such as short-chain fatty acids (SCFA). Generally little soluble fibre is recoverable from faeces. Insoluble fibre, e.g. cellulose, can bind water but does not form a solution. It is more resistant to fermentation and is thus excreted in larger amounts, producing a greater laxative effect. The main sources of fibre in the diet are non-starch polysaccharides (NSP) although fibre supplements such as ispaghula, methylcellulose and sterculia are frequently used as laxatives. About 10–20 g of NSP reaches the caecum daily, the rest of the fibre in the diet coming in the form of resistant starch. Most starch in the diet is digested by amylase but 1–5% is resistant, reaches the caecum and is fermented. Starch may be resistant because it is physically inaccessible in grains or seeds, because it is present in resistant granules as in raw banana and potato or following cooking. Cooking may disrupt the crystalline structure (gelatinisation). On cooling the crystals reform (retrogradation), a process which increases resistance to digestion by amylase.

However, there appears to be little discernible difference in the fibre intake of healthy individuals and IBS sufferers. Furthermore, in a review examining the outcome of 13 trials in which fibre was used to supplement the diet of IBS patients, only 1 out of 6 trials using bran reported an improvement in symptoms (Hammonds & Whorwell 1997). Indeed supplements of insoluble fibre, particularly wheat bran, may make IBS worse because they lead to increased fermentation and gas production. Fibre supplements are now generally reserved for cases when IBS is associated with constipation.

Other forms of IBS may involve food intolerance. Twenty-five unselected IBS patients were invited to follow an extremely restricted diet of lamb, rice and pears for 7 days; 21 agreed to do so and 14 reported that gastrointestinal symptoms had satisfactorily cleared. Reintroducing foods back singly, and avoiding any that provoked symptom recurrence, enabled the establishment of diets on which patients gained long-term symptom relief (Parker et al 1995). Double-blind placebo-controlled (DBPC) challenges were performed in 11 and revealed increased prostaglandin E_2 release in the rectum after active challenge. Prostaglandin production correlated significantly with faecal weight.

A number of workers have repeated this work and all have found IBS patients with objectively demonstrable food intolerance. The incidence varied between 10% and 67% and depended on patient selection and the stringency of diets used.

The gastrointestinal tract is continuously exposed to a wide range of foreign bacteria, chemicals and foods, many of which have the capability of acting as antigens and provoking immune responses (see Section 26.7 in Ch. 26). The gastrointestinal immune system is a major factor in the defence of the organism against these agents. Luminal antigens taken up by specialised cells in the Peyer's patches of the small intestine pass to the lymphatic system and stimulate the formation of specific lymphocytes which migrate to reside in the intestinal mucosa. These lymphocytes are of two types, B and T. B-lymphocytes in the gastrointestinal tract produce antibodies which are predominantly immunoglobulins A and M (IgA and IgM). T-helper lymphocytes may be Th1, which are primarily involved in cell-mediated protection against infection, or Th2, which may be involved in producing immunoglobulin E (IgE) – responsible for allergic responses. If the balance between Th1 and Th2 is upset, excessive IgE production may lead to the development of allergies. Genuine IgE-mediated food allergy is relatively uncommon, probably occurring in only 1% of the population. It is now believed that non-IgE-mediated reactions to food may also be clinically important. These may be mediated by many different mechanisms, including direct pharmacological effects (e.g. caffeine, ethanol) and enzyme deficiencies (e.g. alactasia, monoamine oxidase inhibitors). These are referred to as food intolerances rather than food allergies, as no immune mechanism is involved.

No evidence of classical food allergy has been demonstrated in IBS. Serum IgE concentrations in these patients are normal. The radioallergoabsorbent (RAST) test, which measures the amount of specific IgE antibodies in blood to various environmental and food allergens, and skin prick tests, which rely on the presence of circulating IgE antibodies, are therefore of no value in identifying the foods concerned.

In contrast to classical IgE-mediated allergy, where small quantities of allergens provoke symptoms of pain, diarrhoea and vomiting within an hour, food reactions in patients with IBS are provoked by much larger quantities of food and may take several hours or days to begin. This has prompted a search for other mechanisms of food intolerance. Some foods such as coffee, tea and wines may provoke symptoms because of chemicals which they contain such as caffeine and ethanol. This is not true of the vast majority of food intolerances in IBS and it has now been suggested that abnormal colonic fermentation may underlie these reactions.

Prospective studies have shown that the development of IBS is much more likely after bacterial gastroenteritis or a course of antibiotics. The relative risks are 3.9 and 11.9, respectively. These events may damage the colonic flora. It is now known that the colonic flora in IBS contains reduced numbers of *Lactobacillus* and *Bifidobacter* with overgrowth of facultative anaerobic organisms such as *Streptococcus*, *Proteus* and *E. coli,* which although normally requiring oxygen for growth, are able to survive in the colon, where oxygen concentrations are very low. Such a gastrointestinal flora may produce abnormal fermentation of food residues entering the caecum.

A study of fermentation was performed in previously untreated IBS patients and normal controls who were asked to follow a standard British diet for 2 weeks. At the end of that time they spent 24 hours in a purpose-built calorimeter. Hydrogen and methane, both products of bacterial fermentation, were measured in air drawn from the calorimeter and compared to that of the surrounding room. Hydrogen production and the maximum rate of gas production were significantly increased in IBS patients compared to controls. The subjects were then invited to follow a standard exclusion diet which was carefully matched to contain the same amounts of substrates for fermentation as the standard diet and after 2 weeks calorimetry was repeated. Whilst there was no significant change in gas production in controls, hydrogen and maximum gas excretion fell dramatically in the patients, with symptomatic improvement (King et al 1989). Subsequent studies have confirmed increased colonic gas production and when this was reduced by antibiotics or after an enteral feed, symptomatic improvement again followed.

Treatment – nutrition

There is no evidence to suggest that nutritional deficiencies occur as a result of untreated IBS. However, nutrient deficiencies may develop secondary to individuals excluding specific foods or food groups from their diet. Reviews of dietary intakes have identified calcium and vitamin D as commonly occurring deficiencies and this is often secondary to individuals avoiding dairy products. In the case of IBS thorough investigation of the diet is essential to establish if the individual may be at risk of developing a deficiency state.

As there is no single cause of IBS it follows that there is no single treatment. This review will be limited to the value of diet and nutritional supplementation in the management of IBS.

Manipulation of fibre in the diet may provide significant relief to individuals with IBS. The use of a high fibre diet in IBS is limited to treatment of simple constipation. Fibre is an important substrate for fermentation. Reducing the fibre content of the diet to less than 10 g per day may reduce gas production and symptoms in patients who present with diarrhoea, bloating urgency and pain (Woolner & Kirby 2000). In many cases the patient may experience constipation or an alternating bowel habit instead of diarrhoea. The low fibre diet supplemented by a synthetic, non-fermentable fibre provides a diet that can increase stool bulk without the side effects of excess fermentation often experienced with a high fibre diet.

A specific exclusion diet has been developed for the treatment of food-intolerant IBS (Table 23.1). Before any therapeutic dietary manipulation is undertaken a thorough review of eating habits is essential to detect and correct any abnormal eating patterns or food aversions. The core exclusion diet is followed for a period of 2 weeks, for which patients whose symptoms significantly improve may reintroduce a food every 2 days. Foods that have not triggered symptoms may be reintroduced into the diet. Exclusion diet studies at Addenbrooke's Hospital, Cambridge, UK, have shown that approximately 50% of compliant patients respond successfully to the exclusion diet. However, although the exclusion diet may be an extremely successful intervention it is not without problems. Patients may experience symptoms of headache, nausea and fatigue 2–4 days after commencing the diet. Lifestyle implications may mean it is not a realistic treatment option for some.

Approximately 25% of Europeans with symptoms of IBS test positive for lactose intolerance. In a recent study less than 40% of people with IBS who had positive hydrogen breath test for lactose intolerance responded to a low lactose diet. Of those that failed to respond several went on to trial an exclusion diet, identifying milk as a cause of symptoms. It has therefore been suggested that there is little value in treating IBS patients for hypolactasia as many appear to be upset by constituents of cow's milk other than lactose (Parker et al 2001).

As diets are always restrictive and difficult to follow, considerable interest has arisen in the possibility of improving symptoms in IBS by manipulating the gastrointestinal flora. Probiotics are living microorganisms which, when consumed, exert health benefits beyond basic inherent nutrition. It has been suggested that restoring the 'normal' colonic microflora using probiotic supplementation may be an effective method of treating the condition. Unfortunately, because of a phenomenon known as colonisation resistance, it is not easy to change the intestinal

Table 23.1 **Addenbrooke's Hospital exclusion diet for IBS**

Foods not allowed	Foods allowed
Pork and meat products	All other lean meat and poultry
Fish in batter/crumb, fish tinned in oil/tomato	All other types of fish, shellfish
Cow's, sheep's and goat's milk, dairy products, eggs and chocolate	Soya milk and products; soya margarine in moderation
Wheat, rye, barley, corn, oats, yeast	Rice, rice cakes, Rice Krispies, tapioca, sago, arrowroot
Corn oil, vegetable oil	Sunflower, olive oil, etc.; oils in moderation
Pulses, onion, tomato, sweetcorn	Potato and all other vegetables, two portions per day, no skins or seeds
Citrus, apple, banana, dried fruit	All other fruit, two portions per day, no skins or seeds
Tea, coffee, alcohol, squash, cola, etc.	Fruit and herbal teas, tap and mineral water, blackcurrant squash, non-citrus fruit juice
Gravy mixes, salad dressings, etc.	Salt, pepper, herbs and spices
Nuts, seeds	Sugar, jam, honey, mint cake (glucose)

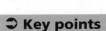

microflora and most probiotic bacteria, like pathogens, disappear rapidly from the gastrointestinal tract when their administration ceases. Although some patients have reported benefit, there is no conclusive evidence that any bacterial preparation thus far available is reliably effective, and further research is needed to clarify the role of probiotics in the treatment of IBS. Similarly, probiotics are now under trial in IBD, and one mixture of eight separate species, VSL-#3, may have value in UC. This field is in its infancy and may develop rapidly. (See Further reading on the CD-ROM for review articles.)

⊃ Key points

- ⊃ Chronic disorders of the intestine are associated with complex interactions between diet, the intestinal microflora and intestinal mucosal immunity.

- ⊃ Diet may be of significant value in modifying intestinal damage and the clinical course of these diseases.

- ⊃ Manipulation of the gastrointestinal flora may provide a future means of treating these disorders.

References and further reading

References

Hammonds R, Whorwell P J 1997 The role of fibre in IBS. International Journal of Gastroenterology March: 9–12

Kelly S M, Thuluvath K, Fotherby J et al 1989 Elemental diet is an effective treatment of acute Crohn's disease. Scandinavian Journal of Gastroenterology 24(Suppl 158):149

King T S, Elia M, Hunter J O 1989 Abnormal colonic fermentation in irritable bowel syndrome. Lancet 352:1187–1189

Parker T J, Naylor S J, Riorden A M et al 1995 Management of patients with food intolerance in irritable bowel syndrome: the development and use of an exclusion diet. Journal of Human Nutrition and Dietetics 8:159–166

Parker T J, Woolner J T, Prevost A T et al 2001 Irritable bowel syndrome: is the search for lactose intolerance justified? European Journal of Gastroenterology and Hepatology 3:219–225

Riorden A M, Ruxton C H S, Hunter J O 1998 A review of associations between Crohn's disease and consumption of sugars. European Journal of Clinical Nutrition 52:229–238

Shoda R, Matsueda K, Yamato S, Umeda N 1996 Epidemiological analysis of Crohn's disease in Japan: increased dietary intake of n-6 polyunsaturated fatty acids and animal protein relates to the increased incidence of Crohn's disease in Japan. American Journal of Clinical Nutrition 63(5):741–745

Woolner J T, Kirby G A 2000 Clinical audit of the effects of low-fibre diet on irritable bowel syndrome. Journal of Human Nutrition and Dietetics 13:249–253

Further reading

Brostoff J, Challacombe S 2002 Food allergy and intolerance, 2nd edn. Saunders, London

Camilleri M, Spiller R 2002 Irritable bowel syndrome diagnosis and treatment. WB Saunders, Edinburgh

Feldman M, Scharschmidt B, Sleisenger M 1998 Sleisenger & Fordtran's Gastrointestinal and liver disease: pathophysiology/diagnosis/management, 6th edn. WB Saunders, London

Forbes A 2001 Inflammatory bowel disease, a clinician's guide. Arnold, London

Gibson P 1997 Baillière's clinical gastroenterology, ulcerative colitis. Vol 11, No 1. Baillière Tindall, London

Howdle P 1995 Baillière's clinical gastroenterology, coeliac disease, Vol 9, No 2. Baillière Tindall, London

Thomas B 2001 Manual of dietetic practice, 3rd edn. Blackwell Science, London

Woolner J T, Kirby G A 1998 The development and evaluation of a diet for maintaining remission in Crohn's disease. Journal of Human Nutrition and Dietetics 11:1–11

CD-ROM contents

Tables

Table CD 23.1 Suitable foods for a gluten free diet
Table CD 23.2 Nutrient deficiencies, deficiency states and mechanisms of occurrence in Crohn's disease

Table CD 23.3 Nijmegen questionnaire

Further reading

Review articles: probiotics

Further reading from the book

Useful web links

24

Nutrition and the skeleton

Margo E. Barker and Aubrey Blumsohn

Objectives

By the end of this chapter you should:
- understand the dynamic nature of skeletal metabolism
- be able to define osteomalacia, rickets and osteoporosis
- be able to discuss the role of vitamin D and calcium nutrition in skeletal health
- appreciate the role of other nutrients in skeletal health.

24.1 INTRODUCTION

Osteoporosis and osteomalacia or rickets are the two main skeletal disorders related to nutrient supply. Of these, osteoporosis has the greatest public health importance in contemporary society. This chapter examines the evidence for the importance of nutritional factors in the pathogenesis of these disorders. Classically, dietary deficiencies of calcium and vitamin D have been implicated as causative in the development of osteoporosis, but recent research has implicated lack of or excess of many other nutrients and food components. Deficiency of vitamin D is the most frequent cause of osteomalacia (adults) and rickets (children).

The chapter begins with a review of bone structure and skeletal remodelling and how bone mineral mass changes throughout the life-course. An understanding of bone physiology is basic to evaluating how diet may impact on skeletal health. An awareness of the strengths and weaknesses of different designs of nutritional studies, and the value of different end-points as indices of skeletal health, is also important in evaluating the role of diet in influencing skeletal health.

24.2 BONE STRUCTURE AND REMODELLING

Bone composition and cells

Although the primary role of the skeleton is to provide mechanical support and protection for internal organs, bone also serves several other functions. The skeleton is involved in the homeostatic regulation of several minerals, plays a role in acid–base homeostasis and serves as an important defence against some toxins such as lead, which can be adsorbed to bone. Bone marrow is involved in haematopoiesis (production of blood cells).

The human adult skeleton weighs approximately 3 to 4 kg and consists of an organic matrix, minerals and bone cells. By weight, bone comprises about 10% water, 60% inorganic material, and 30% organic matrix. The organic matrix consists largely (95%) of a single protein, type I collagen. Other organic components include non-collagenous proteins, lipids and proteoglycans. The mineral phase of bone consists chiefly of calcium, phosphate and carbonate in a crystalline form called hydroxyapatite. Bone also serves as a reservoir for other minerals (Table 24.1). Deficiency or excess of these components in bone may contribute to loss of bone strength and to fractures.

The two main types of bone cells, osteoclasts and osteoblasts, have opposite functions. Osteoclasts are multinucleated cells responsible for bone resorption. These cells attach to the mineralised bone surface and secrete protons and enzymes. Osteoblasts produce bone matrix and are responsible for bone formation. Other cells called osteocytes are found embedded within the bone and may function to regulate changes in bone structure in response to mechanical loading.

Table 24.1 Some important minerals in bone

Element	Total bone content (g)	% bone weight
Calcium	1000	25
Phosphate	400	10
Sodium	200	5
Magnesium	80	2
Zinc	8	0.2
Potassium	4	0.1
Strontium	0.8	0.02
Boron	1.6	0.04
Aluminium	0.8	0.02
Lead	0.4	0.01
Copper	0.08	0.002

Types of bone

The skeleton is composed of two types of bone:

1. Cortical bone (sometimes called compact bone). This dense form of bone comprises about 80% of skeletal mass.
2. Trabecular bone (also called spongy or cancellous bone). This type of bone consists of an intricate structural mesh of trabeculae that form the interior scaffolding of bone. The spaces between the trabeculae and the centres of the bones (marrow cavities) contain red and yellow marrow and other tissue. Red marrow is responsible for the formation of blood cells (haematopoiesis).

Although trabecular bone accounts for only 20% of total bone mass, it accounts for as much as 70% of bone surface area and metabolic activity. Trabecular bone constitutes most of the bone tissue of the axial skeleton (skull, ribs and spine). The ends of long bones also contain a variable proportion of trabecular bone. Regions of the skeleton which contain a high proportion of trabecular bone such as the hip, spine and wrist are most susceptible to fracture in patients with osteoporosis.

Bone remodelling

Bone is a metabolically active tissue. In the adult skeleton most metabolic activity occurs by the process of bone 'remodelling' or bone turnover. This metabolic activity serves to maintain the structure and homeostatic functions of the skeleton. Although the total amount of bone tissue in an adult is relatively static, there is a continuous turnover of bone mineral and organic matrix. About 5–10% of existing bone is replaced through remodelling each year. Remodelling involves a defined sequence of events (Fig. 24.1). The process of bone formation occurs at sites at which bone resorption has recently occurred. This integration between bone formation and bone resorption is termed 'coupling'.

In the long term, a change in bone mineral content reflects an imbalance between the processes of bone formation and resorption. Incomplete refilling of resorption cavities will result in a net loss of bone, and overfilling of these cavities will result in a net gain of bone. In the short term (<1 year) changes in bone mass can arise simply from a change in the rate of remodelling and hence the amount of 'remodelling space' (space taken up by remodelling cycles currently in progress). Therefore, short-term changes

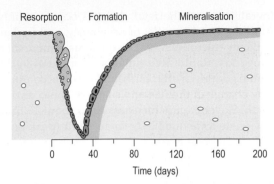

Figure 24.1 Schematic view of bone remodelling. Activated osteoclasts attach themselves to the bone surfaces, and tunnel into the bone. Osteoblasts are attracted to the new cavities and secrete collagen strands (fibrils), which combine to form unmineralised matrix called osteoid. This osteoid is subsequently mineralised.

in bone mass do not necessarily reflect an imbalance between the fundamental rates of bone formation and resorption.

Bone growth and change in bone shape in children occurs by a different mechanism called 'modelling'. In contrast to remodelling, the processes of bone formation and resorption are dissociated in time and space, so that a change in shape or size of the bone can occur.

A variety of so-called 'calciotropic hormones' regulate the process of bone formation and resorption. These include parathyroid hormone (PTH), vitamin D and its metabolites, sex steroids, glucocorticoids, growth hormone, insulin-like growth factors and many more. PTH stimulates bone resorption, but can also stimulate bone formation (anabolic action). Vitamin D metabolites affect bone metabolism directly and indirectly by influencing mineral supply. Sex steroids (oestradiol and testosterone) decrease bone remodelling. The effect of testosterone in men is mediated mainly by peripheral conversion to the female sex steroid, oestradiol. Growth hormone, insulin-like growth factor 1 (IGF-1) and thyroid hormones increase bone remodelling. The predominant effect of glucocorticoids is to inhibit bone formation.

Bone mineral content during growth, ageing, pregnancy and lactation

By 10 weeks of gestation the human fetal skeleton is composed mainly of unmineralised cartilage.

Mineralisation of the fetal skeleton occurs mainly during the last 10 weeks of pregnancy, and by late pregnancy calcium accrual by the fetus is more than 100 mg/day. Rapid accumulation of mineral in the skeleton continues after birth, and this is accompanied by change in the size and shape of bones during growth. Skeletal mass increases from about 100 g in the neonate to about 3000 g in an adult (peak bone mass). Peak bone mass is achieved at about age 35. The rate of change in bone mass increases during puberty, and more than 90% of peak bone mass is achieved by age 18. Bone mineral content declines in the elderly, and is particularly rapid in women after the menopause. It is important that adequate amounts of bone mineral are acquired during growth because that contributes to bone mineral content later in life. Because much of peak bone mass is attained by age 20, children and adolescents are a particularly important target for interventions to increase bone mass.

With ageing, individuals tend to maintain their ranking within the population distribution of bone mineral content. In other words peak bone mass is the most important predictor of bone mineral content in later life. Although some individuals do lose bone faster than others, these differences are less important, although rapid bone loss may be important in some people. After attainment of peak bone mass, there is a gradual loss of bone mineral in both men and women. Bone remodelling increases after the menopause in women and this is associated with accelerated loss of bone mineral. This is caused in large part by a reduced ovarian production of oestradiol. Oestrogen production is also an important determinant of bone mineral loss in older postmenopausal women as well as in men.

Genetic and lifestyle factors influence bone mineral accrual during growth. Lifestyle factors influencing peak bone mass include exercise, calcium intake, general nutritional status, smoking and use of medications such as corticosteroids and some contraceptives. Many studies comparing bone mineral content in members of the same family or in twins have shown that up to 75% of the difference in peak bone mass between individuals might be explained by genetic factors. In general, peak bone mass is greater in Blacks than in Whites. Although interventions such as exercise and calcium supplementation may increase bone mineral accrual during puberty, it is not clear whether these interventions will result in greater bone mineral content in adult life. Genetic factors are likely to be relatively less important as determinants of bone loss with ageing.

Pregnancy and lactation increase calcium requirements, and these demands are met by a combination of increased efficiency of maternal calcium absorption from the diet as well as maternal bone mineral loss. The amount of calcium required by the fetus is relatively small (approximately 30 g) in comparison with the much greater calcium demand imposed by lactation (up to 1 g of calcium per day for milk production). This additional calcium requirement for milk production is largely obtained as a result of skeletal mineral loss. Lumbar spine bone mineral content decreases by about 4% during pregnancy, and decreases progressively during lactation. Despite the substantial short-term impact of pregnancy and lactation on the skeleton, these physiological changes do not appear to have any long-lasting effect on bone mineral content or on later fracture risk.

Bone remodelling and disease

A wide variety of genetic and acquired diseases such as collagen disorders, cancer and infections can influence the skeleton. Other diseases may affect the skeleton by altering the normal regulation of bone remodelling. For example, endocrine disorders may involve excessive or defective secretion of a calciotropic hormone resulting in loss of bone mineral. The two most common diseases affecting the skeleton are (a) osteoporosis, and (b) osteomalacia or rickets due to vitamin D deficiency. Nutrient supply plays a role in the pathogenesis of these disorders.

Disorders which influence intake or gastrointestinal absorption of nutrients (such as anorexia nervosa, coeliac disease and inflammatory bowel disease) may also cause skeletal disease. Low bone mineral content is common in patients with newly diagnosed coeliac disease, and bone mass improves in most patients when started on a gluten-free diet. Although these diseases influence nutritional status, the loss of bone mineral in these disorders is due to many factors in addition to deficient nutrient supply. These factors include drug therapy, immobility, endocrine disturbances and the response to inflammation.

24.3 TYPES OF EVIDENCE LINKING DIET TO SKELETAL HEALTH

Study design

Individual case reports

There are many reports of individual patients or groups of patients who have developed skeletal disease due to markedly excessive or deficient intake of a particular nutrient. For example, individuals with vitamin A toxicity develop hypercalcaemia (elevated concentration of calcium in plasma) and skeletal disease. However, it is usually not possible to conclude from these studies that the nutrient is either harmful or beneficial to the skeleton within the general population. These case reports are, however, of considerable scientific interest and may help to guide further research into the role of the nutrient.

Cross-sectional studies of fracture risk

It is possible to relate the intake of a particular nutrient to fracture risk within the general population. It is also possible to relate a biomarker of nutrient exposure to fracture risk. For example, it has been found that consumption of carbonated beverages is associated with a substantially increased risk of fracture in adolescent girls. There are a number of pitfalls associated with cross-sectional observational studies. Intake of different nutrients may be strongly related to one another, and it may be difficult to be certain that any particular nutrient is important. It is also likely that nutrient intake is strongly related to other lifestyle and social factors such as smoking, exercise and social class. It is also possible that fracture risk could be associated with past intake of the nutrient rather than current intake.

Effect of dietary intervention on fracture incidence

Experimental studies relating a change in intake of a nutrient to fracture incidence provide very strong evidence that the nutrient is of relevance to skeletal health. Ideally such studies require appropriate placebo controls with randomisation to nutrient or placebo. However, placebo-controlled designs may be difficult for some nutrients, and participants may not be blind to the treatment allocation. The nutrient dose is also important. If the magnitude of supplementation is greater than could be achieved by alterations in diet, then the study is pharmacological rather than nutritional.

Unfortunately, because fractures are infrequent, it is necessary to study a large number of people for a long period of time in order to demonstrate an effect where one exists. For example, to demonstrate a 50% reduction in the rate of fracture it may be necessary to study several thousand individuals for several years. Since the effect of individual nutrients may be small, randomised fracture intervention trials are not feasible for most nutrients. When trials are carried out, the results cannot be assumed to apply to individuals who are very different from those studied. For example, nutritional interventions shown to be beneficial in elderly institutionalised women may not be beneficial in younger women or in men.

Surrogate indicators of fracture risk

Because nutrient intervention trials with a fracture end-point are difficult and expensive, much attention has been paid to the use of other 'surrogate' end-points, which might be presumed to relate to fracture risk. These surrogates include bone mineral content, ultrasound properties of bone, structural analysis of bone using other imaging techniques, and biochemical assessment of bone remodelling.

Bone densitometry

Bone mineral content (BMC) or bone mineral density (BMD) can be assessed by measuring the attenuation of X-rays by a skeletal region of interest. By using two different energies of X-ray beam it is possible to distinguish between X-ray attenuation due to fat, lean tissue or bone (dual energy X-ray absorptiometry, DEXA). The precision of DEXA (reproducibility typically about 2%) is poor in comparison with the rate of change in bone mineral content in response to an intervention. It is therefore necessary to study the response to intervention for at least one year, but preferably for several years in many individuals.

Bone mineral density measured by DEXA is strongly related to fracture risk. However, there are substantial pitfalls associated with reliance on bone densitometry in studies with nutrients or other therapies. Change in body weight can cause spurious underestimation or overestimation of BMD depending on the instrument used. This may confound nutritional studies. Other pitfalls have been brought to light by examination of change in BMD with drugs designed to prevent fracture. Several recent studies have drawn attention to the fact that change in BMD with antiresorptive drug therapy (such as bisphosphonates or oestrogen replacement therapy) explains less than a quarter of therapeutic fracture risk reduction. Many other factors (such as change in bone remodelling) explain the fracture benefit of these drugs. Other supportive evidence is therefore required, and bone densitometry cannot serve as a sole surrogate for fracture risk.

Other techniques for assessing bone structure

Several enhanced radiographic techniques may add to information provided by traditional densitometry. These include ultrasound assessment (generally at the heel), radiographic 'texture' analysis of bone or quantitative tomography. It is even possible to assess fracture risk using detailed mathematical analysis of three-dimensional computer reconstruction of whole bones from individual patients. These techniques are likely to be of increasing importance.

Measurement of bone remodelling

The rate of bone formation and resorption can be assessed using several techniques including quantitative histology, radiotracer kinetics and measurement of biochemical markers in blood or urine. Most markers reflect the synthesis or degradation of bone collagen. Differences in the rate of bone remodelling between individuals might be related to fracture risk, although these relationships are weak. However, the change in bone remodelling following bisphosphonate drug therapy in adults is more predictive of the reduction in fracture risk than is the change in bone mineral density. The time-course of fracture risk reduction following these treatments is also similar to the time-course of change in bone remodelling, and not to change in bone density. Whether these principles apply to nutritional interventions, or to other populations (such as children) is uncertain. However, there is reason to question the use of bone densitometry as a sole surrogate of fracture risk in nutritional studies.

24.4 OSTEOPOROSIS, OSTEOMALACIA AND RICKETS

The epidemiology of skeletal fracture

Fractures are most common in children and in the very elderly. Fractures in children involve mainly long bones, tend to be more common in males than in females, and are only weakly associated with bone mineral content. By contrast, osteoporotic fractures in the elderly classically occur in bones which have a high proportion of trabecular bone (the wrist, hip and spine), are more common in women, and are strongly associated with low bone mineral content. The healthcare costs and morbidity associated with these fractures is substantial. The rate of osteoporotic fracture increases with age. About 30% of women and about 10% of men will experience an osteoporotic fracture at some point in their lifetimes.

The lifetime risk of hip fracture in North America and Europe is approximately 15%. The incidence of hip fracture differs substantially between countries for reasons that are not fully explained. X-ray screening studies of populations in these countries have shown that about 15% of women between the age of 50 and 80 have one or more vertebral (spine) fractures. Many vertebral fractures are not associated with back pain or other symptoms. In general, fracture rates are higher in northern European countries than in southern European countries. These differences may reflect differences in race and ethnicity, habits such as smoking, nutrition, body weight, exercise, and risk of falling.

The incidence of osteoporotic fractures is also increasing with time, due in part to increased life expectancy. However, the risk of fracture also appears to be increasing for reasons unrelated to increased lifespan. The most important reason for this is likely to be reduced physical activity, which could influence both bone mineral content and the risk of falling. It has been estimated that the number of hip fractures will increase approximately three-fold in European countries over the next 50 years.

Osteoporosis

Osteoporosis has been defined as a disease characterised by low bone mass and 'microarchitectural' deterioration of bone, resulting in an increased risk of fracture. Included in this definition is the concept that bone mineral content is not the only skeletal factor resulting in increased fracture risk. Changes in the internal 'microarchitecture' of bone (such as the way in which trabeculae in cancellous bone are connected) can also influence fracture risk without influencing bone mineral content.

Although many factors influence fracture risk, bone mineral density (BMD) is a strong predictor of fracture. Fracture risk in adults is approximately doubled for each standard deviation reduction in BMD at a variety of measurement sites (spine, hip and wrist). What this means is that fracture risk in individuals with BMD in the lowest 20% of the population is about five times higher that that of other individuals of the same age and sex. The World Health Organization (WHO) has emphasised the role of BMD measurement in the definition and diagnosis of osteoporosis. According to this definition, an individual is designated as having osteoporosis at a BMD value 2.5 standard deviations below that expected for young adults. The WHO define an individual as having osteopenia when BMD is between 1 and 2.5 standard deviations below the young adult mean. Because BMD is not a perfect indicator of fracture risk, many osteoporotic fractures occur in individuals who do not fulfil these criteria for a diagnosis of osteoporosis.

At least 30% of postmenopausal women in Western countries are defined as having osteoporosis according to WHO criteria. However, these criteria for diagnosis of osteoporosis and osteopenia were not intended to be used as a simple therapeutic threshold. Differences in skeletal geometry (length and width of bones) as well as non-skeletal factors (such as frequent falling, poor muscle strength, low body mass and poor vision) also influence fracture risk. Many of these risk factors may be influenced by nutritional status. Previous osteoporotic fractures greatly increase the chance of subsequent fractures irrespective of BMD. It is possible to estimate fracture risk given information about these clinical risk factors, BMD and age.

Risk factors for osteoporosis can be divided into those resulting in low peak bone mass, and those resulting in an increased rate of bone loss. Genetic factors are likely to play an important role in determining peak bone mass, but non-genetic factors during childhood are also likely to be important. These non-genetic factors include intake of calcium and other nutrients, exercise, and delayed puberty. Risk factors for age-related bone loss include early menopause in women, low body mass, a low residual concentration of serum oestradiol after the menopause, poor nutritional status and lack of exercise. A variety of other diseases can result in loss of bone mineral, and it is important to exclude these secondary causes of osteoporosis in patients.

The aim of treatment in osteoporosis is to reduce the risk of fracture. This can be achieved by increasing BMD, by reducing bone remodelling, and by decreasing the risk of falls. Lifestyle measures include avoidance of smoking, increasing dietary intake of calcium, ensuring adequate vitamin D status, and exercise. A variety of drugs such as bisphosphonates, oestrogens, selective oestrogen receptor modulators and intermittent parathyroid hormone have been shown to reduce fracture risk.

Osteomalacia

Osteomalacia is a skeletal disorder resulting from defective mineralisation of bone matrix (osteoid). This results in accumulation of unmineralised osteoid. The commonest cause of osteomalacia is vitamin D deficiency. However, osteomalacia does have a number of other causes such as disorders of phosphate metabolism, genetic defects, and excessive intake of nutrients such as fluoride.

Rickets

Historically vitamin D deficiency was predominantly a disease of childhood. Where osteomalacia occurs in children prior to skeletal maturity, this results in deformities and the clinical features of rickets. Rickets is osteomalacia that occurs when bones are still growing. Rickets has been an important cause of childhood illness and deformity for many centuries. Following the industrial revolution, the combination of urbanisation, pollution and poor diet resulted in increased prevalence of the disease in England. Rickets continues to be an important disease in the developing world, and is still seen in developed countries particularly in non-Whites.

Whistler described the clinical features of rickets in 1645. Children with rickets classically present with knock-knees or bowed legs, muscle weakness, and short stature. In breastfed infants, rickets can develop within the first few months of birth, particularly when the mothers of these infants have vitamin D deficiency. These infants may have craniotabes (soft areas of the skull causing a 'ping-pong' ball sensation on pressure), thickening of the wrists and ankles, and enlargement of the costochondral junctions (rachitic rosary). Fractures and other deformities can occur. Children with rickets also have poor muscle development and tone. The skeleton is poorly mineralised, and the growth plates are widened (cupped) and irregular on X-ray. As in adult osteomalacia, there is an excess of unmineralised osteoid. The concentration of alkaline phosphatase is elevated in the blood of children with rickets, and the concentration of phosphate may be lower than expected. The concentration of calcium in the blood is generally maintained within the normal range. Infants with rickets may develop respiratory infections, and are more likely to have tuberculosis. Many of the clinical features of rickets resolve within a short period after administration of adequate amounts of vitamin D. Rickets may result in pelvic deformities that can lead to difficulties during labour and increased perinatal morbidity in subsequent generations (see Figs CD 28.19, 28.20).

The importance of sunshine and diet in the aetiology of rickets was not defined until the early part of the twentieth century. It was discovered that a fat-soluble nutrient or sunshine exposure could cure the condition. An unfortified infant diet contains a very small amount of vitamin D, although there are small amounts in milk and egg yolk. A vegetarian diet or a high intake of phytate also predispose to the development of rickets.

Although rickets is commonly due to vitamin D deficiency, this is not the only cause. Since sunshine is plentiful in tropical countries, other factors are likely to explain the high prevalence of rickets in some of these countries. Increased skin pigmentation or traditional dress may account for some cases of vitamin D deficiency in sunny countries. However, studies in South Africa and Nigeria have suggested that calcium deficiency alone may cause rickets. Genetic or acquired disorders of phosphate metabolism or vitamin D metabolism, and deficiency of the enzyme alkaline phosphatase can also cause osteomalacia and rickets.

24.5 CALCIUM AND VITAMIN D

Evolutionary perspectives

Although the genetic constitution of modern humans has changed little over the past 10 000 years, environmental and nutritional influences on the skeleton have altered markedly over that time. It has been argued that human skeletal metabolism has adapted to conditions which are very different from those encountered by most modern humans. Cultivated plant foods such as cereal grains have far less calcium than do other vegetable food sources. Dietary calcium intake was probably twice as great in pre-agricultural humans, and this was largely of vegetable origin rather than of dairy origin. In most modern humans in Western industrialised countries about half of dietary calcium is derived from dairy foods. Cereals and cereal products provide up to 25% of dietary calcium. Other sources of calcium include green leafy vegetables such as spinach and broccoli, but the oxalate content of these foods may limit calcium bioavailability. Calcium fortification of some foods such as fruit juice and white bread differs between countries.

Modern humans get less exercise and far less sunshine exposure than did our evolutionary ancestors. Dietary sources of vitamin D in prehistoric humans are likely to have been minimal in comparison with the abundant supply from sunshine. There is very little vitamin D in the unsupplemented diet of most modern humans.

Body weight and the skeleton

Body weight is a strong predictor of osteoporotic fracture. Many factors contribute to excess fracture risks in lean individuals. Fractures may relate in part to an increased incidence of falls due to poor muscle strength. In individuals with more body fat, fracture may be prevented by fat 'padding' during falls. Obese individuals also have higher bone mineral density. This is related in part to increased production of oestrogens in fatty tissue, and to mechanical strains induced by excess body weight.

Extreme weight loss associated with anorexia nervosa results in marked loss of bone mineral content due to nutritional deprivation and amenorrhoea. Patients with anorexia nervosa are at increased risk of fracture during later life.

Calcium and dairy foods

An acute effect of oral calcium on bone metabolism is well recognised. A reduction in bone resorption is observed within 2 hours of a single oral calcium dose. Studies using dairy foods show a similar effect. Longer-term studies have also shown that calcium or dairy supplementation for several weeks decreases serum PTH and bone resorption.

Numerous studies have addressed the effect of calcium intake on bone mineral density and fracture risk. The extent to which the skeletal effects of dairy foods can be attributed to increased calcium intake is not certain. A variety of calcium-supplemented food products are also available, but the skeletal benefits of these supplements cannot necessarily be assumed from their calcium composition. Several other components of dairy foods may have beneficial or deleterious effects on the skeleton. These include protein, phosphate, other minerals or specific proteins such as milk basic protein. Dairy foods may also result in modulation of endocrine systems such as the growth hormone–IGF-1 axis.

There have been many observational studies, incorporating cross-sectional, case-control and cohort designs, which have shown a positive association between calcium intake and bone mineral density or fracture risk. However, a substantial number of studies have found no association.

Randomised controlled trials of calcium or dairy food supplementation provide a better insight into the relationship. The participants investigated in studies fall into two age groups: (a) older men and women and (b) growing children. The results of randomised controlled trials of calcium supplementation are summarised in the sections below.

Calcium bioavailability

Bioavailability is the proportion of ingested calcium that is absorbed from the diet. This can vary between individuals and depends on the food source of calcium. Lactose in milk may increase calcium bioavailability from dairy foods. Dietary protein and non-digestible oligosaccharides may increase calcium absorption. Several other components of the diet such as phytates and oxalic acid can inhibit calcium absorption. Supplemental calcium can also alter the absorption of other nutrients such as iron, phosphorus and zinc.

Calcium and dairy intervention studies in postmenopausal women and men

Older people may have a greater calcium requirement than young adults. This greater need may result from impaired intestinal calcium absorption because of an age-related decline in intestinal mucosal mass, decreased dermal synthesis of vitamin D and a decline in renal synthesis of $1,25\text{-}(OH)_2$ vitamin D. At least five studies have addressed whether non-dairy calcium supplementation reduces risk of osteoporotic fracture. The classic study of Chapuy et al (1994) in elderly women stands out by virtue of study size and the large number of fracture cases over the 3-year study period. This trial of over 3000 institutionalised women with a mean age of 84 years reported a substantial (29%) reduction in hip fracture with supplementation in comparison with placebo. The supplement in this trial was 1200 mg of calcium, as calcium phosphate, combined with 20 µg of vitamin D. The results of this study cannot necessarily be applied to other populations, younger women or men. The women studied were institutionalised, with generally poor mobility, and had low dietary calcium intake (mean 500 mg/day). However, Dawson-Hughes et al (1997) showed a reduction in incidence of non-vertebral fractures in elderly men and women living at home with a combined calcium and vitamin D supplement (500 mg/day calcium, 17.5 µg of vitamin D). There have been a few small supplementation trials using calcium alone with fracture as an end-point. Whilst these have shown a positive effect of calcium in reducing fracture risk, the small number of fractures in these studies limits interpretation. The effects of increasing consumption of dairy foods on fracture incidence have not been tested in older men or women.

A larger number of studies, reviewed by Heaney (2000), have examined the effect of supplemental calcium (with or without vitamin D) using BMD as a surrogate end-point. Almost all studies show a positive effect on BMD, although the size of effect is modest. The response to calcium supplementation may depend on habitual calcium intake. For example, one 3-year study observed no effect of supplemental calcium and vitamin D (1000 mg calcium, 25 µg vitamin D) on bone loss in men (Orwoll et al 1990). However, these men had high habitual calcium intakes (1160 mg/day) and were heterogeneous in age.

Several controlled trials of dairy supplementation in older women have also demonstrated a reduction in the rate of bone loss. A recent 2-year study of milk supplementation in postmenopausal Chinese women on a low calcium intake (about 400 mg/day) showed that women receiving a milk powder supplement (calcium content about 1 g/day) had a lower rate of bone loss at the total body, lumbar spine and total hip compared to a control group (Lau et al 2001).

Calcium supplementation appears to have less influence on bone loss in the years immediately after the menopause. This may be due to the overriding importance of oestrogen deficiency during this time.

Calcium and dairy intervention studies in children and adolescents

Since a large proportion of peak bone mass is attained during childhood and puberty, children and adolescents are a particularly important target for interventions to increase bone mass. To this end, there have been a number of randomised controlled trials of calcium or dairy supplementation in children (see Table CD 24.1 for a summary of studies). The level of daily supplementation varied from 500 to 1000 mg of calcium for periods up to 3 years. These studies found that calcium supplementation resulted in greater bone mass accrual. The magnitude of the increase in bone acquisition has been of the order of 1–7%. The increase in bone mineral content with calcium supplementation during childhood may be due in part to a reduction in the rate of bone remodelling and reduced remodelling space.

Although calcium or dairy supplementation has been shown to accelerate bone mineral accrual in children and adolescents during the period of supplementation, the long-term effects of supplementation are unclear. The possible beneficial effects of nutritional supplementation during puberty may relate to an effect on skeletal size rather than bone mineral density. Some studies have examined whether the benefits of supplementation are maintained after the intervention is withdrawn. The majority have failed to show a persistent effect, although larger studies are necessary to confirm this.

Concerns have been expressed that policies to increase intake of milk and dairy products could result in cardiovascular disease and obesity. However, recent studies have shown that milk supplementation is likely to result in a lowering of body mass and body fat rather than an increase.

The role of calcium supplementation in management of osteoporosis

Low calcium intake is only one factor contributing to loss of bone mass in patients with osteoporosis. Although calcium supplementation is important in many patients with osteoporosis, ensuring adequate protein intake is also likely to be of benefit. Maintenance of body weight is critical, since moderate weight loss and low body weight are associated with loss of bone mass and risk of fracture. Although a number of micronutrients, such as vitamin D and K and antioxidant vitamins, have been linked with increased risk of bone mineral loss, only vitamin D has recognised therapeutic value. Combined supplements of calcium and vitamin D are often recommended to patients with osteoporosis and dietary advice to increase intake of dairy products is commonplace. Excessive calcium intake may occasionally result in hypercalcaemia, may result in renal insufficiency or renal stones, and may impair absorption of other nutrients such as iron, phosphorus and zinc.

Recommended calcium intakes

The UK reference nutrient intake (RNI), which is the intake deemed sufficient to satisfy 97% of the population's requirements, is set at 700 mg per day for adults including elderly people. The reference nutrient intake for teenagers is 1000 mg/day for males and 800 mg/day for females, and 550 mg/day for children aged 7 to 10 years. In the USA recommended calcium intake is greater. For children and teenagers aged 9 to 18 years the reference intake is 1300 mg/day, whilst for adults it is 1000 mg/day and for the elderly 1200 mg/day. Most calcium supplementation studies which have shown a skeletal effect have used intakes of at least 1000 mg per day.

Vitamin D hormone

Vitamin D and its metabolites play an important role in calcium and phosphate homeostasis and skeletal development. Vitamin D also plays a role in muscle function, control of cell proliferation and in the immune system.

The unfortunate designation of vitamin D as a 'vitamin' is derived largely from the important findings of Mellanby in 1919. He showed that oral administration of cod liver oil was able to cure rickets. Vitamin D is a sunlight-derived hormone precursor, and is not an essential nutrient in sunlight-exposed humans. Fatty fish such as sardines contain vitamin D, and there is also some vitamin D in eggs. Interesting experiments involving sailors in submarines have shown that individuals who are not exposed to ultraviolet light rapidly develop vitamin D insufficiency despite consuming a usual diet.

The main causes of vitamin D deficiency (Table 24.2) can be understood based on an appreciation of vitamin D metabolism (Fig. 24.2). Vitamin D is derived in large part from conversion of 7-dehydrocholesterol (provitamin D_3) to vitamin D_3 when skin is exposed to ultraviolet B (UV-B) irradiation from sunlight. Vitamin D generated in skin is termed vitamin D_3 (cholecalciferol). Some vitamin D supplements are of plant origin (ergocalciferol or vitamin D_2). Production of vitamin D in skin is reduced in wintertime, and in individuals with increased skin pigmentation. Individuals who do not venture out of doors, who wear clothing that covers a large proportion of body surface, or who live in countries with limited sunshine are also predisposed to vitamin D deficiency.

Endogenous vitamin D_3 and dietary D_3/D_2 are converted to 25-(OH) vitamin D (25-(OH)D) in the liver. 25-(OH)D is the main storage form of vitamin D and is commonly measured in serum to assess vitamin D status. The concentration of 25-(OH)D in serum shows a seasonal variation (Fig. 24.3). Anticonvulsant drug therapy is a risk factor for vitamin D deficiency because of increased conversion of 25-(OH)D to inactive metabolites in the liver. 25-(OH) vitamin D is converted to the hormone 1,25-dihydroxy vitamin D (1,25-$(OH)_2$D) in the kidneys. Renal conversion to 1,25-$(OH)_2$D is stimulated by PTH and suppressed by phosphate. In patients with chronic renal failure, the ability of the kidney to synthesise 1,25-$(OH)_2$D is reduced.

The physiological actions of 1,25-$(OH)_2$D are mediated by binding to specific nuclear vitamin D receptors (VDR). In the gastrointestinal tract the action of 1,25-$(OH)_2$D results in increased intestinal absorption of calcium and phosphorus. In severe vitamin D deficiency fractional dietary calcium absorption is generally less than 20% and occurs through a vitamin D independent mechanism. When vitamin D supply is sufficient, fractional calcium absorption is generally greater than 35%. The overall

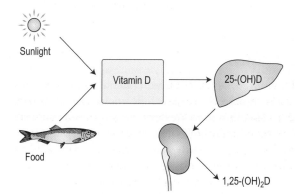

Figure 24.2 Schematic view of vitamin D metabolism.

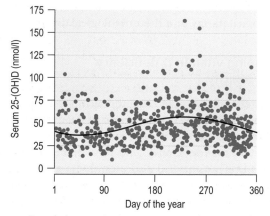

Figure 24.3 Effect of season on the concentration of 25-(OH) vitamin D in serum of postmenopausal women in five European cities. (Adapted from J Bone Miner Res 2003;18:1274–1281 with permission of the American Society for Bone and Mineral Research.)

Table 24.2 Factors contributing to vitamin D hormone insufficiency
1. *Deficiency of sunlight-derived vitamin D* Failure to go out-of-doors Limited UV-B exposure in wintertime Countries with limited UV-B exposure Decreased skin exposure due to traditional dress Use of sunscreen creams Ageing Darker skin colour
2. *Gastrointestinal disease* Pancreatic disease (fat malabsorption) Coeliac disease Other malabsorption syndromes
3. *Anticonvulsant drug therapy*
4. *Defective renal production of 1,25-(OH)₂D* Renal insufficiency Genetic vitamin D pseudodeficiency rickets

effect of 1,25-$(OH)_2$D is to increase the concentration of calcium and phosphate in the plasma, and this allows mineralisation of newly formed bone matrix. 1,25-$(OH)_2$D also acts via the VDR to activate osteoblasts, to stimulate bone resorption by osteoclasts.

It is commonly assumed that 25-(OH)D is biologically inert, and that the physiological actions of vitamin D are mediated only via renal production of 1,25-$(OH)_2$D. This dogma has been increasingly questioned. Although 1,25-$(OH)_2$D is far more potent as an activator of the VDR, the concentration of 25-(OH)D is at least 100-fold greater. Plasma 25-(OH)D is an important determinant of skeletal disease in patients with renal failure in whom renal 1,25-$(OH)_2$D production is impaired. Several tissues other than the kidney express the enzyme required to convert 25-(OH)D to 1,25-$(OH)_2$D and this local conversion may be important. For further discussion of vitamin D metabolism see Section 11.2.

Skeletal consequences of vitamin D deficiency

In children, severe vitamin D deficiency causes rickets. Although vitamin D deficiency rickets is becoming less common in Western industrialised countries, childhood vitamin D deficiency remains a significant problem, particularly in Black and Asian children, and in children who are exclusively breastfed. Breast milk contains only small amounts of vitamin D.

The clinical features of osteomalacia in adults are often more subtle. Patients with severe vitamin D deficiency often have generalised bone pain, muscle pain and muscle weakness. This may be misdiagnosed as 'chronic fatigue' or a rheumatological disorder.

Defining vitamin D deficiency and toxicity

It is generally accepted that the serum concentration of 25-(OH)D is the best indicator of vitamin D status. Plasma 1,25-$(OH)_2$D may be low, normal or increased in vitamin D deficiency, and measurement of 1,25-$(OH)_2$D is not a useful indicator of vitamin D status.

However, it has been difficult to define precise thresholds of plasma 25-(OH)D associated with deficiency, insufficiency or toxicity. It is possible to define thresholds by examining the relationship between plasma 25-(OH)D and fracture risk. However, plasma 25-(OH)D may be low in individuals with other risk factors for fracture (such as lack of exercise or poor general health), and the relationship between low 25-(OH)D and fracture may therefore not be causal.

Vitamin D insufficiency results in an elevated concentration of PTH in plasma (secondary hyperparathyroidism). Serum PTH is a sensitive indicator of vitamin D deficiency. It is possible to define thresholds for vitamin D deficiency based on cross-sectional studies of association between plasma 25-(OH)D and plasma PTH.

Individuals with plasma 25-(OH)D less than 50 nmol/l tend to have elevated serum PTH in comparison with vitamin D replete individuals. This secondary hyperparathyroidism is responsive to modest doses of exogenous vitamin D. It has therefore been suggested that individuals with plasma 25-(OH)D below 50 nmol/l should be regarded as vitamin D insufficient. Approximately half the population in most Western industrialised countries would be regarded as vitamin D insufficient using this criterion. Plasma 25-(OH)D below 15 nmol/l is often associated with overt osteomalacia or rickets.

Vitamin D toxicity is unusual. Individuals regularly exposed to intense sunlight may have plasma 25-(OH)D concentrations up to 200 nmol/l throughout the year, and these individuals do not have any disturbance in skeletal metabolism. Plasma 25-(OH)D greater than 250 nmol/l may be consistent with vitamin D toxicity. The symptoms of vitamin D toxicity include nausea, vomiting, anorexia, fatigue and changes in mental state, such as confusion and nervousness. Serum calcium levels are elevated, which may result in calcium deposition in soft tissues such as arteries, kidney and heart. Heart arrhythmias may be a consequence of raised serum calcium.

Vitamin D and fracture risk

There is an association between plasma 25-(OH) vitamin D and bone mineral density in older people. Several studies have shown that combined calcium and vitamin D supplementation reduces fracture incidence particularly in elderly subjects with a low calcium intake. The independent role of vitamin D deficiency as a determinant of fractures in older people is less certain. In one important study, Trivedi et al (2003) examined the effect of vitamin D supplementation (2500 μg every 4 months for 5 years) in non-institutionalised elderly men and women. They found that there was a 22% reduction in the incidence of first fracture in comparison with placebo. However, some other randomised trials of vitamin D alone have not shown benefit in terms of fracture.

The efficacy of vitamin D may depend on habitual calcium intake and the dose of vitamin D used.

If vitamin D does prevent fracture, it is very likely that some of the benefit could be due to a reduction in the incidence of falls rather than increased bone mineral content. Vitamin D deficiency is common in elderly people who fall, and is associated with poor muscle strength and impaired motor function in the elderly.

Vitamin D status may also influence skeletal growth and bone mineral density during childhood and puberty. There is also some evidence to support the idea that vitamin D status during fetal development and the first year of life may result in long-lasting changes in skeletal function by 'programming' physiological function.

Recommended vitamin D intake

Vitamin D is only an essential nutrient in the absence of sunshine exposure. It is also difficult to determine the amount of vitamin D normally obtained from diet and from sunshine. This depends on a large number of variables including sunshine exposure, latitude and skin pigmentation. Foods containing vitamin D (such as oily fish and egg) may contain very different amounts depending on their source. For adults living a normal lifestyle, the panel on dietary reference values in the UK did not therefore recommend an RNI for oral vitamin D intake in adults. For adults confined indoors, the panel agreed an RNI of $10 \mu g/day$. This amount of vitamin D is, however, not sufficient to prevent vitamin D deficiency in the absence of any sunshine exposure, although it is likely to prevent overt osteomalacia. For infants up to 6 months of age, the panel recommended an intake of $8.5 \mu g/day$. For individuals not exposed to sunshine, the United States Food and Nutrition Board recommended daily allowance (RDA) of vitamin D is $5 \mu g/day$ for infants, children and adults. The RDA is set at $10 \mu g/day$ for older adults (age 50 to 70 years) and at $15 \mu g/day$ for those over the age of 70.

24.6 PROTEIN, AND ACID–BASE BALANCE

Protein intake and skeletal health

Bone matrix is composed largely of protein, and amino acid supply is therefore an essential requirement for bone formation. Early studies in humans and animals found that a diet high in protein results in increased urinary calcium excretion. This effect was thought to reflect increased bone resorption, possibly as a result of skeletal buffering of the net acid load associated with protein catabolism. More recent studies suggest that the increased calcium excretion with high intake of animal protein may be due in large part to increased efficiency of dietary calcium absorption, rather than bone resorption. The source of protein may also be important. Animal proteins may increase urinary calcium excretion, in contrast to plant proteins, which may have the opposite effect. Catabolism of plant protein results in less acid production and because of their alkalinity it has been suggested that they may be less harmful. However, evidence that intake of animal protein is harmful to the skeleton is not strong. Increasing protein intake may increase bone mineral density and decrease the risk of falling in some populations, particularly in the elderly.

Protein intake may alter skeletal health through several mechanisms in addition to the well-described effect on net acid intake. These mechanisms include improved dietary calcium absorption, increased serum IGF-1, and possible beneficial effects of specific proteins on the skeleton. IGF-1 stimulates osteoblast proliferation and differentiation, and enhances bone collagen and matrix synthesis. It is also possible that particular milk proteins, such as milk basic protein (MBP), may have a direct antiresorptive effect on the skeleton. Low serum IGF-1 has been associated with increased fracture risk. It is overly simplistic to consider animal protein as a single nutritional entity. Although many early studies showed that intake of purified protein products (such as casein) results in increased urine calcium loss, these proteins may not reflect the effect of common food proteins. More recent studies using meat as a protein supplement have shown little effect on urinary calcium excretion.

Cohort studies relating protein intake to bone mineral density and fracture have also not provided consistent evidence of a harmful effect of dietary animal protein (see Table CD 24.2 for summary references). The majority of studies report that a high intake of animal protein decreases bone loss or fracture risk. Extreme protein excess may increase skeletal risk.

The relevance of protein intake may also vary by age and nutritional status. Elderly persons with osteoporotic hip fracture are often undernourished, particularly with respect to protein, and tend to have a reduced concentration of albumin in serum. Low body weight is an important risk factor for fracture. Randomised controlled trials of patients who have already sustained a hip fracture have shown that protein supplementation improves clinical outcome, increases muscle strength and improves BMD. In these trials the protein supplement was given in conjunction with calcium. Correction of protein undernutrition could reduce fractures by increasing muscle mass, increasing bone mineral density, and by reducing the risk of falls. No controlled studies have investigated the effect of protein supplementation on fracture risk.

Fruit and vegetable intake

There is substantial evidence that a diet high in fruit and vegetables may be associated with a slightly reduced fracture risk. The relationship between the alkalinising effect of fruit and vegetable intake on the one hand and the acidifying effect of meat intake on the other hand has received considerable attention. However, as discussed above, the effect of animal protein on bone is controversial. Conclusions relating to the beneficial effect of fruit and vegetable intake currently rely on observational cross-sectional studies and a few cohort studies. Some studies use indirect indices of fruit and vegetable intake, such as potassium intake, magnesium intake, or estimated net dietary acid load. These studies suggest that individuals who consume a diet rich in fruit and vegetables relative to animal protein have less bone mineral loss. Some cohort studies have failed to find such an association, and in other studies the effects are not gender-consistent. For example, one study reported that men with a high intake of fruit and vegetables had less bone loss at one site, but this did not apply to women. Most studies have not shown significant differences in skeletal health or fracture risk between vegetarians and meat-eaters.

The evidence relating to a possible beneficial role of fruit and vegetables is of variable quality and is potentially confounded by colinearity of nutrient intake. The intake of fruit and vegetables is associated with lifestyle factors such as smoking, alcohol consumption and exercise. Adequate statistical correction for these confounders may not be possible. Even if fruit and vegetable intake is beneficial, the effect size is likely to be modest. One meta-analysis showed that less than 1% of the variance in bone mineral density is attributed to potassium intake, although this was statistically significant. It is premature to draw conclusions about the role of fruit and vegetables in the prevention of fracture risk until the results of randomised intervention trials are available.

24.7 OTHER VITAMINS

Vitamin A
It has been known for many years that very excessive intake of vitamin A causes hypercalcaemia (increased concentration of calcium in the blood), increased bone resorption and skeletal disease. A number of investigators have recently suggested that vitamin A intake might be an important determinant of bone health within the general population. Given currently available evidence it is not clear whether vitamin A intake within the general population is related to skeletal health (see Table CD 24.3 for a summary of such studies). Studies are difficult to compare due to the use of different dietary instruments and laboratory methods, and differing mean retinol intake between studies. Vitamin A intake may be associated with intake of other nutrients which affect skeletal health (such as vitamin D and protein).

B vitamins
There has been some interest in the possibility that dietary supply of B vitamins, particularly folate, riboflavin and vitamin B_6, may impact on bone health. This may be due to increased plasma homocysteine in individuals with deficiency of these vitamins. There are some data to suggest that elevated plasma homocysteine may be associated with low BMD and increased fracture risk.

Vitamin C
Vitamin C is necessary for collagen synthesis and cross-linking. Extreme vitamin C deficiency (scurvy)

is associated with bone disease, especially in children. Scurvy is associated with bone pain, subperiosteal haemorrhages and fractures around the growth plates. Scurvy is now rare except in food faddists or in extreme malnutrition. However, there is some evidence that milder vitamin C deficiency may affect skeletal health, particularly in smokers. Some observational studies have reported an association between moderate vitamin C insufficiency and fracture risk, but the evidence for this is insubstantial.

Vitamin K
Vitamin K influences bone metabolism, at least in part by post-translational carboxylation of bone proteins such as osteocalcin. Supplementation with vitamin K_2 has been reported to increase bone mineral density and reduce the rate of osteoporotic fracture. The importance of dietary vitamin K as a determinant of fracture risk is uncertain. One study found that hip fracture risk is higher in elderly women in whom osteocalcin is undercarboxylated.

24.8 MINERALS

Sodium
Numerous studies have shown that a diet high in sodium increases urinary calcium excretion. An increase in sodium intake equivalent to one teaspoon of salt increases urinary calcium excretion by about 1.5 mmol per day. Short-term experimental studies in postmenopausal women have shown that a low sodium diet reduces bone remodelling. However, studies of dietary sodium intake in relation to BMD are less convincing, and there are no data to suggest that altering sodium intake would reduce fracture risk. Nevertheless, given the important effect of sodium intake on renal calcium handling, avoidance of excessive sodium intake does seem prudent in individuals at increased risk of fracture.

Phosphorus
Phosphorus is the sixth most abundant element in the body. Bone mineral consists largely of calcium phosphate, and phosphorus supply is therefore essential for skeletal development. A reduced concentration of inorganic phosphorus in the extracellular fluid results in impaired skeletal mineralisation. Typical dietary intake of phosphorus is about 1500 mg/day. It is sometimes claimed that phosphorus intake in the typical adult diet is excessive, and that the molar ratio of dietary calcium to phosphorus should be about 1:1 for optimal skeletal health, although there is little evidence to support this. Excess phosphorus intake lowers urinary calcium excretion and impairs absorption of calcium from the diet. Phosphorus is present in a wide variety of foods, and is also added to foods and cola drinks as polyphosphates or phosphoric acid.

The effect of high phosphate intake on the skeleton has been assessed by measuring bone mineral density, and by calcium balance studies. Some studies have shown an inverse relationship between phosphorus intake and bone mineral density. However, phosphorus intake is closely associated with intake of other nutrients (such as meat) as well as lifestyle factors, which may affect the skeleton. Cross-sectional studies of dietary phosphorus in relation to skeletal health are likely to be misleading. The possible harmful effect of a high phosphorus diet on the skeleton may be more relevant when calcium requirements are high during puberty.

The form of ingested phosphorus is also important. Polyphosphates may have a greater deleterious effect on calcium balance than orthophosphates. There is little information on the independent relationship between phosphorus intake and fracture risk.

Magnesium
Severe magnesium (Mg) deficiency results in disturbed calcium homeostasis, impaired PTH secretion, end-organ resistance to PTH, and hypocalcaemia. The implications of more subtle Mg deficiency are less clear. Some studies have shown that Mg intake is positively correlated with bone mineral density or quantitative ultrasound properties of bone in both adults and children.

Fluoride
Fluoride increases the activity of osteoblasts. A number of studies have addressed the effect of fluoride in drinking water on fracture risk. These studies have shown either a small increase in risk, a small beneficial effect, or no detectable effect. However, fluoride in drinking water accounts for a relatively small proportion of total fluoride intake, and these studies do not imply that the effect of dietary fluoride is unimportant. Substantially increased fluoride intake is associated with severe skeletal disease (fluorosis). Fluoride therapy in patients with osteoporosis increases trabecular bone mineral density, but this is associated with an increased rate of fracture rather than a decrease.

Zinc

There is very limited evidence that dietary zinc is important for the skeleton. Most empirical research has been orientated towards investigation of the effect of dietary zinc on bone growth in undernourished children. Some studies of children and adolescents have reported that zinc supplementation increases linear growth. The effects of dietary zinc on growth may be mediated through changes in serum IGF-1.

Zinc undernutrition has been proposed as a risk factor for osteoporosis, especially since many elderly people consume zinc-deficient diets. Several studies have reported that women with postmenopausal osteoporosis had elevated urinary zinc levels compared to healthy controls, and that in this population group urinary zinc excretion was associated with bone resorption. One small randomised, controlled trial reported reduced bone loss with zinc supplementation, but the supplement contained other trace elements as well as calcium.

Copper

Copper is required for normal cross-linking of collagen in bone. Very severe copper deficiency is associated with osteoporosis, but the role of copper deficiency as a determinant of fracture risk within the general population is unknown. One study found that low serum copper was associated with lower bone mineral density in an apparently healthy postmenopausal population.

Boron

A possible role for boron in bone metabolism is controversial, although boron supplements are widely sold for their putative skeletal benefits. Human studies are rare and contradictory. Possible effects of boron supplementation on urinary calcium excretion have been found in some studies but not in others. Boron is also reputed to increase serum oestradiol, which could benefit bone health.

Aluminium

Aluminium toxicity generally occurs in the context of either chronic renal failure or patients receiving parenteral nutrition. In aluminium toxicity, osteoblast function is impaired, and there is reduced bone remodelling and osteomalacia.

Chromium

It has also been hypothesised that chromium is required for bone health. One study showed that urinary excretion of hydroxyproline (a non-specific indicator biochemical marker of bone collagen resorption), as well as calcium excretion decrease following chromium supplementation in healthy women. However one recent study using more specific markers showed that chromium supplementation had no effect on bone remodelling.

24.9 OTHER DIETARY COMPONENTS

Phytoestrogens

Phytoestrogens are widely promoted as a 'natural' alternative to oestrogen replacement therapy. Isoflavones are phytoestrogens which are found in high concentrations in foods such as soya. These compounds have weak oestrogen-like properties. It is important to distinguish between the nutritional effects of dietary phytoestrogens and pharmacological intake of these compounds.

A possible beneficial role of phytoestrogens for skeletal health has been demonstrated in several animal studies but the doses used have been very high and the relevance of these to human nutrition is uncertain. Human studies of isoflavone supplementation are conflicting. It has been argued that the dose of isoflavone in these human studies relative to body weight is only about 10% of that used in animal studies. Several studies have reported a positive association between BMD and intake of soya foods in Chinese and Japanese postmenopausal women. However, the association between soya food intake and bone mass has not been easy to demonstrate in populations with lower habitual soya intake.

Alcohol

Alcohol abuse and dependence may compromise bone quality and increase risk of fracture. The skeletal effects of excess alcohol intake are due to a direct toxic effect of alcohol on bone osteoblasts, insufficient intake of other nutrients, vitamin D deficiency, decreased sex hormone secretion and increased risk of falls. There is less evidence that moderate alcohol consumption is associated with fracture risk. Some studies have shown that modest alcohol intake is associated with increased BMD rather than a decrease.

Caffeine

Many observational epidemiological studies have investigated the association between intake of caffeine-containing beverages and fracture risk. The majority have found no association or a weak increase in risk with excessive consumption. The largest prospective study of caffeine intake and fracture risk showed that there was a three times greater risk of hip fracture for women consuming more than 817 mg caffeine per day (approximately five cups of coffee). However, in this study the number of hip fractures was small. It is possible that the association may not be causal, and may be due to other confounding associations such as an inverse association between caffeine intake and milk intake. In studies which separated tea-drinkers from coffee-drinkers the former were shown to have a better bone mass and a reduced odds for fracture. Although caffeine ingestion leads to a slight decrease in the efficiency of calcium absorption, it has been estimated that this would be offset entirely by addition of two tablespoons of milk to a cup of coffee.

Carbonated beverages

Two observational studies in teenagers have reported that a high intake of carbonated cola-type drinks is associated with a low bone mineral density and a higher prevalence of fracture. The mechanism for this is not clear, and may be due to other associated lifestyle or dietary factors. The phosphorus content and caffeine content of some carbonated drinks may contribute to risk.

○ Key points

- The skeleton is composed of two types of bone: cortical bone, which is a dense form of bone comprising about 80% of skeletal mass, and trabecular bone, which consists of an intricate structural mesh of trabeculae that form the interior scaffolding of bone.

- Bone is a metabolically active tissue. In the adult skeleton most metabolic activity occurs by the process of bone 'remodelling' or bone turnover. This metabolic activity serves to maintain the structure and homeostatic functions of the skeleton.

- Osteoporosis is a disease characterised by low bone mass and microarchitectural deterioration of bone, which results in an increased risk of fracture.

- Observational studies relating fracture risk to intake of calcium and other nutrients have yielded conflicting results. Where relationships are shown in cross-sectional studies, these may not be causal. Surrogate measures of fracture risk (such as bone mineral density and measures of bone turnover) provide useful supportive information, but do not provide definitive evidence of either benefit or harm. Nutritional intervention studies with fracture as an end-point provide much stronger evidence, but are impractical for most individual nutrients.

- It seems possible that nutritional intervention during childhood and puberty could increase peak bone mass and reduce the risk of fracture in later life. Controlled studies of calcium or dairy food supplementation in children and adolescents show short-term benefit in increasing bone mineral mass. However, this benefit may be lost following the cessation of supplementation.

- The majority of observational studies report that low intakes of animal protein are associated with lower bone mineral density and increased fracture risk. However, protein supplementation has not been tested in a controlled study with fracture as an outcome. It is possible that extremely elevated protein intake could result in bone loss. The evidence for this is, however, not substantial.

- Randomised controlled trials of a combined supplement of vitamin D and calcium show a reduction in fracture incidence in elderly people. The independent effect of vitamin D status on risk of fracture is unknown, although vitamin D deficiency is common in older adults even in countries which have plenty of sunshine.

of high caries risk. Information on other cariogenic bacteria is given in Section CD 25.3 and a more detailed account of the role of microbial aspects of dental caries is given by Russell (2003).

Bacteria associated with periodontal disease include *Actinobacillus actinomycetemcomitans*, an aerobic Gram-negative coccus associated with juvenile periodontitis and adult chronic periodontitis. Other anaerobic Gram-negative bacteria (e.g. *Porphyromonas gingivalis*, *Tannerella forsythensis*, *Prevotella intermedia* and *Fusobacterium nucleatum)* may be isolated from periodontal pockets and are associated with periodontal disease, dental abscesses and root canal infections. However, these bacteria are not strictly speaking infectious and form part of the normal oral flora. The specific species responsible for the destruction of the periodontal structures is unclear as periodontal disease is a mixed anaerobic infection. The diet does not directly influence the composition of the subgingival flora, with the exception of food impaction which may cause localised microbial expansion.

The caries process

Dietary sugars diffuse into the dental plaque where they are metabolised by plaque microorganisms to acid. Most of the acid produced is lactic, with some acetic, formic and propionic acids also being produced. The acid produced reduces the pH of dental plaque, the mineral phase of enamel is dissolved by the plaque acids, and the caries process has begun. Enamel hydroxyapatite usually begins to dissolve around pH 5.5, which is sometimes referred to as the 'critical pH'. When the pH rises above this value, remineralisation of enamel may occur. Saliva promotes remineralisation as it contains bicarbonate which increases pH and encourages deposition of mineral in porous areas where demineralisation of enamel or dentine has occurred. A demineralised lesion may therefore be remineralised; however, this is a slow process that competes with factors causing demineralisation. If the pH in the mouth remains high enough for sufficient time then complete remineralisation may occur. However, if demineralisation dominates, the enamel becomes more porous until finally a carious lesion forms. The rate of demineralisation is affected by the concentration of hydrogen ions (i.e. pH at the tooth surface) and the frequency with which the plaque pH falls below the critical pH. Another relevant point is the amount of calcium and phosphate in plaque, since high levels

of these minerals in plaque will help resist dissolution of the enamel. Overall, caries occurs when demineralisation exceeds remineralisation. The development of caries requires sugars and aciduric bacteria to occur, but is influenced by the composition of the tooth (the structure of the enamel can be altered by the diet while the teeth are forming), the quantity and composition of saliva (e.g. calcium and phosphate content and buffering power) and the time for which dietary sugars are available for fermentation.

The Stephan curve: the effects of different food combinations on plaque pH

Stephan, in the 1940s, pioneered work on the pH of dental plaque using microelectrodes. This work indicated that the resting pH of plaque was around 6.5 to 7 but, on exposure to sugars (glucose or sucrose), fell rapidly within a few minutes, to around pH 5. The rapid fall was followed by a slow recovery to baseline pH over the next 30–60 minutes. Stephan plotted pH against time and this time/pH graph is commonly referred to as a 'Stephan curve'. An example of a Stephan curve is shown in Figure 25.2. The Stephan curve has been commonly used to measure the acidogenic potential of a range of foods and this provides an indirect measure of the cariogenic potential of the food. However, it must be noted that measures of plaque pH alone must not be taken as a direct measure of cariogenic potential since these measurements take no account of protective factors in foods, the resistance of enamel and salivary factors that influence the caries process. In order to determine the cariogenic potential of a food, data from plaque pH studies need to be interpreted alongside data from other types of study including animal studies and epidemiological surveys.

Consumption of different food combinations results in different patterns in plaque pH. This was clearly illustrated in a study that looked at the effect on plaque pH of consuming a sugary snack followed by either sweetened coffee or a 15 g piece of cheese (Fig. 25.2). Consumption of cheese following a sugary snack almost abolishes the fall in plaque pH that usually results from sugars consumption. This effect of cheese is probably due to the stimulation of saliva by this highly flavoured food and its low carbohydrate (lactose) content. Other foods that are good stimuli to salivary flow include peanuts and sugar-free chewing gum, and these also reduce the pH fall if consumed following a sugar-containing item.

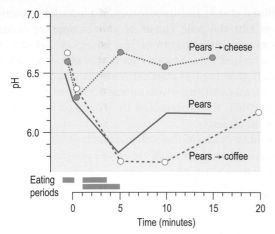

Figure 25.2 Stephan curves produced by eating either cheese or sugared coffee after tinned pears in syrup. Adapted from Rugg-Gunn et al (1975), with permission.

When sugars are consumed with other foods, the effect on pH is reduced, probably due to a diluting effect and the increased salivary flow due to mastication of other foods. This is one reason why it is often recommended to consume sugary foods at mealtimes only (another reason is that limiting sugars to mealtimes reduces the frequency of consumption). A study that examined the effect of consuming breakfast items in a different order on plaque pH illustrates this diluting effect. The breakfast items were sugar-containing coffee, a boiled egg and crispbread with butter. The smallest drop in pH was observed when all three items were consumed together and the largest drop in pH was observed when the sugared coffee was consumed alone. So consumption of one food may affect the acidogenicity of another.

Chewing sugar-free chewing gum following a sugars-containing snack has also been shown to increase the rate at which plaque pH returns to baseline. This has led to the advice to chew sugar-free gum following a sugary snack or meal.

> ⮑ **Key points**
>
> ⮑ Dental caries occurs due to demineralisation of the dental mineralised tissues by acids derived from the bacterial metabolism of dietary sugars to acids.
>
> ⮑ Plaque on the tooth surface is largely composed of bacterial cells and extracellular glucans.
>
> ⮑ Mutans Streptococci have an important role in dental caries since they can produce acid from sugars at a low pH.
>
> ⮑ Changes in plaque pH on consumption of a food provide a measure of acidogenic potential, which is an indirect measure of cariogenic potential.

25.4 PROMOTING AND PROTECTIVE FACTORS

There are many factors that have the potential to promote dental decay: poor oral hygiene, high MS counts and an excess intake of dietary sugars among them. Likewise there are several factors known to be protective against decay, most notably fluoride exposure (both dietary and non-dietary) and restricted intake of sugars. However, there are also a number of other dietary factors that protect against dental caries, including milk, cheese and xylitol, and knowledge of these factors assists in making dietary advice for dental health more positive.

Diet

Diet can affect the teeth while they are forming, before they erupt into the mouth (a pre-eruptive effect) and, once erupted, by a local direct effect. Much research was undertaken in the first half of the twentieth century on the pre-eruptive effect of diet on tooth structure. Deficiencies of vitamin D, vitamin A and protein energy malnutrition (PEM) have been associated with enamel hypoplasia. This is an enamel developmental defect characterised by pits, fissures or larger areas of missing enamel that become stained post eruption and which render the tooth more susceptible to decay. PEM and vitamin A deficiency also cause salivary gland atrophy, reducing the quantity and affecting the composition of saliva, ultimately reducing the mouth's defence against plaque acids. However, in developing countries, in the absence of dietary sugars, undernutrition is not associated with dental caries. Undernutrition coupled with a high intake of sugars results in levels of caries greater than expected for the level of sugars intake. Despite considerable past interest in the pre-eruptive effect of diet on tooth decay, today, the post-eruptive local effect of diet in the mouth is considered to be much more important. The aforementioned studies of Kite and colleagues showed that the presence of food in the mouth was a prerequisite for dental caries formation. There is a wealth of evidence for the association between diet and dental caries and most attention has focused on the important role of dietary sugars in the aetiology of caries.

The frequency of eating sugars, the amount eaten and the cariogenicity of different dietary sugars have all to be considered. The cariogenicity of starches, the relative cariogenicity of naturally occurring and 'free' sugars (sometimes called 'added' sugars), the possible effect of factors in foods that may protect against dental caries are important issues for health professionals and nutritional and dental scientists. The evidence relating diet to dental caries comes from a number of types of experiments, including human observational studies and human intervention studies, animal experiments, aforementioned plaque pH studies and in vitro laboratory experiments. The strongest evidence comes from human epidemiological studies; however, it is important to consider collative evidence from all types of study in order to obtain an overall picture regarding cariogenicity of a product.

The role of dietary sugars

In the past, when sugar intake and levels of dental caries have been compared on an inter-country basis using food balance data and WHO data on caries levels of different countries, a positive correlation has been found. Today, the relationship is not so evident in countries that have a high sugars intake since the relationship between sugars intake and dental caries is thought to be sigmoid with countries having a high level of intake on the upper flattened part of the curve. However, sugar availability still accounts for over a quarter of the variation in dental caries levels.

Evidence for an association between sugars intake and dental caries also comes from observations of the marked increase in dental caries that has occurred in populations that have undergone the 'nutrition transition', that is they have moved away from their traditional diets that were low in free sugars and adopted a Westernised diet high in free sugars. The incidence of dental caries in Eskimos was very low before the introduction of a high sugars diet but dental caries subsequently increased rapidly. It is sometimes argued that in such populations the change in diet also included an increased consumption of

refined starch and therefore increased sugars intake was not the sole cause of the change in caries. However, inhabitants of the island of Tristan da Cunha had a traditional diet that was low in sugars but high in cooked starch (potato) but had low levels of caries until sugar was introduced into the diet in the 1940s, which resulted in a marked increase in dental caries.

Other epidemiological studies have observed the level of dental caries in groups of people that habitually consume high or low amounts of sugars in their diet. Examples of high sugars consumers in which higher than average levels of dental caries have been reported include confectionery workers, sugar cane cutters and children taking long-term sugared liquid medicines. A low level of caries has been reported in groups of people with a low sugars intake, including children in institutions where strict dietary regimens low in sugars are followed and also in children with hereditary fructose intolerance, a condition in which fructose, and therefore sucrose, must be avoided.

During the Second World War there was a reduction in sugar availability in many countries. Data exist from 11 European countries showing that a reduction in caries accompanied reduced sugar availability. Takahashi studied levels of dental caries and sugar intake before, during and after the Second World War in Japan. Sugar consumption fell from 15 kg/year before the war to only 0.2 kg/year in 1946 and the annual dental caries increment in the first permanent molars mirrored the changes in sugar availability.

Cross-sectional studies correlating sugars consumption with dental caries experience have been popular as they are easy to do, but they can be misleading. This is because simultaneous measurements of diet and dental caries levels may not provide a true reflection of the role of diet in the development of the disease. Dental caries takes time to develop and therefore it is the diet several years earlier that may be responsible for current levels of dental caries. Cross-sectional studies are of most use in young children where diet has not changed radically since the eruption of the teeth. Such studies have shown, for example, dental caries development to be closely related to prolonged and frequent use of sugar-containing soft drinks in bottles and use of sugared medicines by children.

When investigating the association between diet and the development of dental caries it is best to relate sugars consumption to changes in dental caries over time in a longitudinal design; however, this type of study is relatively rare. Two famous longitudinal studies are that of Rugg-Gunn et al (1984) in northeast England and Burt et al (1988) in Michigan, USA. In the study of caries and diet of over 400 English adolescents (aged 11 to 12 years) a small but significant correlation existed between sugars intake and caries increment over 2 years. The top 10% of sugars consumers developed significantly more dental caries than the 10% with the lowest sugars intake. The Michigan study (Burt et al 1988) investigated the relationship between sugars intake and dental caries increment over 3 years in children initially aged 10 to 15 years and also found a significant relationship between the amount of dietary sugars and dental caries. Intake of sugars was generally high for all subjects in this study, with only 20 out of 499 children consuming less than 75 g/day.

Human intervention studies

There have been two human intervention studies of importance. First, the Vipeholm study was conducted in a mental institution in Sweden shortly after the Second World War. The 964 patients (80% of whom were male) were divided by wards into one control group and six test groups. Groups were given high sucrose intakes at meals only, or at and between meals, in non-sticky (sucrose solution, chocolate) or sticky forms (caramels, toffees, sweet bread). The study was complicated but from the results it was concluded that: sugars consumption even at high levels is associated with only a small increase in caries increment if taken up to four times a day as part of meals; consumption of sugars between meals as well as at meals is associated with a marked increase in caries; and caries activity disappears on withdrawal of sugars from the diet. The highest caries increment was observed in the group that consumed 24 sticky toffees throughout the day. However, subtle differences between types of sugars were largely overridden by the effect of frequency. It

would not be possible to repeat such a study today, as it would be unethical to prescribe high sugars diets knowing of the association between sugars and dental caries.

The second human intervention study took place in Turku, Finland, in the 1970s. The aim of this 2-year study was to investigate the effect on dental caries of nearly total substitution of sucrose in a normal diet with either fructose or xylitol. When only cavities were counted the results showed 56% fewer cavities in the xylitol group than in the sucrose group but a similar number of cavities formed in the sucrose and fructose groups. The diet containing xylitol was therefore less cariogenic than the sucrose or fructose diets, but fructose is no less cariogenic than sucrose. The inability of plaque microorganisms to metabolise xylitol to acids probably explains this cariostatic effect.

Frequency and amount of sugars

The strong correlation between frequency and amount of sugars is clearly seen in many animal experiments (Table 25.2). The results of experiments in rats have shown caries severity to increase with increasing sugars concentration up to a concentration of 40% (see Fig. CD 25.3). The frequency of intake was similar in the groups of rats so the weight and concentration of sugars eaten related to the severity of caries. Evidence from studies in humans also shows that the two variables are strongly associated (see Fig. CD 25.4).

Some studies in humans have shown that frequency of sugars intake is related to caries development, including the aforementioned Vipeholm study. Studies conducted since the introduction of fluoride have also shown caries development to be lower when intake of sugars does not exceed four times a day: for example, in a study of 5-year-old Icelandic children, those consuming sugars four or more times a day or three or more times between meals per day had significantly more caries compared with children who consumed sugars less frequently. Therefore it

Table 25.2 **The mean number of carious fissure surfaces and daily food intake in four groups of rats fed at different frequencies per day; six animals per group (König et al 1968)**

Group	Eating frequency	No. of carious fissures	Daily food intake (g)
1	12	0.7	6.0
2	18	2.2	6.0
3	24	4.0	6.0
4	30	4.7	6.0

the early twentieth century and its effectiveness has now been demonstrated in over a hundred surveys in more than 20 countries including the UK. The first area in the UK to have an artificially fluoridated water supply was Birmingham in 1964, an area that consequently has seen a dramatic improvement in levels of dental caries. The reduction in treatment arising from fluoridation results in considerable savings to health costs, due to the fall in the number of extractions and general anaesthetics. There are examples where water fluoridation has been discontinued and subsequently levels of dental caries have increased, for example areas of Scotland including Kilmarnock, Wick and Stranraer where dental caries levels increased, despite the fact that fluoride toothpastes were available. A 25% increase in dental caries was observed in some areas of Scotland over 5 years after removal of water fluoridation.

Fluoridation of drinking water can substantially decrease dental caries but an excess of fluoride during the development of the teeth may cause 'dental fluorosis', an enamel developmental defect that manifests as small white diffuse opacities with severe pitting and staining of enamel in more severe cases. For permanent teeth the period when there is greatest risk from excess fluoride is between 2 and 5 years. Severe fluorosis is rare in the UK and cases have usually been linked with excessive fluoride ingestion from eating toothpaste or misuse of fluoride supplements. Severe fluorosis is observed particularly in countries that have very high levels of fluoride in water supplies. Enamel fluorosis as well as skeletal fluorosis are found in large areas of India, Thailand, in the Rift Valley of East Africa and in many Arab states. It is important to realise that fluoride is not the only cause of opacities in teeth.

The optimal level of fluoride in water is the level at which a substantial caries reduction is observed with a negligible prevalence of enamel fluorosis. In temperate climates including the UK the optimum concentration of fluoride is 1.0 mg/l, while in warmer climates it might be nearer 0.6 mg/l. Water fluoridation is endorsed by more than 150 science and health organisations including the International Dental Federation, the International Association for Dental Research and WHO. Despite this expert endorsement, there are small groups of people who strongly oppose water fluoridation on the grounds of perceived health risks and imposed treatment of the water supply (see Section CD 25.4).

In conclusion, fluoridation of the water supply is a caries-preventive measure with the potential to reach the sectors of the population that are at highest risk of caries. One could argue that in some areas, where caries levels are very low, water fluoridation might not be a cost-effective measure. However, in some parts of the UK and other countries, including areas of social deprivation, prevalence of caries remains high and dental attendance, oral hygiene practice and dietary habits are poor. For such areas water fluoridation is a highly effective, economical public health measure.

Other sources of fluoride

The recent WHO report 'Diet, nutrition and the prevention of chronic diseases' (WHO 2003) recommended that 'There should be promotion of adequate fluoride exposure via appropriate vehicles, for example affordable toothpaste, water, salt and milk'. Fluorides are widely found in nature in addition to being naturally present in some water supplies. Fluoride is found in seafood (when bones are eaten), tea leaves, some beers and in foods cooked in fluoridated water. In addition to water, suitable vehicles for artificial fluoridation are salt and milk although neither of these is used extensively. Salt fluoridation has been successfully implemented in Switzerland since 1955 and fluoridated salt sits alongside non-fluoridated salt in supermarkets, allowing the consumer choice, which is politically advantageous. Dietary fluoride provides a local effect on the teeth whilst in the mouth and a systemic effect on the teeth after digestion and absorption. Fluoride in toothpaste and mouth rinse provides a mainly topical effect as these are not supposed to be swallowed.

Does refined sugar have the same relationship to dental decay in the presence of fluoride?

Despite a marked effect of fluoride on caries prevalence, a relationship between sugars intake and caries still exists in the presence of fluoride. Longitudinal studies of the relationship between intake of dietary sugars and dental caries levels in children in the UK and USA have shown that the observed relationship between sugars intake and development of dental caries remains even after controlling for use of fluoride. Data from the National Diet and Nutrition Survey of children aged 1.5 to 4.5 years also shows a significant relationship between frequency of sugar-rich snacks and caries levels in young children even after controlling for use of fluoride. A study conducted in northeast England reported on the decrease in dental caries levels during the Second

World War in 12-year-old children from areas with naturally high and low water fluoride. Caries levels were lower in the high fluoride area in 1943 but, following the wartime sugar restriction, dental caries levels fell further by approximately 50%, thus indicating that exposure to fluoride did not totally override the effect of sugar in the diet. A comprehensive literature review on changes in caries prevalence and associated factors (Marthaler 1990) concluded that even in modern societies that make use of preventive measures such as fluoride, a relationship between sugars consumption and caries still exists and free sugars remain the main threat for dental health in some developed and many developing countries. It is likely that, in industrialised countries where there is adequate exposure to fluoride, a further reduction in the prevalence and severity of dental caries will not be achieved without a reduction in the intake of free sugars. Furthermore, a systematic review (Burt & Pai 2001) that addressed whether in the era of extensive fluoride exposure individuals with a high level of sugars intake have greater caries severity compared with those with lower sugars intake concluded that where there is good exposure to fluoride, sugars consumption is a moderate risk factor for caries in most people, but sugars consumption is likely to be a more powerful indicator for risk of caries in persons who do not have regular exposure to fluoride. Overall it was concluded that where there is adequate use of fluoride, reduction of sugars consumption still has a role to play in the prevention of caries but this role is not as strong as it is without exposure to fluoride.

Other dietary factors

Other minerals
Apart from fluoride there are other trace elements that influence dental caries although the influence is of relatively small importance. Dietary molybdenum, strontium, boron and lithium are related to a lower caries experience in humans while higher selenium intakes are related to higher caries prevalence.

Other factors that protect against dental caries
The protective effect of some food components against dental caries has been recognised for decades. In the 1930s Osborn and Noriskin suggested that foods provided substances that protect against decay. Apart from the well-recognised role of fluoride, other dietary components such as phosphates,

calcium, casein and polyphenols may also have cariostatic properties. Milk, despite containing approximately 4% sugars as lactose, was one of the first foods to be described as cariostatic. Although lactose may be fermented to acid, it has been shown to be the least cariogenic of the common dietary sugars. Milk also contains high concentrations of calcium and phosphate and is also rich in casein. Many studies of several types have all indicated that milk is not cariogenic and may even protect against dental caries. The cariostatic nature of cheese is also well established with evidence from animal and human experimental and intervention studies demonstrating its cariostatic nature. Cheese is a strong gustatory stimulus to salivary flow which conveys protection to the teeth. However, cheese has been shown to be cariostatic in animals that have had their salivary glands removed and so the cariostatic effect is not due to saliva alone. A high concentration of calcium and phosphate and the formation of casein phosphopeptides are thought to convey a strong anti-caries effect.

Inorganic phosphates protect against dental caries by increasing the availability of phosphate in plaque so that demineralisation is resisted and remineralisation encouraged. Organic phosphates protect mainly by binding to the tooth surface and reducing enamel dissolution. Phytates are the most effective of these compounds. Despite promising results from incubation and animal experiments for a cariostatic effect of phosphates, studies in humans showed them to be less effective, possibly due to the higher phosphate concentration of human compared with rat saliva. Phytates also reduce the absorption of some micronutrients, e.g. iron and zinc, and are therefore unsuitable as caries-preventive food additives.

Other foods such as honey, chocolate and liquorice all contain factors that protect against dental caries but the benefits of these factors is overridden by the negative effect of the high sugars content of these foods or in the case of liquorice the dark staining effects.

Sugar-free foods that stimulate salivary flow can be classed as caries protective and include sugar-free chewing gum. Plaque pH studies have shown that chewing sugar-free gum increases plaque pH (see Fig. CD 25.5). Results of several clinical trials have shown that sugared gums are cariogenic when compared with sugar-free gum or no gum and sugar-free gums are caries preventing compared with no gum. The most impressive results have been obtained with gums containing the non-sugar sweetener xylitol.

26

Immune function, food allergies and food intolerance

Stephan Strobel and Anne Ferguson*
with a contribution by Andrew Tomkins

---

*Anne Ferguson died in 1998.

infants and animals. Larger antigen doses may cause T-cell deletion and anergy, whereas smaller doses lead to suppression through induction of IL-4/IL-10-secreting Th2 cells and cells secreting TGF-β. Thus food allergic diseases can be envisaged as being due to a breakdown in the usual physiological downregulation of immunity to dietary and other gut-derived antigens.

Allergic sensitisation

Patients are clinically sensitised when they have generated high enough specific IgE levels that permit elicitation of an allergic reaction. A number of individuals may have circulating antigen-specific IgE antibodies without clinical symptoms on ingestion of this particular food. This is one of the reasons why it is not possible to establish clinical diagnoses on the level of antigen-specific IgE alone. IgE antibody binds to high affinity receptors on the surface of mast cells and basophils in such a manner that contact between only a few membrane-associated molecules and the inducing antigen will trigger the release of highly active mediators of inflammation, including histamine, proteolytic enzymes, leukotrienes and prostaglandins, from the granules of these cells.

Aberrant immunity, malabsorption and infection

A range of dietary antigens, eaten every day, reach the organised lymphoid tissues in sufficient amounts to induce a variety of mostly harmless humoral and cellular immune responses. If an active immune response is induced, then the entry of that same antigen in a further meal may result in a local immune reaction, which may cause immediate or delayed reactions including tissue damage.

Severe immunodeficiency states, where infants lack all or most important aspects of their immune system (e.g. X-linked severe combined immunodeficiency), do not cause primary nutritional or morphological mucosal abnormalities. However, some intestinal and systemic infections resulting in failure to thrive states are common in the children.

26.3 AN APPROACH TO CLINICAL INVESTIGATION OF THE IMMUNE SYSTEM

Protocols for the clinical evaluation of systemic immunity are widely used by clinical and laboratory immunologists for the investigation and management of patients with primary, acquired and iatrogenic immunodeficiency syndromes; these are continuously evolving with the discovery of new immunodeficiency states and a better understanding of existing ones. Patients can normally be classified by the type of effector mechanism involved, for example T-cell-mediated immunity, immunoglobulin isotype, polymorphonuclear function or reticuloendothelial system (Bonilla & Geha 2003) (Table 26.1).

Commonly used diagnostic procedures for immunodeficiency states

The history of responses to immunisation, particularly with live vaccines (BCG), is valuable and can indicate earlier normal cell-mediated immunity. An aberrant immune status can usually be deduced from a history of atopy, for example rhinitis, eczema and asthma. Important features to note on general clinical examination include presence of palpable lymph nodes, size of tonsils, splenomegaly, and thymic shadow on the chest X-ray of an infant.

Blood examination

Examination of blood films should be the first investigation, with total white cell count, an accurately performed differential analysis and inspection of cell morphology. The absolute lymphocyte count in peripheral blood is an important but often neglected test. The final diagnosis of an immunodeficiency is based on specialised laboratory tests that must be interpreted by specialists in this area.

Table 26.1 Immunological changes observed in malnutrition and micronutrient deficiencies

Observation or test	Effect
Weight of lymphoid organs	↓
Bactericidal capacity (neutrophils)	↓
Susceptibility to infections	↑
Delayed-type hypersensitivity	↓
T-lymphocyte proliferation	↓
T-lymphocyte numbers	↓
Cytokine production (IFN-γ, IL-1, IL-2, IL-6, TNF-α)	↓
Natural killer cell activity	↓

Other parameters of the immune system can be affected, for example antibody responses, but these effects are less predictable.

Lymphocytes and specific cell-mediated immunity

Evidence of the existence of specific cell-mediated immunity (implying both normal afferent and efferent limbs) can be obtained by in vivo tests of delayed-type hypersensitivity, using a range of antigen to which the body will usually have been exposed. These 'recall' antigens include tuberculin, tetanus antigen, and candida.

Many in vitro tests of antigen-reactive T-cell function are available, ranging from antigen-driven blast transformation to the secretion of cytokines in culture with antigen. Usually, these tests are carried out using blood lymphocytes in specialised laboratories.

Immunoglobulins and antibodies

Assays of total immunoglobulins can be readily carried out on serum, by a variety of techniques. Immediate skin prick tests and serum RAST tests are used for the in vivo and in vitro detection of IgE antibodies. More precise information on the induction and expression of humoral immunity is obtained by studying the primary and secondary immune responses to defined killer vaccine antigens.

Other more specialised assessment of polymorphonuclear leukocyte and other non-antigen-specific functions may be needed.

Gastrointestinal mucosal immunity

It is difficult to study the immune system of the gastrointestinal tract in detail. Clinical tests of gastrointestinal immune function have been slow to develop and require mucosal biopsies and often short-term organ culture systems. Some guidelines for investigation of an individual patient or of a group of patients in whom intestinal mucosal immunodeficiency or hypersensitivity states may be present are given below.

Attention must be paid to the potential roles of non-immunological digestive factors. These may act not only as alternative mechanisms of disease, mimicking immunological disorders (e.g. certain infections), but also as factors that will alter immunity in general (e.g. malnutrition) or change intestinal antigen patterns (e.g. pancreatic insufficiency).

Assessment of specific immunity

In general, methods available concern non-antigen-specific functions such as helper activity, suppressor inducer, suppressor cytotoxic B-cell and natural killer cell functions. Short-term antigen-specific culture systems evaluating the mucosal immunity after in vitro challenge with toxic allergens have been described in coeliac disease patients and milk allergies. The existence of an ongoing delayed-type hypersensitivity (DTH) reaction in the small intestinal and/or the colonic mucosa can be inferred by a cluster of features defined on the basis of work on experimental animals. These include villous atrophy, crypt hyperplasia and a high intraepithelial lymphocyte count.

Mucosal hypersensitivity reactions

Normally it appears that pathogenic antigen-specific immunity of T-cell origin does not develop in the intestine to enterically encountered antigens such as foods. Whether this is true tolerance, antigen-specific suppression, or whether it is merely the absence of this limb of the immune response at gut level, is unknown.

The three jejunal mucosal histopathological features of villous atrophy, crypt hyperplasia and high intraepithelial lymphocyte count may imply the existence of a cell-mediated inflammatory immune reaction within the mucosa. In antibody-mediated hypersensitivity, the diagnosis of an IgE-mediated immune response may require demonstration of mucosal mast cells and eosinophilic infiltration and evidence of mucosal mast cell degranulation.

26.4 NUTRITION AND IMMUNODEFICIENCY DISORDERS

Virtually any component of the immune system, specific or non-specific, can be absent or abnormal; the consequent immunodeficiency states vary in severity from trivial to fatal. Immunodeficiency can also result from acquired diseases. This is well illustrated in severe form in the acquired immunodeficiency syndrome (AIDS). Acquired immunodeficiency may also be iatrogenic, for example as a result of corticosteroid or other immunosuppressive treatment. In addition to causing susceptibility to infection, immunodeficiency may be associated with abnormally regulated immune reactions, as in allergy or autoimmunity.

In general, an immunodeficiency itself has no effect on the nutritional capacity of the gut. Secondary effects often occur on the basis of diarrhoea and

Keusch G T 2003 The history of nutrition: malnutrition, infection and immunity. Journal of Nutrition 133(1):336S–340S

Newell M L 2001 Prevention of mother-to-child transmission of HIV: challenges for the current decade. Bulletin of the World Health Organization 79(12):1138–1144

Sampson H A 2003 9. Food allergy. Journal of Allergy and Clinical Immunology 111(2 Suppl):S540–547

Strobel S 2002a Oral tolerance, systemic immunoregulation, and autoimmunity. Annals of the New York Academy of Sciences 958:47–58

Strobel S 2002b Clinically validated diagnostic tests and non-validated procedures of unproven value. In: Buttriss J (ed) Adverse reactions to foods. Blackwell Scientific, London, p 131–137

Tomkins A 2000 Malnutrition, morbidity and mortality in children and their mothers. Proceedings of the Nutrition Society 59(1):135–146

Wills-Karp M, Santeliz J, Karp C L 2001 The germless theory of allergic disease: revisiting the hygiene hypothesis. Nature Reviews Immunology 1:69–75

Further reading

Bhaskaram P 2002 Micronutrient malnutrition, infection, and immunity: an overview. Nutrition Reviews 60(5 Pt 2):S40–45

Brandtzaeg P 2003 Mucosal immunity: integration between mother and the breast-fed infant. Vaccine 21(24):3382–3388

Braun-Fahrländer C 2000 Allergic diseases in farmers' children. Pediatric Allergy and Immunology 11(Suppl 13):19–22

Brostoff J, Challacombe S J 2002 Food allergy and intolerance, 2nd edn. Saunders, London

Burks A W, Sampson H A 1999 Anaphylaxis and food allergy. Clinical Reviews in Allergy and Immunology 17(3):339–360

Calder P C, Field C J, Gill H S (eds) 2002 Nutrition and immune function. Culinary and Hospitality Industry Publication Services (CHIPS), Weimar, TX

Chin A P M J, de Jong N, Pallast E G et al 2000 Immunity in frail elderly: a randomized controlled trial of exercise and enriched foods. Medicine and Science in Sports and Exercise 32(12):2005–2011

Halken S, Host A 2001 Prevention. Current Opinion in Allergy and Clinical Immunology 1(3):229–236

Heine R G, Elsayed S, Hosking C S, Hill D J 2002 Cow's milk allergy in infancy. Current Opinion in Allergy and Clinical Immunology 2(3):217–225

Hill D J, Hosking C S 2000 Infantile colic and food hypersensitivity. Journal of Pediatric Gastroenterology and Nutrition 30(Suppl):S67–76

Høst A 2002 Frequency of cow's milk allergy in childhood. Annals of Allergy, Asthma, and Immunology 89(6 Suppl 1):33–37

Høst A, Andrae S, Charkin S et al 2003 Allergy testing in children: why, who, when and how? Allergy 58(7):559–569

Hourihane J O, Warner J O, Bock S A et al 2000 Definitive diagnosis of nut allergy. Archives of Disease in Childhood 82(1):88

Lesourd B 2004 Nutrition: a major factor influencing immunity in the elderly. Journal of Nutrition, Health and Aging 8(1):28–37

Sampson H A 2000 Food anaphylaxis. British Medical Bulletin 56(4):925–935

Strobel S, Lessof M, Kimber I 2002 Manifestations of food intolerance. In: Buttriss J (ed) Adverse reactions to foods. Blackwell Science, London, p 89–103

van Odijk J, Kull I, Borres M P et al 2003 Breastfeeding and allergic disease: a multidisciplinary review of the literature (1966–2001) on the mode of early feeding in infancy and its impact on later atopic manifestations. Allergy 58(9):833–843

Waser M, Schierl R, Von Mutius E et al 2004 Determinants of endotoxin levels in living environments of farmers' children and their peers from rural areas. Clinical and Experimental Allergy 34(3):389–397

CD-ROM contents

Further reading from the book

27

Eating disorders

C. G. Fairburn and A. J. Hill

Objectives

By the end of this chapter you should be able to:

- define eating disorders and name the main types
- describe the main features of anorexia nervosa and bulimia nervosa
- outline the characteristics of other eating disorders.

27.1 INTRODUCTION

An eating disorder may be defined as a persistent disturbance of eating (or eating-related behaviour) which impairs physical health or psychosocial functioning, or both, and which is not secondary to any general medical disorder or any other psychiatric disorder. The best-recognised eating disorders are anorexia nervosa and bulimia nervosa. These disorders share many features and together they are a major source of ill health among young women in Western societies. In addition, there are eating disorders in which the person does not meet the diagnostic criteria for anorexia nervosa or bulimia nervosa. These are the 'atypical eating disorders'. (See also Section CD 27.1.) In this chapter, the characteristics and management of these three groups of eating disorder will be described. Though important, the prevention of eating disorders is beyond the scope of this chapter. Reading on this and other key issues is included in the further reading list at the end of this chapter and on the CD-ROM. (Also see Ch. 14: Infancy, childhood and adolescence, and Ch. 20: Obesity.)

27.2 ANOREXIA NERVOSA

Definition

Three features are required to make a diagnosis of anorexia nervosa. The first is active maintenance of an unduly low weight. The definition of what constitutes low weight varies: 15% below a person's expected weight for their age, height and sex is the common cut-off. A body mass index below 17.5 is a similarly used threshold.

While low weight and emaciation are the most obvious features of anorexia nervosa, the most distinctive is the set of attitudes and values concerning body shape and weight. This cognitive disturbance is sometimes referred to as the core psychopathology of the disorder. It has been described in various terms, including 'relentless pursuit of thinness' and a 'morbid fear of fatness'. Thinness and weight loss are idealised and sought after, and strenuous attempts made to avoid weight gain and any possibility of fatness. The heart of the cognitive disturbance is the tendency to judge self-worth largely, or even exclusively, in terms of shape and weight. Whereas it is usual to judge self-worth on the basis of performance in a variety of domains (such as relationships, work performance, sporting activities), people with anorexia nervosa evaluate themselves primarily in terms of their shape and weight. This level of shape and weight concern is far more intense than the dissatisfaction regarded as normative for young women.

The third diagnostic feature is amenorrhoea (in postmenarcheal females not taking an oral contraceptive). The defining low weight of anorexia nervosa is achieved in several ways, including strict dieting, excessive exercising, and in some, self-induced vomiting or laxative misuse. The DSM-IV (Diagnostic and Statistical Manual) psychiatric classificatory system distinguishes between two subtypes of the disorder based on the presence of bulimic or purging symptoms (see Section CD 27.1 for full DSM-IV criteria for anorexia nervosa and bulimia nervosa). The restricting subtype excludes regular binge-eating or purging behaviour. A person with anorexia nervosa can alternate between restricting and bulimic subtypes at different times in their illness, and can migrate into a different eating disorder such as bulimia nervosa (see below).

Epidemiology

Estimates of the incidence or prevalence of eating disorders in Western societies vary according to the assessment method, the population sample and the context of sampling. A typical estimate of the incidence of anorexia nervosa in females is 8 per 100 000 of the population per year. For males, it is less than 0.5 new cases per 100 000 per year. Incidence is highest in women aged 15–24 years. As these figures suggest, anorexia nervosa is more common in females at a male:female prevalence ratio of from 1:6 to 1:10.

The average point prevalence of anorexia nervosa (actual number of cases at a certain point in time) is 280 per 100 000 young females (i.e. 0.28%). The 1-year period prevalence rate is 0.16% in primary care. This is the number of young women who their doctors consider to have an eating disorder. Since many patients deny or hide their eating disorder, the comparable community 1-year prevalence rate is estimated to be higher at 0.37% (Hoek & van Hoeken 2003). Furthermore, the lifetime prevalence of anorexia nervosa in women ranges from 0.5% for strictly defined to 3.7% for more broadly defined anorexia nervosa.

Some incidence figures have suggested an increase in young females with anorexia nervosa over recent decades, but alternative explanations cannot be ruled out. These include changes in diagnostic practice, improved recognition of the disorder, wider availability of services, and changes in the demographic structure of the population.

Certain groups in the population show higher than expected prevalence rates of anorexia nervosa. Female dancers and athletes, such as distance runners and gymnasts, are especially vulnerable. They share highly competitive subcultures where it may be common to manipulate eating and weight to improve aesthetics of appearance and maximise performance. This pressure is intense for athletes competing in sports with strict weight restriction or those requiring a lean body or low weight for reasons of performance or appearance.

Anorexia nervosa has long been considered confined to Western culture and in particular to Caucasians. Recent cross-cultural work has challenged this view. Careful consideration of Chinese and Japanese 'anorexic' patients shows around half to display food refusal or emaciation without the usual intense fear of fatness but, instead, to attribute food refusal to stomach bloating. One explanation is that they come from subcultures where stomach bloating is a more effective local idiom for distress than fat phobia. This suggests that anorexia nervosa, and eating disorders in general, are culturally bound disorders. Alternatively, eating disorders may simply vary in form from culture to culture.

Development

The onset of anorexia nervosa is generally in adolescence, although childhood-onset or pre-pubertal cases are observed. In children, boys represent 20–25% of referrals. Occasionally, anorexia nervosa does not begin until adulthood. Usually it starts as normal dieting which then gets out of control. As the dieting intensifies, body weight falls and the physiological and psychological features of semi-starvation develop. Additional methods of controlling shape and weight may be used at any stage. The characteristic concerns about shape and weight may not be finally expressed until later on. In some cases, the initial weight loss has some other origin such as a general medical illness. However, the low weight is then actively maintained.

Clinical features

Weight loss in anorexia nervosa is primarily achieved through a severe reduction in food intake. The amount consumed may be very small and some patients fast at times. To understand this behaviour, two questions need to be addressed. Do they know what to eat, and do they feel hungry? Several studies have shown that people with anorexia nervosa have greater knowledge about the caloric and macronutrient content of foods but lack awareness of micronutrient and vitamin contents. Their diets are certainly inadequate in energy. However, diet histories are compromised by the over-reporting typical of anorexic patients. Laboratory studies show that restricting anorexics consume 60–70% less energy than age-matched controls. Interestingly, vitamin and mineral deficiencies are rarely seen. This may reflect a decreased metabolic need for micronutrients or an adequate intake of vitamins and minerals.

In most cases hunger persists and for this reason the term 'anorexia' is misleading. However, the perception and reporting of hunger are often distorted. Experimental investigations have revealed abnormal hunger–satiety curves relative to controls. It is also suggested that anorexics learn to control or suppress normal hunger signals. This denial of hunger may be experienced as rewarding and a mark of personal self-control. In addition, the physiological consequences of starvation, such as a slow rate of gastric emptying, can make food intake unpleasant as eating only a little results in bloating. Normalising the amount and pattern of eating helps to rehabilitate hunger and satiety.

Frequent intense exercising is common and also contributes to the low body weight. Laxative and diuretic misuse and self-induced vomiting may also be practised, especially by those patients whose control over eating occasionally breaks down. This is true of about a third of patients with anorexia nervosa, but the amount eaten during these binges is often not truly large.

Accompanying the disordered eating is the disturbance of body image. This includes a perceptual component such that all, or parts, of the body may be seen as larger than their actual size, and the cognitive disturbance described earlier. Judging the body to be larger than it really is may justify the relentless pursuit of thinness. However, neither feature improves as weight is lost: indeed, both tend to get worse. Early in the course of illness, patients often have limited recognition of their disorder and experience their symptoms as ego-syntonic, meaning they are not viewed as a problem and patients do not want to get rid of them.

A range of other psychological symptoms commonly accompany anorexia nervosa, many of which are known to result from semi-starvation. These include depressed mood, irritability, social withdrawal, loss of sexual libido, preoccupation with food, and eventually, reduced alertness and concentration. Dysphoria (unhappiness) is particularly important and often misunderstood by clinicians who make an inappropriate second diagnosis of a mood disorder. Similarly, severe obsessional symptoms, usually related to eating and food, are common in anorexia nervosa. Often, these symptoms improve with weight gain.

A wide range of physical complications is encountered in anorexia nervosa. Earlier last century the disorder was mistakenly attributed to pituitary insufficiency. More recently it was suggested there might be an underlying primary hypothalamic disorder. The balance of evidence, however, strongly suggests that the endocrine disturbance is secondary to abnormalities in eating and weight rather than being a cause of them.

On examination, the degree of emaciation is often striking. Growth may be stunted in patients with a pre-pubertal onset and there may be a failure of breast development. Often patients present with no physical complaints. However, systematic inquiry may reveal heightened sensitivity to cold and a variety of gastrointestinal symptoms such as constipation, fullness after eating, bloatedness and vague abdominal pain. Other symptoms include restlessness, lack of energy and early morning wakening.

In females who are not taking an oral contraceptive, amenorrhoea is (by definition) present. Amenorrhoea, if sustained, is associated with osteopenia, possibly progressing to osteoporosis and risk of bone fractures. Amenorrhoea that starts in early teenage years and persists into young adulthood presents the greatest risk to bone health as patients not only lose bone mass but fail to form bone at a critical phase of development. The resulting osteoporosis is often irreversible.

The physical complications of anorexia nervosa affect each main organ system of the body. Acute complications include dehydration, electrolyte disturbances (due to purging), cardiac compromise with various arrhythmias, gastrointestinal mobility disturbances, renal problems, infertility, hypothermia, and other evidence of hypometabolism.

Causation

Dieting is firmly installed as a general vulnerability factor for both anorexia nervosa and bulimia nervosa. Longitudinal studies have shown that female teenagers who dieted were 5–18 times more likely to develop an eating disorder, depending on the severity of their dieting (Patton et al 1999). However, a simple linkage is problematic for two reasons. First, while many young women diet, relatively few develop an eating disorder. Second, dieting is more likely in those who are heavier and dissatisfied with their body. Dieting may therefore be a relatively non-specific marker of other individually-variable vulnerability factors. Accordingly, retrospective, case-controlled studies show women with anorexia nervosa to have high levels of exposure to a broad range of risk factors, many of which are shared with other psychiatric disorders. These include personality traits of perfectionism, negative self-evaluation, pre-morbid psychiatric disorder, and adverse childhood experiences such as victimisation or abuse.

Most descriptions of the pathogenesis of anorexia nervosa distinguish between groups of vulnerability or predisposing factors. Genetic factors are implicated by family studies showing a 7–12-fold increase in the rates of anorexia nervosa and bulimia nervosa in relatives of eating-disordered probands compared with controls. Since first-degree relatives share both genes and environment, twin studies have been used to disentangle the two (Bulik et al 2000). Clinic samples show concordance for anorexia nervosa of around 55% in identical twins and 5% in non-identical twins. In addition, studies show that 58–76% of the variance in anorexia nervosa is accounted for by genetic factors (Klump et al 2001). These are very similar heritability estimates to those found in schizophrenia and bipolar disorder. There is also evidence of shared transmission between anorexia nervosa and bulimia nervosa. This suggests the existence of a broad eating disorder phenotype with possible shared genetic predispositions. There is still some way to go to revealing how genes are involved in eating disorders, especially in terms of influencing pathological behaviour, affect and cognition. Similarly, the push for molecular genetic studies to identify underlying loci and genes has still to yield consistent findings.

Accounts of the contribution of sociocultural factors to eating disorders seek evidence of the environmental transmission of pathology. Eating disorders show cultural specificity, being largely confined to countries that have an abundance of food, that hold a thin body shape as ideal, and in which dieting is commonplace. The media are often blamed for their blanket use of naturally (and unrepresentative) or unnaturally thin models and celebrities, driving others to achieve thinness themselves. This probably overstates the influence of the media. Exposure to thin bodies in the media can induce body dissatisfaction, but mainly in those already dissatisfied. In turn, they may seek out such images for comparison or motivational purposes. The derogation of fatness, by exclusion or mockery, sits alongside the idealisation of thinness in producing shape and weight dissatisfaction. This dissatisfaction is a common precursor, and continuing accompaniment, of eating disorders.

Peers and family are important contributors to the sociocultural perspective. Negative peer influence is recognisable in the adolescent friendship cliques that are bound by mutual body image concerns. Peers may also be influential in victimising those not conforming to shape or weight ideals or aspirations. Family dynamics (enmeshment, intrusiveness, hostility) and abnormal attachment processes have been proposed as eating disorder causes. Some of these features may be secondary to the presence of an ill family member. However, research suggests that adolescents who perceive parental caring and expectations as low and those who report physical or sexual abuse are at risk for developing eating disorders.

Maternal influence has also been argued as a negative contributory factor in some cases, the mother conveying her own weight and shape concerns by acting as a role model, directly by critical comments, or through inappropriate feeding interactions. Less attention has been paid to the ways in which other family members contribute in similar ways. Nor have researchers looked closely at how families and peers show their positive and protective function in respect of eating disorder vulnerability. Overall, it is difficult to conclude how large a contribution is made by, or the relative importance of, families or peers to anorexia nervosa or bulimia nervosa. What sociocultural factors do appear to do is to channel women's dissatisfaction and distress towards a focus on body shape and size, providing an outlet for individual pathology. The result is thinness being relentlessly pursued by those who see no better way to solve their problems (Polivy & Herman 2001).

Individual risk factors range from personality traits such as perfectionism to personal experiences such as abuse. Trauma, teasing and sexual abuse have all been linked with bulimic behaviour, as has negative affect and low self-esteem (see below). Perfectionist and obsessive features are characteristic of many with anorexia nervosa. The fact that they do not disappear on weight restoration suggests that perfectionism in particular is a trait that predisposes to anorexia nervosa.

Individual factors also encompass life stresses and difficulties encountered. It is common for people to identify a single event that triggered their dieting or intensified their pursuit of thinness but without recognising the range of risk or vulnerability factors in operation. Several of the changes characteristic of anorexia nervosa act to perpetuate the disorder. So it is important to recognise that many of the physical and psychological responses to reduced food intake and low body weight act as maintenance factors. The fullness and bloating resulting from the slowing in gastric emptying, even after eating small amounts of food, makes eating unpleasant. Similarly, the preoccupation with food and eating intensifies the difficulties with eating, encouraging social withdrawal. This isolates the person from his or her peers, encouraging further self-preoccupation. Those who have been overweight in the past are understandably pleased with the weight loss and may be complimented on it. Many patients report that exerting strict control over eating is in itself intensely rewarding. However, the most potent maintaining factor is likely to be cognitive disturbance, the extreme concerns about shape and weight. Given its presence, most other features of the disorder are comprehensible.

recovery. The techniques used include the daily self-monitoring of relevant thoughts and behaviour, often in diaries used to record food intake, binge-eating and purging; education about eating, shape and weight; the use of behavioural procedures to help establish a pattern of regular eating; the gradual reintroduction of avoided food; and cognitive procedures designed to identify and challenge problematic thoughts and attitudes.

Pharmacological treatment has been used more in bulimia nervosa than in anorexia nervosa. Of the several drugs trialled, only antidepressants (tricyclics, monoamine oxidase inhibitors (MAOI) and fluoxetine) have any beneficial effect. They result in a decline in the frequency of binge-eating and an improvement in mood, but the effect is not as great as that of cognitive behaviour therapy. Importantly, the improvement is generally not maintained. The monitoring of patient compliance is recommended since many patients are reluctant to take medication and may stop without consulting the clinician. These drugs cannot be recommended as first-line treatment.

There is increasing evidence that a modest subgroup of patients respond to self-help programmes based on cognitive behavioural principles (e.g. Fairburn 1995). These programmes are either administered on their own or with a modest amount of support and encouragement from a non-specialist therapist (guided self-help). As a result, a proportion of patients can either treat themselves or can be successfully treated in primary care. There is still some work necessary to identify who will benefit from self-help programmes.

The effectiveness of self-help has led to the suggestion that a stepped care approach to treatment should be adopted. Step one is guided self-help (unless the patient has already followed such a programme). Those who do not respond are referred to a trained therapist to receive cognitive behaviour therapy (step 2). In this way trained therapists focus their efforts on those patients who truly need their help, while patients whose eating disorder is responsive to self-help procedures are saved from receiving an unnecessarily elaborate form of treatment. Step three may involve extending the cognitive behavioural therapy, an alternative psychotherapy, or the addition of medication. Such an approach has the advantage of apparent economy but runs the risk of increasing dropouts from treatment as patients feel they are failing. An alternative argument is that patients should be selected for particular therapies

on the basis of the psychological, social and biological factors that underpin the individual case. In reality, this choice is nullified by the lack of choice of available treatment alternatives.

Course and outcome

The evidence base on the course of bulimia nervosa is relatively small. Of the studies with a follow-up of at least 5 years, between a third and a half of those with bulimia nervosa at outset still had an eating disorder, and 10–25% still had bulimia nervosa. There is also considerable flux within samples. For example, in a community sample, each year about a third of patients remitted and a further third relapsed. Studies also report very low rates of spontaneous remission. Given this background, the favourable outcome to properly administered cognitive behavioural therapy is striking. Predictors of poor response to treatment include childhood obesity, low self-esteem, and personality disturbance.

The crude mortality rate for bulimia nervosa is low at 0.5% (Nielsen 2001). Although the standardised mortality rate is higher, it is based on a small number of studies followed up over shorter time periods than in anorexia nervosa. The likelihood is that this will fall as more information is gathered.

➲ Key points

- ➲ Bulimic episodes (bouts of out of control over-consumption) are accompanied by compensatory behaviour (such as self-induced vomiting).

- ➲ The prevalence is increasing and is characteristic of females in their late teens and early twenties.

- ➲ While sharing some clinical features with anorexia nervosa, patients with bulimia nervosa differ in respect of body weight and frequency of bulimic episodes.

- ➲ Increased exposure to dieting and general risk for psychiatric disorder contribute to the development of bulimia nervosa.

- ➲ Reducing and eliminating binge-eating and purging are primary treatment goals.

- ➲ Cognitive behavioural therapy is a very effective therapeutic approach.

27.4 ATYPICAL EATING DISORDERS

It often gets forgotten that around half of the cases of eating disorders in the community are neither anorexia nervosa nor bulimia nervosa. These patients are said to have an atypical eating disorder. DSM-IV describes this as eating disorder not otherwise specified (EDNOS) (see Section CD 27.1). Within EDNOS is binge-eating disorder, a diagnosis currently with research diagnostic criteria.

Eating disorder not otherwise specified (EDNOS)

Many patients with EDNOS have symptoms similar in form to anorexia nervosa and bulimia nervosa but fail to meet their diagnostic criteria either because a particular feature is missing (partial syndrome) or because they do not quite meet the specified level of severity (sub-threshold case). These variants of anorexia nervosa and bulimia nervosa are likely to have similar risk and maintaining factors to those described above, and they appear to respond similarly to treatment.

A diagnosis of EDNOS should not be considered a low-grade disorder or one undeserving of thorough treatment. Instead, EDNOS presents the opportunity to intervene early in the course of a serious disorder at a stage when it might be more amenable to treatment, although in reality many patients are chronic and have had anorexia nervosa and/or bulimia nervosa in the past. The very limited available data on the course of EDNOS supports this view, since the eating disorder either persists or, in around half the cases, evolves into anorexia nervosa or bulimia nervosa.

An associated point is that patients with eating disorders tend to migrate between the diagnostic categories of anorexia nervosa, bulimia nervosa, and the atypical eating disorders (Fairburn & Harrison 2003). The main pathways are shown in Figure 27.1. This movement, together with the fact that they share the same distinctive and core psychopathology, suggests that common mechanisms are involved in their persistence. However, the fact that eating disorders do not evolve into other conditions shows the distinctiveness of the diagnostic category as a whole.

Binge-eating disorder (BED)

The research diagnostic criteria for binge-eating disorder differ from those of bulimia nervosa in several

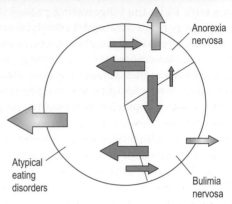

Figure 27.1 The temporal movement between the eating disorders. The size of the arrow indicates likelihood of movement in the direction shown. Arrows that point outside of the circle indicate recovery. (Adapted from Fairburn & Harrison 2003.)

respects (see Section CD 27.1). First, the frequency specification for BED is for binge episodes to occur on 2 days per week rather than 2 episodes per week. In bulimia nervosa a binge is normally terminated by some form of purging. In BED, binges are sometimes difficult to separate into discrete episodes. Indeed, some may last an entire day. Associated with this is an extended time frame: 6 months, rather than the 3 months for bulimia nervosa. This conservative requirement to show a key behaviour over a longer period is controversial but certainly acts to reduce the prevalence of BED. Second, BED does not include the core psychopathology of shape and weight overconcern, so important to understanding anorexia nervosa and bulimia nervosa. The only cognitive component in the diagnostic criteria is the significant distress over the binge-eating. Third, the regular use of inappropriate compensatory behaviours is an exclusionary criterion. Purging is 'recurrent' in the criteria for bulimia nervosa but no indication is available for how frequently the use of fasting or self-induced vomiting should be to define 'regular' for BED.

Estimates of the prevalence of BED vary widely, according to the implementation of these diagnostic criteria and the target sample. The better community studies suggest rates of 2–3% in the adult population. Not surprisingly these figures are higher in obese samples, with BED present in 5–10% of those seeking treatment for obesity in the USA. However, the association between BED and obesity is not invariable and many questions remain regarding the relationship. For example, in nearly half of patients with BED, the binge-eating preceded first dieting; these patients also report obesity at an earlier age than those who dieted before the eating disorder. Overall, the aetiology of binge-eating disorder has been barely studied. It would appear that these patients have lower exposure to the eating disorder risk factors noted above for anorexia nervosa and bulimia nervosa.

Most patients with binge-eating disorder are concerned about their shape and weight, certainly compared with those of an obese control group. But these concerns generally do not have the same intensity and personal significance as those seen in the other eating disorders. Another difference is that patients with binge-eating disorder eat relatively normally outside their binges, tending to under-eat rather than over-eat. Their binge-eating appears to be more of an habitual response to negative moods than a breakdown of rigid dietary restraint. In addition, binge-eating disorder is seen in an older age group (most presenting between age 30 and 50), and is more common in men than either anorexia nervosa or bulimia nervosa (20–25% of cases are male).

The early signs are that binge-eating disorder is very responsive to treatment (Stunkard & Allison 2003). Both cognitive behaviour therapy and interpersonal psychotherapy appear extremely effective in reducing binge-eating and maintaining this relief, although the response may be non-specific unlike in bulimia nervosa. Importantly, this treatment success occurs without any significant weight loss. Pharmacotherapy, primarily antidepressants, also reduces the frequency of binge-eating. Most of the trials are short term and there is some evidence of a recurrence of binge-eating when medication is stopped. Several studies have shown that weight loss programmes that ignore the issue of binge-eating may be as effective as those designed purely to reduce binge-eating. This strengthens the idea that dietary restriction is not responsible for binge-eating in this group, as dietary restriction is a major part of these interventions. Furthermore, such programmes both reduce binge frequency and lead to modest weight loss. Also promising is guided self-help, indeed more so than for bulimia nervosa.

The non-specificity of treatment in binge-eating disorder is in part related to the high placebo responsiveness and spontaneous remission of the disorder. For the latter, the longer the duration of follow-up the greater the improvement, with in one study 90% no longer presenting with BED 5 years after initial diagnosis.

⊃ Key points

⊃ Atypical eating disorders represent around half of the cases of eating disorders in the community.

⊃ Patients with eating disorders tend to migrate between the diagnostic categories of anorexia nervosa, bulimia nervosa, and the atypical eating disorders.

⊃ Patients with binge-eating disorder (BED) do not have intense concern about shape and weight nor do they use purging behaviours after bingeing.

⊃ Many different approaches show success in treating BED.

References and further reading

References

American Psychiatric Association 2000 Practice guidelines for the treatment of patients with eating disorders. American Journal of Psychiatry 157(Suppl 1): 1–39. Available at: http://www.psych.org/clin_res/guide.bk-2.cfm

Bulik C M, Sullivan P F, Wade T D, Kendler K S 2000 Twin studies of eating disorders: a review. International Journal of Eating Disorders 27:1–20

Fairburn C G 1995 Overcoming binge eating. Guilford Press, New York

Fairburn C G, Harrison P J 2003 Eating disorders. Lancet 361:407–416

Hoek H W, van Hoeken D 2003 Review of the prevalence and incidence of eating disorders. International Journal of Eating Disorders 34:383–396

Klump K L, Kaye W H, Strober M 2001 The evolving genetic foundations of eating disorders. Psychiatric Clinics of North America 24:215–225

Nielsen S 2001 Epidemiology and mortality of eating disorders. Psychiatric Clinics of North America 24: 201–214

Patton G C, Selzer R, Coffey C et al 1999 Onset of adolescent eating disorders: population based cohort study over 3 years. British Medical Journal 318:765–768

Polivy J, Herman C P 2002 Causes of eating disorders. Annual Review of Psychology 53:187–213

Stunkard A J, Allison K C 2003 Two forms of disordered eating in obesity: binge eating and night eating. International Journal of Obesity 27:1–12

Further reading

American Academy of Pediatrics Committee on Adolescence 2003 Identifying and treating eating disorders. Pediatrics 111:204–211 *(policy statement on paediatric identification and management of eating disorders)*

American Dietetic Association 2001 Nutrition intervention in the treatment of anorexia nervosa, bulimia nervosa, and eating disorders not otherwise specified (EDNOS). Journal of the American Dietetic Association 101:810–819 *(position statement with regard to involvement of registered dieticians in eating disorder treatment)*

Fairburn C G, Brownell K D (eds) 2002 Eating disorders and obesity. A comprehensive handbook, 2nd edn. Guilford Press, New York *(112 short summary chapters give a good introduction to many issues covered in this chapter)*

Lask B, Bryant-Waugh R (eds) 2000 Anorexia nervosa and related eating disorders in childhood and adolescence, 2nd edn. Psychology Press, Hove

Nasser M, Katzman M, Gordon R (eds) 2001 Eating disorders and cultures in transition. Brunner-Routledge, London

National Collaborating Centre for Mental Health. Eating Disorders 2004 Core interventions in the treatment and management of anorexia nervosa, bulimia nervosa, and related eating disorders. National Clinical Practice Guideline CG9. British Psychological Society, Leicester; http://www.bps.org.uk/eatingdisorders/files/ED.pdf

CD-ROM contents

Expanded material
Section CD 27.1 DSM-IV diagnostic criteria

Tables
Table CD 27.1 Measures for the detection and assessment of eating disorders

Additional references related to CD-ROM material

Further reading

Further reading from the book

Useful websites

28
Deficiency diseases

Maureen Duggan and Barbara Golden

Objectives

By the end of this chapter you should be able to:

- describe the major deficiency diseases, where they occur, and their association with poverty and infection
- recognise the current and older terminology and classifications of malnutrition, and their limitations
- discuss the immediate and underlying causes of the main deficiency diseases, recognising the importance of their interactions
- be aware of the deficiencies that may occur in situations of particular risk
- give examples of particular 'at risk' groups in different situations
- identify the long- and short-term consequences of simple and multiple deficiencies
- be aware of the general principles of treatment and prevention.

28.1 INTRODUCTION

The major deficiency diseases are here described in their global context, with emphasis on pathogenesis and principles of management. The epidemiology is covered in more detail in Chapter 33. Nutritional deficiency is common in poor regions of the world, where there is a vicious cycle of endemic food insecurity and structural injustice (see Ch. 32), and where the spread of infections such as malaria and diarrhoea is favoured by poverty and the tropical climate. Population movements forced by war and economic migration have also favoured the spread of HIV, which interacts with malnutrition to deadly effect.

Migrants and refugees are at increased risk of malnutrition, as are broken families, female-headed households (see also Section 32.3) and the elderly. In regions living with HIV, many elderly people are also caring for orphaned grandchildren. The demographic shift in industrialised countries has led to increasing numbers of isolated elderly and there exist pockets of poverty and undernutrition, for example among inner city dwellers, patients in hospital, immigrants and refugees, drug addicts and the homeless.

WHO (2003a) reported that general nutritional status, evidenced by food availability and by anthropometric indicators of malnutrition in women and children, was improving in South and Southeast Asia and in Central America and the Caribbean, but worsening in sub-Saharan Africa. They reported improvements in two of the three major micronutrient deficiencies, iodine and vitamin A status, except for East Africa, but widespread deterioration in iron status. The strong link between nutrition and child survival suggests that child nutrition is a particularly useful proxy indicator of public health delivery. In Western countries and in cities in the developing world, the diseases of 'affluence' are paradoxically seen among the poor, with micronutrient deficiency coexisting with obesity. The problem of detrimental fetal programming, first recognised in Western countries, is already evident in Asia and South America, as individuals underfed in fetal life are later exposed to high energy intakes and reduced levels of activity. (See also Section CD 28.1.)

For other deficiencies, see Section CD 28C, D, and Chapters 10, 11, 12 and 24.

28.2 UNDERNUTRITION

Definitions

Malnutrition has been defined as a change in nutritional status that carries the penalty of illness, dysfunction or death. Strictly speaking, that definition includes dietary excess but in this section the term malnutrition is taken to mean undernutrition. Commonly used descriptive terms, e.g. chronic energy deficiency (CED) or protein energy malnutrition (PEM), may imply causality in a way that is now recognised as simplistic or false. Other terms are simply archaic, e.g. *marasmus* and *cachexia*. Since children are the earliest victims of food insecurity, many classifications were devised with childhood malnutrition in mind. For practical reasons they initially focused on growth, by measuring weight for age.

Length measurement (until the age of 2 years, and height thereafter) was introduced more recently. Growth failure is marked by 'thinness and shortness', which reflect the distinction between the determinants of ponderal and linear growth. 'Nutritional' growth faltering is not always due to simple under-feeding. Infection is a major contributory factor. Not only does nutrient intake fall, but nutrient requirements are increased to supply the costs of infection-related biosynthesis (see 'The pathogenesis of weight loss and wasting, kwashiorkor and stunting', below and Ch. 26). Borderline malnutrition may be common enough to escape notice, but syndromes with clear physical signs and high fatality are well recognised. A stunted underweight child, living among similarly sized age-mates, might well appear to be thriving.

In Section CD 28.2(a) we follow a typical village infant of a relatively short teenage mother through the nutritional experiences of her first year. This case study of an apparently healthy mother and baby being 'stunted' with reference to international 'standards' illustrates the conundrum of biological variability: how can we compare the nutritional status of the short stocky Alaskan Inuit with that of a lanky East African cattle keeper? Following millennia of biological and cultural adaptation, the physique of each demonstrates 'good fit' with his environment. Adaptation takes other forms; e.g. metabolic adaptation to low protein and energy intakes respectively includes reduction in protein turnover and basal metabolic rate. Stunting has been described as an adaptation to longstanding underfeeding. In acute malaria, where host and pathogen compete for iron, it has even been claimed that malnutrition might confer an adaptive advantage (see Section 28.5). Clearly there are limits to such adaptation beyond which health suffers. As for height, growth often falters in response to repeated infection as well as nutrient depletion. It is also true that variation in height, especially during the early years of life, owes more to nutritional and socioeconomic than to ethnic variability.

Biological variation in height and body build is generally accepted, with the proviso that extremes are likely to be detrimental. In practice we assume that anthropometric variables are normally distributed, the normal range extending from -2.0 to 2.0 standard deviations from the mean. Malnutrition is defined in terms of negative deviation $>2.0\,\mathrm{SD}$ from the reference mean. However, a greater degree of deviation may be needed before the risk of an adverse outcome rises significantly.

Anthropometric indicators, classifications and reference standards

Indicators of nutritional status vary in their ability to predict functional outcome. There is a link between deficiency and malfunction that holds true for all nutrients. Lack of fuel compromises basal metabolism, activity and storage. Repair, growth and structural support fail in the absence of substrate (e.g. nitrogen and bulk minerals), as do enzymatic processes when micronutrients are deficient. The major fuel stores are in adipose tissue and lean body mass, with a minor contribution from glycogen. Anthropometry offers a simple way of estimating their magnitude. Total weight is often used as an indicator but includes skeletal and essential organ weight, which have slow tissue turnover. Inclusion of height in the indicator allows a better estimate of 'disposable' mass, i.e. the lean and fat bulk extra to that in essential structures. An estimate of the partition of fuels between superficial adipose and fat-free mass can be made by measuring skinfold thickness. Indicators involving stature, e.g. weight for height in children, are better short-term prognostic predictors than weight for age alone, which was first used as a functional indicator by Gomez in 1956.

Deficiency of fuel stores, identified by anthropometry, is known in children as protein energy malnutrition (PEM), and in adults by the more recent and less satisfactory term 'chronic energy deficiency' (CED). The term 'protein' is excluded from the descriptive term in adults on the basis that protein requirements are relatively less important after growth has ceased. Since several of the descriptive terms applied to PEM have become deeply embedded in the jargon of many isolated field workers, we need to be aware of them. Marasmus is one example; it describes extreme thinness and was defined as weight $<60\%$ of the reference weight for age. However, if an underweight child is also severely stunted he may paradoxically appear plump. 'Wasting' is another confusing term. Its original meaning was similar to 'marasmic', but was defined as weight $<80\%$ of reference weight for a given height. 'Clinical wasting' and terms such as 'baggy pants' are used to describe recent severe fat loss (over the buttocks). Wasting is held to indicate that malnutrition is recent, whether weight loss is due to illness or simple under-feeding. The corollary that stunting indicates long-term malnutrition is open to simplistic misinterpretation.

Table 28.1 **Classification of malnutrition (WHO 1999)**

	Moderate malnutrition	Severe malnutrition
Symmetrical oedema	No	Yes
Weight for height	SD score >−3.0 and <−2.0 ≥70% and <80% reference	SD score <−3.0 <70% reference
Height for age	SD score >−3.0 and <−2.0 ≥85% and <90% reference	SD score <−3.0 <85% reference

The term 'kwashiorkor' indicates nutritional oedema which carries a poor prognosis, and all oedematous children are defined as severely malnourished (WHO 1999, Table 28.1). The child with typical kwashiorkor also has variable underweight, 'psychosis' and dyspigmented skin and hair. (Figs CD 28.2 to CD 28.8 show examples of kwashiorkor and wasting; Fig. CD 28.1 shows a healthy child for comparison). The typical history is of recent weaning or exposure to infection or other stress. Among other common features are dry or moist skin peeling, and enlargement of the liver. Nutritional oedema (kwashiorkor) is a complication of malnutrition rather than a different 'type' or part of a spectrum. Stunting is considered as distinct in aetiology and outcome from uncomplicated PEM (CED) due to reduced protein energy stores. Children with severe wasting plus oedema (marasmic kwashiorkor) or severe wasting plus stunting are particularly vulnerable.

Anthropometric assessment describes the appearance of individuals with reduced energy stores and quantifies that deficiency against reference standards to facilitate comparisons over time or between individuals, groups or regions (see Section 31.3 and Section CD 28.2(b) and Section CD 28A) Table 28.2 illustrates indicators used for assessment of children and adults, together with the cut-off points (COP) that define moderate malnutrition, and their validation or evidence basis.

The pathogenesis of weight loss and wasting, kwashiorkor and stunting

The main features of uncomplicated PEM and CED are weight loss and wasting caused by negative energy balance, in which available metabolisable energy is less than energy expenditure, due to factors such as malabsorption, increased energy losses in urine and increased energy expenditure from the biosynthetic costs of infection or malignancy, and from fever. In practice the major causes of negative balance are low intakes of low energy-dense foods, exacerbated by infection-related anorexia. The energy shortfall is made up from energy stored in adipose and lean mass (usually muscle) leading to underweight and wasting. As adipose tissue is more energy-dense than lean tissue, a plump individual loses less weight for a given level of negative balance. An increased intake is needed to restore lost weight and to provide the essential amino acids that are required to resynthesise lost muscle mass. This is more difficult on a low energy-dense diet.

Nutritional oedema is commonly triggered by infection. The body's protective response, particularly if it is already malnourished, is nutritionally costly (see Ch. 26). Furthermore, reactive oxygen species, which are toxic, are generated during the cellular response to infection. Their adverse effect on intracellular metabolism is normally held in check by a number of antioxidant mechanisms, many of which require nutrients such as vitamins A, C and E, zinc, selenium and copper. Iron, especially free iron, may act as a pro-oxidant (see Ch. 12). In PEM, oxidative stress to structural lipids causes cell membranes to become permeable to sodium and potassium, which leak with water into the extracellular space causing oedema. At the same time reduced hepatic synthesis of export proteins, due to an insufficient supply of amino acids from the diet or to catabolism of endogenous protein, leads to a lower concentration of circulating plasma proteins including albumin and retinol-binding protein (Waterlow 1992). Hypoalbuminaemia, which lowers intravascular oncotic pressure, was considered to be the main cause of nutritional oedema but Golden and his co-workers have demonstrated the importance of imbalance between the actions of free radicals and protective antioxidants in the genesis of oedema. Micronutrient deficiencies therefore play a critical role in predisposing the child with PEM to kwashiorkor. Oedema may supervene at different degrees of wasting, even in apparently normal children.

Table 28.2 Commonly used anthropometric indicators, the cut-off points for a diagnosis of 'moderate' malnutrition, and evidence base for use, where available

Indicator	Cut-off point (COP) for diagnosis of malnutrition	Evidence base for use as indicators
Weight for age[a]	80% of reference mean ~−2.0 SD	Risk of death rises when weight for age <70% and further at <60%[b,c]
Weight for height[a]	80% of reference mean ~−2.0 SD	Risk of death rises at weight for height <70%[c]
(Length) height for age	90% of reference mean ~−2.0 SD	Risk of death rises at length for age <90%[b], rarely used as single index
Body mass index wt ÷ ht^2 (kg/m^2)	18.5 and 17 for men and women in developing countries[d]	Used in adults; borderline values usually supported by evidence of physical incapacity
Mid-upper arm circumference (MUAC) (see also **Figs CD 28.9, CD 28.10**) Age 1 to <5 years	<12.5 cm[e]: the Shakir strip is coloured red, yellow and green to discriminate MUAC <12.5, 12–<14, and ≥14 cm respectively	Low MUAC <12.5 cm correlates with weight for age <80%, i.e. MUAC used as a swift screening test
MUAC in adults	<23 and <19 cm in men and women in developing countries	Evidence base less convincing, is used as a proxy for low BMI[f]
Height and MUAC	For heights between 70 and 130 cm COP for MUAC is 13.25 to 17.5	Screening in emergencies, RR death rises as MUAC falls[g]
Symmetrical oedema	At any weight for age or weight for height[h]	Associated with increased risk and therefore defines severe malnutrition

[a]Jelliffe & Jelliffe 1989; [b]Chen et al 1980; [c]Kielman & McCord 1978; [d]WHO 1990; [e]Shakir 1975; [f]James et al 1994; [g]Sommer & Loewenstein 1975; [h]WHO 1999. For full reference details see **Further reading** on the CD-ROM ('Anthropometric indicators, classifications and reference standards' section).

Stunting is extremely common, affecting around 45% of children in developing countries, with an even higher prevalence in Asia, and may be evident from an early age. The nutritional determinants of linear growth act at the growth plate of long bones, together with growth hormone (GH) and insulin-like growth factor (IGF-1). Certain amino acids, specifically leucine, and various micronutrients such as zinc, copper, molybdenum and possibly vitamin A exert an influence on linear growth. Beneficial effects of zinc supplementation on stunted children have been reported from the USA and developing countries. Interaction between micronutrients and possible confounding due to multiple concurrent deficiencies limit the conclusions from single nutrient supplementation studies. In a major multinational growth study, dietary 'quality' (implying dairy produce, fruits and green vegetables) had a greater positive influence on growth than any specific nutrient. Stunting and underweight have also been reported in young European children on alternative (macrobiotic) diets. Various cytokines produced in the acute phase response to infection may slow bone growth. Cohort studies have demonstrated cessation and faltering in growth due to frequent or chronic infections including HIV, or to worm infestation. Nutritional stunting is commonly multifactorial in origin. Catch-up in linear growth during nutritional rehabilitation rarely starts until weight recovery is well under way. It may occur immediately, after an interval, or never.

Global trends in malnutrition

Much of our information on the prevalence and trends in malnutrition comes from measurements in under-five children who are both vulnerable and accessible (see also Ch. 33). Comparative national data on underweight in adult women correlate strongly with low birthweight and underweight in children, emphasising the intergenerational effect of female malnutrition. There are few data on pregnancy weight gain, which when linked with fetal birthweight give important information on pregnancy stress. There appears to have been a general improvement in the weight for age of young children except in sub-Saharan Africa, although improvement had slowed by the turn of the century. There has been a fall in overall prevalence of stunting over twenty years.

There is little information on the community prevalence of severe or oedematous malnutrition. Surveys in Africa show rates of severe PEM between 3% and 7%. The pattern of malnutrition seen in hospitals is selectively biased towards more severe illness, although 'malnutrition' may be an unrecorded second diagnosis. Kwashiorkor constituted 35% to 50% of malnutrition in Indian and African hospitals (Waterlow 1992). Kwashiorkor (plus marasmic kwashiorkor) constituted 51% (59%) of 5855 recent admissions with PEM to an urban unit in Malawi with an overall case fatality of 18% during the 4-year study period (Walford & Duggan personal communication). A high prevalence of PEM persists in Africa although the under-five death rate has fallen following various public health initiatives such as immunisation, oral rehydration and provision of vitamin A. Mortality rate is falling less rapidly in areas with high rates of malnutrition, which indicates that malnutrition is a marker for poor programme coverage in such areas. Oedematous malnutrition which is much less common, carries a persistently high case fatality of around 20%.

Causes of malnutrition

The risk of underfeeding begins in fetal life, and is commoner during the last trimester of pregnancy. Risk situations in the first few years of life include lactation failure, a low energy-dense weaning diet, and infection. Maternal death increases risk at any age. Underfeeding may result from insufficient breast milk when the mother is ill with HIV, for example, or has twins. Breast milk substitutes may be unsuitable because of a high renal solute load, as with fresh cow's milk, or low energy density as with diluted cow's milk or incorrectly reconstituted formula (see Section CD 28B). Contaminated water is also important.

When kwashiorkor was first described, it was thought to be due to the low protein content of maize weaning porridge. The common history of infection was neglected. It later became clear that low energy intakes, from low energy-dense foods, were also implicated. The current view is that nutrient density (energy density, protein energy % and micronutrient composition) plays a part in determining the adequacy of a weaning diet. A traditional porridge often has much lower energy density than breast milk,

with a low chemical protein score due to low levels of certain essential amino acids, virtually no vitamin A, and poorly available iron and zinc (WHO 1998). PEM is commonly seen in weanling children during the second year of life, children with kwashiorkor being somewhat older than children with simple wasting. Oedematous malnutrition is commonly triggered by infection, particularly by measles and diarrhoea accompanied by under-feeding. HIV has altered the pattern and now kwashiorkor is seen both in breastfed babies and in older children. In these children, who are sometimes relatively affluent, PEM is associated with frank malabsorption and secondary infection which may be linked to HIV immune failure.

Sporadic CED is often linked to HIV, the African nickname of which was 'slim disease'. HIV has an important cross-generational effect with high rates of orphans, who risk malnutrition and early death, even when seronegative. Malnutrition is highly prevalent in hospitals in developing countries, in association with other severe infections such as typhoid or tuberculosis, with malignancy, or lack of access to suitable feeds by postoperative or badly burned patients. In affluent countries toddlers with PEM usually present with faltering weight gain; oedema is extremely rare. The euphemism for the malnutrition of deprivation is 'non-organic failure to thrive'. Children refusing food or eating alternative diets may also present with marginal PEM. Anorexia nervosa and bulimia present in adolescence with weight loss which may be attributed to dieting (see Ch. 27). CED may also occur in deprived groups such as the homeless and the isolated elderly.

The aetiology of childhood malnutrition was reviewed by UNICEF in 1998. Among many interacting causative factors are urban and rural poverty (see Ch. 32, Section 32.4) which is linked to high fertility, land-hunger, insufficient and contaminated water, and persistent gender inequality. The fundamental problem of food insecurity varies in magnitude in different regions (see Section 32.4). Other acute causes of insecurity are drought and war, which can lead to famine and malnourished refugees (see 'Famines' and 'Refugees', below).

Effects on health and growth: short and long term

The magnitude of effect of malnutrition on health depends on the timing and duration of nutritional stress. The immediate effects, when low birthweight is due to intrauterine growth retardation, are a high neonatal death rate, due to hypoglycaemia, hypothermia and infection. Malnutrition increases a child's vulnerability to other illnesses, especially infection. It is rarely recorded as a cause of death, although it contributes to the case fatality of many illnesses. Waterlow (1992) notes that 'child (1 to 5 years) mortality' rates give a better indication of the link with malnutrition than infant mortality (0–12 months), which includes birth hazards. Meta-analysis of Asian and African studies demonstrates that the relative risk of death due to diarrhoea, respiratory infection, malaria varies with nutritional status.

Severe malnutrition especially if accompanied by oedema has a high case fatality (from 20% for all severe PEM to >50% in kwashiorkor) related both to infection and to metabolic complications of the disease itself. It is difficult to disentangle the long-term effects of an episode of severe malnutrition from those of persistent socioeconomic deprivation. This applies both to PEM and to micronutrient deficiency. There is evidence of an adverse effect of prolonged stunting on cognitive development. In the longer term, the survivor of early malnutrition may recover completely, remain stunted, or have a delayed adolescent growth spurt. Delayed growth and final short stature in women contribute to obstruction in labour, and thereby to high maternal mortality. Adult stunting is also associated with low birthweight. If the pendulum then swings towards nutritional excess in adult life, the survivor is at increased risk of chronic diseases, e.g. diabetes, heart disease. The long-term impact of early malnutrition may be affected by the nutritional transition that is occurring in several developing countries, characterised by rising intakes of fat and sugar and by reduction in physical activity (see Ch. 1, Section 1.4, Ch. 32, Section 32.4, WHO 2003a). An individual who suffered nutritional deprivation in fetal and early life, followed by rapid catch-up growth in childhood due to the nutrition transition, might easily become an overweight adult with increased risk of chronic disease. Because the pace of economic and lifestyle transition has varied in different parts of the world, the distribution of people with increased risk of chronic disease will vary with the stage of 'development'.

Treatment of malnutrition

Treatment of malnutrition is covered in Section CD 28.2(c).

Prevention of malnutrition

Healthy eating is easier to advocate than to achieve. Fetal nutrition, which is obviously important, depends not only on maternal intake but also on expenditure. Since pregnancy stress is greater during the planting season in agricultural societies, women should be encouraged to avoid heavy work, or be targeted for nutritional supplementation at this time. Exclusive breastfeeding is recommended for 6 months, except when milk supply fails to meet the growth requirements of the infant. The tradition of prolonged breastfeeding persists in developing countries with 40% to 50% of mothers still breastfeeding 20–23 months after birth.

A current dilemma is the early infant feeding of babies whose mothers are HIV positive or dead. The pros and cons of feeding with breast milk substitutes (BMS) are discussed in Section CD 28B. In summary, although artificial feeding seems logical, in resource-poor situations where the risks of contamination and other infection are high, there is a strong argument for 'safe suckling', even when a mother knows she is HIV positive, and if she has access to antiretroviral drugs. Breastfeeding has been reported to have adverse effects on the health of the HIV-positive mother. It is also reported that mucosal damage to the baby's gut caused by mixed feeding may increase the risk of mother-to-child transfer of HIV during suckling. Such reports have important implications for infant feeding policies in countries with high rates of HIV. At such a time caution is needed in interpreting new information, especially if it is likely to lead to sudden changes in long established practice. General guidelines from WHO need to be continually reviewed and adapted to the local situation.

When women know they are HIV positive, and have opted for 'safe suckling', it seems prudent to avoid mucosal damage to the infant gut while the baby is still breastfeeding. Thus the interval between starting solids and cow's milk, until suckling stops should be as short as possible. This also makes sense for mothers on antiretroviral treatment, even though the risks are less. The aim at this time is to ensure frequent intakes of palatable food of high nutrient density. Dietary diversification depends not only on access to a variety of foods, but also on willingness to adapt dietary and culinary traditions. Even if amylase-rich flour quadruples the energy density of porridge, there is often a time lag before such a technology is implemented. Local manufacture of commercial weaning foods in urban Kenya and Latin

such as cataract and malignancy. In summary, the role of retinol in epithelial differentiation in the gut and respiratory tract as well as cornea, and its immune function, explains why vitamin A deficiency contributes to morbidity and mortality in many childhood infections. Other effects of deficiency are less well understood. Remodelling of bones during linear growth may be adversely affected by deficiency. And some nutritional anaemia responds to repletion of vitamin A deficiency.

Toxicity is rare in situations where the main dietary source of vitamin A is β-carotene and when self-medication is rare. However, the risks of teratogenicity due to accidental overdosage have influenced public health policies in many countries. Despite the fact that many women in the reproductive age group are at risk of deficiency, women are rarely given prophylactic treatment with vitamin A except during lactation when, it is argued, the risks of teratogenicity are virtually absent. Studies in Nepal and India , using respectively low dose medication and a 'dose' of red palm oil, have shown reduction in maternal mortality and anaemia respectively.

Treatment and prevention

Acute and symptomatic vitamin A deficiency usually presents as keratomalacia. If the cornea is affected, e.g. by measles or exposure keratitis, the eye is kept closed and antibiotic and mydriatic ointment applied. Vitamin A is given by intramuscular injection when possible. Otherwise oral treatment with 50 000 IU is given on days 1, 2 and 28. It is now common policy to give 'prophylactic' supplementation to children at risk of exacerbating viral or other infection. All children with cystic fibrosis should receive daily multivitamin supplements.

Ideally, in countries with endemic vitamin A deficiency, healthy children are supplemented with vitamin A at 6-monthly intervals until the age of 5 years, and opportunistically during childhood infections. WHO recommends doses of 50 000, 100 000 and 200 000 IU respectively for infants less than 6 months, 6 to 12 months and 1 to 5 years. Lactating mothers are similarly supplemented with 200 000 IU within 2 months of delivery. Reduction in morbidity has been linked to such policies. In practice, however, it is not easy to achieve the intended coverage. Toxicity of these empirical high doses is rarely reported.

Fortification is the most appropriate long-term preventive strategy in regions at risk, in view of the fact that sufficient intakes in industrialised countries are largely due to fortification. Fortification (see also Ch. 33) has been implemented successfully in Central America where, legally enforced for more than a decade, fortified sugar now provides, for those over 2 years old, more than 50% of the RDA. Various other vehicles have been assessed in pilot or voluntary programmes including noodle seasoning in Thailand, and margarine in the Philippines. Combined fortification of maize meal with vitamin A, iron, and B complex vitamins, and fortification of sugar with vitamin A are under consideration in several southern African countries. Sustainability is threatened if increasing hard currency costs of the fortification process have an adverse impact on the otherwise acceptable cost of a locally processed food.

Additional strategies, which are likely to produce general benefit, include increasing the agricultural production of high β-carotene strains of cereals and tubers, including transgenic 'golden' rice. Dietary diversification, e.g. by encouraging the consumption of otherwise neglected green leaves, or improving the year-round availability of β-carotene by sun-drying mangoes or tomatoes are also options. Education about cooking methods which conserve the vitamin, the benefits to bioavailability of a higher fat diet, and the development and social marketing of vitamin-rich snacks are also relevant. Other beneficial policies are aimed at reduction of diarrhoeal and respiratory diseases.

⊃ Key points

- ⊃ β-Carotene, which is the major source of vitamin A in areas of endemic deficiency, is more bioavailable in fruit than leaves.
- ⊃ Marginal deficiency, without clinical signs of xerophthalmia, is linked with increased morbidity in measles, other respiratory infections and diarrhoeal disease.
- ⊃ Vitamin A requirements are increased in infection.
- ⊃ Regular supplementation is generally given to young children at risk of deficiency.
- ⊃ Global control of deficiency will depend on fortification of foods.

28.4 IODINE DEFICIENCY DISORDERS

Definition

Iodine deficiency disorders (IDD) result in partial or absolute failure to synthesise thyroid hormone. IDD may be evident as 'endemic cretinism', which is characterised by delayed motor and cognitive development and growth failure in children, and also by a slow rate of general cellular metabolism at all ages. Goitre, present in variable severity, represents reactive hyperplasia of the iodine-deficient thyroid gland, which is often exacerbated by the action of coincidental goitrogens. Deficiency is inferred from clinical signs including presence of goitre, in an area of IDD, and confirmed by a low ($<50\,\mu g/24$ hours) rate of urinary excretion of iodine. (See Figs CD 28.15–16.)

Prevalence and trends

IDD is widely distributed in the world, with regional prevalence ranging from 5% to 35% (WHO 1999). Africa, Asia and the eastern Mediterranean regions are more affected than the Pacific and the Americas. Paradoxical increases in prevalence may result from improved case finding. Since IDD is due to geographical deficiency of the micronutrient iodine, this deficiency does not respond to general socio-economic improvement and will always require specific intervention. At present this is best achieved through iodine fortification of foods.

Causes

With the exception of seafood, the iodine content of all foods, whether flesh or vegetable in origin, depends on that of the soils in which they grew. Iodine deficiency occurs when people subsist on food grown on iodine-deficient soils and have no access to food from elsewhere. There is an iodine cycle in the environment in which iodine present in soil and sea water as iodide is oxidised to elemental iodine and then evaporates. Iodine is also leached out of soil by heavy rain and flooding, and river water is often relatively high in iodine in the tropical rainy season. Iodine reaches the sea, increasing its iodine concentration, and that of marine plants and fish. Recycling of volatile iodine in rainwater is insufficient to replenish iodine-poor soils, which results in geographical variability of iodine in soils and consequently in plants and animals reared in those areas. Poverty and isolation are characteristic of areas of IDD. Up to 100 million people living in the highlands bordering the Rift Valley stretching from Ethiopia via Kenya, Tanzania, Uganda, Democratic Republic of the Congo (DRC), south to Malawi are at risk of IDD. In such areas, notably the DRC, the problem is aggravated by consumption of the tuber cassava, which contains a toxin *linamarin*. This goitrogen is hydrolysed to release cyanide which, after further metabolism to thiocyanate, inhibits uptake of iodine by the thyroid gland, which hypertrophies further, increasing the size of the goitre. Other goitrogens occur in cabbage, bamboo shoots and bacteria in contaminated water.

Effects on growth and health: short and long term

Failure to iodinate tyrosine, precursor to the active thyroid hormones tri- and tetra-iodothyronine (T3 and T4), has consequences which vary with the maturity of the affected individual. Iodine deficiency in fetal life results in failure to myelinate the central nervous system, especially the cerebellum. There is high fetal and neonatal loss, and survivors show hypertonia, poor coordination of movement and delay in cognitive development, 'learning difficulty', sometimes accompanied by deafness. The slowly growing infant is also slow to reach neurological developmental milestones.

In areas where IDD is complicated by consumption of goitrogens, goitre becomes visible in mid childhood. It is even more prominent in adult life, women being affected more than men. Biological variability in iodine requirements probably explains the varying expression of IDD in an affected community. Furthermore, the size and position of the goitre in relation to the trachea and mediastinum may produce debilitating and even life-threatening complications.

The process of making a community diagnosis of IDD is as follows. Anecdotal information that goitre is common leads to a pilot survey of goitre, usually in a primary school, where healthy children are easy to access. If goitre prevalence >10% confirms the likelihood of a public health problem, the entire community is surveyed. The size of goitre is used as a proxy indicator and the urinary iodine:creatinine ratio is determined on a spot sample (the cut-off point for a diagnosis of deficiency is urinary excretion of less than $50\,\mu g/day$ of iodine). Goitre is graded from 0 to 3, grades 1a and 1b requiring palpation or close examination while grades 2 and 3 (visible goitre) refer to goitres easily visible at close and distant range respectively.

Treatment and evaluation of progress

Treatment is offered to affected individuals and then to entire communities. Iodine-containing oils were at first given by intramuscular injection, providing a bolus from which iodine was gradually released. Oral treatment is now preferred. An oral dose of 0.5 to 1.0 ml of lipiodol is repeated at 3-yearly intervals, for women throughout reproductive life, and for men until the age of 40. Even where the benefits of such treatment are literally visible by reduction in goitre size, compliance remains a problem.

Reduction in the degree and prevalence of goitre is used to evaluate progress in individuals and communities, though interval checking of urinary iodine is a more effective 'impact indicator'. Screening of newborns for thyroid-stimulating hormone (TSH) concentration is also useful, using the same blood spot method used in screening for sporadic cretinism in Western countries (WHO 2003b).

Prevention

Iodine fortification of salt is the preferred long-term strategy, salt being universally eaten and more often subject to large-scale processing than most other foods. The level of fortification is decided after determining the level of individual salt consumption in the region. Local small-scale manufacture may interfere with implementation as can cross-border smuggling of cheaper non-iodised salt. The success of fortification programmes in poor countries depends on effective health education, enforceable legislation, maintenance of the fortification equipment in working order, and sustained availability of testing kits. Unexpectedly high salt intakes may result in high levels of urinary iodine. Inequalities persist: despite evidence of lesser risk of IDD, virtually all households in the Americas have access to iodised salt compared with around two-thirds in Africa (WHO 1999).

> ## ➲ Key points
>
> ➲ Although geographical deficiency of iodine is common, IDD usually affects isolated communities consuming their own produce.
>
> ➲ IDD does not respond to measures aimed at improving general health and nutrition.
>
> ➲ Interval dosage with iodine-containing oil (lipiodol) is effective but long-term compliance is poor.
>
> ➲ Iodisation of salt is the preferred strategy and >60% of households in affected regions now have access to fortified salt.

28.5 IRON DEFICIENCY AND IRON DEFICIENCY ANAEMIA

Definition

Anaemia is a late manifestation of iron deficiency (ID). Iron deficiency anaemia (IDA) is defined by a haemoglobin concentration below the age-appropriate range for healthy individuals, due to iron deficiency and responding to iron repletion. Since iron is essential to the synthesis of the oxygen carrier haemoglobin, the size and haemoglobin density of the red cell (*erythrocyte*) is reduced by deficiency. IDA is, therefore, characterised by small, pale (*microcytic, hypochromic*), red blood cells. These small corpuscles have a low mean volume (MCV) and lower mean concentration of haemoglobin (MCHC).

The rate of production of red cells (erythropoiesis) is not affected by iron deficiency. By contrast, in deficiency of folic acid and vitamin B_{12}, which are both necessary for cell proliferation, the process of erythropoiesis is faulty and circulating red cells are fewer in number and unusually large (macrocytic). A disturbance in globin synthesis can occur in riboflavin deficiency, which is manifested by fewer circulating red cells of normal size and haemoglobin concentration. The rare anaemia of copper deficiency is microcytic and hypochromic. In multiple deficiency a mixed picture is common. (See Section CD 28C for additional information on nutrient deficiency anaemias other than IDA.)

The earliest sign of iron deficiency in an otherwise healthy individual is reduced stores, with low bone marrow iron, and low serum ferritin. As iron status deteriorates, the rate of iron transport falls, but red cell function remains satisfactory for a while. Uncomplicated iron deficiency produces an adaptive rise in transferrin synthesis and in total iron binding capacity (TIBC) due to a fall in saturation of circulating transferrin. Anaemia is evidence that iron has failed to reach the red blood cells. Physical signs such as reduced work capacity or breathlessness on exertion are seen in severe IDA.

Some indicators of iron status give confounding results. The ferritin apoprotein behaves like an acute phase protein so that, in acute infection or inflammation, its serum concentration may rise to normal or elevated levels, even when the body is iron deficient. High values for serum ferritin may also coexist with anaemia in children with oedematous PEM (see 'The pathogenesis of weight loss and wasting, kwashiorkor and stunting', above). Ideally, combined indicators of iron metabolism and infection are recommended to assess iron status. By contrast, hepatic synthesis of the binding protein transferrin may fall in PEM. Hereafter we shall refer to iron deficiency as IDA implying severe iron deficiency (ID).

Prevalence and trends

ID is the commonest nutritional deficiency worldwide, particularly affecting young children and women of reproductive age (WHO 1992). The areas worst affected include sub-Saharan Africa, South and Southeast Asia and the West Pacific. Rates of IDA in women range from around 40% in Africa to 65% in South Asia. ID is also associated with poverty in the USA and UK but even when the adult diet is high in flesh foods, the weaning diet may be deficient in iron. ID in young children may be due to avoidance, for religious reasons, of commercial weaning foods containing meat. Macrobiotic vegetarian diets have also been causally linked with iron deficiency, although reports are conflicting. 'Junk food' diets have been incriminated in iron deficiency in adolescents.

Causes

As with other nutrients, iron status depends on the balance between intake and losses. Dietary ID is especially common where the main dietary source is non-haem iron in plant foods, which is absorbed less well than haem iron, and is exacerbated by blood loss. Avoidance of meat by adults is more commonly due to poverty than culture, flesh foods being eaten on special occasions. In meat-free diets, cereals, especially millet, are a major iron source with a small contribution due to contamination from soil or iron pots, and dark green vegetables and pulses are other main dietary source of iron. Diets are classified by WHO according to bioavailability of iron, with nominal values of 5%, 10% and 15% for low, medium and high bioavailability respectively, according to their content of iron absorption inhibitors (such as phytate, calcium, tannin and oxalates) and enhancers (such as by ascorbic acid, other fruit acids and a factor in flesh foods) ID is typically associated with diets of low bioavailability due to high phytate and little haem.

Blood loss is an important cause of ID. Menstrual losses explain the increased allowance for women in the reproductive age group, and heavy losses may cause ID. The RDA in the USA includes an increment in iron intake during pregnancy and lactation but other published dietary reference values, including those of WHO, allow for an increased requirement during lactation but not in pregnancy. The cumulative effect of perinatal blood loss and short birth interval increases the risk of ID. In the humid tropics, persistent low grade blood loss due to intestinal parasites, such as hook-worm and whipworm, may also be a factor as well as less dramatic blood loss from (urinary or intestinal) schistosomiasis.

The major iron store in the newborn is in haemoglobin itself, and babies are born with a high haemoglobin concentration. A baby born with a low birthweight has a lower blood volume and a smaller iron store. Low birthweight babies who are also born before term have even smaller stores. Catch-up growth, during the early months of suckling, on a diet that is naturally low in iron, leads to an increased risk of ID in infancy. This risk is increased if the baby is introduced early to unmodified cow's milk, which may cause microscopic intestinal blood loss. In practice such babies are ideally fed on breast milk, the low iron content of which is highly bioavailable, or on iron-fortified formulae. Weanling children with behavioural feeding problems, as well as those eating a low iron diet, are at risk of ID. ID is also seen in conditions such as coeliac disease where the gut absorptive area is reduced, and in chronic inflammatory bowel disease. IDA due to insidious blood loss may also be the mode of presentation of intestinal tumours.

Effects

At all ages IDA results in reduced oxygen carriage to the tissues with an adverse effect on oxidative metabolism. The reduction in work capacity due to

ID has been quantified in agricultural labourers performing standard tasks. Experimental studies on iron-depleted animals show reduced oxidative capacity of muscle mitochondria. In studies of humans under-performing when iron deficient, iron treatment resulted in improved exercise performance before muscle mitochondrial function had recovered. This suggests that reduced delivery of oxygen to muscle rather than reduced muscle function is the major limiting factor in humans. In developing countries women are also engaged in hard physical work, even when pregnant. In these harsh environments anaemia in pregnancy is commonly associated with higher rates of low fetal birthweight and perinatal death. Furthermore an anaemic mother is more likely to die from haemorrhage at the time of delivery. However, the contribution of ID to such severe anaemia is uncertain because these women are at risk from multiple deficiencies and also malarial anaemia.

Iron is also active in neurotransmitter systems in the brain and the effects of deficiency depend on the maturity of the affected individual. Animal studies suggest that different areas of the developing brain have different iron requirements and therefore different sensitivities to iron deprivation. Reversibility of the effects of experimental iron deprivation in animals varies with the stage of brain development, early deprivation being more resistant. Children with ID in infancy demonstrate delay in developmental milestones with 'catch up' after iron repletion. Information on the long-term outcome of early ID or the benefits of repletion has been conflicting. It appears that repletion of deficiency in older children has more effect on cognitive development than if deficiency occurred when very young. There are difficulties in obtaining and interpreting information: there may be confounding due to coincidental nutrient deficiencies or psychosocial disadvantage; secondly, ethical considerations will inevitably limit the scope of case-controlled studies; and lastly, psychometric testing in longitudinal studies is difficult to interpret.

The role of iron in infection is complex, since it is a nutrient for both host and pathogen, especially for intracellular organisms such as malaria, and also a potential toxicant. Studies in iron-deficient but otherwise healthy humans have shown reduced production of myeloperoxidase (a precursor to bacterial killing) by neutrophils, reduced bactericidal activity of macrophages, and also a reduction in T-lymphocyte number and proliferation. These abnormalities are corrected by iron repletion. The adverse effect of ID on the cellular response is more marked than its effect on humoral immunity.

There have been reliable reports that bacterial infection is exacerbated by iron therapy, especially if given by injection, which is followed by a brief period of hyper-ferraemia. It seemed that this excess of free iron became available to bacteria in the bloodstream. It was postulated that iron supplementation of formula milks, which do not contain lacto-ferrin, might also increase infection risk, although contamination during preparation was also likely. More importantly, anaemic children with malaria were reported to deteriorate if given oral iron. Iron is not given currently by injection, and iron supplementation of formula milks is more modest. The question whether iron treatment during acute malaria increases the severity of illness has not been resolved. Prudence, however, dictates that iron treatment to anaemic children be postponed until malaria has been treated, and that community supplementation should be postponed until after the malaria season.

Treatment

People with confirmed ID are generally treated with oral iron as a ferrous salt. Treatment should continue until stores are replete, estimated to be 3 months after normalisation of haemoglobin concentration. Supplementation is generally recommended in pregnancy with a daily dose of 60 mg of elemental iron for 6 months, and higher dosage for mothers presenting late for antenatal care. There is some evidence that the effect of iron depends on the total dose, so that frequency of treatment may not be critical. Disappointing results of supplementation programmes may be due to multifactorial anaemia as well as poor compliance. In high risk areas combined treatment with folic acid is more effective, especially in Asia and Africa, and multiple micronutrient supplementation is also promoted, despite some reports of a reduced haematological response, e.g. when iron supplementation is combined with zinc. An enhanced response to iron supplementation has been attributed to synchronous vitamin A supplementation in vitamin A deficient subjects. Iron deficiency may coexist with malnutrition and infection in young children. A cautious approach to management is described in Section CD 28.5.

Prevention

In areas at risk of ID, fortification of staple foods is a cost-effective strategy. The same principles apply as to fortification with other micronutrients – the level of need is assessed, a suitable vehicle is identified, ideally a cheap food with similar levels of consumption by all population groups. The iron should be in a bioavailable form, stable when stored, and with an acceptable taste. Central processing facilitates the technical process of fortification, though low technology systems have been developed for fortification during small-scale milling of maize. A number of vehicles for iron fortification have been assessed including sugar, milk powder, maize and wheat flour. A number of iron salts are listed as safe by the US Food and Drugs Administration, but they vary in cost, solubility in water or gastric acid, and in the metallic taste they impart to food. Milk has been satisfactorily fortified with ferrous sulphate and wheat flour with ferrous fumarate. High extraction (low phytate) wheat flour is a particularly suitable vehicle. Even when fortification appears to be effective and cost beneficial, the long-term success of the strategy depends on legislation and active participation of an informed community. In Western countries, the majority (omnivore) consumes a diet in which iron is highly bioavailable. For groups at risk, postponing of drinking raw milk until the end of the first year, education about sources of dietary iron, including Halal sources, and about enhancers of absorption are basic points in nutrition education. Fortification of bread flour and commercial breakfast cereals is long established and accepted, although it has been suspended in some European countries.

See Section CD 28D for additional information on other mineral and vitamin deficiencies.

⊃ Key points

- ⊃ Iron deficiency is strongly linked with diets low in haem iron and high in phytate, which have low (~5%) bioavailability of iron.

- ⊃ Dietary iron deficiency is exacerbated by blood loss due to intestinal parasites.

- ⊃ Severe iron deficiency results in anaemia and is its major cause in deficient populations.

- ⊃ Oxidative metabolism and therefore work capacity are reduced by iron deficiency.

- ⊃ In young infants and children iron deficiency is also associated with motor and cognitive delay though long-term sequelae are unclear.

- ⊃ Iron fortification of staple foods is a cost-effective preventive strategy.

28.6 SPECIFIC SITUATIONS AND POPULATION GROUPS AT RISK OF MALNUTRITION

Famines

Famine is defined as a sharp increase in mortality due to diseases related to acute starvation (see Section CD 28.6(a) for fuller discussion, and Section 32.4) Famine was thought to be a direct and inevitable consequence of sudden and severe crop failure, sometimes exacerbated by isolation and transport problems. This traditional paradigm was overturned when Sen (1982) demonstrated that widespread starvation could occur even when food was available.

In the mid-nineteenth century, potato blight affected much of northern Europe, but Ireland alone was struck by famine. The potato had flourished in Ireland, giving high energy yields per cultivated area. Early warnings about rotting crops were met by a combination of forward planning and legislative inertia. Efforts were made to provide employment and hold down food prices, but a powerful political lobby strove to maintain high prices for wheat farmers. Ireland continued to export wheat, while the unfamiliar maize was imported as food aid. Delay in releasing the 'Indian corn' led to soaring food prices and starvation. People began to leave home, and scurvy and famine oedema were reported. Many succumbed to louse-borne typhus and relapsing fever, or emigrated in conditions of appalling squalor. Death and emigration were together responsible for a major fall in population, although the actual death toll remains uncertain.

More recent examples are from Bengal, Bangladesh and Ethiopia. Floods and cyclones in wartime (1943) Bengal resulted in some crop losses. Meanwhile an urban boom, fuelled by armament production, had led to inflation of grain prices. Factory workers were little affected by this, but the service economy and food producers, specifically barbers and poor fishermen, found they could no longer buy sufficient rice for their needs. Sharp increase in price and some hoarding of rice further disrupted exchange conditions and there was widespread hunger. A similar natural catastrophe occurred in 1974 in (then) Bangladesh, resulting in rural unemployment, plus an uncontrolled rise in rice price. National statistics proved that per capita grain production actually peaked in the famine year. A drought in Ethiopia in the mid-1980s resulted in a failed harvest for subsistence farmers working exhausted land and using poor equipment. Their plight was exacerbated by a forced famine levy, plus continued pressure to remit a grain quota to the government as part of a strategy to hold down urban food prices. Farmers were forced to sell livestock, exacerbating the food shortage in drought affected areas. Sen and other writers agree that famine is less likely in a functioning democracy, since the administration will be goaded by the media and political opposition into some effective response to an emergency.

Four stages of progression to famine have been identified: dearth or food shortage; privation and coping strategies; and social collapse with dispersal and migration. When a calamity affects food stocks, early coping strategies include foraging for wild foods, gradual selling of possessions, and reduction of activity, including changes in health-seeking behaviour. Young men move away to find work. A sign that coping mechanisms have failed is when destitute people begin to leave home. This process is accompanied by gradual deterioration of general nutritional status and falling immunisation rates. By the time starving people begin to congregate in camps they are vulnerable to infectious diseases, and mortality begins to rise.

Early intervention aims to interrupt this baleful progress before irrevocable damage has been done. In countries at risk, vulnerability mapping is undertaken, using satellite images, climatic, and agricultural data including crop estimates, census and health information and anthropometric assessment. At the domestic level, information on food availability from production, labour or barter takes note of seasonal variation, of recent 'shocks' and traditional coping strategies. Baseline information is continually updated and re-analysed to compare predicted and actual outcome, and as part of a sophisticated warning system. This proactive data collation is an example of effective partnership between government and international agencies. There is a global and national responsibility to avert famine, by facilitating development, encouraging good governance and preventing war.

Refugees

Global statistics indicate that conflict has overtaken climatic disaster as the trigger for large-scale population movements. People migrate within their own or to another country, fleeing from danger or seeking food and security. Global estimates suggest that around 10.4 million people are currently refugees. If asylum seekers, internally displaced and returned refugees are included, more than 20 million people are insecure.

Food distribution to refugees or in emergency situations may take several forms: general or complementary rations and supplementary or therapeutic feeding programmes. A general ration supplies total nutritional requirements, using acceptable foods as far as possible; the term 'basic' applies to a ration of staple only. Rations are supplied dry and collected at intervals. Complementary rations such as pulses and oil may be supplied separately from the basic ration. They are also collected in bulk and prepared by the family. This is the preferred method of feeding since it respects autonomy, prevents cross-infection and reduces stress.

On site ('wet') feeding may be required for at-risk groups, especially young children. Appropriate balanced meals are prepared on site and fed in a canteen manner. There are risks associated with gathering children together, when some are incubating, and others not immunised against childhood infections. Clean water must be ensured and measles immunisation must be well under way. Therapeutic feeding of malnourished children follows the usual principles. When general rations and supplementary feeding are based on dry foods, there is a risk of micronutrient deficiency, especially when refugees are unable to forage or grow vegetables. Clinical deficiency of thiamin, niacin and vitamin C has been reported in refugees in Africa and Asia. Vitamin A supplementation is critical. Information on the daily and monthly amount and composition of a balanced general ration is available on the websites of experienced aid organisations. Fortification of dry rations with niacin, thiamin and vitamin C is recommended, followed by early facilitation of access to fresh foods. See Section CD 28.6(b) regarding the safe management of refugee camps.

Hospital malnutrition

Nutritional status at admission to hospital has implications both for management and for outcome. Undernutrition, when evidenced by loss of lean body mass, is associated with prolonged admission (see Section 28.2 on CED). The high prevalence of undernutrition in hospital patients in the USA forty years ago initiated research into the nutritional cost of infection, surgery and burns. Early estimates of the energy and protein requirements in critical illness were too high, because values obtained during acute illness were assumed to apply during convalescence. Furthermore, hyper-metabolism of infection is less common due to more aggressive management of sepsis and necrosis, and general improvements in intensive care. Enteral and parenteral over-feeding, which led to hepatic steatosis, is much less common. Nevertheless there are drawbacks associated with estimating energy and protein requirements simply in terms of weight, because the ratio of active lean body mass to total weight is not constant. This is an argument for caution in interpreting current guidelines. The trend towards supplementation with n-3 fatty acids and glutamine, in order to modulate the infection response, is a proactive approach to surgical undernutrition. Nutrition therapy at the level of intensive care is usually efficient.

Some conditions, e.g. renal failure, are associated with increased risk of micronutrient deficiency due to dietary restriction, exacerbated by interaction between uraemic toxins and nutrients, and nutrient losses during dialysis. Folate deficiency may present as failure of anaemia to respond to treatment with erythropoietin. Micronutrient supplementation is recommended. Surgical patients are also at increased risk of deficiency when, for example, nutrient absorption has been compromised by gastric bypass or gut resection. Vitamin and mineral supplementation is indicated, allowance being made, in the latter case, for competition between minerals for absorption. Malnutrition may slow down the metabolism of drugs, and also affect the response to treatment of infection. Supplementation with antioxidant vitamins and minerals may act by repletion of deficiency or by immune modulation. Folate, B_6 and B_{12} have been used for their pharmacological effect on disturbed homocysteine metabolism (see also next section). The prevention of malnutrition (before entry to hospital) is part of primary care for the elderly and other vulnerable groups. Those at risk should be comprehensively assessed at admission, and all attempts to improve the quality of hospital meals encouraged.

Alcoholism

Alcoholism is a global problem, the nutritional consequences of which are worse when superimposed on an already impoverished diet (see Ch. 9). A daily intake of 5 to 7 units of alcohol supplies up to 10% of energy requirements as 'empty calories'. For the heavier drinker, meals may be nutritionally inadequate, or omitted due to forgetfulness or poverty. Signs of CED will be evident when protein energy intake is compromised. Micronutrient deficiency is common; folic acid, thiamin, pyridoxine and vitamin A deficiency may be accompanied by low serum concentrations of magnesium, zinc and calcium. Micronutrients with antioxidant action protect against the effects of alcohol on intracellular redox reactions including lipid peroxidation. Since alcohol inhibits the conversion of retinol to retinal, alcoholics may become night-blind. Other clinical signs of vitamin A deficiency are uncommon.

Thiamin deficiency is common, and it can be predicted from recorded behaviour plus clinical signs of undernutrition. Chronic thiamin deficiency may result in polyneuropathy or the complexities of the Wernicke–Korsakoff syndrome, which are due to ischaemic changes in the brainstem. The risk of sensory neuropathy depends on the duration of alcohol abuse. The Wernicke–Korsakoff syndrome presents with signs mimicking those of acute alcohol toxicity such as unusual eye movements, an ataxic gait, memory failure and finally stupor and coma. Treatment with thiamin is effective if given in time; otherwise the changes are irreversible. Thiamin is given by infusion together with riboflavin, nicotinamide and vitamin C at a dose of 250 mg 8-hourly, reducing gradually to a daily oral dose of 200 to 300 mg if the patient recovers.

Cyanide toxicity due to consumption of cassava, in an otherwise deficient diet, is particularly prevalent in indigent alcoholics in West Africa. The condition, known as tropical ataxic neuropathy, presents with peripheral neuropathy accompanied by typical changes in the retina. Treatment with vitamin B_{12} and riboflavin has been tried.

Groups with a high risk of malnutrition in affluent countries

Poverty is linked with malnutrition in affluent countries, but there may be divergence between macro- and micronutrient status. In the USA, micronutrient deficiency is commonly associated with obesity both in children and in the elderly, in the latter being

(iron). The fetal demand for iron increases during gestation and failure to take adequate dietary iron may lead to maternal iron-deficient anaemia and an increased risk of premature birth. In recent years, evidence has accumulated to support a link between fetal nutritional status and adult morbidity and mortality. This is known as the 'fetal origins' or thrifty phenotype hypothesis, which states that inappropriate levels of nutrition at critical times during fetal development can result in disproportionate growth, with the programming of the adult onset of several diseases including coronary heart disease, type 2 diabetes and hypertension. Such a phenomenon implies a long-term reprogramming of gene expression.

The amount of fat in the diet has received much emphasis in relation to the aetiology of major 'Western' diseases, such as coronary heart disease, cancer and obesity. Current recommendations for the amount of dietary fat are 30% or less of total energy intake, but the proportions of the different types of fat are just as important. There is a strong association with elevated levels of low-density lipoprotein (LDL) and the increased risk of cardiovascular disease (CVD). LDL is the main route for cholesterol delivery to peripheral tissues and contains the apoprotein B_{100} (apo-B_{100}) which acts as a ligand for the LDL receptor. Excess lipids (dietary and endogenous) in the liver divert apo-B_{100} from a degradation pathway to the assembly of very low-density lipoprotein (VLDL), the precursor for LDL, by a post-transcriptional mechanism. Diets high in saturated fatty acids (laurate, myristrate and palmitate, but not stearate) are associated with increased secretion of VLDL and elevated LDL levels. Furthermore, these saturated fatty acids have also been shown to decrease the LDL receptor affinity, thus raising the levels of plasma LDL. The inclusion and replacement of saturated fatty acids with monounsaturated (MUFA) and polyunsaturated fatty acids (PUFAs) in the diet have been found to provide health benefits with respect to reducing the risks of CVD by various direct and indirect mechanisms, including reduced apo-B_{100} secretion.

One of the additional health benefits from an increased intake of n-3 PUFAs, namely eicosapentaenoic (EPA) and docosahexaenoic (DHA) acid, is a reduction in cytokine synthesis, a mediator in the immune response. The release of the cytokines interleukin-1 (IL-1) and tumour necrosis factor-alpha (TNF-α) from macrophages is decreased in the presence of n-3 PUFAs. Lymphocyte synthesis of interferon-γ (INF-γ) and IL-2 is also decreased. The decrease in IL-2 synthesis can occur directly by the suppression of IL-2 transcription, or indirectly by (i) the reduction in IL-1 synthesis, and/or (ii) suppression of the eicosanoid, leukotriene B_4 (LTB_4) synthesis. EPA inhibits the synthesis of LTB_4 at the expense of producing the less active LTB_5. The observed reduction in immune response by n-3 PUFAs has led to their therapeutic application in treating inflammatory diseases such as rheumatoid arthritis and psoriasis.

29.5 POLYMORPHISMS AND THEIR EFFECTS ON NUTRIENT METABOLISM

Comparison of the genome of any two individuals will show genetic variation of some 0.1%. These differences underlie individual and population diversity in factors such as height, hair and skin colour, as well as disease susceptibility and the response to drug therapy. The most abundant and simplest form of variation is a result of mutations at individual points along the DNA sequence, termed single nucleotide polymorphisms (SNPs, pronounced 'snips'). Following completion of the draft of the human genome sequence, some 1.4 million SNPs were assigned to the genome map at an average density of 1 in 1000–2000 bases (see Sachidanandam et al 2001). The location of SNPs within the genome dictates the extent of their influence on phenotype. Most SNPs are found in the non-coding regions of genes, some of which may be in the regulatory regions, affect mRNA stability, or disrupt exon–intron boundaries. Of the SNPs that are found within the gene coding sequences, the resultant polymorphism can be either synonymous (no amino acid substitution occurs) or non-synonymous (amino acid substitution – which may alter the function of the encoded protein) (Fig. 29.3). This is because some polymorphisms do not alter the encoded amino acid, while others do (see 'Principles of gene expression', above).

Gly	Ser	Asn	Arg	
G G A	T C G	A A T	C G T	Individual A
G G *C*	T C G	A A *A*	C G T	Individual B
Gly	Ser	**Lys**	Arg	

Figure 29.3   Single nucleotide polymorphisms (SNPs) within a gene. The figure shows how a polymorphism within the coding region of a gene may result in either no change in the encoded amino acid or in an amino acid substitution – synonymous and non-synonymous polymorphisms, respectively.

Mutations that alter protein structure and function to a substantial extent generally result in an end-point disease – an inborn error of metabolism. These can range from single loss-of-function mutations such as the rare condition, glucose-galactose malabsorption (a defect in an intestinal glucose transporter), to loss of enzyme activity such as in phenylalanine hydroxylase in the well-known inborn error of phenylketonuria (Table 29.2). Both these cases may be alleviated by dietary intervention. By deciphering the association between genetic variation and disease, the possibility of designing specific diets – or providing dietary advice – tailored to the genotype of an individual can be envisaged.

As always, the ability to realise such a scenario depends upon appropriate technological advances so that SNPs can be readily identified. DNA microarrays or variant detector arrays have recently been developed to support the favoured direct DNA sequencing approach to SNP detection, both being high-throughput technologies.

Table 29.2 **Examples of common inborn errors of metabolism related to nutrition**

Disorder	Clinical features	Dietary management
Biotinidase deficiency	Ketoacidosis, eczema, retardation, alopecia	Responsive to biotin treatment
Cystinuria	Cystine stones	Dietary reduction of methionine
Familial hypercholesterolaemia	Elevated cholesterol levels, xanthomas, atherosclerosis	Low cholesterol, low saturated fat diet
Fructose intolerance	Keto and lactic acidosis, hypoglycaemia	Fructose-free diet
Galactosaemia	Cataracts, enlarged liver, enlarged spleen, mental retardation	Galactose-free diets
Glycogen storage diseases: e.g. von Gierke's disease, Pompe's disease, Cori's disease, McArdle's disease	Enlarged liver, easy muscle fatigue	High carbohydrate diets
Gout	Arthritis, tophi, hyperuricaemia	Protein, purine and alcohol restriction
Hartnup disease	Dermatosis, cerebellar ataxia, aminoaciduria	Responsive to nicotinamide treatment
Lactose intolerance	Nausea, cramps, bloating, gas, and diarrhoea	Dietary restriction of lactose
Leigh's disease	Degeneration of the central nervous system	Responsive to thiamin treatment
Lipoprotein lipase deficiency	Abdominal pain, pancreatitis, xanthomas	Low fat diet
Maple syrup urine disease (MSUD)	Retardation, ketoacidosis, seizures	Dietary reduction of the amino acids, leucine, isoleucine and valine. Responsive to thiamin treatment
Phenylketonuria (PKU)	Mental retardation, growth failure	Dietary restriction of phenylalanine
Refsum's disease	Retinitis pigmentosa, peripheral neuropathy, ataxia, impaired hearing, and bone and skin changes	Dietary restriction of chlorophyll and foods containing phytanic acid

Adapted from McLaren (1992).

Genes and disease

Most common diseases such as diabetes, obesity and cardiovascular disease are a consequence of complex interactions between multiple genes and environmental/lifestyle factors – particularly diet and exercise. The development of such diseases as the result of a mutation in a single gene can occur, but it is rare (see section below on obesity). An individual's susceptibility to complex diseases is underpinned by the unique combination of SNPs distributed throughout their genome (see Shastry 2002). As most SNPs are synonymous rather than non-synonymous, research will need to go beyond the candidate-gene approach, i.e. examining particular genes because of an a priori basis for considering an association.

One strategy for looking at polygenic disorders is that of an association study in which patterns of SNPs (haplotypes) are identified and compared between a disease-carrying population and a control group. Profiles of disease-related genes can be compiled to provide diagnosis and intervention strategies. There is now a considerable focus on the identification of SNPs and understanding their role in nutrition-related disease conditions. Outlined below are three specific examples of SNPs in different genes and their consequences.

MTHFR

The enzyme 5,10-methylene tetrahydrofolate reductase (MTHFR) is involved in folate metabolism. Its reaction product, 5-methyltetrahydrofolate, serves in the remethylation of homocysteine (Hcy) to the essential amino acid methionine, required for protein synthesis. A common SNP, resulting in a C to T change at position 677 (commonly referred to as C677T), causes an amino acid substitution of alanine to valine at position 222 (Ala222Val). The frequency of the homozygous *TT* genotype ranges from around 1% in African-Americans, through to about 10% in Caucasians and 20% in some Italian populations. This polymorphism has the effect of reducing the activity of the enzyme, which results in increased plasma levels of homocysteine, particularly in folate-deficient conditions (see Ueland et al 2001).

The hyperhomocysteinaemia caused by the presence of the Ala222Val polymorphism increases the risk of neural tube defects (NTD) during pregnancy and may be associated with cardiovascular disease and colorectal cancer. Conversely, at high folate status, the *TT* genotype is thought to protect against colorectal neoplasias. Increasing the intake of folate appears to override the deleterious effects of the TT genotype. During pregnancy, increasing the daily intake of total folate from 200 to 600 µg has been shown to halve the risk of NTD. Furthermore, daily supplements of 5 mg of folic acid have been recommended for women wishing to conceive who have had a previous pregnancy affected by NTD.

A second common SNP has been described in MTHFR, A1298C, and this results in a glutamate to alanine substitution. Individually, the *CC* genotype has no effect on MTHFR activity. However, combined heterozygosity for both the C677T and A1298C polymorphisms can result in hyperhomocysteinaemia, although the presence of both mutations on the same allele is rare.

The UK Government's Committee on Medical Aspects of Food and Nutrition Policy (COMA) has recommended the fortification of staple foods (flour, cereals) with folic acid. However, care is needed as too much folate can lead to complications by masking the effects of vitamin B_{12} deficiency. This highlights the need for individualised nutritional assessments – which is one of the goals of nutritional genomics.

Vitamin D receptor (VDR)

The steroid hormone 1,25-dihydroxyvitamin D_3 (cholecalciferol, $1,25-(OH)_2D_3$), elicits its biological action through binding to the vitamin D receptor (VDR). This receptor is a transcription factor and when it binds the vitamin D ligand in the nucleus transcription is activated in a wide range of tissues through responsive elements in the promoter regions of target genes. The principal action of vitamin D is to maintain calcium homeostasis to assist in the growth and integrity of bone. Other roles have been suggested and these include those in the immune system and in cell differentiation. A number of loss-of-function mutations of the VDR gene have been identified which result in hereditary vitamin D-resistant rickets.

Several subtle allelic polymorphisms have been identified in the VDR gene, which have been linked to diseases such as osteoporosis, a prevalent metabolic bone disorder characterised by reduced bone density (see Uitterlinden et al 2002). However, the effects of these SNPs are not well understood. Many of the polymorphisms being studied are either found in intronic or non-coding regions (3'UTR) or are in the coding region, however, their change does not result in an amino acid substitution (synonymous SNP), making it difficult to assign a functional role to the individual variations. Nevertheless, due to the large size of the VDR gene it is expected that many more SNPs will be identified and assessed for their susceptibility to disease states.

One polymorphism that does result in an amino acid change is found in exon 2. The T to C transition results in the removal of a start codon. Translation of this protein product begins at the next available start site, three amino acids further along. Whilst both protein products are known to exist, transcriptional activity appears to be higher for the shorter protein. The longer protein may be associated with lower bone mineral density. While it may be difficult at present to associate individual SNPs with bone disorders, the combination of different SNPs may produce varying levels of expressed VDR protein and therefore account for variation in individual responses to levels of circulating vitamin D. Knowledge of the vitamin D response would consequently allow for the appropriate adjustment in dietary calcium intake.

Gluten sensitivity (coeliac disease)

Gluten intolerance (coeliac disease) is one of the most common genetic diseases in Europe with about 1 in 130 to 1 in 500 of the population being affected. It is rare in African, Japanese and Chinese populations. Contrary to what was initially thought, however, coeliac disease is also common in the USA, where it is now estimated to occur at a rate of 1 in 133. It is a digestive disorder in which the presence of gluten found in wheat and certain cereals causes

damage to the mucosa of the small intestine, resulting in the malabsorption of nutrients from the diet. The symptoms of coeliac disease range from classic features, such as diarrhoea, weight loss and malnutrition, to latent symptoms such as isolated nutrient deficiencies, though no gastrointestinal symptoms.

Coeliac disease is an immune-mediated response associated with the major histocompatibility complex (MHC) – one of the most gene dense regions in the human genome, consisting of 264 human leukocyte antigen (HLA) genes. These genes are noted for their large number of polymorphisms, which presently number 1556 alleles (see Table CD 29.1). Coeliac disease patients belong to either the DR3 (or DR5/DR7 heterozygous) genotype (95%) and express the HLA-DQ2 α, β heterodimer, or to the DR4 genotype (5%) and express the HLA-DQ8 α, β. However, the broad range of symptoms presented with this disease implies that it is a multifactorial disorder with SNPs found on either HLA-related or other closely related genes (see Guandalini & Gupta 2002).

Dietary intervention in this disease requires total exclusion of gluten-containing products. It is known that intolerance to gluten is highly variable between coeliac disease sufferers, implying that some individuals could accommodate small amounts of dietary gluten. However, no data are available to support this, which is why a total exclusion of dietary gluten is recommended. SNP typing and assignment of particular haplotypes to various symptomatic disease states is an achievable goal, potentially resulting in the safe inclusion of small amounts of gluten back into the diet.

29.6 DIET, GENOTYPE AND SUSCEPTIBILITY TO DISEASE: THE EXAMPLE OF OBESITY

As is evident from what has been said earlier, the susceptibility to a number of diseases involves an interaction between environmental factors and the genotype. Obesity is a good example of such a disease and one in which nutritional genomics has had some early successes. Although there is no doubt that the recent rapid escalation in the incidence of obesity in Western countries – and increasingly in the developing world – is the result of environmental factors, it is widely accepted that there is a genetic predisposition to the development of the disorder (see Arner 2000). The environmental factors relate, of course, to diet (what and how much we eat) and to a declining level of physical activity. Easy access

to cheap, palatable, high fat 'fast foods' and increasingly sedentary lifestyles through the widespread use of cars and the substantial amounts of time being spent watching television, videos and computer screens are overwhelming our genetically determined regulatory mechanisms for energy balance.

There are several single gene mutations in laboratory animals which lead to frank obesity – *ob*, *db*, *fat*, *tub* and agouti genes in mice, and the *fa* gene in the rat – which have proved invaluable in obesity research. These genes have now each been cloned and the protein product identified. There are also a number of transgenic models in which obesity, mild or substantial, has been identified as a consequence of the knock-out of a single gene, e.g. UCP-1 knock-out (the UCP-1 gene encodes the protein responsible for heat dissipation, or thermogenesis, in brown adipose tissue). The identification of the mutant genes in *ob/ob* and *db/db* mice and in the fatty *fa/fa* rat has revolutionised our understanding of the control of energy balance. A physiological regulatory loop has been identified with the *ob* gene encoding a hormone – leptin – and the *db* gene encoding its receptor. The *fa* gene is the rat homologue of the *db* gene.

Leptin is synthesised in several tissues but the major site quantitatively, and the main source of the circulating protein, is white adipose tissue. This hormone is now recognised to have a very wide range of functions, but a central function is as a signal from adipocytes to the hypothalamus in the control of appetite (which is inhibited) and energy expenditure (which is stimulated). Mutations in the leptin gene or in its receptor result in either no protein product or a dysfunctional hormone, and a profound obesity of early onset ensues (see Montague et al 1997). There are human analogues to the mouse mutants, with mutations in both the leptin and the leptin receptor gene having been identified in a handful of human subjects. These individuals are obese and the adults show reproductive dysfunction, closely paralleling the phenotype of the mouse mutants. Although this demonstrates how a mutation in a single gene can lead to human obesity, its main significance lies in demonstrating that a functional leptin system is as important for the normal control of energy balance and body weight in humans as in rodents. Additional mutations causing obesity in humans include that reported for the melanocortin 4 receptor – now regarded as the most common monogenetic effect causing human obesity.

Such overt mutations as those for leptin and its receptor are rare in humans and do not inform the generality of obesity. Polymorphisms in specific genes or clusters of genes are, however, increasingly being linked to increased body fat and obesity. The most discussed such association is with the Trp64Arg polymorphism in the β3-adrenoceptor. A number of studies have observed a linkage between this polymorphism and indices of fatness or fattening, while others, often in different populations or ethnic groups, have not. Similar associations have also been made with the Gln27Glu polymorphism in the human β2-adrenoceptor and again there are apparent differences between studies or population groups.

This illustrates the problem in trying to find a consistent association between a single polymorphism and a complex phenotype such as body weight where many genes will be involved. Clearly, several different polymorphisms may have an additive effect, or different polymorphisms (linked to leanness) may have opposing effects thereby cancelling one another out. There is also the likelihood that dietary interactions modulate the effects of specific polymorphisms. The interaction between particular gene polymorphisms can be illustrated by the synergistic effect of the Trp64Arg polymorphism in the β3-adrenoceptor gene with the A(-3826)G polymorphism in the 5′-flanking region of the uncoupling protein-1 gene. The two polymorphisms together strengthen the association with fattening.

The complexity of the number of genes involved in determining the amount of body fat is shown by reference to a recent study on the worm *Caenorhabditis elegans*. By applying genome-wide RNA-mediated interference (RNAi), 305 gene inactivations that cause reduced body fat and 112 that cause increased fat have been identified, there being a total of 16 757 genes in this worm. Many of these *C. elegans* genes have clear human homologues, thereby providing a focus for further studies on the genes underlying the predisposition to obesity. Overall, this provides a potent example of the integrative power of nutritional genomics.

⊃ Key points

- ⊃ The concepts and techniques of molecular biology are being increasingly applied to nutritional science, and the interaction between an organism and nutrients examined at the level of the genome and of gene products – the field of nutritional genomics, or *nutrigenomics*, has recently been established.

- ⊃ It is now thought that there are just 23 000 genes in humans, most genes consisting of coding regions (*exons*), regulatory sequences (*promoters*), and non-coding internal regions (*introns*).

- ⊃ The primary control of gene expression occurs at the level of transcription from DNA to mRNA through modulation of the regulatory promoter region. Nutrients can influence gene transcription by interacting with transcription factors, and by interactions at the post-transcriptional, translational and post-translational levels.

➲ New technologies allow global gene transcription and protein expression to be determined in a cell, tissue or organism, through DNA microarrays and proteomics, respectively.

➲ The genome of any two individuals shows approximately 0.1% variation and this is the basis for individual and population differences; the most common form of variation is the result of single base changes along the DNA sequence, termed single nucleotide polymorphisms (SNPs).

➲ Most common nutrition-related diseases such as coronary heart disease and obesity are the consequence of an interaction between the genome and the environment – only rarely do they result from a major mutation in a single gene, SNPs being central to determining the individual susceptibility to a disease.

References and further reading

References

Arner P 2000 Obesity – a genetic disease of adipose tissue? British Journal of Nutrition 83(Suppl 1):S9–16

Guandalini S, Gupta P 2002 Celiac disease: A diagnostic challenge with many facets. Clinical and Applied Immunology Reviews 2:293–305

Hannon G J 2002 RNA interference. Nature 418:244–251

McLaren D S 1992 A colour atlas and text of diet-related disorders, 2nd edn. Wolfe, London

Montague C T, Farooqi I S, Whitehead J P et al 1997 Congenital leptin deficiency is associated with severe early-onset obesity in humans. Nature 387:903–908

Moreno-Aliaga M J, Marti A, Garcia-Foncillas J et al 2001 DNA hybridization arrays: a powerful technology for nutritional and obesity research. British Journal of Nutrition 86:119–122

Sachidanandam R, Weissman D, Schmidt S C et al 2001 A map of human genome sequence variation containing 1.42 million single nucleotide polymorphisms. Nature 409:928–933

Shastry B S 2002 SNP alleles in human disease and evolution. Journal of Human Genetics 47:561–566

Tyers M, Mann M 2003 From genomics to proteomics. Nature 422:193–197

Ueland P M, Hustad S, Schneede J et al 2001 Biological and clinical implications of the MTHFR C677T polymorphism. Trends in Pharmacological Sciences 22:195–201

Uitterlinden A G, Fang Y, Bergink A P et al 2002 The role of vitamin D receptor gene polymorphisms in bone biology. Molecular and Cellular Endocrinology 197:1

Further reading

Berg J M, Tymoczko J L, Stryer L 2002 Biochemistry, 5th edn. Freeman, New York

Kendrew J, Lawrence E 1994 The encyclopaedia of molecular biology. Blackwell Science, Oxford

Lewin B M 2000 Genes VII, 7th edn. Oxford University Press, Oxford

Lodish H F, Baltimore D, Berk A et al 1995 Molecular cell biology, 3rd edn. Scientific American Press, New York

McLaren D S 1992 A colour atlas and text of diet-related disorders, 2nd edn. Wolfe, London

CD-ROM contents

Tables
Table CD 29.1 Websites of interest

Figures
Figure CD 29.1 Examples of post-transcriptional and translational nutrient regulation

Figure CD 29.2 Schematic view of nutrient–gene interactions

Further reading from the book

Part 6

Public health nutrition

Edited by Lawrence Haddad

30

The science of epidemiology

Annhild Mosdøl and Eric Brunner

important types of outcome measurements: incidence, prevalence and mortality rates. *Incidence* is defined as the number of new cases appearing in the study population during a specified period of time. If the study population is roughly constant, the incidence is:

$$\frac{\text{Number of new events in a defined period}}{\text{The population at risk at the beginning of the period}}$$

In many cases, the assumption of a constant study population holds true because birth, death, migration and immigration balance each other out. This rough estimation is also typically used in routine health statistics. If a population of 100 000 people saw 190 cancer cases over a period of one year, the cancer incidence would be 0.0019 per person year. By convention this figure is often presented per 1000 person years in order to get a figure closer to 1, here giving 1.9 cancer cases per 1000 person years.

The most accurate way of measuring incidence is to divide the number of new cases by the *person time at risk*. Person time is calculated by summing up the time each individual is at risk during the measurement period. This measure takes into account that when a person becomes a case he is no longer part of the population at risk and should not contribute to the observation time.

$$\text{Incidence rate} = \frac{\text{Number of new cases}}{\text{Total person time at risk}}$$

The British Whitehall II study of civil servants recruited 10 308 participants between 1985 and 1988. In 1999, 355 of the participants had died (mean follow-up time of 12.7 years). A rough estimate of total observation time would be 10 308 persons × 12.7 years = 130 912 person years. However, as no new participants entered the study after 1988 the total number of participants decreases as they drop out or die. The exact observation time was calculated to be 130 613 person years of follow-up, giving an incidence rate of 355 deaths/130 613 person years or 2.7 deaths per 1000 person years.

The *prevalence* is the proportion of a population that is cases at a given point in time. A prevalence figure has no dimension of time, giving it several limitations in its application. Prevalence is typically used to estimate the disease burden in a population, for instance to plan health services. The relationship between incidence and prevalence depends on the nature of the disease and the effectiveness of

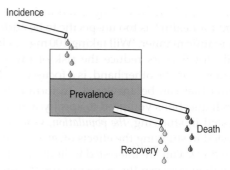

Figure 30.1 The relationship between incidence, the prevalence pool and duration of the disease.

treatment. For diseases with shorter duration the prevalence will be low and vice versa. There are three prospects for the diseased: to continue being ill, to recover or to die. The risk of death among the diseased is described by the *case-fatality rate*, which is the incidence of death among the cases. Figure 30.1 illustrates how the prevalence pool is related to incidence, recovery and death. It is a paradox that efforts to improve the survival of those with a disease without curing it will increase the prevalence. Diabetes is a typical example. In populations with good health services, diabetes patients will live a long time with their disease before they die of it or even of other causes. Inevitably, the burden on the health services will increase.

Mortality rates are a special form of incidence rates, the incidence of death, and can have different forms. When presented as crude mortality rates they relate to the population as a whole. Mortality rates of specific diseases can be calculated the same way by using only deaths from this specific cause.

$$\text{Crude mortality rate} = \frac{\text{Number of deaths in a year}}{\text{Mid-year population}}$$

Crude mortality rates may hide useful information needed to understand the health and disease patterns of different populations. Crude cancer death rates are much lower in Mexico than in the UK. Is the Mexican population less exposed to risk factors for cancer? It may be so, but another very likely explanation is that the difference in cancer mortality rates is not genuine but due to different age distribution in the two countries. Cancer rates are higher in older people. The higher the proportion of older persons in a population, the higher the cancer mortality overall, even given the same age-specific cancer

Box 30.1 *Definitions of incidence rate, prevalence and mortality rates*

Incidence rate
= number of new cases / total person time at risk

Prevalence
= number of existing cases at one point in time / population at same place and time

Crude mortality rate
= number of deaths (defined place and time) / mid-period population (same place and time)

Age-specific mortality
= number of deaths to people in a particular age group (defined place and time) / mid-period population (same age group, place and time)

Cause-specific mortality
= Number of deaths due to a particular cause (defined place and time) / mid-period population (same place and time)

death rates. Breaking down mortality rates for specific groups, most commonly by gender and age, will contribute to a better understanding of death rates over time and between different populations. Crude and specific rates may be applied to measures of disease in the same way as measures of death. Box 30.1 provides definitions of the terms used in this section.

The exposure

An *exposure* is any factor suspected to modify the risk of the outcome of interest. Exposures include a broad range of factors, from microbiological or chemical agents to all kinds of physical, social or psychological variables. An exposure can be based on observations of what happens naturally in a population or of what happens when the study participants are assigned to a certain exposure in an experimental setting. Common exposures in nutritional epidemiology include biochemical markers, nutrients, foods or food patterns, and socioeconomic variables. You may have noticed that some of the examples of exposure variables could also be outcome variables. In a study of stroke, blood pressure may be the exposure of interest, but in another setting blood pressure may be the outcome of interest with specific food habits as the exposure. What functions the variables have depend on the objective of the study and the relationship being examined.

As with outcome variables, exposure variables often take binary forms with the population divided into exposed and unexposed, or they are continuous variables. In nutritional epidemiology, many exposure variables appear on continuous scales, although categorisation into two or more groups with graded levels of exposure is common. The way the exposure is measured depends on the question being asked. If the outcome is a food-borne disease, it may be sufficient to know whether or not the study participants have eaten shellfish from a certain shop the previous week. When studying thyroid cancer, the average shellfish consumption over time may be more relevant.

There is, however, one very important requirement applying to all exposure variables: the exposure must vary in the population that is to be studied. In a population where everyone eats exactly the same amount of fruit and vegetables, we would not be able to show any positive or negative effects on the risk of cancer – no matter how strong the real effect is. You are more likely to discover the real effects of an exposure in a population where this variable has a wide range than in a population where the range of exposure is narrow.

Many of the diseases we would like to study, such as coronary heart diseases and cancer, have a long lag between the onset of the relevant exposure to manifest stages of the disease. This is called the *latency period*. It will normally take many years for healthy cells to turn malignant and then a single cancer cell may again take years to develop into a detectable tumour. The relevant dietary exposure affecting the risk of developing cancer may therefore be 10–20 years back in time. Exposures could also exert their effect during critical periods. This appears to be the case with neural tube defects, where the mother's folate status during the first 4–6 pregnancy weeks is the critical time. Thus, it can be relevant to gather information on both the exposure during a certain part of the lifespan, for instance calcium intake during childhood, and the average intake of a nutrient, say saturated fat, over the most recent years.

When would be the correct point in time to get information about exposures? Researchers need to have a theory of the time dimensions relevant to the study outcome to handle these challenges properly. The chosen interval for measuring the exposure is sometimes called the *window of measurement*. One option is to decide on a window of measurement thought to be important back in time and gather information about past exposures. It was possible to examine aspects of Barker's hypothesis that low birthweight increases the risk of cardiovascular diseases in adult life because a large amount of anthropometrical data on babies had been gathered for other purposes in the early 1900s. Later these individuals could be identified for an examination of their cause-specific death rates (Barker 1998).

Without such historical data sources giving information on past exposures, it sometimes is assumed that measurements at a later period may serve as reasonable alternatives. If we believe that dietary habits are stable over time, data on present food intakes may give some indication of intakes in the past. Recall of past exposures is also an option, although this often turns out to be problematical. Measurements of current exposures are preferred as they are much easier to quality control, but if we want the time aspect to unfold, there is nothing for the researchers to do but wait.

In an experimental setting where the exposure is assigned to the participants, the exposure is often called an *intervention*. Usually this is hypothesised to be a protective factor, such as a treatment or a drug, as it would be unethical to expose participants to suspected harmful factors apart from over very short periods. Exposures can also be called risk factors. When established, a risk factor is a characteristic that, based on epidemiological evidence, is known to increase the probability of a particular disease or malign condition developing. Risk factors can also be factors that are only suspected to be harmful.

Measures of association and effect

In general, an *association* refers to the statistical link between two variables or factors. The epidemiologist is primarily interested in causal associations or effects, which address questions of disease causality, prevention or treatment. Several measures of association are used to summarise exposure–outcome relationships, each with its special applications. The choice of suitable measures for a given study will depend on the format of the exposure and outcome variables, whether they are binary or continuous.

Binary exposure – binary outcome
Relative risk (abbreviated RR) is the measure of effect most commonly used by epidemiologists when both the exposure and the outcome are binary variables. This is given by the ratio of risk, or incidence, in the exposed group to the risk in the unexposed group. A relative risk of one indicates that there is no difference in incidence between the exposed and the unexposed. When the relative risk is higher than one, the exposure poses a hazard, while a relative risk lower than one means that the exposure is protective. Another commonly used measure is the attributable risk (abbreviated AR), which is the incidence among the exposed minus the incidence among the non-exposed. Attributable risk estimates the proportion of disease incidence that may be due to a particular exposure or risk factor.

Dedicated gamblers have an advantage when introduced to the *odds ratio* (abbreviated OR). This measure is frequently used to describe associations in epidemiology, and is an alternative to the relative risk outlined above. The term *odds* refers to a measure of probability based on a ratio rather than a proportion. Consider the relationship between obesity (the exposure) and gestational diabetes (the outcome). If 50 of 100 women with gestational diabetes were obese compared with 20 of 100 non-diabetics, the odds of obesity among the diabetics are 50:50 (odds = 1), and the odds of obesity among the non-diabetics are 20:80 (odds = 0.25). The odds ratio is calculated by dividing the odds of exposure among the cases by the odds of exposure in the non-cases. In our example the odds ratio is $(50:50)/(20:80) = 1/0.25 = 4$. The odds of being obese among the women with gestational diabetes are four times greater than among the healthy women (Box 30.2).

When the relative risk and odds ratio can be calculated on the same set of data, these will often be similar. How closely they match depends on the

---

Box 30.2 *Calculating relative risk (RR), attributable risk (AR) and odds ratio (OR)*

	Cases	Non-cases	Total
Exposed	a	b	a + b
Non-exposed	c	d	c + d
Total	a + c	b + d	

$$RR = Risk_{exposed}/Risk_{unexposed} = (a/(a + b))/(c/(c + d))$$

$$AR = Risk_{exposed} - Risk_{unexposed} = (a/(a + b)) - (c/(c + d))$$

$$OR = (a/c)/(b/d) = ad/bc$$

ratio of cases compared to the controls, in other words the outcome prevalence. When the number of cases is small compared to the non-cases, the relative risk and the odds ratio will be similar. This is illustrated in Box 30.3.

Binary exposure – continuous outcome

If the exposure variable is binary and the outcome is a continuous variable, the effect due to the exposure can be expressed as the mean difference in outcome between the two groups. An example is the mean difference in serum homocysteine level among participants given a supplement containing a vitamin B complex compared to the participants given placebo tablets.

Box 30.3 *Example of how RR and OR differ according to the outcome prevalence*

A high prevalence of cases in the study population:

	Cases	Non-cases	Total
Exposed	a	b	a + b
	90	410	500
Non-exposed	c	d	c + d
	30	470	500
Total	a + c	b + d	a + b + c + d
	120	880	1000

Prevalence = (a + c)/(a + b + c + d)
        = 120/1000 = 12%
RR = (a/(a + b))/(c/(c + d)) = (90/500)/(30/500)
   = 3.0
OR = (a/c)/(b/d) = ad/bc = (90 × 470)/(30 × 410)
   = 3.44

A low prevalence of cases in the study population:

	Cases	Non-cases	Total
Exposed	a	b	a + b
	9	491	500
Non-exposed	c	d	c + d
	3	497	500
Total	a + c	b + d	a + b + c + d
	12	988	1000

Prevalence = (a + c)/(a + b + c + d)
        = 12/1000 = 1.2%
RR = (a/(a + b))/(c/(c + d)) = (9/500)/(3/500) = 3.0
OR = (a/c)/(b/d) = ad/bc = (9 × 497)/(3 × 491)
   = 3.04

Continuous exposure – continuous outcome

When both the exposure and the outcome variables are continuous, the two data for each individual in the sample can be plotted against each other. Statistical methods such as correlation and regression analyses are used to describe such relationships in numerical terms. When we compare the level of exposure versus the level of outcome, the most important characteristic is the relative position of each individual compared to other individuals in the sample. Thus, in many instances it is less important to know the exact exposure level of each respondent as long as the method used to measure the exposure manages to rank individuals correctly.

Continuous exposure – binary outcome

The combination of continuous exposure and binary outcome is seen frequently in nutritional epidemiology, for instance where the exposure is the serum homocysteine and the outcome is a myocardial infarction event. The statistical technique used in these situations is logistic regression and the results are presented as odds ratios. Although the odds ratio in this case is created through a different technique than the 2 × 2 table described above, it may be interpreted in the same way.

The above approaches to the quantification and description of epidemiological associations are among the most commonly used, but are not the only ones available (see Bland 1995).

Quality of the measurements

The foundation of any scientific study is valid and reproducible measurements. Poorly measured variables, either exposure or outcome, can lead to misleading results and incorrect conclusions. Validity is an expression of the degree to which a measurement assesses the aspect it is intended to measure. For example, a 1-day diet record is unlikely to assess habitual dietary intake, and a 7-day diet record will be more valid. Reproducibility indicates if the method is capable of producing the same result when used repeatedly under the same circumstances. Validity is a concept that not only refers to individual measurements such as the exposure and outcome measurements, but is also used to describe the degree to which results from a study represent the truth. Figure 30.2 uses target and bullet holes to illustrate the difference between the validity and reproducibility for measurements of a variable. The

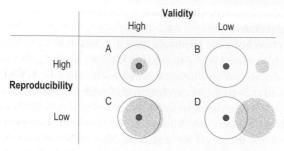

Figure 30.2 Illustration of the terms validity and reproducibility by using a target where the gunshots, shown as bullet holes (the measurements), have been aimed at the bull's eye (the truth). When all the bullet holes are positioned closely to each other, the shooting gives a highly reproducible result, if positioned over a wider area reproducibility is low. If the shooting is systematically drawn to one side of the target, the validity is poor, while hits symmetrically around the bull's eye indicate high validity.

bull's eye is the true value we are aiming at. Picture A is our goal – high validity and reproducibility as the hits are positioned closely and the average is close to the truth. In Picture B, each shot arrives closely to each other, giving a high reproducibility, but the target is missed every time. Picture C shows a situation where the hits are scattered symmetrically around the bull's eye, meaning the average is valid but the reproducibility is poor. Situation D has both poor reproducibility and validity.

Poor reproducibility may be due to errors in the measurement tool or because of natural biological variation. Many variables have a natural variation over time, while others are more stable. A stable measure is for instance adult height – apart from a slight decrease over many years we would expect to find the same value every time it is measured. Blood glucose on the other hand varies naturally over the course of a day. When a study variable shows natural variability, it is important to decide what aspect of the variable we think is relevant and carefully standardise the measurements to this aspect. By deciding to measure fasting blood glucose, the amount of error due to fluctuations after meals could be minimised. Part of the standardisation process in this case would be to define criteria for what is meant by fasting. Repeat measurements of the same variable also provide a better estimate of the true average and a quantification of its reproducibility. Thus, repeatability is both a feature of the variable itself and associated with the technical error of its measurement.

Any measurement will to some extent include deviations from the truth. The size of these errors varies with each variable and the survey test method. For any measurement, the errors should be minimised as much as possible before the study is performed by choosing the best-suited method and by careful data collection. It is, on the other hand, important to measure and describe the size of any unavoidable errors if possible, so that they may be taken into account when analysing and discussing the results.

Often the most valid measurement methods are the most burdensome and expensive. For practical or economic reasons, investigators may choose to use a less valid method for measuring the variables of interest. How large the errors that can be tolerated will vary with the study objective, but this needs to be decided on before the study is carried out. To establish how valid a measurement is we need to compare it with an absolute or gold standard. The gold standard of a measurement is usually the best test we have so far for the measure of interest. The more practical or cheaper measurement method is here called the test method while the gold standard is called the reference method.

For variables in binary form, whether it is exposure or outcome, the validity of its measurement is determined by classifying the subjects first by the test method and secondly by the reference method. For instance, waist–hip ratio greater than 0.95 as a measure of excess abdominal fat in adult men may be validated against a cut-point derived from a dual-energy X-ray absorption (DEXA) scan. It is conventional to use the expressions positive and negative test to denote the two test results. The possible combinations of the repeat measurement are presented in Box 30.4. Four quality measures of the test method can be derived from this table. *Sensitivity* indicates the proportion of true positive results detected by the test method. The *specificity* indicates whether the test method correctly identifies negative results and has few false positive results. The *positive predictive value* gives the proportion of the test positive results that are truly positive, and the *negative predictive value* presents the proportion of the test negative that are truly negative. While the sensitivity and specificity are properties of the test method, the positive and the negative predictive value will vary according to the outcome prevalence. If a condition is rare in a given population, the positive predictive value will be lower than in another population where the condition is more common.

Box 30.4 *Calculating important quality characteristics of a test method*

Test method	Reference method		
	Positive	**Negative**	**Total**
Positive	a	b	a + b
Negative	c	d	c + d
Total	a + c	b + d	

Sensitivity = a/(a + c)
Specificity = d/(b + d)
Positive predictive value = a/(a + b)
Negative predictive value = d/(c + d)

For variables in a continuous form, the validity is also estimated by comparing results from the test method with a standard reference method. The important aspect of this comparison is the degree of association between the methods, predominantly by giving a picture of the ranking ability of the survey test method compared to the standard reference method. Such data are often presented as correlations and contingency tables; for instance by cross-tabulation according to quartiles of the distribution for each of the methods. This is an important aspect of validating dietary intake data.

An estimate of validity as above requires a gold standard. In some instances, no superior standard exists because all the available reference test methods have considerable limitations themselves. Instead, the preferred reference method is one that is thought to be the best test available and that preferably has different types of errors than the survey test method. When the reference method has notable limitations, it is more appropriate to call the comparison of the test method and the reference method a *relative* validation. This is the case for validation of dietary assessment methods when another dietary assessment method is used as a reference method. Validation of dietary measures is thought to be so complex that it is recommended even to include a second reference method that is unrelated to the first two as part of the validation procedure, usually a biological marker of energy or nutrient intake (Margetts & Nelson 1997, Willett 1998).

⊃ Key points

⊃ Population – the population of interest for a particular study question.

⊃ Outcome – the disease or health-related variable being studied.

⊃ Exposure – any factor that may influence the risk of the outcome.

⊃ Measures of association and effect – the quantified relationship between exposure and outcome.

⊃ Validity – the degree to which a measurement assesses the aspect it is intended to measure.

⊃ Reproducibility – the degree to which a measurement produces the same result when used repeatedly under given conditions.

30.3 INTERPRETATION OF RESULTS

The survey is completed and the measures collected, but how should the results be interpreted? And how do you interpret studies reported in scientific journals? If an association between exposure and an outcome is observed, this may be due to four different reasons: bias, chance, confounding or a true causal relationship. Before we even start to consider the possible importance of the results observed, the first three options should be considered carefully.

Bias

Bias refers to measurement errors or misclassification that lead to results that consistently deviate from the truth. Many sources of bias have been identified, but all of them fit into two broad categories: selection bias and information bias. When study participants have been selected to the study in a way that gives distorted results, we have *selection bias*. This can arise in many different ways. In a clinical setting, terminally ill patients may be more willing to try out a novel treatment with unknown risks attached to it than patients with good prospects may. If the new treatment performs badly it is impossible to know whether this is because the treatment really was poor or because the patients would have died anyway. Important questions to ask when facing a study sample can be: how were the subjects selected for investigation and how representative were they of the population at risk with regard to the study question?

Another example applies to studies where a group of people is invited to participate, but only a subset is willing to take part. The size of this sample relative to the original group is described as the *response rate*. Almost without exception, participants who volunteer to take part in studies are likely to be more educated and health conscious than the general population. The prevalence of a condition may be different among responders than among the population from which they came from. Likewise, volunteers to nutritional studies may have better diets. Faced with such studies you might ask: what was the response rate and are the responders and non-responders likely to have differed in important ways? It is easier said than done to make sure that study groups are comparable and that they are representative of the population at risk. However, not all differences pose a problem; it depends on the study objective. If a study sample is not fully representative of the study population, the results may misrepresent the true disease burden. However, the relationship between an exposure and an outcome may be correctly estimated even when there is considerable selection bias.

If the information we have collected on either the exposure or the outcome varies systematically between groups, we have *information bias*, the other main form of bias. Dietary assessment studies repeatedly show that obese subjects tend to underestimate their energy intake more than non-obese subjects do. Thus, it may be wise to avoid self-reports of diet in a study of obesity. Another example of information bias arises when asking people about past exposures. A mother who has recently given birth to a child with neural tube defects will seek to understand her unfortunate situation by asking herself what could have caused it. She may recall supplement use and diet much more carefully than a mother with a healthy baby. This type of information bias is also called recall bias. As with selection bias, information bias is potentially important if its magnitude differs in relation to the presence or absence of the study outcome.

Bias is caused by imperfections in the design or the implementation, and usually it is difficult or even impossible to remove its effects at a later stage. Almost all studies are somewhat biased. This does not mean that they are scientifically unacceptable or that their results should be disregarded. If a study has been analysed and interpreted carefully, the investigators will have addressed this question themselves. There are no simple formulas for measuring biases and quantifying their effects. Each study must be judged by assessing the probable impact of biases on the study question and then allowing for them when drawing conclusions.

The role of chance

When do we know that a numerical difference is meaningful? If a group of children who had been breastfed for at least 4 months had an average primary school reading test score of 67 while children who never had been given breast milk had a score of 65, are they really different? What do we mean by different, and when is a difference most likely to be caused by chance? This is the realm of statistics. Chance can be thought of as variation due to errors, bias, biological differences and other unknown factors. Chance cannot be eliminated, but we should seek to confirm that chance is an unlikely explanation for the study results. Statistics provide measures to quantify the element of chance and account for the uncertainty in the results of our study.

Hypothesis testing is a common approach used to test for chance effects. If we estimate the mean level of a parameter in a population, say mean fasting blood glucose, by measuring this variable in a small sample, we would get a slightly different result just by chance if the procedure was repeated in another sample drawn from the same population. The procedure called hypothesis testing starts by defining a *null hypothesis*, which usually is a statement saying that there is no real difference (only differences by chance) between the two groups we are studying. The *p-value* gives the probability of getting the observed or a more extreme result if the null hypothesis is true, or rephrased: what is the likelihood that we observe this difference between two groups if they really are similar? Usually a *p*-value less than 5% ($p < 0.05$) is considered to give a statistically significant result leading to rejection of the null hypothesis. Note that failing to reject the null hypothesis is not the same as saying that it is true. A similar example is performed daily in court. Until it is proven beyond reasonable doubt that the suspect is guilty, the court will assume his innocence. Although the evidence fails to convict the suspect, he may still be the guilty person.

Thus, significance testing is a method for assessing whether a result, such as differences between groups, is likely to be due to chance or some real effect. It cannot prove that it is one or another. With a *p*-value of 0.05, the investigator runs a risk of falsely rejecting the null hypothesis on average 5% of the time. Two possible errors can be made when using the *p*-value to make a decision: to conclude that a difference exists when it does not is called a *type I error* (false positive or alpha error). Conversely, concluding that a difference does not exist when in fact it does by failing to reject a false null hypothesis is called a *type II error* (false negative or beta error). The *p*-values depend on the numerical difference between the groups, but also the sample size and the variation in the observations. Larger studies will be able to identify more subtle differences between groups than smaller studies. Failure to achieve a specified significance level will have different interpretations according to the sample size.

Confidence interval is another measure of the uncertainty in our data by giving a lower and upper confidence limit where the true value in question is likely to be. The intervals have a given probability, usually 95% or 99%, that the true value in the underlying population is included. A 99% confidence interval includes a higher proportion of possible values than the 95%. We would want confidence intervals to be narrow because this means that the estimate is more precise than with a wide confidence interval. Since confidence intervals combine information about chance effects and precision, it is preferred against hypothesis testing alone. It also avoids the arbitrary cut-point in significant testing where a *p*-value of 0.049 is regarded very differently from 0.051. When an estimated 95% confidence interval for a relative risk or odds ratio includes the value 1, which indicates no effect, the association is not statistically significant at the 0.05 level. For instance, if two different studies both gave relative risks of 2.1 but their 95% confidence intervals were 1.9 to 2.3 and 0.8 to 3.4 respectively, you would recognise that only the first study had a statistically significant result.

Confounding

A *confounder* is any factor that can cause or prevent the outcome of interest and at the same time is associated with the exposure in a way that distorts the observed exposure–outcome association. Let us assume we have recorded the coffee-drinking habits in a study population and monitored them for years. During the observation period the heavy coffee drinkers have a higher rate of bladder cancer than the participants drinking little or no coffee at all. An important question to consider is whether the relationship between bladder cancer and coffee drinking

can be due to another risk factor for this type of cancer that is also associated with coffee intake. Smokers being more likely to be heavy coffee drinkers may for instance create such an observation. If smoking was the real risk factor for bladder cancer, it is called a confounder of the relationship between coffee and bladder cancer. To shed light on the relationship between coffee and bladder cancer we may look at the association between coffee drinking and bladder cancer separately in smokers and non-smokers to overcome the confounding effect. A confounding factor may produce spurious effects as in the example above, but can also hide real ones.

Confounding may be regarded as a subcategory of bias, but while it is difficult or even impossible to adjust for many types of bias after the study has been completed, confounding can often be adjusted for. In the example above, the data could be analysed separately for smokers and non-smokers. Analysis by subgroups is called a *stratified analysis*. Another method is *standardisation*. Age is a common confounder in many studies since the risk of diseases usually increases with age. Two populations with different age distributions can be compared if the outcome is standardised to a general age distribution. Confounders can also be controlled in statistical models. However, these modifications are possible only if the relevant confounding factor has been measured. If confounding is considered at the design stage, it can be controlled by *exclusion of subgroups* that may cause interpretation problems. In experimental settings, random allocation of participants to two treatment groups (*randomisation*) will minimise confounding.

Causality

Smoking as a risk factor for lung cancer produces one of the strongest relative risks demonstrated for any lifestyle disease. Still, we have all heard about the old men smoking 40 cigarettes a day that are living happily into their nineties. How can we regard smoking as a cause of lung cancer when many smokers never get the disease? Causation can rarely be proven without doubt. Epidemiology is the science that takes a health-related hypothesis into the real world and attaches a probability to it. When considered together with other types of evidence, such as that derived from laboratory-based studies, epidemiology is a powerful tool for testing whether a proposed disease mechanism is important for population health.

Medical journals publish thousands of studies every year and most put forward associations between an exposure and the risk of a health outcome. Many also claim that these reflect causal effects. What guidelines should be used for judging the evidence? The question of causality can be approached in different ways. A set of criteria proposed by Sir Austin Bradford Hill (Hill 1974) is often used to judge whether one or a series of studies strongly suggest a causal association between a risk factor or intervention and an outcome. However, before appraising the evidence according to this list, the presence of chance, bias or confounding should have been assessed carefully.

Hill's criteria for causality, discussed below, are:

- strength of the association
- consistency
- specificity
- temporal sequence of cause and effect
- biological gradient
- biological plausibility and coherence
- experiment (reversibility).

Strength of the association

A strong association, as measured by relative risks, increases the likelihood that it reflects a causal relationship. Confounding may also create strong associations but, if an association is to be completely explained by confounding, the confounder must carry an even higher risk for the disease under study. This argument does not work the other way around though, as weak associations may also be causal. Many factors determine the strength of associations observed, including measurement errors and the range of exposure in the study sample. Some weak causal factors may be important factors for understanding disease aetiology.

Consistency

While tabloid newspapers may make headlines of a study showing that eating carrots is associated with increased risk of stroke, the scientific community is usually very slow to accept such findings as important. Only when a body of studies consistently points in the same direction over time and across populations is the association accepted as likely to be causal. If similar results are obtained from different studies, the evidence is strengthened. As studies giving no significant results often fail to be published, the available studies may not represent the full span of evidence concerning the phenomenon. This is also called publication bias. Thus, consistency is a desirable criterion, but not a necessary one.

Specificity

The idea of specificity is that one particular exposure always should lead to a specific disease and that one disease always is triggered by the same cause. This criterion seems less relevant as we increasingly discover that many diseases have multiple causes and some factors may contribute to more than one condition.

Temporal sequence of cause and effect

If a statistically significant association is found between two variables but the presumed cause occurs after the effect rather than before it, the association cannot be causal. Logical temporal sequence of events, with the exposure appearing before the outcome, is an absolute criterion for causality.

Biological gradient

A dose–response relation where the risk increases progressively with higher exposure is generally strong support for a causal interpretation. However, it cannot be an absolute criterion for a relationship to be causal. A dose–response curve may have many different forms and we do not always know where on this curve the observed range of exposure is situated.

Biological plausibility and coherence

As with consistency, the biological plausibility and coherence with present knowledge can only be fully appraised when the relationship has been thoroughly studied. Epidemiological studies have repeatedly pointed to proposed causal risk factors for disease that could not be explained by biological knowledge at the time they were published. Such findings often spark off studies using different scientific approaches to examine possible mechanisms in more depth.

Experiment (reversibility)

When an epidemiological association can be reversed it is strong confirmation that the link most likely is causal. Reversal of the effect appears when reduction in a factor that previously has been shown to increase the disease risk gives a corresponding drop in disease risk. An example is in patients who manage to lower their total serum cholesterol level through a controlled diet and who later present a reduced risk of coronary heart diseases compared with those who had stable and high serum cholesterol.

There are clearly different levels of cause. This is more comprehensively understood with many

Box 30.5 *Levels of cause*

Sufficient cause: If the exposure (cause) is present, the outcome (disease) will always occur

Necessary cause: If the exposure (cause) is absent, the outcome (disease) cannot occur

Risk factor: If the exposure is present and active, the probability that the outcome (disease) will occur is increased

non-communicable diseases where several causal factors are involved. If a factor triggers a disease every time it is present, it is called a *sufficient cause* (Box 30.5). Apart from some genetic abnormalities, there are very few conditions where this holds true. Even food poisoning or other infections will depend on the vulnerability of the person exposed. The bacteria are, on the other hand, a *necessary cause* of the food poisoning. If a necessary cause is absent, the disease cannot occur. We have already defined a *risk factor* as a characteristic that is known to increase the probability that a particular disease or malign condition will develop. Risk factors are neither sufficient nor necessary causes of disease. Smoking is a good example, as many smokers never get lung cancer while a small number of non-smokers do. Still smoking is thought of as being the most important cause of lung cancer. Nutritional exposures are very often risk factors; they increase the likelihood of diseases to occur but are neither sufficient nor necessary causes.

Only in a very few cases, such as serious injuries, will a causal factor trigger off a disease or a health outcome directly. For most health outcomes, there will be *causal pathways* between the exposure and the outcome. Fruit and vegetable intake is believed to exert part of its protective effect on development of cancers by increasing the circulating antioxidant level, which again protects DNA from oxidative damage and prevents cells from becoming malignant. For someone interested in the biochemical aspects of nutrition, the intake of specific nutrients and the molecular mechanisms involved are the most interesting aspects of this causal pathway. In a clinical or a one-to-one nutritional advice situation, the dietary aspect of preventing cancer is most relevant. Among community nutritionists, there may be particular interest in the social, cultural and psychological determinants of food habits. These explanations operate at different levels, but are complementary. Each level is necessary to understand the causal pathways of disease at the population level. Epidemiological studies have contributed considerably to present scientific understanding of the relationships between dietary habits and health.

⊃ **Key points**

- ⊃ An observed exposure–outcome association can be due to four factors: bias, chance, confounding or because there is a true causal relationship.

- ⊃ Bias – systematic deviation of results from the truth – takes two main forms: selection bias (related to the sample) and information bias (related to the data).

- ⊃ Chance – random variation – may produce a plausible or implausible finding.

- ⊃ Confounding – confusion between two processes – may distort study findings.

- ⊃ Causality can rarely be proven, but if bias, chance and confounding have been considered and the Hill criteria are broadly met, then causal inference is appropriate.

30.4 EPIDEMIOLOGICAL STUDY DESIGNS

Some elements of planning and designing studies

When someone starts planning an epidemiological study, the most important task is to formulate the essential question the study seeks to answer. If there are any relevant additional questions, these should also be considered. These questions will guide the decisions that need to be taken regarding the study sample, how exposure and outcome are measured and the preferred study design. It is at this stage that potential biases can be best controlled or minimised. If a relevant variable is missed during the implementation, for instance a confounder, it can rarely be made up for after the data collection is completed.

Who should be included in the study sample and how many participants need to be included? These two questions are very important. The goal for most studies is to generate results that have a wider application beyond the study participants, in other words to get results that are *generalisable* to the whole target population or, as it also has been called here, the population at risk. If we could include all members of the target population in our studies, the question of generalisability would not be an issue. Usually this is neither feasible nor desirable, and a smaller study sample is selected. The generalisability of a study is the same as the *external validity*. Validity has earlier been defined as the degree to which a measurement assesses the aspect it is intended to measure. The external validity considers to what extent the study captures accurately the phenomenon as it exists in the target population.

Often the final study sample is formed in two steps. A subset of the target population is selected on certain criteria to form the study population; it can for instance be through random selection from the general population or by choosing an accessible group that can be followed up over time. The study sample is the subset of the study population that actively participates in the study.

Target population → study population → study sample

It is usually desirable to get a sample that is representative of the population at risk in terms of age,

sex and other demographic factors. Other important characteristics of external validity will differ with the study question. For instance, in a study exploring causal relationships it is important that the exposure–outcome relationship found in the study sample represents the association in the larger population. If prevalence is important, the level of risk factors or outcome should be representative of the target population.

In the Oslo health study carried out 2000/01, the aim was to investigate the social inequalities in health in the Norwegian capital. All adult Oslo citizens were the target population. From these, citizens born in certain years were selected to create the study population. The study population included all individuals living in Oslo County that were born in 1970, 1960, 1955, 1940/41 and 1924/25. In total 46% of the invited participants attended the initial screening. How representative was this final study sample of the target population? It was possible to examine aspects of this question because official registers with basic socioeconomic data on all citizens were available to the investigators.

The other crucial task when selecting a study sample is to determine the necessary number of participants. It is vital that the sample size is big enough to detect as statistically significant any true differences between the study groups. Performing studies that are too small to answer the main objective

			Time				Example
		Past	Present		Future		
		Retrospective			Prospective		
Observational studies:							
Ecological		Observe exposure and outcome at population level, at single or multiple points in time					Average per capita fruit and vegetable intake plotted against CHD mortality in different countries
Cross-sectional		Observe exposure and outcome at individual level					Associations between estimated vitamin K intake and bone mineral density among a group of women
Case control	Record past ← exposure	Select sample by outcome status					Comparison of fatty acid composition in adipose tissue among patients with myocardial infarction and a group of matched controls
Cohort		Select on or observe exposure status	**Follow up** →	Record outcomes			The relationship between plasma ascorbic acid level in a large group of people and all cause mortality 4 years later
Experimental studies:							
Trials		Assign exposure to individuals, groups or communities	**Follow up** →	Record outcome			Comparison of subsequent mortality in a group of people given antioxidant supplementation and a control group given placebo

Figure 30.3 A schematic overview of epidemiological study designs and their main characteristics. (See also Section CD 30.4(a).)

Box 30.6 *Advantages and disadvantages of different epidemiological study designs*

Studies	Advantages	Disadvantages
Ecological studies	Quick and easy to carry out Hypothesis generating	Cannot be used for causal investigations since the data are on groups rather than individuals Not good for hypothesis testing
Cross-sectional studies	Quick and easy to carry out Gives prevalence of condition in population Hypothesis generating	Cannot differentiate temporal sequence Unsuited for rare conditions or conditions of short duration Not good for hypothesis testing
Case-control studies	Quick and easy to carry out Can study many risk factors Require relatively few participants Suited for studies of rare diseases	Cannot provide measures of risk, only odds ratios Subject to recall bias, difficult to validate the measurements Poor differentiation of temporal sequences Only one outcome can be studied
Cohort studies	Can provide measures of risk Can study many exposures and outcomes Permits quality control of the exposure measurements	Time-consuming and costly, many participants required Can only examine the exposures that were measured at the onset of the study, relevant factors to study may change Can only be used for common outcomes It may be difficult to keep track of the study sample
Randomised controlled trials	The gold standard for evaluating treatments or interventions Allow the investigators to have strong control of the parameters (minimises bias and confounding)	Can be time-consuming and costly Only one exposure can be studied Can have problems with participants not complying or dropping out of the study The generalisability may be limited Unethical if exposure is suspected to pose a hazard

is a waste of resources and can be considered unethical. If we want to demonstrate that drug A is superior to drug B in lowering blood pressure, we first need to define what we mean by superior. Is a real difference in systolic blood pressure reduction of 2 mmHg relevant or should the difference be at least 5 mmHg? The next step is to specify the probability we would like to have of achieving a specific statistical significance level, for instance a *p*-value of 0.05. This probability is called the *power* of a study and is usually aimed at being between 85% and 95%. In the example above, we may want a study sample that is large enough to demonstrate a difference in reducing systolic blood pressure of 5 mmHg between drug

A and B with a 90% probability. Power increases with the number of persons included in the sample and can be modified by characteristics of the variables including the magnitude of measurement errors. (For power and sample size calculations see Kirkwood 1988, Altman 1991).

Again, the best study design in a particular situation depends on the question being asked. Figure 30.3 gives a schematic overview of the main study designs, and in the subsequent two sections we will describe their features, strengths and weaknesses (see Section CD 30.4(a) for examples) (see also Box 30.6). Study designs differ according to whether the researchers observe natural processes (*observational*

⊃ Key points

- ⊃ The effects of diet can be studied at a number of levels: nutrients, non-nutrients, foods and food patterns. This is a challenge of nutritional epidemiology.

- ⊃ Dietary variables are strongly interrelated. It may be difficult to single out the relevant variable.

- ⊃ Between-population comparisons offer a useful means for investigating dietary effects on health by widening the range of exposures.

- ⊃ Great care is needed in dietary assessment and in the capture of the relevant period of exposure.

References and further reading

References

Altman D G 1991 Practical statistics for medical research. Chapman & Hall, London

Barker D J P 1998 Mothers, babies and health in later life, 2nd edn. Churchill Livingstone, Edinburgh

Bingham S A 2002 Biomarkers in nutritional epidemiology. Public Health Nutrition 5:821–827

Bland M 1995 An introduction to medical statistics, 2nd edn. Oxford University Press, Oxford

Brunner E, Rayner M, Thorogood M et al 2001 Making public health nutrition relevant to evidence-based action. Public Health Nutrition 4:1297–1299

de Onis M, Blössner M 2000 Prevalence and trends of overweight among preschool children in developing countries. American Journal of Clinical Nutrition 72:1032–1039

Egger M, Schneider M, Smith G D 1998 Meta-analysis: Spurious precision? Meta-analysis of observational studies. British Medical Journal 316:140–144

Hill A B 1974 Principles of medical statistics, 9th edn. The Lancet, London

Kirkwood B 1988 Essentials of medical statistics. Blackwell Scientific Publications, Oxford

Margetts B M, Nelson M 1997 Design concepts in nutritional epidemiology, 2nd edn. Oxford University Press, Oxford

Pryer J A, Nichols R, Elliott P et al 2000 Dietary patterns among a national random sample of British adults.

Journal of Epidemiology and Community Health 55:29–37

Willett W 1998 Nutritional epidemiology, 2nd edn. Oxford University Press, New York

Further reading

Introduction to epidemiology

Coggon D, Barker D J P, Rose G 1997 Epidemiology for the uninitiated, 5th edn. BMJ Publishing Group, London

Last J M 2001 A dictionary of epidemiology, 4th edn. Oxford University Press, New York

Nutritional epidemiology

Margetts B M, Nelson M 1997 Design concepts in nutritional epidemiology, 2nd edn. Oxford University Press, Oxford

Willett W 1998 Nutritional epidemiology, 2nd edn. Oxford University Press, New York

Introduction to medical statistics

Altman D G 1991 Practical statistics for medical research. Chapman & Hall, London

Bland M 1995 An introduction to medical statistics, 2nd edn. Oxford University Press, Oxford

Kirkwood B 1988 Essentials of medical statistics. Blackwell Scientific Publications, Oxford

CD-ROM contents

Expanded material

Section CD 30.4(a) Examples of epidemiological study designs

Section CD 30.4(b) Example of systematic review

Figures

Figure CD 30.1 CHD mortality by fruit and vegetable intake in EU countries

Figure CD 30.2 A case-control study design

Figure CD 30.3 A cohort study design

Figure CD 30.4 Example of systematic review

Further reading from the book

31

Nutritional assessment methods

Christopher J. Bates, Michael Nelson and Stanley J. Ulijaszek

Objectives

By the end of this chapter you should be able to:

- summarise the purposes for which each of the currently used measures of nutritional status has been developed, and the scope of their individual usefulness and their limitations.

- outline the broad choices of different types of available measures, comprising (a) dietary estimation; (b) anthropometric measurements; (c) biochemical status indices; and to a lesser extent, (d) functional and clinical evidence of adequacy.

- summarise the common criteria for usefulness and reliability of these indices and measures, and to list some of the common pitfalls that must be avoided during planning, practical work and interpretation.

31.1 INTRODUCTION

Measures of nutritional status are usually valuable inasmuch as they may be predictive of health outcomes. The practical requirements for assessment of nutritional adequacy arise from the need to intervene, either by advice or by more aggressive strategies, to improve the nutrition of individuals or populations, and thereby to reduce the risks and the burdens of those diseases that have, or may have, a nutritional component. Such diseases may range from the classical 'single nutrient' deficiency diseases such as beriberi or scurvy, to multifactorial diseases such as vascular diseases or cancer, where nutrition is thought to play a modulating role as one of many aetiological factors.

The major categories of nutritional assessment strategies include: (a) dietary, (b) anthropometric, (c) biochemical status and (d) functional and clinical status (Gibson 1990).

Dietary assessment can be performed by weighed or household measures-intake records, usually for 4 or 7 days. It can be done by diet recall histories, usually for the previous 24 hours, or by a food frequency questionnaire to probe the frequency with which specified food items are usually eaten, per week for instance.

Anthropometry measures typically include weight and height (with body mass index being calculated from these); mid-upper arm circumference, and perhaps others such as demispan and skinfold thicknesses.

Biochemical status measures or indices are selected and tailored for each nutrient, and are often the concentration of the nutrient or its derivatives in a body fluid such as serum or plasma. Thus plasma retinol is an index of vitamin A status; 25-hydroxy-vitamin D is an index of vitamin D status, and the activation of the flavin-dependent red cell enzyme, erythrocyte glutathione reductase, is an index of riboflavin (vitamin B_2) status.

Functional indices assess the integrity and efficiency of metabolic processes that are nutrient dependent. Thus plasma homocysteine concentration is influenced by several B vitamins and is a functional index for their adequacy. Dark adaptation is influenced by vitamin A and zinc. Blood clotting is influenced by vitamin K.

Clinical indices comprise clinical signs or symptoms of nutrient deficiency: thus rickets is a sign of vitamin D deficiency and impaired blood clotting is a symptom of vitamin K deficiency. To some extent these indices may overlap: for instance, some biochemical indices are based on nutrient concentrations in body fluids which are, in turn, highly dependent on recent dietary intake, whereas others are based on related biochemical functions and metabolic-pathway-adequacy, which are more dependent on tissue status and are more closely related to functional adequacy.

In this chapter, the main focus will be on the first three categories, (a) to (c), although the importance of category (d) is always implicit in the discussion. The functional tests are most useful as research tools to investigate causal links, whereas the biochemical indices are most useful in population surveys and individual nutritional investigations. Clinical signs may be less specific for particular nutrients than are biochemical tests (see Ch. 28).

One of the most important growth areas in current nutritional research effort is the development of useful 'intermediate markers' between diet and health outcomes, since many of the latter may develop over long periods, and indeed over a lifetime. Where it is possible to demonstrate, experimentally, the influence of a change in dietary patterns on an intermediate marker, coupled with a strong relationship between that marker and a longterm health outcome, it is then possible to conduct population intervention studies, using the intermediate markers, to help identify those high risk groups that could benefit from aggressive nutritional interventions.

In this chapter, the three assessment categories, (a) to (c), will be compared and contrasted for their advantages and disadvantages, and their pitfalls and associated need for precautions. The contrasting approaches to the nutritional assessment of individuals and of populations will be considered, with respect to feasibility, validity and reproducibility (see Ch. 30). Validity measures the closeness of the estimate to the true value (its accuracy).

Reproducibility measures the spread (or precision) of estimates. High validity and reproducibility means that a measure has a closer approximation to the truth. The requirements and precautions for reliable assessment methodologies will be discussed, together with the criteria for the choice of indices for different types of questions.

For some population studies, a single type of assessment may permit the deployment of resources to large numbers of participants. However, a combination of several categories of assessment may provide more reliable information, and help to avoid the pitfalls of confounders. Thus the balance between simplicity of design and robustness of conclusions is a challenge, requiring care and astuteness at the planning stage. (Many more references for this chapter are provided on the accompanying CD-ROM; see Additional references and further reading.)

31.2 METHODS OF DIETARY ASSESSMENT

Objectives

On completion of this section, the student should:

- understand why dietary assessment needs to be carried out
- be able to describe the various methods of dietary assessment used at national, household and individual level
- be aware of the strengths and weaknesses of the different approaches to dietary assessment at national, household and individual level
- recognise the contexts in which it is appropriate to use specific methods
- understand how to take into account the measurement errors associated with dietary assessment when interpreting results from dietary surveys.

The aim of this section is to explore the reasons for undertaking dietary assessment, to outline the different techniques that are available, to clarify which techniques are appropriate for specific purposes, and to consider the errors that arise when measuring diet and how to cope with them. Further information on the CD-ROM includes detailed definitions of different methods (see Section CD 31.2(a)), how to describe the methods when reporting findings from dietary investigations (see Section CD 31.2(b)), an extended section on identifying and dealing with measurement error in dietary assessment (see Section CD 31.2(c)) and more on individual dietary assessments (see Section CD 31.2(d)).

The objectives of dietary assessment

Before undertaking dietary assessment, it is necessary to consider the exact purpose of the assessment, what is to be measured, in whom, over what time period, and how the measurements are to be collected. This will determine which technique is most appropriate for a given purpose, and avoid wasting resources using a technique that does not provide an appropriate measure.

What is the underlying purpose?

All dietary assessments aim to measure food consumption or to estimate the intake of nutrients or non-nutrients (Cameron & van Staveren 1988). There

Table 31.1 Strengths and limitations of measurements of individual food consumption

Method	Strengths	Limitations
Prospective methods		
General features	Current diet Direct observation of what is eaten Duration of survey can be varied to meet requirements for precision of estimates of food consumption or nutrient intake	Labour intensive Require literacy and numeracy skills Subjects need to be well motivated Usual consumption pattern may change due to: inconvenience of recording; choice of foods which are easy to record; beliefs about which foods are 'healthy' or 'unhealthy' Overweight subjects tend to under-report true consumption levels Coding and data entry errors are common
Duplicate diet	Direct analysis of nutrient content of food (not dependent upon food composition tables) Required in metabolic balance studies	Very expensive Intense supervision needed Usual diet may not be consumed
Weighed inventory	Widely used, facilitates comparisons between studies Precision of portion sizes	Food composition tables used to estimate nutrient intake
Household measures	No scales needed	Loss of precision compared with weighed inventory
Retrospective methods		
General features	Inexpensive Quick Lower respondent burden than required for prospective methods Can assess current or past diet	Biases caused by: errors in memory, perception and conceptualisation of food portion sizes; presence of observer Daily variation in diet not usually assessed Dependent on regular eating habits Food composition tables used to estimate nutrient intake
Diet history	Assesses 'usual' diet	Over-reporting of foods believed to be 'healthy' (e.g. fruit)
24-hour recall	Very quick Can be repeated to gain measure of daily variation and improve precision	Prone to underestimate intake due to omissions Single observation provides poor measure of individual intake
Food frequency and amount questionnaire	Suitable for large-scale surveys Can be posted Short version can focus on specific nutrients with few food sources	Requires validation in relation to reference measure Literacy and numeracy skills needed if self-completed

the type and amount of all individual items consumed over a specified period of time (e.g. 24-hour recall), or creating a mental construct of 'usual' consumption involving recollection of both the frequency of consumption of specific foods or food groups and the amounts consumed. The main advantages of the retrospective methods are that they are quick to administer compared with prospective methods. They are also less expensive in terms of equipment and (except for repeat 24-hour recalls, see below) the time taken for interviewers to see

subjects. A further advantage is that because there is a lower respondent burden than required for prospective methods, the chances of obtaining a more representative sample of all consumers is increased. They can also be used to assess diet in the past, which may be relevant to studies where the underlying causes of chronic diseases such as heart disease or cancer may lie in past rather than current diet.

Many sources of bias affect retrospective dietary assessments. Errors in memory result in the omission of foods from the assessment. This may be a problem for some elderly subjects and for children under the age of about 12. Subjects *and* interviewers must have good skills relating to the perception and conceptualisation of food portion size (the ability to develop an accurate mental construct of the amount of food consumed and to translate that construct into a description which corresponds to the amount actually consumed). Amongst respondents, this is a problem especially in children under 12 years of age. The presence of an observer (interviewer) may cause subjects to over-emphasise what they perceive as the 'good' aspects of their diet and to minimise the 'bad' aspects ('social desirability' and 'social approval' bias). Daily variation in diet is less readily assessed using retrospective methods (unless repeat 24-hour recalls are collected from each subject). Subjects who do not have regular eating habits will have difficulty describing the 'usual' frequency of consumption. And, as with most prospective methods, the use of food composition tables will introduce error into the estimates of energy and nutrient intake. (See Section CD 31.2(b) for more detail on each method.)

Prospective methods

- *Duplicate diet method*. This technique requires subjects to weigh and record their food consumption at the time of eating. At the same time, they weigh and put aside an exact duplicate portion of each food consumed. These samples are then analysed chemically for their energy and nutrient content. The main advantage of the duplicate diet method is that it is independent of errors associated with the use of food composition tables. It is the method best suited to metabolic balance studies in free-living populations.

- *Weighed inventory method*. The weighed inventory is one of the most widely used techniques. It was first described by Elsie Widdowson in 1936. Subjects keep a record of all food and drink consumed. Each food item is weighed immediately prior to consumption using portable food weighing scales. Battery operated scales with a large digital read-out make the recording process easier and reduce problems associated with the misreading of dials on analogue (mechanical) scales.

- *Household measures technique*. The method is similar to the weighed inventory, except that subjects record portion sizes in household measures (cups, bowls, spoonfuls, etc.) rather than weighing their

food. In practice, most weighed inventories include a proportion of items recorded in household measures. Records in household measures have the advantage of simplifying the recording process for subjects. (Use of cups and spoonfuls is common in the USA where recipe books often give volume measures rather than weights. Results from surveys carried out in different countries may therefore vary to some extent according to the familiarity of the population with the measuring technique being used.)

- *Food checklist method*. Respondents are provided each day with a pre-printed list of foods and asked to tick a box each time an item is consumed. Foods eaten but not listed can be described in blank spaces provided at the bottom of the printed list. Standard portion sizes may be indicated, or portion descriptions entered. The method is simple to use and well liked by respondents, but the information collected is less detailed than with other prospective methods (for example, time of consumption is not recorded).

Retrospective methods

- *24-hour recall*. In the 24-hour recall (originally attributed to Wiehl in 1942), a trained interviewer asks subjects to recall and describe every item of food and drink consumed over exactly 24 hours. The information is obtained through systematic repetition of open-ended questions. Amounts are described in household measures. Interviewers must be thoroughly familiar with both the local diet and the food composition tables to be used to estimate nutrient intakes, in order to obtain adequate detail for subsequent coding of data. The 'multi-pass' 24-hour recall is now in widespread use (consisting of a 'quick list' of uninterrupted recall by the respondent; a detailed interview elaborating the quick list; and a thorough review of the detailed interview).

- *Diet history*. The diet history is used to assess 'usual' diet over the recent past. Typically, an interviewer trained in the diet history technique begins by carrying out a 24-hour recall of diet. This is then elaborated in an interview lasting up to 2 hours. For each meal, subjects are asked to describe the range of foods that would be likely to be consumed, the frequency of their consumption, and typical amounts. Differences between weekdays and weekends are clarified, and seasonal variations elaborated. In its original inception by Burke in 1947, the 'diet history method' included a 'cross-check food frequency list' and a 3-day record in household measures. These were used to improve the validity of the history and to check for inconsistencies. In practice, the three components are rarely used together, although recent data suggest that multiple assessments can improve the accuracy of classification of subjects according to level of nutrient intake.

- *Food frequency questionnaire.* Food frequency questionnaires (FFQ) are pre-printed lists of foods on which subjects are asked to indicate the typical frequency of consumption and to state in household measures the average amount consumed on the days when the food is eaten. An example of a segment of an FFQ is shown in Figure CD 31.3.

Conclusions regarding individual dietary assessments

The wide variety of techniques for assessing individuals' diets reflects both the difficulties and frustrations associated with attempts to measure diet without bias, and the importance attached to the need to obtain accurate measurements in many different circumstances. The failure to demonstrate associations between diet and disease may in many instances be due to the imprecision of the measures of diet rather than to the absence of an association. Improvement in techniques of dietary assessment has been hampered by the lack of a readily measured absolute standard of intake against which to assess the precision of other measures. The situation has improved to some degree in recent years as a result of better understanding of how to identify mis-reporting (see 'Validity and measurement error', below). Nevertheless, many of the problems regarding objective assessment of individuals' diets remain. The need to measure diet requires us to appreciate (and not ignore!) our present limitations, and to continue to develop and improve methods of dietary assessment.

Appropriate uses of dietary survey methods

Techniques for dietary assessment are summarised in Table 31.2. It is clear that certain techniques are limited to particular applications. For example, food balance sheets are appropriate for assessing diet at the country level, facilitating comparisons between countries and mapping trends in consumption within a country over time. Weighed inventory data can be used to assess diet at individual level and to build up pictures of regional or national consumption based on representative samples, but they may be too labour intensive for looking at distribution of food in families and cannot be used for metabolic studies. The footnotes given in Table 31.2 clarify the specific problems, limitations or advantages of using a particular technique in a particular setting.

Validity and measurement error

In the last 10 years, there has been a growing awareness of the sources of bias in *any* measure of diet. Dieticians, clinicians, epidemiologists and researchers no longer accept that their particular measure of diet is 'good enough'. Instead, they seek to determine the biases in their measurements in order to adjust for them when assessing the relationships between diet and health. The work often requires the assistance of a statistician to disentangle the many threads of truth and error that are present in any dietary measurement.

The main problems arising from inaccurate measurements are of two types:

- incorrect *positioning* of a country, household, or person in relation to the truth or some external reference measure (e.g. dietary reference values)
- incorrect *ranking* of countries, households or persons in relation to one another.

The first type of error can result in inappropriate investigations or actions being taken to remedy an apparent dietary deficit or excess that does not really exist. Alternatively, no action may be taken when some is needed (e.g. a true deficit is not detected because diet is overestimated). The second type of error tends to undermine the ability to assess relationships between diet and health (e.g. someone who properly belongs in the top quarter of the distribution of intake is classified in the bottom quarter, or vice versa). Again, this can lead either to inappropriate recommendations for improving health in the population or, more often, a failure to take action because the true relationship between diet and health is obscured by measurement error. Measurement error and their effects are described by Nelson & Beresford (2003).

Section CD 31.2(c) lists some of the sources of measurement error, their principal effects, some ways of taking errors into account in analysis, and ideas for dealing with them in practice. A summary is given in Table CD 31.4.

Table 31.2 Appropriate uses of dietary survey methods (+++ very suitable, ++ moderately suitable, + limited application, − not suitable)

Level of dietary measurement	Dietary survey method		Surveys of individuals					
			Prospective			Retrospective		
	Food balance sheets	Household surveys	Duplicate diet[a]	Weighed inventory	Household measures	Diet history	24-hour recall	Questionnaires
National	+++	+++	+[b]	+[b]	+[b]	+[b]	++[b]	+[b]
Regional	−	+++	+[b]	+[b]	+[b]	+[b]	++[b]	+[b]
Institution/group	−	+++	+[b]	++[b]	++[b]	++[b]	++[b]	++[b]
Household	−	++[c]	++[d]	++[d]	++[d,e]	++[d]	++[d]	++[d]
Individual	−	[f]	+++[g]	+++[g]	+++[g]	+++[g]	+++[g]	+++[g]
Type of study								
Epidemiological	+++[h]	+++[h]	+[i]	+++[i]	+++[i]	++[i]	+++[i]	+++[i]
Clinical	−	−	++	+++	+++	+++	+++[j]	+++
Metabolic	−	−	+++	+[k]	−	−	−	−

[a]Includes other techniques of direct analysis (see text).
[b]Requires sample representative of population, institution or group, or analysis weighted to reflect balance of subgroups.
[c]Requires larder inventory. Short-term measures (e.g. one week) may not reflect usual diet in individual households.
[d]The need for data from all household members may distort usual household food consumption patterns.
[e]Semi-weighed method reduces total respondent burden within household.
[f]Requires complex mathematical modelling of within-household food and nutrient distribution.
[g]Important to screen out individuals whose responses may not be valid (see text).
[h]Appropriate for ecological studies.
[i]See Margetts & Nelson (1997) for detailed discussion of use of dietary survey methods in epidemiological studies.
[j]Requires repeat 24-hour recalls for valid classification of subjects according to levels of intake (see text).
[k]Useful only if range of foods is of limited variation in composition, allowing reliable use of food composition tables.

⊃ Key points

⊃ There is a wide variety of methods for assessing diet. The method chosen should be appropriate for the purpose and circumstances of the work being carried out.

⊃ All methods for dietary assessment include errors. It is important:
  – not to take the measurements of food consumption and nutrient intake at face value;

  – to understand the likely sources of error; and
  – to appreciate how the errors may influence the interpretation of apparent associations (or apparent lack of associations) between diet and health.

⊃ When reporting findings on dietary assessment, it is important to provide a full description of the sample characteristics (e.g. age, height, weight, body mass index), number of subjects or households and number of days of measurement collected.

31.3 ANTHROPOMETRIC ASSESSMENT

Objectives

- To understand the different uses of various anthropometric measures used to assess nutritional status.
- To appreciate how inaccuracies in their recording can be minimised.
- To be able to compare the measures to the most appropriate reference.

Anthropometry is a relatively quick, simple, and cheap means of assessment of nutritional status. This involves the physical measurement of some or several aspects of human body size, which when related to normative values are taken to be outcomes of nutritional experience (World Health Organization 1995).

Uses, advantages and limitations

The reasons why anthropometry is the most commonly used method of nutritional assessment globally include the relative cheapness and portability of equipment needed, the high accuracy and precision relative to dietary methods, and the relatively low level of training required. Although a wide range of anthropometric measurements can be made for ergonomic, anthropological, physiological, medical and sports purposes, a rather more limited list is appropriate to nutritional anthropometry (Table 31.3). All of the measurements given in this table are appropriate for the assessment of undernutrition, while waist and hip ratios are useful in the assessment of overnutrition in addition to weight and height.

The most common anthropometric measures of undernutrition in children are weight and height, either individually or combined, relative to reference

Table 31.3 Recommended measurements for nutritional assessment

Age group (years)	Practical field observations	More detailed observations
0–1	Weight, length	Head and arm circumference Triceps and subscapular skinfolds
1–5	Weight, length, height, arm circumference	Triceps and subscapular skinfolds
5–20	Weight, height, arm circumference	Triceps, subscapular and medial calf skinfolds Calf circumference
Over 20	Weight and height	Arm and calf circumference Triceps, subscapular and medial calf skinfolds Waist and hip circumferences (overnutrition only) Demispan (elderly subjects)

values. The two preferred indices are height for age and weight for height, since they can be used to discriminate between acute and chronic undernutrition (Waterlow et al 1977). Table 31.4 summarises the usefulness of weight for age, height for age and weight for height in nutritional assessment in children. Weight for height can also be used to assess overnutrition in children, and the body mass index (BMI: weight (kg) divided by height (m)^2) is now the most widely used measure for this purpose, although it is a less sensitive marker of body fatness than are skinfold thicknesses.

The most commonly used measure of undernutrition and overnutrition in adults is the BMI. Adult undernutrition has been labelled chronic energy deficiency, and BMI cut-offs for this are: 17–18.5, grade I CED (chronic energy deficiency); 16–17, grade II CED; below 16, grade III CED. BMI cut-offs of 25, 30 and 40 are used internationally to define mild, moderate, and severe obesity respectively (Shetty & James 1994), although various nations may have differently defined criteria. The cut-off of 25 is called overweight by some. In addition, waist circumferences and waist–hip ratio are simple measures of central distribution of body fatness.

The major limitation of anthropometry is the extent to which measurement error can influence interpretation of nutritional status. Potential anthropometrists need good training, although the relative simplicity of measurement can encourage investigators to skimp on training. It is important that anthropometrists achieve good levels of precision and accuracy. Precision reflects the extent to which repeated measures give the same value, while accuracy reflects the extent to which measurements represent 'true' values.

If all anthropometric nutritional assessments are made by one person, there is only within-observer measurement error to consider. However, large studies of nutritional status as well as nutritional screening and surveillance may require a number of anthropometrists, adding to potential measurement error, especially if there is between-observer bias as well. This principle applies equally to other methods of assessment. In choosing the instrument to assess anthropometric nutritional status, workers often elect to measure only height (or length, in the case of infants) and weight. These measures are quick, simple and require only limited training. More comprehensive measurement sets which include skinfolds and circumferences require more training and carry different degrees of error with them.

Types of anthropometric measurements

The most basic measurements, *height (or length) and weight*, are fundamental to all nutritional anthropometric studies, since they give the simplest measure of attained skeletal size (height or length), and of soft tissue mass (weight). *Arm and calf circumferences* are used as proxies for soft tissue mass. In each case the assumption is made that the cross-sectional area of bone in the upper arm and lower leg respectively is standard across populations, and is unaffected by acute undernutrition. This is broadly acceptable, given that the size and relative proportions are largely inherited characteristics that show as much variation within populations, as between them. Furthermore, although skeletal growth is plastic, responding both to nutritional circumstances and to physical activity, it is less plastic than soft tissue

Table 31.4 **The usefulness of weight and height measures relative to reference data**

	Weight for age	Height for age	Weight for height
Usefulness in populations where age is unknown or inaccurate	4	4	1
Usefulness in identifying wasted children	3	4	1
Usefulness in identifying stunted children	2	1	4
Sensitivity to weight change over a short time frame	2	4	1
Ease of accurate collection	2	3	2

Key: 1: excellent; 2: good; 3: moderate; 4: poor.
After Gorstein et al (1994).

mass. Decline in height with increasing age among the elderly has been noted in studies throughout the world. Demispan (distance between index–middle finger web and the sternal notch) has been shown to be a reliable and reproducible alternative measure of stature in the elderly.

Skinfolds are used as proxies for body fatness although they are measures of subcutaneous fatness only; since body fatness is largely comprised of both subcutaneous and visceral fat, the use of skinfolds assumes that the partitioning of subcutaneous to visceral fat does not vary across nutritional states. This assumption is likely to be wrong, given that visceral fat and subcutaneous fat have recently been shown to be biologically distinct. Total fat loss among obese subjects involves different reductions in size between the two tissues. The acquisition of the two abdominal fat compartments is likely to involve different physiological mechanisms, given that the expression of 40 genes involved in glucose homeostasis, insulin action, and lipid metabolism has been shown to differ significantly between them.

The use of *waist and hip circumferences* gives a composite measure of fatness, both subcutaneous and visceral. *Lower limb skinfold and circumference* measures are valuable, since it cannot be assumed that measures of the upper body are also representative of the lower body; upper body–lower body differences in fatness and muscularity are possible in individuals performing hard work on a regular basis. This may not be true for young children, and older children not engaged in child labour; in this case, upper body measures alone are useful in nutritional assessment. In practice, measures of upper arm circumferences may be both accurate and useful only in children below the age of 6 years.

Section CD 31.3(e) describes the equipment needed, standardised methods used and indices created.

Accuracy of measures

Even poorly conducted anthropometry is far more reproducible (precise) and valid (accurate) than the majority of techniques used to measure individual dietary intake. However, there is a need to measure accurately, and be aware of the pitfalls of anthropometry. This set of techniques is more simply carried out than many other measures of nutritional status, and there is often a tendency to delegate measurement to less-qualified individuals. Although there is nothing wrong with this, all potential anthropometrists should receive adequate training from an expert or supervisor to reach a measurable level of expertise prior to survey, and maintain this level of expertise throughout. Depending on the number of individuals involved, this can often be done in two days for measures of weight and height. Initial rounds of measurement and remeasurement are used to determine the technical error of measurement of each trainee anthropometrist. Individuals with poor technique can thus be identified for additional help. Once criterion levels of technical error of measurement are achieved, the anthropometrist can be considered trained.

Even where experienced anthropometrists are employed, small differences in technique can occur over time, and this should be controlled for. Once trained, an estimate of measurement error is needed for any particular study or series of observations. The most commonly used indices of this are the technical error of measurement (TEM) and reliability (R). The TEM is obtained by carrying out a number of repeat measurements on the same subject, either by the same observer, or by two or more observers, taking the differences and entering them into an appropriate equation (see Table CD 31.5). R is a related measure that compares TEM to the total inter-subject variance for the study in question. Reference values for acceptable TEM according to age and sex for height, weight, arm circumference, triceps and subscapular skinfold thicknesses are given in Ulijaszek & Kerr (1999). Examples of the calculations of TEM and R are given in Sections CD 31.3(a) and CD 31.3(b). Studies that do not bother to present this type of information carry unknown levels of measurement error.

It is important to assess, where possible, interobserver differences between anthropometrists and there should be a designated criterion anthropometrist engaged both in training new anthropometrists, and subsequently in the course of work, to maintain quality of measurement. This serves to identify and correct systematic errors in newly trained anthropometrists, and maintain quality of measurement among already trained anthropometrists. The determination of accuracy is problematic, since the correct value of any anthropometric measure is impossible to know. Operationally, accuracy is determined by comparison of measurements made against those of a criterion anthropometrist, an individual who has internalised, as far as is humanly possible, the rules of anthropometric measurement as delineated in the literature, and has received training to the highest level and compares well in anthropometric measurement against other criterion anthropometrists.

It is important to note that error may be introduced if the reporting of age is inaccurate, especially for young children, and all steps should be taken to use available records, or local events calendars, to get as good an estimate of age as possible.

Reference standards for anthropometric nutritional assessment

Large-scale anthropometric surveys associated with public health surveillance in industrialised nations first led to the generation of growth curves for children, and distribution curves for adults, for use in health monitoring. Such normative population-based constructs subsequently came to be used in nutritional assessment globally, normative growth curves being generated subsequent to anthropometric survey in a number of less-developed countries. The use of indigenously produced growth references for the monitoring of the growth performance of members of the same population is uncontroversial, as long as the reference data fulfil the criteria given in Table 31.5.

In order to estimate nutritional status of children from anthropometry, values of measures such as height and weight must be related to normative values. This is done by comparing individual values using percentiles, percentage of the mean or median reference value for age, and/or Z (standard deviation) scores. Whichever of these comparators is used, the distribution of the anthropometric measure against the reference values can be determined, or the

---

Table 31.5 **Minimal criteria for anthropometric reference data in nutritional evaluation**

1. The population should be well nourished
2. Each age/sex group of the sample should contain at least 200 individuals
3. The sample should be cross-sectional
4. Sampling procedures should be defined and reproducible
5. Measuring procedures should be optimal
6. Measurements should include all variables used in nutritional evaluation
7. Raw data and smoothing procedures should be available

Source: Waterlow et al (1977).

---

proportion of the population falling below cut-offs defining the normative range stated. There is rough correspondence between Z scores, centiles, and percentage of median reference value. As a very general rule of thumb, 90% of median reference value for height for age is roughly similar to the 3rd percentile, and $-2\,Z$ scores height for age. Similarly, 80% of median weight for age is roughly equivalent to the 5th percentile, and $-1.5\,Z$ scores of weight for age, while 80% of median reference value of weight for height is roughly equivalent to the 3rd centile and $-2\,Z$ scores of weight for height.

The use of growth references developed in industrialised nations for the use of nutritional assessment of individuals in less developed nations has been widely debated. Studies showing that the growth patterns in height of well-fed, healthy preschool children from globally diverse populations are broadly similar have led to the acceptance by the WHO of the US National Center for Health Statistics 1977 reference curves for height and weight for international use in the late 1970s. These internationally adopted growth curves have served many useful purposes across the years, but have been challenged on both technical and biological grounds. A new international growth reference based on well-off children from six developed and developing countries (Garza & de Onis 1999) is at an advanced stage of development by the WHO at the time of writing.

There are reference centile values for all the major anthropometric measures of nutritional status, as well as for indices such as BMI. Many of these are summarised in Gibson (1990) and Ulijaszek et al (1998). The following growth references should be added to this list: the British 1990 reference values for weight, height, and BMI; the Eurogrowth references for weight, length, and arm circumference of young children, and the CDC reference values for height, weight and BMI for the USA, and the international references for child overweight and obesity. The proliferation of growth references probably reflects the growing realisation that nutritional assessment is an important component of any nationally-based child health strategy. Possession of nationally- or regionally-based growth references is also a matter of political pride.

Nutritional anthropometric data may be compared directly with normative reference values, or be standardised for age using Z scores (also known as standard deviation scores) relative to reference data, if such information is to be combined across a range of ages. Cut-offs of -1, -2 and $-3\,Z$ scores can then be used as estimates of the level of under-nutrition in children, at either individual or population level. For international comparison, the growth references adopted by the WHO for international use are the most appropriate. However, these do not provide a comprehensive set of reference data for a variety of measures, and for those wishing to examine or use more than weight and height or length in children, or make comparisons of adult and child anthropometric status, there is a choice of using data from a variety of sources, samples and populations, or to limit the comparison of measurements to the variables and age groups represented in the set of reference data chosen (see Section CD 31.3(c)) There are various software programs for the assessment of anthropometric nutritional status (see Section CD 31.3(d)).

○ Key points

- ○ Anthropometry is the most frequently used means of assessing nutrition status of a population.

- ○ Each age group has its own most appropriate anthropometric measures.

- ○ The ease of collection of anthropometric measures should not mask the considerable potential for error in collection, but these errors are manageable if anticipated.

- ○ The measurements are typically compared to measurements obtained for 'healthy' populations. These normative reference standards are continually being updated and reviewed and care must be taken to use the most appropriate one and to cite its use.

31.4 BIOCHEMICAL ASSESSMENT

Objectives

- To summarise the available choices of tissue and body fluid samples that may be selected and collected for biochemical status assessment.

- To summarise the necessary precautions to be taken during sample selection, storage and analysis, and to provide an outline of essential fieldwork and laboratory methodologies.

- To highlight the common problems of interpretation, and the inter-relationships between the biochemical and other indices of nutritional status, to be used in conjunction with each other for a composite and integrated picture of status and nutritional adequacy.

As explained in Section 31.1, biochemical assessment ideally forms part of a coordinated set of nutritional investigations that may also include diet estimates, anthropometry, functional and clinical investigations. These are used to distinguish between deficiency, adequacy and overload of one or more nutrients (see Bates et al 1997, Bates 1997, and Sauberlich 1999). The design of the biochemical part of the investigation depends on there being an available and suitable sample of body fluid or tissue for analysis, and biochemical tests to estimate concentrations of key nutrients. The results must then be interpreted in the light of established normal ranges. Therefore, it is essential to have access to suitable analytical equipment, and relevant expertise for the collection, storage, analysis and interpretation of the tests.

Biochemical markers of nutritional intake and status

The following section will describe the biochemical markers, i.e. the specific diagnostic analytes that can be measured in accessible human body fluids and tissues such as blood, urine, saliva, hair and nails. They are selected on the basis that they can be used as predictors for the different levels of nutrient intake and of tissue status adequacy that occur in human individuals and populations.

Biochemical markers are potentially useful for the following reasons:

- They can be measured with high specificity, and excellent accuracy and objectivity, without reliance on information being provided by the individual(s) being studied.

- They can represent the integral effect of dietary intakes of nutrients from food and supplements over a period of time, ranging from hours up to months or even years before the sample is taken.
- Different types of index for each nutrient can specifically reflect either recent nutrient intakes or long-term intakes and status, and thus the accumulating risk of functional inadequacy and disease risk. 'Functional ' indices (such as plasma homocysteine or dark adaptation for instance) may provide links with the risk of disease or of physiological malfunction which, in turn, can provide a goal for the definition of nutrient adequacy or optimal nutrition for individual nutrients.
- Unlike clinical signs and symptoms of deficiency disease, biochemical markers are usually nutrient-specific and are rapidly and predictably responsive to the correction of nutrient deficiencies.
- In a few cases, dietary nutrient intakes can in practice be predicted more accurately from biochemical indices than from diet assessment. This is particularly the case for urinary sodium, potassium and nitrogen as markers for sodium, potassium and protein intakes, and for urinary fluoride and iodide as markers for fluoride and iodine intakes.

Although biochemical marker measurements can be informative on their own, they are even more powerful when combined with nutrient intake estimates and clinical assessments of nutritional adequacy. These three approaches can be likened to different windows providing different complementary viewpoints on a landscape, or different forensic tools combining to build an irrefutable legal case. In combination they can define both 'nutritional adequacy', i.e. freedom from deleterious effects of malnutrition which can threaten health and lead to deficiency disease, and 'optimum nutrition', for which the concept of minimum nutritional adequacy is enhanced by the concept of variable tissue stores, whose repletion can provide additional insurance against future dietary shortage or increased tissue demand.

The concept of 'optimum nutrition' remains controversial, insofar as some scientists argue that an optimum intake is harder to define than the minimum that is required to reach a definite titratable end-point. Such an end-point occurs where the index values vary across the deficiency range, but reach a constant or plateau value once adequacy is achieved. Most recommended or reference intakes

of nutrients consider both of these concepts. Population surveys rely heavily on the information that is provided by intake estimates and by status measurements, and these, in turn, permit the identification of 'high risk' groups within a population, e.g. older people living in nursing homes, people with low incomes or low socioeconomic status, etc. It is important to recognise that the 'normal ranges' for status indices may differ between different age groups, between the two sexes, between different physiological states (e.g. pregnant versus non-pregnant) and between different ethnic and genetic subgroups. The study of genetic subgroups, and how these can be affected differentially by nutrition, comprises part of the study of gene–nutrient interactions, which is at an early and very exciting stage of research.

Nutrient indices measured, and feasibility of predicting intakes from indices

Biochemical status indices for individual nutrients

Protein and essential amino acids

There are no good indices for tissue protein status (in the sense of reflecting the adequacy of dietary protein as distinct from metabolic processes). The most commonly used index is serum (or plasma) albumin. It is lowered in conditions such as kwashiorkor, partly attributed to low protein intakes or poor protein quality. However, serum albumin is also reduced by the acute phase reaction, and severely malnourished children commonly have infections. Serum albumin is measured by a dye-based assay, or by a more specific and reliable immunoassay. An alternative, possibly more reliable index of inadequate protein supply is the plasma amino acid profile, since the 'essential' amino acids, notably the branched-chain amino acids, are lowered when dietary protein is inadequate. Protein intakes can be monitored fairly accurately by nitrogen excretion rates.

Essential fatty acid status (and fatty acid profiling)

Serum or plasma is frequently used for fatty acid profiling, and hence for monitoring of essential fatty acid (EFA) intakes. However, interpretation is complicated by variability of lipoprotein profiles and by diurnal variation. More promising, but less explored, are new techniques for fatty acids in red cell membranes, fat biopsies (reflecting long-term fat stores composition), etc. Research into relationships

32

Food supply, factors affecting production, trade and access

Marc J. Cohen

Objectives

By the end of this chapter, you should be able to:

- compare world food supply with population needs

- give examples of past scares about the adequacy of world food supply, and the reasons for their resolution

- discuss the socioeconomic, agroecological, and health constraints on future food production

- explain the factors impeding access to food

- show how globalisation relates to food security

- demonstrate the multiple functions of agricultural and rural development in achieving equitable and sustainable food security

- elucidate the role of various approaches to agricultural research, including biotechnology, in achieving food security

- make clear the relationship between sustainable natural resource management and food security

- define the terms food security, food insecurity, food supply, food demand, hunger, famine, Green Revolution, and entitlements.

32.1 INTRODUCTION

At the 1996 World Food Summit, high-level representatives of 186 nations and the European Union, including over 100 heads of state and government, agreed to the Rome Declaration on World Food Security, which states,

We consider it intolerable that more that 800 million people throughout the world, and particularly in developing countries, do not have enough food to meet their basic nutritional needs. This situation is unacceptable. Food supplies have increased substantially, but constraints on access to food, instability of supply and demand, as well as natural and man-made disasters, prevent basic food needs from being fulfilled.

In the years since, these problems have persisted stubbornly. Absolute food shortages are much less of a concern today than in the past, with access to food the critical problem. Nevertheless, many analysts continue to worry that human population growth will outpace the earth's ability to produce adequate food supplies. This concern, voiced by Thomas R. Malthus in 1798, remains a preoccupation two centuries later (Brown et al 1998), notwithstanding the successful role of science, technology, and public policy in addressing this dilemma in the twentieth century. Growing demand for animal products in the developing world (Rosegrant et al 2001) further fuels concern about overburdening the earth's 'carrying capacity'.

At the dawn of the twenty-first century, the paradoxical nature of contemporary food insecurity is all too clear: India's parliamentarians debate what to do with a 50 million tonne grain surplus while some 233 million of their fellow citizens go to bed hungry each night (FAO 2002). Furthermore, the overwhelming majority of the world's hungry people live in rural areas and depend on food production and other agricultural activities for their livelihood. Growing integration of global markets, combined with revolutionary advances in transportation and communications, holds great promise for better matching food supplies and needs. But rich-country farm subsidies and trade barriers make it difficult for poor farmers in developing countries to reap potential gains.

This chapter will examine whether technological and institutional innovation will continue to allow food production to keep pace with population growth and rising food demand, as well as the environmental costs that this will entail. It will also focus on the critical problem of *access* to food and the bearing that globalisation has on food security. The chapter concludes by looking at the policy actions needed to achieve food security in developing countries – particularly the importance of broad-based agricultural and rural development – while assuring sustainable management of the natural resource base upon which food production depends. For review publications on food supply see Section CD 32.1.

32.2 DEFINITION OF FOOD SECURITY

'Food security', according to one widely accepted definition, 'exists when all people, at all times, have physical and economic access to sufficient, safe, and nutritious food to meet their dietary needs and food preferences for an active and healthy life'. This definition is in keeping with the principle that everyone has a right to adequate food, to be free from hunger, and to enjoy general human dignity, enshrined in the International Bill of Human Rights. *Food insecurity*, then, is the absence of food security. *Hunger*, a condition in which people lack the basic food intake to provide them with the energy and nutrients for fully productive, active lives, is an outcome of food insecurity.

The availability of adequate food is a necessary condition for achieving food security, but it is not sufficient. Of equal importance are *access to food* and *appropriate utilisation of food* (see Ch. 33). Thus, even when food supplies are satisfactory, food insecurity may persist because people lack access, whether by means of production, purchase, public social safety net programmes, private charity, or some combination of these, to available food. In addition, people may fail to consume sufficient quantities of food or a balanced diet even when supplies are ample (see Section CD 32.2 on food insecurity in sub-Saharan Africa).

⮑ Key points

⮑ Food security requires more than just adequate food availability; it also is a matter of access to the food that is available and of its appropriate utilisation.

32.3 WORLD FOOD SUPPLY

Past trends and current supply situation

Scholars and policy-makers alike have long worried about how to balance food supplies with the demands of a rapidly growing population. Malthus claimed that population increases by a geometric ratio, whereas food production only increases by an arithmetic ratio, and thereby exerts a natural 'check' on population growth. Malthusian worries may have reached their apogee in the late 1960s and early 1970s. Then, analysts wrote off much of Asia as 'a hopeless basket case'. The threat of famine gripped West and Central Africa, Ethiopia and Bangladesh, and it seemed as though Malthus's 'check' had kicked in with a vengeance. The popular press in the industrialised countries turned out tomes on 'lifeboat ethics' and 'triage'.

The Green Revolution
In fact, food availability rose dramatically between 1970 and 1997, and by the latter year, global harvests and stocks offered more than enough calories per person per day to meet minimum requirements, if the food were distributed according to need. The key factor controverting Malthusian predictions was a rapid increase in the output of cereals, the main source of calories in developing countries, as farmers in Asia and Latin America widely adopted high-yielding varieties, and governments, especially in Asia,

implemented policies that supported agricultural development. Between 1967 and 1997, per capita cereal production in the developing world increased 28% (Rosegrant et al 2001). By 2002, developing-country cereal harvests, at 1.2 billion tonnes, were triple those of 40 years earlier, while the population was a little over twice as large. Daily per capita calorie supplies in the developing world jumped from 2140, below the minimum requirement of 2350, in 1970 to 2667 in 1997 (Fig. 32.1). However, calorie availability per person remained below minimum requirements in sub-Saharan Africa and barely above the threshold in South Asia (Rosegrant et al 2001).

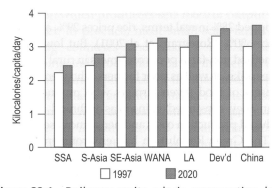

Figure 32.1 Daily per capita calorie consumption, by region, 1997 and 2020. SSA, sub-Saharan Africa; WANA, West Asia–North Africa; LA, Latin America.
Source: Rosegrant et al (2001).

strategies that result in improved soil organic matter, and by making the use of nitrogen and water more efficient. Planting trees, integrating tree and crop cultivation, and reduced deforestation all offer potential carbon gains.

Health constraints

Infectious disease has a significant bearing on food production, especially in sub-Saharan Africa. About 36 million people are currently living with HIV/AIDS, two-thirds of them in sub-Saharan Africa, and it is spreading dramatically in Asia. It has contributed to labour shortages (from those afflicted and those affected, i.e. caring for the afflicted), a decline in the transfer of farmer knowledge across generations, weaker collective action, weaker property rights, a declining asset base, breakdown of social bonds, loss of livestock, and reliance on crops that are easier to produce but less nutritious and economically valuable. Because malaria often strikes during harvest time, it also threatens food output.

In order to cope with the effects of HIV/AIDS on agriculture and food security, as labour becomes depleted, new cultivation technologies and varieties need to be developed that do not rely so much on labour, yet allow crops to remain drought-resistant and nutritious. Innovations such as farmer field schools can facilitate the transfer of community-specific and organisation-specific knowledge within and between generations. Making institutions, including agricultural research centres, more client-focused can help natural resource management remain effective in the presence of weakened social capital (i.e. the norms and networks that allow collective action, especially at the community level) and property rights. For example, where there are large numbers of women widowed by AIDS, gender-equitable land ownership rights are ever more important.

It is also critical to explore integrated efforts to address development problems across sectors. For example, the use of drip irrigation can make agricultural water use more efficient while denying habitat to malaria mosquitoes.

> ## ⮫ Key points
>
> ⮫ Technological and institutional innovation has permitted food production to more than keep pace with population growth.
>
> ⮫ Projections to the year 2020 indicate that food supplies will remain adequate.
>
> ⮫ Poor farmers frequently engage in a mix of subsistence and commercial activities.
>
> ⮫ Small-scale farmers face many constraints, including lack of access to productive resources, natural resource degradation, and health crises.

32.4 WORLD FOOD DEMAND AND ACCESS TO FOOD

Demand for food

Food demand derives primarily from income growth, population growth (see 'Population growth', above), and urbanisation. IFPRI projects income growth (as measured by growth of gross domestic product) in all developing regions between 1997 and 2020 at levels exceeding those of the world as a whole and the developed countries. Growth rates will be highest in Asia and lowest in sub-Saharan Africa (Table 32.1) (Rosegrant et al 2001).

Urban population in developing countries is expected to more than double between 2000 and 2030, when 56% of the developing world's population will live in urban areas. Over 90% of the increase in global population during these three decades will occur in the rapidly expanding cities and towns of the developing world.

When people move to cities, their lifestyles become more sedentary, and women experience

Table 32.1 Income growth, 1997–2020

Region	GDP growth, 1997–2020 (%/year)
Developed countries	2.4
Developing countries	
Latin America	3.8
Sub-Saharan Africa	3.6
West Asia/North Africa	3.8
South Asia	5.5
Southeast Asia	4.9
East Asia	5.7
World	2.9

Source: Rosegrant et al (2001).

higher opportunity costs on their time. As a result, urban dwellers tend to shift consumption to foods that require less preparation time (e.g. from sorghum, millet, maize, and root crops to rice and wheat), and to more meat, milk, fruit, vegetables and processed foods.

IFPRI projects a 49% increase in cereal demand in developing countries between 1997 and 2020. Demographic shifts are expected to drive increased demand for meat and the feed to produce it. Maize will overtake rice and wheat in accounting for 30% of total cereal demand in 2020, compared to 26% in 1997. Most of the increased maize demand, especially in Asia, will be for livestock feed associated with rising meat demand, which will grow 57% globally and 92% in developing countries, led by China. Cereal production will grow 1.3% annually over 1997–2020, but production increases in developing countries will not meet rising demand. The USA and European Union will boost their exports to fill in the gap. Expansion of cultivated area will account for just 15% of increased cereal production in

developing countries, with yield gains responsible for 85%. But yield growth has slowed since the mid-1970s, and yields will grow a bit less than 1% per year globally over 1997–2020 (Fig. 32.2). Only sub-Saharan Africa will experience improving yield growth rates during the period. Slowing rates of yield growth will result from increasing input requirements in order to sustain yield gains in Asia, as well as slowed public investment in agricultural research and irrigation infrastructure (Rosegrant et al 2001).

International cereal prices are expected to decline over 1997–2020, but at a slower rate than in the 1980s and 1990s. Wheat prices will decline 8%, rice prices will fall 13%, and maize prices will remain flat, due to strong feed demand. Moreover, prices will only begin to decline significantly after 2010, with increases of 3% for wheat and constant prices for maize and rice over 1997–2010 (Rosegrant et al 2001).

Current state of food insecurity and future outlook

Chapter 33 details the current state of world food insecurity. According to the Food and Agriculture Organization of the United Nations (FAO), as of 1999 (the last year for which data are available), there were 799 million food-insecure people in the developing countries (Table 32.2). Food insecurity can also be found in the countries in transition from centrally planned to market-oriented economies and in the industrialised countries. However, the problems are more severe and affect a far greater proportion of the population in developing nations. The world has made progress – albeit slowly and unevenly – in reducing hunger. Since 1970, the number of food-insecure people in developing countries has

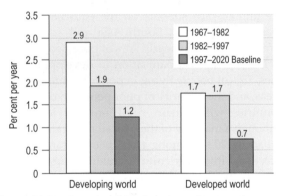

Figure 32.2 Cereal yields: slowdown in growth. Source: IFPRI IMPACT simulation (August 2001).

Table 32.2 Food insecurity in developing countries, 1980, 1999 and 2015 (millions of people and percentage of population)

Region	1970		1999		2015	
	Number	%	Number	%	Number	%
Developing world	959	37	799	17	610	11
Sub-Saharan Africa	88	34	196	33	205	23
West Asia and North Africa	45	25	40	10	37	7
Latin America and the Caribbean	54	19	55	11	40	6
East and Southeast Asia	504	43	192	10	135	6
South Asia	267	37	315	23	195	12

Source: FAO.
Note: *Food security* exists when all people, at all times, have physical and economic access to sufficient, safe, and nutritious food to meet their dietary needs and food preferences for an active and healthy life.
Food insecurity is the absence of food security.

Box 32.1 *A profile of hunger*

Kone Figue is a mother of six in Ponoundogou in northern Côte d'Ivoire, West Africa. She and her husband farm six hectares of government-owned land. They grow cotton and groundnuts, mostly for sale, and maize (to eat and feed to their two cows) on about half the land, along with some yams and cassava. They plant the rest of the land to rice, their family's main staple food.

But the rice crop does not stretch out to provide a whole year's worth of meals, so the family ends up consuming the yams and cassava, even though they much prefer rice (preferably spiced up with some of the groundnuts).

Kone weeds and harvests the rice by hand, with the aid of simple tools like a hoe and a sickle. Her husband clears the land and sows the seeds. It is backbreaking work. Kone cannot afford to buy fertiliser or chemical weedkillers, and even with manure from her cows, her yields are meagre.

Adapted from Schiøler (1998).

---

declined by about 17%, and the food-insecure percentage of the population has dropped dramatically, from 37 to 17%. Today, South Asia and sub-Saharan Africa are home to over three-fifths of all food-insecure people. Progress against hunger slowed considerably in the 1990s, and FAO projects that in 2015, the food-insecure population of the developing world will only decline to 610 million people. This is far short of the World Food Summit goal of reducing the number of people living in hunger by 50% – to 400 million people or fewer – by no later than 2015. Hunger's centre of gravity will remain squarely in South Asia and sub-Saharan Africa (FAO 2002).

Real people with names and faces stand behind these numbers (see Box 32.1).

Access to food

The large numbers of people who remain food insecure and the slow progress in reducing hunger may seem paradoxical in light of adequate food availability (see 'Past trends and current supply situation', above). However, current food availability is sufficient to provide everyone with their minimum calorie requirements *if the food were distributed according to need*; food is *not* so distributed.

People obtain access to the food that is available through *entitlements*, i.e., the amount of food or other necessities that they can command based on their income and assets, given the legal, political, economic and cultural context in which they live. Thus, a farmer may produce food, but may have to deliver some of her harvest to a landlord before she can consume what remains. Likewise, a wage earner's income permits her to command a certain amount of food. Government programmes and private charity are other forms of entitlement (Drèze & Sen 1989).

Poverty drives food insecurity

Food insecurity persists primarily because of poverty. Low-income people cannot afford to buy all of the food they need, even though poor households typically spend 50–70% of their income on food. In addition, poor people frequently lack access to land and other productive resources, and so cannot produce food for themselves (IFAD 2001). According to the World Bank, 1.2 billion people in developing countries (or about one in four) live on the equivalent of less than US\$1 per day, and are too poor to meet their needs for food and the other necessities of life on a sustainable basis (Table 32.3). Almost half of the human race subsists on the equivalent of less than US\$2 per day. South Asia and sub-Saharan Africa are home to nearly 70% of poor people.

Despite rapid urbanisation in developing countries, 75% of people living in poverty remain in rural areas, and the majority of poor people in developing countries will remain rural until at least 2035, although a majority of the overall population will be urban by 2020. Among rural people, farmers who practise rainfed agriculture, smallholders, pastoralists, artisanal fishers, landless labourers, indigenous people, people in female-headed households and displaced people are most affected by poverty. Worldwide, rural wage labourers, especially landless farm workers, are the most likely to be poor. In sub-Saharan Africa, smallholder farmers are the largest group living in poverty. In West Asia and North Africa, women, children and elderly people bear the brunt of rural poverty, as men of working age tend to out-migrate (IFAD 2001). Globally, women bear a disproportionate share of poverty, and children are more likely to be poor than adults. Cultural practices and official policies that marginalise people on the basis of gender, age, race and ethnicity frequently contribute to food insecurity. For example, in India, tribal people and members of 'scheduled castes' (once called 'untouchables') have a higher risk of poverty.

Urbanisation is expected to increase urban poverty and food insecurity. Poor urban dwellers are more

Table 32.3 **People living on less than $1 per day, 1990, 1998 and 2015 (millions of people and percentage of population)**

	1990		1998		2015 (optimistic)		2015 (pessimistic)	
	No.	%	No.	%	No.	%	No.	%
Developing world	1300	29	1200	23	777	13	1000	16
Sub-Saharan Africa	242	48	302	48	361	40	462	47
East and Southeast Asia	452	28	267	15	65	3	101	5
South Asia	495	44	522	40	297	18	426	25
Latin America and the Caribbean	74	17	61	12	43	7	58	9
West Asia and North Africa	6	2	6	2	5	1	6	2

Source: World Bank.
Note: The optimistic scenario for 2015 assumes moderate, broad-based economic growth worldwide, while the pessimistic scenario assumes slower growth and rising inequality.

dependent on money income, may have fewer opportunities to grow their own food, and require access to childcare in order to pursue income-earning opportunities. The needed resources to address food insecurity may not be land so much as economic opportunities, such as secure employment at a wage adequate to meet basic needs or the chance to own a business, as well as access to social safety net programmes.

Poor and food-insecure people frequently lack political voice and organisations that are accountable to them and capable of articulating their interests to policy-makers and other power holders. As a result, policies tend to benefit people who are already well off, and policy-makers tend to give low priority to the needs of poor and hungry people or programmes that would benefit them. A World Bank report based on extensive interviews of poor people in developing and transition countries found that they regard their situation as one where freedom and the power to control one's life are lacking. A low-income Jamaican woman compared poverty to 'living in jail, living in bondage, waiting to be free'.

The World Bank has projected poverty levels to 2015 under two scenarios: one of slow growth and increasing inequality, and one in which countries adopt policies and interventions that foster inclusion and broad-based growth. Overall poverty declines in both scenarios, but much more substantially in the latter, 'optimistic' one. Poverty will likewise decline in South Asia under both scenarios, although many millions of South Asians will remain poor in either. Poverty will increase substantially in Africa under both scenarios, leaving the region with both the highest poverty rate and the largest number of poor people by 2015.

Transitory food emergencies

From time to time, natural disasters, violent conflicts, economic collapse, political crisis, or some combination of these factors will create food emergencies. Whilst these emergencies are often transitory in duration, they may have long-lasting impacts on the affected people. Research in Africa and Asia indicates that drought can lead to child malnutrition that in turn causes poor school performance and reduced earnings over the course of a lifetime. In April 2003, tens of millions of people in 37 countries faced serious food emergencies. Most of the affected people were in sub-Saharan Africa, but reconstruction following the war in Iraq also required considerable food aid. Needs are generally acute among refugees and internally displaced persons, who often live in camps and depend on humanitarian assistance for survival. Since the end of the Cold War, internal conflicts have proliferated in developing and transition countries, particularly in sub-Saharan Africa. At the end of 2002, 13 million refugees had crossed international borders to escape these struggles, which displaced another 22 million people within their own countries. Even after conflict ends, the costly burden of reconstruction may leave many people food insecure for years. Landmines continue to maim and keep land out of production long after fighting ends. Not only does violent conflict cause hunger, but hunger can also contribute to conflict, especially when resources are scarce and perceptions of economic injustice are widespread, as in Rwanda in 1994 or Central America in the 1970s and 1980s.

Where armed conflicts and civil strife occur, governments and the international community must give priority to conflict resolution and prevention. It is essential to expand and strengthen early warning

Table 32.4 Public agricultural research expenditures in developed and developing countries, 1976–1996 (average annual growth rates; %)

	1976–81	1981–86	1986–91	1991–96
Developing countries	7.0	3.9	3.9	3.6
Sub-Saharan Africa	1.7	1.4	0.5	−0.2
China	7.8	8.9	2.8	5.5
Asia and Pacific (excluding China)	8.2	5.1	7.5	4.4
Latin America and the Caribbean	9.5	0.5	0.4	2.9
West Asia and North Africa	7.4	4.0	4.2	3.5
Developed countries	2.5	1.9	2.2	0.2
World	4.5	2.9	3.0	2.0

Source: Pardey & Beintema (2001).

Agroecology

Although high-yielding Green Revolution technologies have been responsible for enormous productivity increases among small-scale farmers in Asia, many farmers in the region's less-favoured areas have been bypassed. The desire to find ways of assisting these farmers, combined with concerns about excessive dependence on external inputs such as fertilisers, pesticides and irrigation water embodied in the first generation of Green Revolution technologies, has stimulated interest in alternative or complementary approaches, including the so-called 'agroecological approach'. This aims to reduce the amount of external inputs that farmers have to use. Instead, it relies heavily on available farm labour and organic material, as well as on improved knowledge and farm management.

One of the great strengths of the agroecological approach is that it promotes sustainable management of natural resources and active participation by farmers in identifying problems as well as designing and implementing appropriate solutions at the farm and community levels. Such participatory technology development can be extremely effective in finding the most appropriate solutions to production problems.

The potential of modern agricultural biotechnology for food security

(This section draws on ideas in Pinstrup-Andersen & Cohen (2001). See also Section CD 32.6(c) on biotechnology.)

It is possible that the introduction of agricultural biotechnology into developing countries can contribute to increased productivity, lower unit costs and prices for food, preservation of forests and fragile land, poverty reduction and improved nutrition. This depends on whether the research is relevant to poor people, on the economic and social policy environment, and on the nature of the intellectual property rights arrangements governing the technology. By raising productivity in food production, agricultural biotechnology could reduce the need to cultivate new lands and help conserve biodiversity.

Modern agricultural biotechnology offers many potential benefits to developing countries. It may help achieve the productivity gains needed to feed a growing global population, introduce resistance to pests and diseases without high-cost purchased inputs, heighten crops' tolerance to adverse weather and soil conditions, improve the nutritional value of some foods, and enhance the durability of products during harvesting or shipping. Biotechnology research could aid the development of drought-tolerant and pest-resistant crops, to the benefit of small farmers and poor consumers. The development of cereal plants capable of capturing nitrogen from the air could contribute greatly to plant nutrition, helping poor farmers who often cannot afford fertilisers. Biotechnology may offer cost-effective solutions to vitamin and mineral deficiencies, such as provitamin A-rich rice, and be used to develop protein-enhanced crops or edible vaccines. By raising productivity in food production, agricultural biotechnology could reduce the need to cultivate new lands and help conserve biodiversity. Bioengineered products may reduce reliance on pesticides, thereby reducing farmers' crop protection costs and benefiting both the environment and public health. Cotton farmers in China who have adopted insect-resistant cotton have reduced their use of highly toxic insecticides that have been responsible for many deaths.

Except for limited work on rice and cassava, little genetically modified (GM) crop research currently focuses on the productivity and nutrition of poor people. In 2002, North America accounted for 72% of GM crop plantings, with the USA alone accounting for 66%. Additional public and philanthropic resources are needed in support of the appropriate research in developing countries.

Successful adaptation of GM crop technology for the benefit of poor farmers and consumers in developing countries will require the establishment of appropriate institutions to assess and manage public health and environmental risks. In addition, developing countries will need to have appropriate policies in place with respect to industrial competitiveness, international trade and intellectual property if they want to use this technology to help advance food security.

Both food safety and biosafety regulations should reflect international agreements and a given society's acceptable risk levels, including the risks associated with not using biotechnology to achieve desired goals. Poor people should be included directly in the debate and decision-making about technological change.

In addition, developing countries that wish to adopt GM crop technology will need to enact and enforce an appropriate intellectual property rights regime. Poor farmers in developing countries often rely on seed saved from the current year's harvest for planting their next crop. Private companies that have developed GM seeds generally subject them to patents or other forms of intellectual property rights protection. Thus, developing countries need legislation that can balance the desire of seed companies to profit from their innovations with the continuing ability of poor farmers to save, reuse and exchange seed, such as India's 2001 seed law.

Trade issues impinge on developing countries' calculations regarding modern agricultural biotechnology. Given consumer resistance to GM food in the European Union and Japan, developing countries that rely on those markets for agricultural exports would either need to avoid using biotechnology, or would have to adopt and manage a system to differentiate and label GM and non-GM foods. A large share of the food imported by developing countries originates in the USA, and these importing countries must decide whether they wish to insist on product differentiation and labelling in the case of imported food. Rejection of GM crops in Europe and Japan may make such crops cheaper for developing-country importers that are willing to purchase them.

⊃ Key points

- ⊃ Equitable agricultural and rural development is essential to achieve food security.
- ⊃ The development of well-integrated markets is necessary but not sufficient.
- ⊃ Public policies are also essential to ensure that rural poor people have access to resources and services.
- ⊃ At present, developing-country governments and aid donors substantially underinvest in agriculture.
- ⊃ Pro-poor agricultural research, engaging all relevant scientific tools, including, where appropriate, biotechnology, has a critical role to play in efforts to attain food security.

32.7 POLICIES FOR SUSTAINABLE MANAGEMENT OF NATURAL RESOURCES

A high degree of complementarity amongst agricultural development, poverty reduction and environmental sustainability is more likely when agricultural development is broad-based and inclusive of small- and medium-sized farms, market-oriented, participatory and decentralised, and driven by technological change that enhances productivity without degrading natural resources. Policies aimed at achieving sustainable agricultural development must take into account the role of property rights and collective action in natural resource management. Many natural resource management technologies and practices take years to give full returns, e.g. terracing. Without secure rights to

resources, farmers lack incentives to adopt these approaches. Some technologies need to be adopted over a wide area to be effective, e.g. integrated pest management (IPM), so adopting farmers must cooperate with their neighbours in collective action.

Promoting sustainable development in less-favoured areas

Although productivity is lower in less-favoured areas, these zones usually have comparative advantage in some agricultural production or non-farm activities if investment in infrastructure and institutions is adequate. Research has found that public investment in less-favoured areas of China and

India results in high returns that sometimes exceed those to investment in favoured areas in terms of both economic growth and poverty reduction. Investments in agricultural research, education, roads and irrigation have greater incremental impact in less-favoured areas in these two countries, in part because opportunities for investment in these areas have been neglected. In sub-Saharan Africa, where overall agricultural public investment is low, additional investment is needed in both high-potential and less-favoured areas (Pender & Hazell 2000).

Soil fertility management

Low soil fertility and lack of access to reasonably priced fertilisers, along with failure to replenish soil nutrients, must be rectified through efficient and timely use of organic and inorganic fertilisers and improved soil management. Chemical fertiliser use should be reduced where heavy application causes environmental harm. Fertiliser subsidies that encourage excessive use should be removed, but subsidies may remain necessary for less-favoured areas where current use is low and soil fertility is being diminished (Pinstrup-Andersen et al 1999).

Integrated pest management

Until recently, developing-country governments and aid donors encouraged use of synthetic pesticides. Now, consensus is emerging on IPM. IPM has a variety of definitions, but it is generally understood to mean a flexible approach to pest management that draws upon a range of methods to produce a result that combines the greatest value to the farmer with environmentally acceptable and sustainable outcomes. The techniques used for crop protection in IPM may include traditional crop management – crop rotation, intercropping, mulching, tillage and the like. IPM may also use pest-resistant crop varieties (developed through conventional breeding or genetic engineering), biological control agents,

biopesticides and, as a last resort, judicious use of synthetic chemical pesticides. The options used by the farmer depend on the local context – agroecological needs, availability and affordability of the various alternatives (see Section CD 32.7, which describes a case study on biological pest control).

Water policy reform

Comprehensive water policy reform is needed to help save water, improve use efficiency and boost crop output per unit. Such reforms will be difficult, due to widespread practices and cultural norms that treat water as a free good and vested interests benefiting from current arrangements. Reforms might include secure and tradable rights for users, and subsidies targeted to poor water users in place of general subsidies. Devolving irrigation infrastructure and management to user associations, combined with secure access to water, will provide incentives for efficient use. Appropriate technology is needed to support conservation incentives.

> ⊃ **Key points**
>
> ⊃ Efforts to achieve food security must take sustainable natural resource management, including the role of property rights and collective action, into account.
>
> ⊃ Public investments in agricultural and rural development in less-favoured areas often lead to high returns in terms of both economic growth and poverty reduction.
>
> ⊃ Policies must ensure that soil fertility is maintained.
>
> ⊃ Policies should favour integrated pest management strategies, to ensure sustainability.
>
> ⊃ Policies should promote efficient agricultural water use.

32.8 CONCLUSION

Implementing the policy changes outlined in this chapter will be expensive, and will require difficult political choices. But the task is far from impossible. IFPRI forecasts that developing countries will make public investments of about $580 billion in irrigation, rural roads, agricultural research, clean water provision, and education between 1997 and 2020.

Boosting this figure to $800 billion would greatly advance food security, reducing the projected number of malnourished preschool children in developing countries from 132 million to 94 million in 2020. If total developing-country government expenditures remained constant at 1997 levels, the investments needed to achieve this more favourable child nutrition outcome would amount to just 4.9% of government spending. Moreover, on an annual basis, the needed additional public investment represents just 5% of current annual military spending in low- and middle-income developing countries. Accelerated progress toward sustainable food security will depend upon the willingness of developing and developed-country governments, international aid agencies, non-governmental organisations, business and industry, and individuals, to back their anti-hunger rhetoric with action, resources and changes in behaviour and institutions. The research community has a moral obligation to monitor the presence or absence of such changes.

References and further reading

References

Brown L R, Gardner G, Halweil B 1998 Beyond Malthus: sixteen dimensions of the population problem. Worldwatch Paper No. 143. Worldwatch Institute, Washington DC. Accessible at http://www.worldwatch.org

Drèze J, Sen A 1989 Hunger and public action. Clarendon Press, Oxford

FAO (Food and Agriculture Organisation of the United Nations) 2001 Mobilizing resources to fight hunger. Report to the 27th Session of the Committee on World Food Security. Accessible at http://www.fao.org/docrep/meeting/003/Y0006E/Y0006E00.htm

FAO 2002 The state of food insecurity in the world 2002. FAO, Rome. Accessible at http://www.fao.org/docrep/005/y7352e/y7352e00.htm

IFAD (International Fund for Agricultural Development) 2001 Rural poverty report 2001. IFAD, Rome. Accessible at http://www.ifad.org/poverty/index.htm

Pardey P G, Beintema N M 2001 Slow magic: agricultural R&D a century after Mendel. Food Policy Report. International Food Policy Research Institute (IFPRI), Washington DC. Accessible at http://www.ifpri.org/pubs/pubs.htm

Pender J, Hazell P (eds) 2000 Promoting sustainable development in less-favoured areas. 2020 Vision Focus No. 4. IFPRI, Washington DC. Accessible at http://www.ifpri.org/pubs/pubs.htm

Pinstrup-Andersen P, Cohen M J 2001 Modern agricultural biotechnology and developing-country food security. In: Nelson G C (ed) Genetically modified organisms in agriculture: economics and politics. Academic Press, London. p 179–189

Pinstrup-Andersen P, Pandya-Lorch R, Rosegrant M W 1999 World Food prospects: critical issues for the early twenty-first century. 2020 Vision Food Policy Report. IFPRI, Washington DC. Accessible at http://www.ifpri.org/pubs/pubs.htm

Quisumbing A R, Meinzen-Dick R S (eds) 2001 Empowering women to achieve food security. 2020 Vision Focus No. 6. IFPRI, Washington DC. Accessible at http://www.ifpri.org/pubs/pubs.htm

Rosegrant M W, Paisner M S, Meijer S, Witcover J 2001 Global food projections to 2020: emerging trends and alternative futures. IFPRI, Washington DC. Accessible at http://www.ifpri.org/pubs/pubs.htm

Schiøler E 1998 Good news from Africa. IFPRI, Washington DC

Further reading

Knox A, Meinzen-Dick R, Hazell P 2002 Property rights, collective action, and technologies for natural resource management: a conceptual framework. In: Meinzen-Dick R, Knox A, Place F, Swallow B (eds) Innovation in natural resource management: the role of property rights and collective action in developing countries. The Johns Hopkins University Press for IFPRI, Baltimore and London, p 12–44

Messer E, Cohen M J, Marchione T 2001 Conflict: a cause and effect of hunger. Environmental Change and Security Project Report No. 7. Washington DC: Woodrow Wilson International Center for Scholars, Smithsonian Institution, p 1–16

Rosegrant M W, Cai X, Cline S A 2002 World water and food to 2025: averting an impending crisis. IFPRI, Washington DC

Wilson S E 2001 Global warming changes the forecast for agriculture. 2020 News and Views (April). IFPRI, Washington DC

World Bank 2001 Poverty trends and voices of the poor. Posted at http://www.worldbank.org/poverty/data/trends/scenario.htm

Yudelman M, Ratta A, Nygaard D 1998 Pest management and food production: looking to the future. 2020 Vision for Food, Agriculture, and the Environment Discussion Paper No. 25. IFPRI, Washington DC

33

Food and nutrition policies and interventions

Lawrence Haddad and Catherine Geissler

Table 33.11 (Continued)

Objective	Direct interventions	Indirect actions
	Children Daily or weekly Fe supplements give improved mental and motor function *Adults* • Fe supplements lead to positive work performance even for iron deficiency/mild anaemia, and tasks with moderate effort • Increased ascorbic acid from local foods not effective • Fe fortification of wheat (Venezuela), salt (+iodine in India), dry milk (Chile) effective • NaFeEDTA (an iron fortificant) shows good potential and increased Fe status when added to salt, soy sauce etc. • Multiple micronutrients may be more effective? • Plant breeding for iron-dense cereals shows some promise, but awaiting efficacy and effectiveness trials • Food-based solutions cannot rely on plant sources – animal sources are critical	
Preventing and treating iodine deficiency	• Salt iodisation is crucial • Prevent cretinism by iodine to the mother during first trimester but no later than second trimester. Supplementation late in pregnancy may improve infant function • Not clear that iodine supplementation in deficient children improves cognition or growth • Iodised oil to 6-week-old infants reduces mortality in first 2 months by 72%	• Improved legislation for fortification
Preventing and treating vitamin A deficiency	*Pregnancy* • Low-dose vitamin A or beta-carotene supplements in pregnancy decrease maternal mortality by 40%; also increases haemoglobin	• Improved legislation for fortification • Agricultural research to be more focused on diet quality and nutrition outcomes

Infants and children

- High-dose maternal supplementation at birth followed by breastfeeding leads to a 64% reduction in mortality under 12 months, 23% reduction in mortality 6–60 age group and major reduction (40%) in HIV mortality
- Can also increase growth of malnourished children
- Urgent need to (a) accelerate food fortification and (b) improve the availability of vitamin A-rich foods
- Continue genetically modified approaches, but with appropriate safety standards

Preventing diet-related chronic disease

Mass media may be able to play a role in nutrition education but not enough experience of what will work in Asia

Dietary guidelines: to explicitly shift the diet towards healthy components, but difficulties when large pockets of undernutrition coexist. China is a good example

Food processing modifications (e.g. changes resulting in differing fat absorption). Shifts in breeding, feeding and market trim practices in the livestock sector can contribute to lower levels of fat in meat over time

School-based efforts: School-based initiatives offer important possibilities for improving diet and activity patterns; however, few initiatives have made a marked improvement in this area and surprisingly few have been carefully evaluated

- Improved status of women for improved intra-household food distribution

- Food price policy to encourage the consumption of healthier foods
- Regulation relative to nutrient content of the diet

Smith L C, Ramakrishnan U, Ndiaye A et al 2003 The importance of women's status for child nutrition in developing countries. IFPRI Research Report 1312

UNICEF (United Nations Children's Fund) 1990 Strategy for improved nutrition of children and women in developing countries. UNICEF, New York

WHO 1998 Obesity – preventing and managing the global epidemic. Report of a WHO consultation on obesity, 3–5 June, 1997. World Health Organization, Geneva

Further reading

Gillespie S, Haddad L 2003 The double burden of malnutrition in Asia and the Pacific. Sage Publications, New Delhi and London

Pinstrup-Andersen P, Pelletier D, Alderman H (eds) Child growth and nutrition in developing countries. Cornell University Press, Ithaca, NY

SCN 2002 Nutrition: A foundation for development. UN Standing Committee on Nutrition (SCN, formerly ACC/SCN). A series of briefs. Posted at http://www.unsystem.org/scn/Publications/foundation4dev/foundation4dev.htm, accessed on 30 July 2003

WHO 1997 Comparative National Nutrition Policies in Europe: an international Expert Conference for the World Health Organization. Nutrition Reviews 55 (11, part 2)

CD-ROM contents

Expanded material

Section CD 33.3(a) Direct interventions to improve nutrition

Section CD 33.3(b) Indirect interventions to improve nutrition (case studies)

Section CD 33.4(a) Nutrition policies in developed countries

Section CD 33.4(b) Interventions for diet-related chronic diseases

Additional references related to CD-ROM material

Further reading

Further reading from the book

Useful websites

Glossary

Note: there is a list of abbrevations on page 695

abrasion – Tooth wear caused by brushing

acceptable daily intake (ADI) – The amount of a food additive that could be taken daily for an entire lifespan without appreciable risk. Determined by measuring the highest dose of the substance that has no effect on experimental animals, then dividing by a safety factor of 100

acetal – Product of addition of alcohol to aldehyde

acetomenaphthone – Synthetic compound with vitamin K activity; vitamin K_3, or menaquinone-0

achlorhydria – Deficiency of hydrochloric acid in gastric digestive juice

acid – Chemically, compounds that dissociate (ionise) in water to give rise to hydrogen ions (H^+); they taste sour

acid foods, basic foods – These terms refer to the residue of the metabolism of foods. The mineral salts of sodium, potassium, magnesium, and calcium are base-forming, while phosphorus, sulphur and chlorine are acid-forming. Which of these predominates in foods determines whether the residue is acidic or basic (alkaline); meat, cheese, eggs and cereals leave an acidic residue, while milk, vegetables, and some fruits leave a basic residue

acidogenicity – Ability to produce acid through bacterial metabolism

acidosis – An increase in the acidity of blood plasma to below the normal range of pH 7.3–7.45, resulting from a loss of the buffering capacity of the plasma, alteration in the excretion of carbon dioxide, excessive loss of base from the body or metabolic overproduction of acids

acrodermatitis enteropathica – Severe functional zinc deficiency due to failure to secrete an as yet unidentified compound in pancreatic juice that is required for zinc absorption

acrodynia – Dermatitis seen in animals deficient in vitamin B_6. There is no evidence for a similar dermatitis in deficient human beings

acrylamide – A chemical that can be generated when the amino acid asparagine is heated above 100°C in the presence of sugars

active transport – Energy-requiring transport of solutes across cell membranes, against the prevailing concentration gradient

acute phase proteins – A variety of serum proteins synthesised in increased (or sometimes decreased) amounts in response to trauma and infection, so confounding their use as indices of nutritional status

acute phase reaction – Increase or decrease in the concentration of certain proteins, or other substances, including micronutrients, in blood serum, following infections or tissue-inflammatory reactions. This reaction represents the body's normal response in counteracting the deleterious effects of a noxious stimulus, but the changes in distributions of proteins and nutrients between body compartments can confound attempts to measure nutrient status by blood assays in those situations where an acute phase reaction is present. Its presence can be monitored, e.g. by measuring C-reactive protein (CRP) or α_1-antichymotrypsin (ACT), both of which are increased by infections or inflammation, in serum or plasma

additive – Any compound not commonly regarded or used as a food which is added to foods as an aid in manufacturing or processing, or to improve the keeping properties, flavour, colour, texture, appearance, or stability of the food, or as a convenience to the consumer. The term excludes vitamins, minerals, and other nutrients added to enrich or restore nutritional value. Herbs, spices, hops, salt, yeast, or protein hydrolysates, air and water are usually excluded from this definition

adenine – A nucleotide, one of the purine bases of the nucleic acids (DNA and RNA). The compound formed between adenine and ribose is the nucleoside adenosine, and can form four phosphorylated derivatives important in metabolism: adenosine monophosphate (AMP, also known as adenylic acid); adenosine diphosphate (ADP); adenosine triphosphate (ATP) and cyclic adenosine monophosphate (cAMP)

adenocarcinoma – Cancer of the glandular epithelium

adenosine diphosphate (ADP) – *See* adenosine triphosphate; *ATP energy metabolism*; energy metabolism

adenosine triphosphate (ATP) – The coenzyme that acts as an intermediate between energy-yielding (catabolic) metabolism (the oxidation of metabolic fuels) and energy expenditure as physical work and in synthetic (anabolic) reactions. *See* energy metabolism

adequate intake – Where there is inadequate scientific evidence to establish requirements and reference intakes for a nutrient for which deficiency is rarely, if ever, seen, the observed levels of intake are assumed to be greater than requirements, and thus provide an estimate of intakes that are (more than) adequate to meet needs

adipocyte – A fat-containing cell in adipose tissue

adiponectin – Hormone secreted by adipose tissue that seems to be involved in energy homeostasis; it enhances insulin sensitivity and glucose tolerance, as well as oxidation of fatty acids in muscle

adipose tissue – Body fat storage tissue, distributed under the skin, around body organs and in body cavities – composed of cells that synthesise and store fat, releasing it for metabolism in fasting. Also known as white adipose tissue, to distinguish it from the metabolically more active brown adipose tissue, which is involved in heat production to maintain body temperature. The energy yield of adipose tissue is 34–38 MJ (8000–9000 kcal) per kg

adiposis – Presence of an abnormally large accumulation of fat in the body – also known as liposis

adipsia – Absence of thirst

adulteration – The addition of substances to foods etc. in order to increase the bulk and reduce the cost, with intent to defraud the purchaser

aerobic – (1) Aerobic microorganisms (aerobes) are those that require oxygen for growth; obligate aerobes cannot survive in the absence of oxygen. The opposite are anaerobic organisms, which do not require oxygen for growth; obligate anaerobes cannot survive in the presence of oxygen. (2) Aerobic exercise is physical activity that requires an increase in heart rate and respiration to meet the increased demand of muscle for oxygen, as contrasted with maximum exertion or sprinting, when muscle can metabolise anaerobically

agalactia – Failure of the mother to secrete enough milk to feed a suckling infant

ageusia – Loss or impairment of the sense of taste

agricultural biotechnology – The application of molecular biology to agriculture, including but not limited to transgenic techniques, in which scientists develop plant and animal varieties that contain genes from other species

AIDS – Acquired immune deficiency syndrome; *see* HIV

alactasia – Partial or complete deficiency of the enzyme lactase in the small intestine, resulting in an inability to digest the sugar lactose in milk, and hence intolerance of milk

alanine – A non-essential amino acid

albumin (albumen) – A group of relatively small water-soluble proteins: ovalbumin in egg-white, lactalbumin in milk; plasma or serum albumin is one of the major blood proteins, which transports certain metabolites including non-esterified fatty acids in the bloodstream. Serum albumin concentration is sometimes measured as an index of protein energy malnutrition. Often used as a non-specific term for proteins (e.g. albuminuria is the excretion of proteins in the urine)

alcohol – Chemically, alcohols are compounds with the general formula $C_nH_{(2n+1)}OH$. The alcohol in alcoholic beverages is ethyl alcohol (ethanol, C_2H_5OH)

alcohol units – For convenience in calculating intakes of alcohol, a unit of alcohol is defined as 8 g (10 ml) of absolute alcohol

aldosterone – A steroid hormone secreted by the adrenal cortex; controls the excretion of salts and water by the kidneys

alkali (or base) – A compound that takes up hydrogen ions and so raises the pH of a solution

alkaline tide – Small increase in blood pH after a meal as a result of the secretion of gastric acid

alkaloids – Naturally occurring organic bases which have pharmacological actions. Many are found in plant foods, including potatoes and tomatoes (the *Solanum* alkaloids), or as the products of fungal action (e.g. ergot), although they also occur in animal foods (e.g. tetrodotoxin in puffer fish, tetramine in shellfish)

alkalosis – *See* acidosis

allele – One of two or more alternative forms of a gene located at the corresponding site on homologous chromosomes

allergen – A chemical compound, commonly a protein, which causes the production of antibodies, and hence an allergic reaction

allergy – Adverse reaction to foods caused by the production of antibodies

allotriophagy – An unnatural desire for abnormal foods; also known as cissa, cittosis, and pica

alpha helix (α-helix) – Common secondary structure in proteins

alpha linkage (α-linkage) – Bond formed by ring closure of a sugar with the hydroxyl group to the right of the chain in the Fischer projection formula (q.v.)

alveolar bone – Spongy part of jaw bone that supports the teeth

amenorrhoea – Cessation of menstruation, normally occurring between the ages of 40 and 55 (the menopause), but sometimes at an early age, especially as a result of severe under-nutrition (as in anorexia nervosa) when body weight falls below about 45 kg

Ames test – An in vitro test for the ability of chemicals, including potential food additives, to cause mutation in bacteria (the mutagenic potential). Commonly used as a preliminary screening method to detect substances likely to be carcinogenic

amines – Formed by the decarboxylation of amino acids. Three are potentially important in foods: phenylethylamine (formed from phenylalanine), tyramine (from tyrosine), and tryptamine (from tryptophan) because they stimulate the sympathetic nervous system and can cause increased blood pressure. In sensitive people they are one of the possible dietary causes of migraine

amino acid profile – The amino acid composition of a protein

amino acids – The basic units from which proteins are made. Chemically compounds with an amino group ($-NH_3^+$) and a carboxyl group ($-COO^-$) attached to the same carbon atom

aminoaciduria – Excretion of abnormal amounts of one or more amino acids in the urine, usually as a result of a genetic disease

aminogram – A diagrammatic representation of the amino acid composition of a protein. A plasma aminogram is the composition of the free amino acid pool in blood plasma

aminopeptidase – An enzyme secreted in the pancreatic juice which removes amino acids sequentially from the free amino terminal of a peptide or protein (i.e. the end that has a free amino group exposed. Since it works at the end of the peptide chain, it is an exopeptidase

aminotransferase – Any enzyme that catalyses the reaction of transamination

amylases – Enzymes that hydrolyse starch. α-Amylase (dextrinogenic amylase or diastase) acts to produce small dextrin fragments from starch, while β-amylase (maltogenic amylase) liberates maltose, some free glucose, and isomaltose from the branch points in amylopectin. Salivary and pancreatic amylases are α-amylases

amylodyspepsia – An inability to digest starch

amylopectin – The branched chain form of starch, with branches formed by α1–6 bonds. About 75–80% of most starches; the remainder is amylose

amylose – The straight chain form of starch, with only α1–4 bonds. About 20–25% of most starches; the remainder is amylopectin

anabolic hormones – Natural or synthetic hormones that stimulate growth and the development of muscle tissue

anabolism – The process of building up or synthesising

anaemia – A shortage of red blood cells, leading to pallor and shortness of breath, especially on exertion. Most commonly due to a dietary deficiency of iron, or excessive blood loss. Other dietary deficiencies can also result in anaemia, including deficiency of vitamin B_{12} or folic acid (megaloblastic anaemia), vitamin E (haemolytic anaemia), and rarely vitamin C or vitamin B_6

anaemia, haemolytic – Anaemia caused by premature and excessive destruction of red blood cells; not normally due to nutritional deficiency, but can occur as a result of vitamin E deficiency in premature infants

anaemia, megaloblastic – Release into the circulation of immature precursors of red blood cells, due to deficiency of either folic acid or vitamin B_{12}

anaemia, pernicious – Anaemia due to deficiency of vitamin B_{12}, most commonly as a result of failure to absorb the vitamin from the diet. There is release into the circulation of immature precursors of red blood cells (megaloblastic anaemia) and progressive damage to the spinal cord (subacute combined degeneration), which is not reversed on restoring the vitamin

anaerobes – Microorganisms that grow in the absence of oxygen. Obligate anaerobes cannot survive in the presence of oxygen, facultative anaerobes grow in the presence or absence of oxygen

anaerobic threshold – The level of exercise at which the rate of oxygen uptake into muscle becomes limiting and there is anaerobic metabolism to yield lactate

aneuploidy – An abnormal number of chromosomes, usually associated with miscarriage, or developmental abnormalities such as Down's syndrome where there are three copies of chromosome 21 instead of two

aneurysm – Local dilatation (swelling and weakening) of the wall of a blood vessel, usually the result of atherosclerosis and hypertension; especially serious when occurring in the aorta, when rupture may prove fatal

angina (angina pectoris) – Paroxysmal thoracic pain and choking sensation, especially during exercise or stress, due to partial blockage of a coronary artery (blood vessel supplying the heart), as a result of atherosclerosis

angio-oedema – Presence of fluid in subcutaneous tissues or submucosa, particularly of the face, eyes, lips and sometimes tongue and throat; may occur during an anaphylactic reaction

angiotensin-converting enzyme (ACE) – Enzyme, in the blood vessels of the lungs, which activates angiotensin. Many of the drugs for treatment of hypertension are ACE inhibitors

angular stomatitis – A characteristic cracking and fissuring of the skin at the angles of the mouth, a symptom of vitamin B_2 deficiency, but also seen in other conditions

anion – A negatively charged ion

anomers – Isomers of a sugar differing only in configuration at the hemiacetal carbon atom

anorectic drugs (anorexigenic drugs) – Drugs that depress the appetite, used as an aid to weight reduction. Apart from sibutramine (Reductil), most have been withdrawn from use; diethylpropion and mazindol are available but not recommended

anorexia – Lack of appetite

anorexia nervosa – A psychological disturbance resulting in a refusal to eat, possibly with restriction to a very limited range of foods, and often accompanied by a rigid programme of vigorous physical exercise, to the point of exhaustion. The result is a very considerable loss of weight, with tissue atrophy and a fall in basal metabolic rate. It is especially prevalent among adolescent girls; when body weight falls below about 45 kg there is a cessation of menstruation

anosmia – Lack or impairment of the sense of smell

anovulation – Failure to ovulate spontaneously

antacids – Bases that neutralise acids, used generally to counteract excessive gastric acidity and to treat indigestion: sodium bicarbonate, aluminium hydroxide, magnesium carbonate, and magnesium hydroxide

anthocyanins – Violet, red, and blue water-soluble colours extracted from flowers, fruits and leaves

anthropometry – Body measurements used as an index of physiological development and nutritional status; a non-invasive way of assessing body composition. Weight for age provides information about the overall nutritional status of children; weight for height is used to detect acute malnutrition (wasting); height for age to detect chronic malnutrition (stunting). Mid-upper arm circumference provides an index of muscle wastage in undernutrition. Skinfold thickness is related to the amount of subcutaneous fat as an index of over- or undernutrition

antibody – Immunoglobulin which specifically counteracts an antigen or allergen (*see* allergen)

antidiarrhoeal – Drug used to treat diarrhoea by absorbing water from the intestine, altering intestinal motility, or adsorbing toxins

antidiuretic – Drug used to reduce the excretion of urine and so conserve fluid in the body

antiemetic – Drug used to prevent or alleviate nausea and vomiting

antienzymes – Substances that inhibit the action of enzymes. Many inhibit digestive enzymes and are present in raw legumes. Most are proteins, and therefore inactivated by heat

antigen – Any compound that is foreign to the body (e.g. bacterial, food, or pollen proteins or complex carbohydrates) which, when introduced into the circulation, stimulates the formation of an antibody

antihistamine – Drug that antagonises the actions of histamine; those that block histamine H_1 receptors are used to treat allergic reactions; those that block H_2 receptors are used to treat peptic ulcers

antihypertensive – Drug, diet, or other treatment used to treat hypertension (high blood pressure)

antilipidaemic – Drug, diet, or other treatment used to treat hyperlipidaemia by lowering blood lipids

antimetabolite – Compound that inhibits a normal metabolic process, acting as an analogue of a normal metabolite. Some are useful in chemotherapy of cancer, others are naturally occurring toxins in foods, frequently causing vitamin deficiency diseases by inhibiting the normal metabolism of the vitamin

antimotility agents – Drugs used to reduce gastrointestinal motility, and hence reduce the discomfort associated with diarrhoea

antimutagen – Compound acting on cells and tissues to decrease initiation of mutation by a mutagen

antioxidant – A substance that retards the oxidative rancidity of fats in stored foods. Many fats, and especially vegetable oils, contain naturally occurring antioxidants, including vitamin E, which protect them against rancidity for some time

antioxidant nutrients – Highly reactive oxygen radicals are formed during normal metabolism and in response to infection and some chemicals. They cause damage to fatty acids in cell membranes, and the products of this damage can then cause damage to proteins and DNA. A number of different mechanisms are involved in protection against, or repair after, oxygen radical damage, including a number of nutrients, especially vitamin E, carotene, vitamin C, and selenium. Collectively these are known as antioxidant nutrients

antirachitic – Preventing or curing rickets

antisialagogues – Substances that reduce the flow of saliva

antivitamins – Substances that interfere with the normal metabolism or function of vitamins, or destroy them

apastia – Refusal to take food, as an expression of a psychiatric disturbance

aphagosis – Inability to eat

apo-carotenal – Aldehydes formed by oxidation of carotenes, other than retinaldehyde

apoenzyme – The protein part of an enzyme which requires a coenzyme for activity, and is therefore inactive if the coenzyme is absent

apolipoprotein – The protein of plasma lipoproteins without the associated lipid

aposia – Absence of sensation of thirst

apositia – Aversion to food

arachidonic acid – A long chain polyunsaturated fatty acid (C20:4 ω6)

arginine – A basic amino acid. Not a dietary essential for adults, but infants may not be able to synthesise enough to meet the high demands of growth

ariboflavinosis – Deficiency of riboflavin (vitamin B_2)

arm, chest, hip index (ACH index) – A method of assessing nutritional status by measuring the arm circumference, chest diameter, and hip width

aromatic ring – Stable ring structure with π electrons delocalised around the ring as in benzene

arterial restenosis – Rate of re-occlusion (narrowing) of arteries after artificial (i.e. mechanical) removal of the accumulated plaque coatings. Used as a measure of susceptibility to atherosclerotic disease; it can be followed non-invasively, e.g. by ultrasound measurements

arteriosclerosis – Thickening and calcification of the arterial walls, leading to loss of elasticity, occurring with ageing and especially in hypertension

arthritis – Painful, swollen and/or inflamed joints

ascites – Abnormal accumulation of fluid in the peritoneal cavity, occurring as a complication of cirrhosis of the liver, congestive heart failure, cancer, and infectious diseases

ascorbic acid – Vitamin C, chemically L-xyloascorbic acid, to distinguish it from the isomer D-araboascorbic acid (isoascorbic acid or erythorbic acid), which has only slight vitamin C activity

ash – The residue left behind after all organic matter has been burnt off, a measure of the total content of mineral salts in a food

asparagine – A non-essential amino acid; the β-amide of aspartic acid

aspartic acid (aspartate) – A non-essential amino acid

asthma – Chronic inflammatory disease of the airways which renders them prone to narrow too much. The symptoms include paroxysmal coughing, wheezing, tightness and breathlessness. Asthma may be caused by an allergic response or may be induced by non-immunological mechanisms

astringency – The action of unripe fruits and other foods to cause contraction of the epithelial tissues of the tongue, believed to result from a destruction of the lubricant properties of saliva by precipitation by tannins

atheroma – The fatty deposit composed of lipids, complex carbohydrates and fibrous tissue which forms on the inner wall of blood vessels in atherosclerosis

atherosclerosis – Degenerative disease in which there is accumulation of lipids, together with complex carbohydrates and fibrous tissue (atheroma) on the inner wall of arteries. This leads to narrowing of the lumen of the arteries

atrophy – Wasting of normally developed tissue or muscle as a result of disuse, ageing or undernutrition

attrition – Tooth wear caused by grinding

auxotrophe – Mutant strain of microorganism that requires one or more nutrients for growth that are not required by the parent organism. Commonly used for microbiological assay of vitamins, amino acids, etc.

availability – (bioavailability or biological availability). In some foodstuffs, nutrients that can be demonstrated to be present chemically may not be fully available when they are eaten, because the nutrients are chemically bound in a form that is not susceptible to enzymic digestion

avitaminosis – The absence of a vitamin; may be used specifically, as, for example, avitaminosis A, or generally, to mean a vitamin deficiency disease

axial position – Substituent in a 6-membered non-aromatic ring is above or below the average plane of the ring

bacteria – Unicellular microorganisms, ranging from 0.5 to 5 μm in size. They may be classified on the basis of their shape: spherical (coccus), rodlike (bacilli), spiral (spirillum), comma-shaped (vibrio), corkscrew-shaped (spirochaetes), or filamentous. Other classifications are based on whether or not they are: stained by Gram's stain; aerobic or anaerobic; and autotrophic or heterotrophic

bacteriophages – Viruses that attack bacteria, commonly known as phages

basal metabolic rate (BMR) – The energy cost of maintaining the metabolic integrity of the body, nerve and muscle tone, respiration and circulation. For children it also includes the energy cost of growth. Experimentally, BMR is measured as the heat output from the body, or the rate of oxygen consumption, under strictly standardised conditions, 12–14 hours after the last meal, completely at rest (but not asleep) and at an environmental temperature of 26–30°C, to ensure thermal neutrality

bdelygmia – An extreme loathing for food

behenic acid – Very long-chain saturated fatty acid (C22:0)

beriberi – The result of severe and prolonged deficiency of vitamin B_1, especially where the diet is high in carbohydrate and poor in vitamin B_1

beta linkage (β-linkage) – Bond formed by ring closure of a sugar with the hydroxyl group to the left of the chain in the Fischer projection formula (q.v.)

beta pleat (β pleat) – Common secondary structure in proteins

beta sheet flattened form – Common secondary structure in proteins

bifidogenic – Promoting the growth of (beneficial) bifidobacteria in the intestinal tract

bifidus factor – A carbohydrate in human milk which stimulates the growth of *Lactobacillus bifidus* in the intestine. In turn, this organism lowers the pH of the intestinal contents and suppresses the growth of pathogenic bacteria

bile – Alkaline fluid produced by the liver and stored in the gall bladder before secretion into the small intestine (duodenum) via the bile duct. It contains the bile salts, bile pigments (bilirubin and biliverdin), phospholipids, and cholesterol

bile salts (bile acids) – Salts of cholic and deoxycholic acid and their glycine and taurine conjugates, secreted in the bile; they enhance the digestion of fats by emulsifying them

bilirubin, biliverdin – The bile pigments, formed by the degradation of haemoglobin

binge–purge syndrome – A feature of the eating disorder bulimia nervosa, characterised by the ingestion of excessive amounts of food and the excessive use of laxatives

bioassay – Biological assay; measurement of biologically active compounds (e.g. vitamins and essential amino acids) by their ability to support growth of microorganisms or animals

bioavailability – Fraction of an ingested nutrient that is absorbed and used for a defined function in the body (*see* availability)

biocytin – The main form of the vitamin biotin in most foods, bound to the amino acid lysine

bio-electrical impedance (BIE) – A method of measuring the proportion of fat in the body by the difference in the resistance to passage of an electric current between fat and lean tissue

bioflavonoids – *See* flavonoids

biofortification – Food fortification achieved by plant breeding or genetic modification to give a higher content of nutrients

bioinformatics – The application of computational techniques to extract meaning from complex biological data

biological value (BV) – The proportion of absorbed nitrogen that is retained for maintenance and/or growth

biotin – A vitamin, sometimes known as vitamin H, required for the synthesis of fatty acids and glucose, among other reactions, and in the control of gene expression and cell division

birth canal – The bony birth canal comprises the passage through the pelvic bones; there is a soft tissue component to the birth canal in the form of the vagina and its supporting tissues

bisfuran polycyclic compounds – Compounds with several rings including more than two 5-membered oxygen-containing rings

Bitot's spots – Irregularly shaped foam-like plaques on the conjunctiva of the eye, characteristically in vitamin A deficiency, but not considered to be a diagnostic sign without other evidence of deficiency

biuret test – A chemical test for proteins based on the formation of a violet colour when copper sulphate in alkaline solution reacts with a peptide bond

black tongue disease – A sign of niacin deficiency in dogs, the canine equivalent of pellagra

bland diet – A diet that is non-irritating, does not over-stimulate the digestive tract and is soothing to the intestines; generally avoiding alcohol, strong tea or coffee, pickles, and spices

blood plasma – The liquid component of blood, accounting for about half its total volume; a solution of nutrients and various proteins. When blood has clotted, the resultant fluid is known as serum

blood sugar – Glucose; normal concentration is about 5 mmol (90 mg)/l, and is maintained in the fasting state by mobilisation of tissue reserves of glycogen and synthesis from amino acids. Only in prolonged starvation does it fall below about 3.5 mmol (60 mg)/l. If it falls to 2 mmol (35 mg)/l there is loss of consciousness (hypoglycaemic coma)

B-lymphocytes – Bursa-equivalent lymphocytes. After maturation into plasma cells they produce antibodies (immunoglobulins) during humoral responses in immunological reactions. They were first discovered in the bursa of Fabricius in the chicken; hence the name

body density – Body fat has a density of 0.90, while the density of fat free body mass is 1.10. Determination of density by weighing in air and in water, or by measuring body volume and weight, permits calculation of the proportions of fat and lean body tissue

body mass index (BMI) – An index of fatness and obesity. The weight (in kg) divided by the square of height (in m). The acceptable (desirable) range is 20–25. Above 25 is overweight, and above 30 is obesity. Also called Quetelet's index

borborygmos – (plural borborygmi); audible abdominal sound produced by excessive intestinal motility

borderline substances – Foods that may have characteristics of medication in certain circumstances, and which may then be prescribed under the National Health Service in UK

botulism – A rare form of food poisoning caused by the extremely potent neurotoxins produced by *Clostridium botulinum*

bovine somatotrophin (BST) – The natural growth hormone of cattle; biosynthetic BST is used in some dairy herds to increase milk production (approved for use in the USA in 1993, prohibited in the EU)

bovine spongiform encephalopathy (BSE) – A degenerative brain disease in cattle, transmitted by feeding slaughter-house waste from infected animals. Commonly known as 'mad cow disease'. The infective agent is a prion; it can be transmitted to human beings, causing early-onset variant Creutzfeldt–Jakob disease

bradycardia – An unusually slow heartbeat, less than 60 beats/min

bradyphagia – Eating very slowly

bromatology – The science of foods

bronze diabetes – *see* haemochromatosis

brown adipose tissue (brown fat) – Metabolically highly active adipose tissue, which is involved in heat production to maintain body temperature, as opposed to white adipose tissue, which is storage fat and has a low rate of metabolic activity

Brunner's glands – Mucus-secreting glands in the duodenum

buffers – Salts of weak acids and bases that resist a change in the pH when acid or alkali is added

bulimia nervosa – An eating disorder, characterised by powerful and intractable urges to overeat, followed by self-induced vomiting and the excessive use of purgatives

butyric acid – A short-chain saturated fatty acid (C4:0)

cachexia – The condition of extreme emaciation and wasting seen in patients with advanced cancer and AIDS. Due partly to an inadequate intake of food and mainly the effects of the disease in increasing metabolic rate (hypermetabolism) and the breakdown of tissue protein

cadaverine – Low molecular weight polyamine with **biological activity**, the decarboxylation product of lysine

caecum – The first part of the large intestine, separated from the small intestine by the ileo-colic sphincter

calcidiol – The 25-hydroxy-derivative of vitamin D, also known as 25-hydroxycholecalciferol, the main storage and circulating form of the vitamin in the body

calciferol – Used at one time as a name for ercalciol (ergocalciferol or vitamin D_2), made by the ultraviolet irradiation of ergosterol. Also used as a general term to include both vitamers of vitamin D (vitamins D_2 and D_3)

calcinosis – Abnormal deposition of calcium salts in tissues. May be due to excessive intake of vitamin D

calciol – The official name for cholecalciferol, the naturally occurring form of vitamin D (vitamin D_3)

calcitriol – The 1,25-dihydroxy-derivative of vitamin D, also known as 1,25-dihydroxycholecalciferol; the active metabolite of the vitamin

calorie – A unit of energy used to express the energy yield of foods and energy expenditure by the body; the amount of heat required to raise the temperature of 1 g of water through 1°C (from 14.5 to 15.5°C). Nutritionally the kilocalorie (1000 calories) is used (the amount of heat required to raise the temperature of 1 kg of water through 1°C), and is abbreviated as either kcal or Cal to avoid confusion with the cal. The calorie is not an SI unit, and correctly the Joule is used as the unit of energy, although kcal are widely used. 1 kcal = 4.18 kJ; 1 kJ = 0.24 kcal

calorimeter (bomb calorimeter) – An instrument for measuring the amount of oxidisable energy in a substance, by burning it in oxygen and measuring the heat produced

calorimetry – The measurement of energy expenditure by the body. Direct calorimetry is the measurement of heat output from the body, as an index of energy expenditure, and hence requirements

canbra oil (canola oil) – Oil extracted from selected strains of rapeseed containing not more than 2% erucic acid

cancer – A wide variety of diseases characterised by uncontrolled growth of tissue

canola – A variety of rape which is low in glucosinolates. Canola oil (canbra oil) contains less than 2% erucic acid

canthaxanthin – A red carotenoid pigment which is not a precursor of vitamin A

capric acid – A medium-chain fatty acid (C10:0)

caproic acid – A short-chain fatty acid (C6:0)

caprylic acid – A medium-chain fatty acid (C8:0)

carbohydrate – The major food source of metabolic energy, the sugars and starches. Chemically they are composed of carbon, hydrogen, and oxygen in the ratio $C_n:H_{2n}:O_n$

carbohydrate by difference – Historically it was difficult to determine the various carbohydrates present in foods, and an approximation was often made by subtracting the measured protein, fat, ash, and water from the total weight

γ-carboxyglutamate – A derivative of the amino acid glutamate found in prothrombin and other enzymes involved in blood clotting, and the proteins osteocalcin and matrix GLA protein (MGP) in bone, where it has a function in ensuring the correct crystallisation of bone mineral. Its synthesis requires vitamin K

carboxypeptidase – An enzyme secreted in the pancreatic juice which hydrolyses amino acids from the carboxyl terminal of proteins

carcinogen – A substance that can induce cancer

cardiomyopathy – Any chronic disorder affecting the muscle of the heart. May be associated with alcoholism and vitamin B_1 deficiency

caries – Dental decay caused by attack on the tooth enamel by acids produced by bacteria that are normally present in the mouth

cariogenic – Causing tooth decay (caries) by stimulating the growth of acid-forming bacteria on the teeth; sucrose and other fermentable carbohydrates

cariogenicity – Ability to cause caries

cariostatic – Preventing tooth decay

carnitine – A derivative of the amino acid lysine, required for the transport of fatty acids into mitochondria for oxidation

exception of tobacco products, cosmetics, and pharmaceuticals

Food and Drug Administration (FDA) – US government regulatory agency; website http://www. fda.gov; website for FDA consumer magazine http://www.fda.gov/fdac

Food and Nutrition Information Center (FNIC) – Located at the National Agricultural Library, part of the US Department of Agriculture; website http://www.nal.usda.gov/fnic

food chain – The chain between green plants (the primary producers of food energy) through a sequence of organisms in which each eats the one below it in the chain, and is eaten in turn by the one above. Also used for the chain of events from the original source of a foodstuff (from the sea, the soil, or the wild) through all the stages of handling until it reaches the table

food exchange – *See* exchange list

food insecurity – The absence of food security

food poisoning – May be due to (1) contamination with harmful bacteria or other microorganisms; (2) toxic chemicals; (3) adverse reactions to certain proteins or other natural constituents of foods; (4) chemical contamination. The commonest bacterial contamination is due to species of *Salmonella*, *Staphylococcus*, *Campylobacter*, *Listeria*, *Bacillus cereus* and *Clostridium welchii*. Very rarely, food poisoning is due to *Clostridium botulinum*, botulism

food pyramid – A way of showing a healthy diet graphically, by grouping foods and the amounts of each group that should be eaten each day, based on nutritional recommendations

food science – The study of the basic chemical, physical, biochemical, and biophysical properties of foods and their constituents, and of changes that these may undergo during handling, preservation, processing, storage, distribution, and preparation for consumption

food security – When all people, at all times, have physical and economic access to sufficient, safe, and nutritious food to meet their dietary needs and food preferences for an active and healthy life. Food security requires more than just adequate food availability; it also is a matter of access to the food that is available and appropriate utilisation

Food Standards Agency (FSA) – Permanent advisory body to UK Parliament through Health Ministers, established in 2000 to protect the public's health and consumer interests in relation to food; website http://www.food.gov.uk

food technology – The application of science and technology to the treatment, processing, preservation and distribution of foods. Hence the term food technologist

Foods for Specified Health Use (FOSHU, Japanese) – Processed foods containing ingredients that aid specific bodily functions, as well as being nutritious (functional foods)

formiminoglutamic acid (FIGLU) test – A test for folic acid nutritional status, based on excretion of formiminoglutamic acid (FIGLU), a metabolite of the amino acid histidine, which is normally metabolised by a folic acid-dependent enzyme

formula diet – Composed of simple substances that require little digestion, are readily absorbed, and leave a minimum residue in the intestine: glucose, amino acids or peptides, mono- and diacylglycerols rather than starch, proteins, and fats

fortification – The deliberate addition of specific nutrients to foods as a means of providing the population with an increased level of intake

fractional test meal – A method of examining the secretion of gastric juices; the stomach contents are sampled at intervals via a stomach tube after a test meal of gruel

free radicals – Highly reactive molecules with an unpaired electron

free sugars – Mono- and disaccharides added to food, plus sugars in fruit juices, honey and syrup

freeze drying – Also known as lyophilisation. A method of drying in which the material is frozen and subjected to high vacuum. The ice sublimes off as water vapour without melting. Freeze-dried food is very porous, since it occupies the same volume as the original and so rehydrates rapidly. There is less loss of flavour and texture than with most other methods of drying. Controlled heat may be applied to the process without melting the frozen material; this is accelerated freeze drying

fructo-oligosaccharides – Oligosaccharides consisting of fructose

fructosan – A general name for polysaccharides of fructose, such as inulin. Not digested, and hence a part of dietary fibre or non-starch polysaccharides

fructose – Also known as fruit sugar or laevulose. A six-carbon monosaccharide sugar (hexose) differing from glucose in containing a ketone group (on carbon-2) instead of an aldehyde group (on carbon-1)

fruit – The fleshy seed-bearing part of plants (including tomato and cucumber, which are usually called vegetables)

fruitarian – A person who eats only fruits, nuts, and seeds; an extreme form of vegetarianism

functional foods – Foods eaten for specified health purposes because of their (rich) content of one or more nutrients or non-nutrient substances which may confer health benefits

galactans – Polysaccharides composed of galactose derivatives

galactose – A six-carbon monosaccharide, differing from glucose only in position of the hydroxyl group on carbon-4

gall-bladder – The organ situated in the liver which stores the bile formed in the liver before its secretion into the small intestine

gallstones (cholelithiasis) – Concretions composed of cholesterol, bile pigments, and calcium salts, formed in the bile duct of the gall-bladder when the bile becomes supersaturated

gastric inhibitory peptide (GIP) – A hormone secreted by the mucosa of the duodenum and jejunum in response to absorbed fat and carbohydrate which stimulates the pancreas to secrete insulin. Also known as glucose-dependent insulinotropic polypeptide

gastrin – Polypeptide hormone secreted by the stomach in response to food, which stimulates gastric and pancreatic secretion

gastritis – Inflammation of the mucosal lining of the stomach; may result from infection or excessive alcohol consumption. Atrophic gastritis is the progressive loss of gastric secretion with increasing age

gastroenteritis – Inflammation of the mucosal lining of the stomach and/or small or large intestine, normally resulting from infection

gastroenterology – The study and treatment of diseases of the gastrointestinal tract

gastroplasty – Surgical alteration of the shape and capacity of the stomach, without removing any part. Has been used as a treatment for severe obesity

gastrostomy feeding – Feeding a liquid diet directly into the stomach through a tube that has been surgically introduced through the abdominal wall. *See also* enteral nutrition; nasogastric tube

gavage – The process of feeding liquids by tube directly into the stomach

gene – Physical and functional unit of heredity. It is the entire DNA sequence necessary for the synthesis of a functional polypeptide or RNA molecule; *see* DNA, RNA

gene expression – Overall process by which information encoded by a gene is converted to an observable phenotype, usually in the form of a protein; *see* phenotype

gene transcription – Conversion of genomic DNA into mRNA; *see* DNA, mRNA

gene translation – The synthesis of protein molecules using the triplet code of mRNA; *see* mRNA

generally regarded as safe (GRAS) – Designation given to food additives when further evidence was required before the substance could be classified more precisely (US usage)

generic descriptor – The name used to cover the different chemical forms of a vitamin that have the same biological activity

genetic polymorphisms – Changes (i.e. variability) in one or more base pairs in the DNA gene sequence encoding a specific protein, which result in the substitution of different amino acids in that protein, which may subtly alter its function. Such polymorphisms, in human populations, are of increasing research interest because in some cases they may alter requirements for certain nutrients

genome – The complete genetic information of an organism; *see* proteome, metabolome

radiation, they are safe for use in labelled compounds given to human beings

isozymes – *See* isoenzymes

jejuno-ileostomy – Surgical procedure in which the terminal jejunum or proximal ileum is removed or bypassed. Was formerly used as a treatment for severe obesity

jejunum – Part of the small intestine, between the duodenum and the ileum

Joule – The SI (Système Internationale) unit of energy; used to express energy content of foods

keratomalacia – Progressive softening and ulceration of the cornea, due to vitamin A deficiency. Blindness is usually inevitable unless the deficiency is corrected at an early stage

Keshan disease – A disease occurring in parts of China where selenium deficiency is believed to be a problem. The cardiomyopathy of the disease is believed to be of viral origin

ketoacidosis – High concentrations of ketone bodies in the blood

ketogenic diet – A diet poor in carbohydrate (20–30 g) and rich in fat; causes accumulation of ketone bodies in tissue

ketone bodies – Acetoacetate, β-hydroxybutyrate and acetone; acetoacetate and acetone are chemically ketones; although β-hydroxybutyrate is not, it is included in the term ketone bodies because of its metabolic relationship with acetoacetate

ketones – Chemical compounds containing a carbonyl group (C=O), with two alkyl groups attached to the same carbon; the simplest ketone is acetone (dimethylketone, $(CH_3)_2-C=O$)

ketonuria – Excretion of ketone bodies in the urine

ketosis – High concentrations of ketone bodies in the blood

Keys score – Method of expressing the lipid content of a diet, calculated as $1.35 \times (2 \times \%$ energy from saturated fat $- \%$ energy from polyunsaturated fat$) + 1.5 \times \sqrt{}$ (mg cholesterol /1000 kcal)

kGy – Kilogray, a unit of radiation intensity

kilo – As a prefix for units of measurement, one thousand times (i.e. 10^3); symbol k

Kjeldahl determination – Widely used method of determining total nitrogen in a substance by digesting with sulphuric acid and a catalyst; the nitrogen is reduced to ammonia which is then measured. In foodstuffs most of the nitrogen is protein, and the term crude protein is the total 'Kjeldahl nitrogen' multiplied by a factor of 6.25 (since most proteins contain 16% nitrogen)

koilonychia – Development of (brittle) concave finger nails, commonly associated with iron deficiency anaemia

Korsakoff's psychosis – Failure of recent memory, although events from the past are recalled, with confabulation; associated with vitamin B_1 deficiency, especially in alcoholics

kosher – The selection and preparation of foods in accordance with traditional Jewish ritual and dietary laws. Foods that are not kosher are traife. The only kosher flesh foods are from animals that chew the cud and have cloven hoofs, such as cattle, sheep, goats, and deer; the hindquarters must not be eaten. The only fish permitted are those with fins and scales; birds of prey and scavengers are not kosher. Moreover, the animals must be slaughtered according to ritual, without stunning, before the meat can be considered kosher

Krebs cycle – Or citric acid cycle, a central pathway for the metabolism of fats, carbohydrates, and amino acids

kwashiorkor (from the Ga language of West Africa) – A disease which occurs frequently in young (weanling) children in some developing countries where weaning foods are of poor quality, and is characterised by oedema (swelling due to extracellular fluid accumulation), failure to thrive, abnormal hair appearance (dyspigmentation), often enlarged liver and increased mortality risk. Associated especially with poor diets that are low in protein and other nutrients, and also with frequent infections; *see* protein energy malnutrition

lactase – The enzyme that breaks down lactose (milk sugar) to galactose-glucose in the small intestine

lactation – The process of synthesising and secreting milk from the breasts

lactic acid – The acid produced by the anaerobic fermentation of carbohydrates. Originally discovered in sour milk, it is responsible for the flavour of fermented milk and for the precipitation of the casein curd in cottage cheese

lacto-ovo-vegetarian – One whose diet excludes meat and fish but permits milk and eggs

lactose – The carbohydrate of milk, sometimes called milk sugar, a disaccharide of glucose and galactose

lactulose – A disaccharide of galactose and fructose which does not occur naturally but is formed in heated or stored milk by isomerisation of lactose. Not hydrolysed by human digestive enzymes but fermented by intestinal bacteria to form lactic and pyruvic acids. Thought to promote the growth of *Lactobacillus bifidus* and so added to some infant formulae; in large amounts it is a laxative

laxative – Or aperient, a substance that helps the expulsion of food residues from the body. If strongly laxative it is termed purgative or cathartic. Dietary fibre and cellulose function because they retain water and add bulk to the contents of the intestine; Epsom salts (magnesium sulphate) also retain water; castor oil and drugs such as aloes, senna, cascara, and phenolphthalein irritate the intestinal mucosa. Undigested carbohydrates such as lactulose and sugar alcohols are also laxatives

lecithin – Chemically lecithin is phosphatidyl choline; a phospholipid containing choline. Commercial lecithin is a mixture of phospholipids in which phosphatidyl choline predominates; *see* choline, phospholipids

lectins – Proteins from legumes and other sources which bind to the carbohydrates found at cell surfaces. They therefore cause red blood cells to agglutinate in vitro, hence the old names haemagglutinins and phytoagglutinins

legumes – Members of the family Leguminosae, consumed as dry mature seeds (grain legumes or pulses) or as immature green seeds in the pod. Legumes include the groundnut, *Arachis hypogaea*, and soya bean, *Glycine max*, grown for their oil and protein, the yam bean *Pachyrrhizus erosus*, and African yam bean *Sphenostylis*

stenocarpa, grown for their edible tubers as well as seeds

leptin – Hormone secreted by adipose tissue that acts to regulate long-term appetite and energy expenditure by signalling the state of body fat reserves

less-favoured areas – Lands that have low agricultural potential because of limited and uncertain rainfall, poor soils, steep slopes, or other biophysical constraints, as well as lands that may have high agricultural potential but have limited access to infrastructure and markets, low population density, or other socioeconomic constraints

lethal dose 50% (LD$_{50}$) – An index of toxicity, the amount of the substance that kills 50% of the test population of experimental animals when administered as a single dose

leucine – An essential amino acid; rarely limiting in foods; one of the branched-chain amino acids

leucocytes – White blood cells, normally 5000–9000/mm^3; includes polymorphonuclear neutrophils, lymphocytes, monocytes, polymorphonuclear eosinophils, and polymorphonuclear basophils. A 'white cell count' determines the total; a 'differential cell count' estimates the numbers of each type. Fever, haemorrhage, and violent exercise cause an increase (leucocytosis); starvation and debilitating conditions a decrease (leucopenia)

leucocytosis – Increase in the number of leucocytes in the blood

leucopenia – Decrease in the number of leucocytes in the blood

leucovorin – The synthetic (racemic) 5-formyl derivative of folic acid; more stable to oxidation than folic acid itself, and commonly used in pharmaceutical preparations. Also known as folinic acid

levans – Polymers of fructose (the principal one is inulin) that occur in tubers and some grasses

Lieberkühn, crypts of – Glands lining the small intestine which secrete the intestinal juice

lignans – Naturally occurring compounds in various foods that have both oestrogenic and anti-oestrogenic activity (phytoestrogens)

lignin (lignocellulose) – Indigestible part of the cell wall of plants (a polymer of aromatic alcohols). It is included in measurement of dietary fibre, but not of non-starch polysaccharide

limosis – Abnormal hunger or excessive desire for food

linoleic acid – An essential polyunsaturated fatty acid (C18:2 ω6)

α-linolenic acid – An essential polyunsaturated fatty acid (C18:3 ω3)

γ-linolenic acid – A non-essential polyunsaturated fatty acid (C18:3 ω6)

lipase – Enzyme that hydrolyses fats to glycerol and fatty acids

lipectomy – Surgical removal of subcutaneous fat

lipedema (lipoedema) – Condition in which fat deposits accumulate in the lower extremities, from hips to ankles, with tenderness of the affected parts

lipids – A general term for fats and oils (chemically triacylglycerols), waxes, phospholipids, steroids, and terpenes. Their common property is insolubility in water and solubility in hydrocarbons, chloroform, and alcohols

lipids, plasma – Triacylglycerols, free and esterified cholesterol and phospholipids, present in lipoproteins in blood plasma. Chylomicrons consist mainly of triacylglycerols and protein; they are the form in which lipids absorbed in the small intestine enter the bloodstream. Very low-density lipoproteins (VLDL) are assembled in the liver and exported to other tissues, where they provide a source of lipids. Lipid-depleted VLDL becomes low-density lipoprotein (LDL) in the circulation; it is rich in cholesterol and is normally cleared by the liver. High-density lipoprotein (HDL) contains cholesterol from LDL and tissues that is returned to the liver. *See also* hypercholesterolaemia; hyperlipidaemia

lipodystrophy – Abnormal pattern of subcutaneous fat deposits

lipofuscin – A group of pigments that accumulate in several body tissues, particularly the myocardium, and are associated with the ageing process

lipoic acid – Chemically, dithio-octanoic acid, a coenzyme (together with vitamin B_1) in the metabolism of pyruvate and in the citric acid cycle. Although it is an essential growth factor for various microorganisms, there is no evidence that it is a human dietary requirement

lipolysis – The hydrolysis of fats to glycerol and fatty acids

lipopolysaccharide (LPS) – Bacterial derived antigenic material that promotes an immune response in animals and humans

liposuction – Procedure for removal of subcutaneous adipose tissue in obese people using a suction pump device

lipotropes (lipotrophic factors) – Compounds such as choline, betaine and methionine that act as methyl donors; deficiency may result in fatty infiltration of the liver

Listeria – A genus of bacteria commonly found in soil of which the commonest is *Listeria monocytogenes*. They can cause food poisoning (listeriosis)

low birthweight (LBW) – Used as shorthand to describe babies born at weight less than 2.5 kg. Average birthweight is close to 3.5 kg (WHO reference mean). LBW can result from delivery before term (preterm) or from intrauterine growth retardation (IUGR) due to many causes including fetal undernutrition

lower reference nutrient intake (LRNI) – Set 2 standard deviations below the EAR for a nutrient. Intakes of nutrients below this point will almost certainly be inadequate for most individuals; *see* reference nutrient intake

lutein – A hydroxylated carotenoid (xanthophyll); not vitamin A active

luxus konsumption – An outdated term for diet-induced thermogenesis

lycopene – Red carotenoid, not vitamin A active

lymph – The fluid between blood and the tissues in which oxygen and nutrients are transported to the tissues, and waste products back to the blood

lymphatics – Vessels through which the lymph flows, draining from the tissues and entering the bloodstream at the thoracic duct

lysine – An essential amino acid of special nutritional importance, since it is the limiting amino acid in many cereals

lysozyme – An enzyme present in tears and body secretions and fluids that helps in the destruction of bacterial cell walls

macrocytes – Large immature precursors of red blood cells found in the circulation in pernicious anaemia and in folic acid deficiency, due to impairment of the normal maturation of red cells; hence macrocytic anaemia

mad cow disease – Bovine spongiform encephalopathy

Maillard reaction – Non-enzymic reaction between lysine in proteins and sugars, on heating or prolonged storage

malnutrition – Disturbance of form or function arising from deficiency or excess of one or more nutrients

malondialdehyde – An oxidation (degradation) product of unsaturated fatty acids, often used as an index of pro-oxidant action and of potential damage to lipids by pro-oxidant species such oxygen free radicals

maltase – Enzyme that hydrolyses maltose to yield two molecules of glucose; present in the brush border of the intestinal mucosal cells

maltodextrin – A polymer of glucose made by acid hydrolysis of starch

maltose – Malt sugar, or maltobiose, a disaccharide consisting of two glucose units linked α1–4

mannosans – Polysaccharides containing mannose

mannose – A six-carbon (hexose) sugar found in small amounts in legumes, manna, and some gums. Also called seminose and carubinose

marasmic kwashiorkor – The most severe form of protein energy malnutrition in children, with weight for height less than 60% of that expected, and with oedema and other symptoms of kwashiorkor

marasmus – An old term still in common use in Anglophone developing countries. The adjective (marasmic) described abnormally small and thin infants. As noun and adjective the term was later used by nutritionists to define a weight less than 60% of the reference mean weight for age. This definition is still used in resource-poor areas where stature is not measured. Now the term protein energy malnutrition (PEM) is more commonly used

market – Any context in which the sale and purchase of goods and services takes place. There need be no physical entity corresponding to the market; it might consist of a global telecommunications network on which company shares are traded

market economy – An economic system in which decisions about the allocation of resources and production are made on the basis of prices generated by voluntary exchanges among producers, consumers, workers, and owners of the factors of production (i.e. land, labour and capital)

mast cells – Cells found predominantly in connective tissue, although a specialised population of mast cells is found in mucosal sites (e.g. the gut). Following degranulation, mast cells release preformed and newly synthesised mediators of inflammation, including histamine

mastication – Chewing, grinding, and tearing foods with the teeth while it is mixed with saliva

maternal death – Death of a woman whilst pregnant or within 42 days of delivery

MaxEPA – Trade name for a standardised mixture of long-chain marine fatty acids, eicosapentaenoic (EPA, C20:5 ω3) and docosohexaenoic (DHA, C22:6 ω3) acids

medium-chain triacylglycerols – Triacylglycerols containing medium-chain (C:10–12) fatty acids, used in treatment of malabsorption; they are absorbed more rapidly than conventional fats, and the products of their digestion are transported to the liver, rather than in chylomicrons

megavitamin therapy – Treatment of diseases with very high doses of vitamins, many times the reference intakes; little or no evidence for its efficacy; vitamins A, D and B$_6$ are known to be toxic at high levels of intake

menadione, menaphthone, menaphtholdiacetate – Synthetic compounds with vitamin K activity; vitamin K$_3$, sometimes known as menaquinone-0

menaquinones – Bacterial metabolites with vitamin K activity; vitamin K$_2$

menarche – The initiation of menstruation in adolescent girls, normally occurring between the ages of 11 and 15. The age at menarche has become younger in Western countries, possibly associated with a better general standard of nutrition, and is later in less-developed countries

menhaden – Oily fish, *Brevoortia patronus*, *B. tyrannus*, from Gulf of Mexico and Atlantic seaboard of the USA, a rich source of fish oils

mesomorph – Description given to a well-covered individual with well-developed muscles. *See also* ectomorph; endomorph

mesophiles – Pathogenic microorganisms that grow best at temperatures between 25 and 40°C; usually will not grow below 5°C

metabolic equivalent (MET) – Unit of measurement of heat production by the body; 1 MET = 50 kcal/hour/m^2 body surface area

metabolic water – Produced in the body by the oxidation of foods; 100 g of fat produces 107.1 g; 100 g of starch 55.1 g; and 100 g of protein 41.3 g of water

metabolic weight – Energy expenditure and basal metabolic rate depend on the amount of metabolically active tissue in the body, rather than total body weight; body weight$^{0.75}$ is generally used to calculate the weight of active tissue

metabolism – The processes of interconversion of chemical compounds in the body. Anabolism is the process of forming larger and more complex compounds, commonly linked to the utilisation of metabolic energy. Catabolism is the process of breaking down larger molecules to smaller ones, commonly oxidation reactions linked to release of energy. There is approximately a 30% variation in the underlying metabolic rate (basal metabolic rate) between different individuals, determined in part by the activity of the thyroid gland

metabolome – The complement of metabolic reactions and metabolic products of an organism

metabolomics – The study of the metabolome

metalloenzyme – An enzyme having a metal (e.g. zinc or copper) as its prosthetic group

metalloproteins – Proteins containing a metal

metaphosphoric acid – A form of phosphoric acid which is used as a preservative for vitamin C (ascorbic acid) because its addition to biological fluids, such as serum or urine, lowers the pH and chelates (i.e. inactivates) the pro-oxidant metal ions such as ferrous and cupric ions

methaemoglobin – Oxidised form of haemoglobin (unlike oxyhaemoglobin, which is a loose and reversible combination with oxygen) which cannot transport oxygen to the tissues. Present in small quantities in normal blood, increased after certain drugs and after smoking; found rarely as a congenital abnormality (methaemoglobinaemia). It can be formed in the blood of babies after consumption of the small amounts of nitrate found naturally in vegetables and in some drinking water, since the lack of acidity in the stomach permits reduction of nitrate to nitrite

methionine – An essential amino acid; one of the three containing sulphur; cystine and cysteine are the other two. Cystine and cysteine are not essential, but can only be made from methionine, and therefore the requirement for methionine is lower if there is an adequate intake of cyst(e)ine

3-methyl-histidine – Derivative of the amino acid, histidine, found mainly in the contractile proteins of muscle (myosin and actin)

methylmalonic acid – An intermediate in the metabolic turnover of succinic acid, this substance typically accumulates in conditions of vitamin B$_{12}$ deficiency, and can be measured in serum or urine, as a functional index of vitamin B$_{12}$ status

micelles – Emulsified droplets of partially hydrolysed lipids, small enough to be absorbed across the intestinal mucosa

micro – Prefix for units of measurement, one millionth part (i.e. 10^{-6}); symbol μ (or sometimes mc)

microbiological assay – Method of measuring compounds such as vitamins and amino acids, using microorganisms. The principle is that the

organism is inoculated into a medium
containing all the growth factors needed except
the one under examination; the rate of growth is
then proportional to the amount of this nutrient
added in the test substance

micronutrients – Vitamins and minerals, which are
needed in very small amounts (micrograms or
milligrams per day), as distinct from fats,
carbohydrates, and proteins which are
macronutrients, since they are needed in
considerably greater amounts

mid-upper-arm-circumference (MUAC) – A rapid
way of assessing nutritional status, especially
applicable to children; *see* anthropometry

migraine – Type of headache, characterised by
usually being unilateral and/or accompanied by
visual disturbance and nausea

milli – Prefix for units of measurement, one
thousandth part (i.e. 10^{-3}); symbol m

mineral salts – The inorganic salts, including
sodium, potassium, calcium, chloride,
phosphate, sulphate, etc. So called because they
are (or originally were) obtained by mining

mineralocorticoids – The steroid hormones
secreted by the adrenal cortex which control the
excretion of salt and water; *see* steroids

minerals, trace – Those mineral salts present in the
body, and required in the diet, in small amounts
(parts per million)

minerals, ultra-trace – Those mineral salts
present in the body, and required in the diet, in
extremely small amounts (parts per thousand
million or less); known to be dietary essentials,
although rarely if ever a cause for concern since
the amounts required are small and they are
widely distributed in foods and water

**Ministry of Agriculture, Fisheries and Food
(MAFF)** – Former UK Ministry now replaced by
DEFRA and FSA

miscarriage – Spontaneous loss of a pregnancy
before 24 weeks of gestation

mitochondrion – (Plural mitochondria). The
subcellular organelles in all cells apart from red
blood cells in which the major oxidative
reactions of metabolism occur, linked to the
formation of ATP from ADP *see* ADP, ATP

monoamine oxidase – Enzyme that oxidises
amines; inhibitors have been used clinically as
antidepressant drugs, and consumption of
amine-rich foods such as cheese may cause a
hypertensive crisis in people taking the
inhibitors; *see* amines

monosaccharides – Group name of the simplest
sugars, including those composed of three carbon
atoms (trioses), four (tetroses), five (pentoses), six
(hexoses), and seven (heptoses). The units from
which disaccharides, oligosaccharides, and
polysaccharides are formed

monosodium glutamate (MSG) – The sodium salt
of glutamic acid, used to enhance the flavour of
savoury dishes and often added to canned meat
and soups

mRNA – An RNA copy of genomic DNA containing
genes for translation into protein *see* RNA, DNA,
genome

mucilages – Soluble but undigested complexes of
the sugars arabinose and xylose found in some
seeds and seaweeds

mucin – Viscous mucoprotein secreted in the saliva
and throughout the intestinal tract; the main
constituent of mucus

mucopolysaccharides – Polysaccharides
containing an amino sugar and uronic acid;
constituent of the mucoproteins of cartilage,
tendons, connective tissue, cornea, heparin, and
blood-group substances; *see* polysaccharides

mucoproteins – Glycoproteins containing a sugar,
usually chondroitin sulphate, combined with
amino acids or peptides; occur in mucin; *see*
glycoprotein

mucosa – Moist tissue lining, for example, the
mouth (buccal mucosa), stomach (gastric
mucosa), intestines, and respiratory tract

mucous colitis – Irritable bowel syndrome (q.v.)

mucus – Secretion of mucous glands, containing
mucin; protects epithelia

mutagen – Compound that causes mutations and
may be carcinogenic; *see* mutation

mutation – a permanent structural alteration in
DNA

mycoprotein – Name given to mould mycelium
used as a food ingredient

mycotoxins – Toxins produced by fungi (moulds), especially *Aspergillus flavus* under tropical conditions and *Penicillium* and *Fusarium* species under temperate conditions

myoglobin – Haemoprotein mainly found in muscle where it serves as an intracellular storage site for oxygen

myristic acid – A medium-chain saturated fatty acid (C14:0)

myxoedema – Low metabolic rate as a result of hypothyroidism, commonly the result of iodine deficiency

nano – Prefix for units of measurement, one thousand-millionth part (i.e. 10^{-9}), symbol n

naphthoquinone – The chemical ring structure of vitamin K; the various vitamers of vitamin K can be referred to as substituted naphthoquinones

nasogastric tube – Fine plastic tube inserted through the nose and thence into the stomach for enteral nutrition

National Center for Health Statistics (NCHS) standards – Tables of height and weight for age used as reference values for the assessment of growth and nutritional status of children, based on data collected by the US National Center for Health Statistics in the 1970s. The most comprehensive such set of data, and used in most countries of the world

National Health and Nutrition Examination Survey (NHANES) – Conducted by the National Center for Health Statistics (NCHS), Centers for Disease Control and Prevention, designed to collect information about the health and diet of people in the United States

natural killer cells (NK) – Specialised T-cells with the continuous task of identifying and eliminating cells recognised as being foreign or non-self

nature-identical – Term applied to food additives that are synthesised in the laboratory and are identical to those that occur in nature

neonatal – Within the first 28 days of life

nephropathy – Diabetic complication that involves the kidney and may lead to chronic renal failure and dialysis

net dietary protein energy ratio (NDpE) – A way of expressing the protein content of a diet or food taking into account both the amount of protein (relative to total energy intake) and the protein quality. It is protein energy multiplied by net protein utilisation divided by total energy. If energy is expressed in kcal and the result expressed as a percentage, this is net dietary protein calories per cent, NDpCal%

net protein ratio/retention (NPR) – Weight gain of a test animal plus weight loss of a control animal fed a non-protein diet per gram of protein consumed by the test animal

net protein utilisation (NPU) – The proportion of nitrogen intake that is retained, i.e. the product of biological value (*see* glossary) and digestibility (*see* glossary)

net protein value (NPV) – A way of expressing the amount and quality of the protein in a food; the product of net protein utilisation and protein content per cent

neural tube defect – Congenital malformations of the brain (anencephaly) or spinal cord (spina bifida) caused by the failure of the closure of the neural tube in early embryonic development

neuropathy – Diabetic complication that involves peripheral and autonomic nervous system

neuropeptide Y – A peptide neurotransmitter believed to be important in the control of appetite and feeding behaviour, especially in response to leptin

niacin – The generic descriptor for two compounds that have the biological activity of the vitamin: nicotinic acid and its amide, nicotinamide. In the USA niacin is used specifically to mean nicotinic acid, and niacinamide for nicotinamide

niacinamide – US name for nicotinamide, the amide form of the vitamin niacin

niacinogens – Name given to protein-niacin complexes found in cereals; *see* niacytin

niacytin – The bound forms of the vitamin niacin, found in cereals

nicotinamide adenine dinucleotide and its phosphate (NAD, NADP) – The coenzymes derived from niacin. Involved as hydrogen acceptors in a wide variety of oxidation and reduction reactions; *see* nicotinamide

nicotinamide – One of the vitamers of niacin

nicotinic acid – One of the vitamers of niacin

night blindness – Nyctalopia. Inability to see in dim light as a result of vitamin A deficiency

ninhydrin test – For the amino group of amino acids. Pink, purple or blue colour is developed on heating an amino acid or peptide with ninhydrin

nitrogen conversion factor – Factor by which nitrogen content of a foodstuff is multiplied to determine the protein content; it depends on the amino acid composition of the protein. For wheat and most cereals it is 5.8; rice, 5.95; soya, 5.7; most legumes and nuts, 5.3; milk, 6.38; other foods, 6.25. In mixtures of proteins, as in dishes and diets, the factor of 6.25 is used. 'Crude protein' is defined as $N \times 6.25$

N-nitroso compounds – are a group of chemicals that occur ubiquitously. They are formed in the environment and can be absorbed from food, water, air and industrial and consumer products, formed within the body from precursors in food, water and air, inhaled from tobacco smoke, and naturally occurring

No Adverse Effect Level (NOAE) – With respect to food additives, equivalent to No Effect Level

No Effect Level (NEL) – With respect to food additives, the maximum dose of an additive that has no detectable adverse effects

Non-digestible oligosaccharide – An oligosaccharide that is not digested (or minimally digested) in the upper gastrointestinal tract

non-esterified fatty acids (NEFA) – Free fatty acids in the blood, as opposed to triacylglycerols

non-starch polysaccharides (NSP) – Those polysaccharides other than starches, found in foods. They are the major part of dietary fibre and can be measured more precisely than total dietary fibre; include cellulose, pectins, glucans, gums, mucilages, inulin, and chitin (and exclude lignin); *see* dietary fibre

nor- – Chemical prefix to the name of a compound, indicating: (1) one methyl (CH_3) group has been replaced by hydrogen (e.g. noradrenaline can be considered to be a demethylated derivative of adrenaline); (2) an analogue of a compound containing one fewer methylene (CH_2) groups than the parent compound; (3) an isomer with an unbranched side-chain (e.g. norleucine, norvaline)

noradrenaline – Hormone secreted by the adrenal medulla together with adrenaline; also a neurotransmitter. Physiological effects similar to those of adrenaline. Also known as norepinephrine (US terminology)

norepinephrine – *See* noradrenaline

Northern blotting – Widely used technique for detecting mRNAs by hybridisation with specific probes following transfer of RNA onto a solid support, such as a nylon membrane; *see* mRNA, RNA, hybridisation

Norwalk-like virus – Viral infection similar to that first reported in Norwalk, USA which causes intestinal illness that occurs in outbreaks

nucleic acids – Polymers of purine and pyrimidine sugar phosphates; two main classes: ribonucleic acid (RNA) and deoxyribonucleic acid (DNA); *see* ribonucleic acid, deoxyribonucleic acid

nucleoproteins – The complex of proteins and nucleic acids found in the cell nucleus

nucleosides – Compounds of purine or pyrimidine bases with a sugar, most commonly ribose. For example, adenine plus ribose forms adenosine. With the addition of phosphate a nucleotide is formed; *see* purines, pyrimidines

nucleotides – Compounds of purine or pyrimidine base with a sugar phosphate

nutraceuticals – Term for compounds in foods that are not nutrients but have (potential) beneficial effects

nutrient density – A way of expressing the nutrient content of a food or diet relative to the energy yield (i.e. /1000 kcal or /MJ) rather than per unit weight

nutrients – Essential dietary factors such as vitamins, minerals, amino acids and fatty acids. Metabolic fuels (sources of energy) are not termed nutrients so that a commonly used phrase is 'energy and nutrients'

nutrification – The addition of nutrients to foods at such a level as to make a major contribution to the diet

nutrition – The process by which living organisms take in and use food for the maintenance of life,

protein quality – A measure of the usefulness of a dietary protein for growth and maintenance of tissues, and, in animals, production of meat, eggs, wool, and milk. It is only important if the total intake of protein barely meets the requirement. The quality of individual proteins is unimportant in mixed diets, because of complementation between different proteins

protein retention efficiency (PRE) – The net protein retention converted to a % scale by multiplying by 16, then becoming numerically the same as NPU

protein score – A measure of protein quality based on chemical analysis

proteinases – Enzymes that hydrolyse proteins

proteolysis – The hydrolysis of proteins to their constituent amino acids, catalysed by alkali, acid, or enzymes

proteome – The protein complement of a cell, tissue or organism translated from its genomic DNA sequence

proteomics – The study of the proteome

prothrombin – Protein in plasma involved in coagulation of blood. The prothrombin time is an index of the coagulability of blood (and hence of vitamin K nutritional status) based on the time taken for a citrated sample of blood to clot when calcium ions and thromboplastin are added

protoporphyrin – Haem molecule minus iron (i.e. the organic ring-structure without the central metal ion), the accumulation of which, in red cells, indicates either iron deficiency or other situations of impaired iron incorporation into haem, e.g. that caused by lead poisoning. Its quantitation in red blood cells can be used as a functional index of iron status

provitamin – A substance that is converted into a vitamin, such as 7-dehydrocholesterol, which is converted into vitamin D, or those carotenes that can be converted to vitamin A

proximate analysis – Analysis of foods and feedingstuffs for nitrogen (for protein), ether extract (for fat), crude fibre and ash (mineral salts), together with soluble carbohydrate calculated by subtracting these values from the total (carbohydrate by difference). Also known as Weende analysis, after the Weende Experimental Station in Germany, which in 1865 outlined the methods of analysis to be used

P/S ratio – The ratio between polyunsaturated and saturated fatty acids. In Western diets the ratio is about 0.6; it is suggested that increasing it to near 1.0 would reduce the risk of atherosclerosis and coronary heart disease

psychrophilic organisms – Bacteria and fungi that tolerate low temperatures. Their preferred temperature range is 15–20°C, but they will grow at or below 0°C; the temperature must be reduced to about −10°C before growth stops, but the organisms are not killed and will regrow when the temperature rises

ptyalin – Obsolete name for salivary amylase

ptyalism – Excessive flow of saliva

pulses – Name given to the dried seeds (matured on the plant) of legumes such as peas, beans and lentils

purines – Nitrogenous compounds (bases) that occur in nucleic acids (adenine and guanine) and their precursors and metabolites; inosine, caffeine, and theobromine are also purines

putrescine – Low molecular weight amine with biological activity

pyridoxal phosphate – 5-Phosphate of the aldehyde form of pyridoxine (vitamin B_6): this is the major form of the vitamin in blood and tissues, and is commonly measured as an index of vitamin B_6 status

pyrimidines – Nitrogenous compounds (bases) that occur in nucleic acids: cytosine, thymidine, and uracil

pyruvate – Salts of pyruvic acid

pyruvic acid – An intermediate in the metabolism of carbohydrates, formed by the anaerobic metabolism of glucose

QUAC stick – Quaker arm circumference measuring stick. A stick used to measure height which also shows the 80th and 85th centiles of expected mid-upper arm circumference. Developed by a Quaker Service Team in Nigeria in the 1960s as a rapid and simple tool for assessment of nutritional status

quantitative ingredients declaration (QUID) – Obligatory on food labels in EU since February 2000; previously legislation only required declaration of ingredients in descending order of quantity, not specific declaration of the amount of each ingredient present

Quetelet's index – *See* body mass index

reciprocal ponderal index – An index of adiposity; height divided by cube root of weight

reducing sugars – Sugars that are chemically reducing agents, including glucose, fructose, lactose, pentoses, but not sucrose

reduction – The opposite of oxidation; chemical reactions resulting in a gain of electrons, or hydrogen, or the loss of oxygen

reference intakes (of nutrients) – Amounts of nutrients greater than the requirements of almost all members of the population, determined on the basis of the average requirement plus twice the standard deviation, to allow for individual variation in requirements and thus cover the theoretical needs of 97.5% of the population

reference man, woman – An arbitrary physiological standard; defined as a person aged 25, weighing 65 kg, living in a temperate zone of a mean annual temperature of 10°C. Reference man performs medium work, with an average daily energy requirement of 13.5 MJ (3200 kcal). Reference woman is engaged in general household duties or light industry, with an average daily requirement of 9.7 MJ (2300 kcal)

reference nutrient intake (RNI) – Defined by COMA (Committee on Medical Aspects of Food Policy for the UK Department of Health), most recently in 1991, as being the amount of each nutrient that is sufficient to meet the needs of the majority (mean +2 standard deviations) of healthy people in a defined population, or subgroup of it. Approximately equivalent (in concept, but not necessarily in magnitude) to the US or WHO RDAs (recommended dietary amounts)

reference standards (international reference standard)/growth standards – These refer to databases recording the linear and ponderal growth of healthy children. They include anthropometric data collected on suitably large samples, and analysed with precise specifications to provide a useful basis for reference

relative protein value (RPV) – A measure of protein quality

renal plasma flow – Rate of passage of plasma through the kidneys, directly related to glomerular filtration rate

renal threshold – Concentration of a compound in the blood above which it is not reabsorbed by the kidney, and so is excreted in the urine

respiratory quotient (RQ) – Ratio of the volume of carbon dioxide produced when a substance is oxidised, to the volume of oxygen used. The oxidation of carbohydrate results in an RQ of 1.0; of fat, 0.7; and of protein, 0.8

respirometer – *See* spirometer

restoration – The addition of nutrients to replace those lost in processing, as in milling of cereals. *See also* fortification

reticulocyte – Immature precursor of the red blood cell in which the remains of the nucleus are visible as a reticulum. Very few are seen in normal blood as they are retained in the marrow until mature, but on remission of anaemia, when there is a high rate of production, reticulocytes appear in the bloodstream (reticulocytosis)

retinal (retinaldehyde), retinene, retinoic acid, retinol – Vitamers of vitamin A

retinal maculopathy – Deterioration of the macula (central region of the retina) which occurs progressively in older people, thus irreversibly impairing vision. Thought to be exacerbated by pro-oxidant action such as by oxygen free radicals

retinoids – Compounds chemically related to, or derived from, vitamin A, which display some of the biological activities of the vitamin, but have lower toxicity; they are used for treatment of severe skin disorders and some cancers

retinol-biding protein – A plasma protein which specifically binds retinol (the alcohol form of vitamin A) and prevents it from being excreted. In vitamin A sufficiency, all the RBP is bound to retinol, in a 1:1 complex, but in vitamin A deficiency the protein may become partially desaturated, so that the ratio of protein to retinol

vegans – Those who consume no foods of animal origin. (Vegetarians often consume milk and/or eggs.)

verbascose – A non-digestible tetrasaccharide, galactose-galactose-glucose-fructose, found in legumes; fermented by intestinal bacteria and causes flatulence

villi, intestinal – Small, finger-like processes covering the surface of the small intestine in large numbers ($20–40/mm^2$), projecting some 0.5–1 mm into the lumen. They provide a large surface area (about $300 m^2$) for absorption in the small intestine

vitafoods – Foods designed to meet the needs of health conscious consumers which enhance physical or mental quality of life and may increase health status

vitamers – Chemical compounds structurally related to a vitamin, and converted to the same overall active metabolites in the body. They thus possess the same biological activity

vitamin – Thirteen organic substances that are essential in very small amounts in food

vitamin Q – Ubiquinone

vitaminoids – Name given to compounds with 'vitamin-like' activity; considered by some to be vitamins or partially to replace vitamins. Includes flavonoids, inositol, carnitine, choline, lipoic acid, and the essential fatty acids. With the exception of the essential fatty acids, there is little evidence that any of them is a dietary essential

waist:hip ratio – Simple method for describing the distribution of subcutaneous and intra-abdominal adipose tissue

wasting/wasted – An old term meaning abnormally thin after weight loss. The term has been used more recently by nutritionists to define weight for height significantly less than the reference range

water activity, a_w – The ratio of the vapour pressure of water in a food to the saturated vapour pressure of water at the same temperature

Waterlow classification – A system for classifying protein energy malnutrition in children based on wasting (the percentage of expected weight for height) and the degree of stunting (the percentage of expected height for age). *See also* Wellcome classification

weaning foods – Foods specially formulated for infants aged between 3 and 9 months for the transition between breast- or bottle-feeding and normal intake of solid foods

Weende analysis – Proximate analysis; *see* proximate analysis

Weight-control Information Network (WIN) – of the National Institute of Diabetes and Digestive and Kidney Diseases; website http://www.niddk.nih.gov/health/nutrit/nutrit.htm

Wellcome classification – A system for classifying protein energy malnutrition in children based on percentage of expected weight for age and the presence or absence of oedema. Between 60 and 80% of expected weight is underweight in the absence of oedema, and kwashiorkor if oedema is present; under 60% of expected weight is marasmus in the absence of oedema, and marasmic kwashiorkor if oedema is present

Wernicke–Korsakoff syndrome – The result of damage to the brain as a result of vitamin B_1 deficiency, commonly associated with alcohol abuse. Affected subjects show clear signs of neurological damage (Wernicke's encephalopathy) with psychiatric changes (Korsakoff's psychosis) characterised by loss of recent memory and confabulation (the invention of fabulous stories). *See also* beriberi

wholefoods – Foods that have been minimally refined or processed, and are eaten in their natural state. In general nothing is removed from, or added to, the foodstuffs in preparation. Wholegrain cereal products are made by milling the complete grain

World Cancer Research Fund (WCRF) – Website http://www.wcrf.org

World Food Programme (WFP) – Part of the Food and Agriculture Organization of the United Nations; intended to give international aid in the form of food from countries with a surplus; website http://www.wfp.org

World Health Organization (WHO) – Headquarters in Geneva; website http://www.who.in

xanthelasma – Yellow fatty plaques on the eyelids, due to hypercholesterolaemia

xanthophylls – Yellow-orange hydroxylated carotene derivatives

xanthosis – Yellowing of the skin associated with high blood concentrations of carotene

xenobiotic – Substances foreign to the body, including drugs and some food additives

xerophthalmia – Advanced vitamin A deficiency in which the epithelium of the cornea and conjunctiva of the eye deteriorate because of impairment of the tear glands, resulting in dryness then ulceration, leading to blindness

xylitol – A five-carbon sugar; said to have an effect in suppressing the growth of some of the bacteria associated with dental caries

Xylitol – sugar-alcohol (polyol)

xylose – Pentose (five-carbon) sugar found in plant tissues as complex polysaccharide; 40% as sweet as sucrose. Also known as wood sugar

zymogens – The inactive form in which some enzymes, especially the protein digestive enzymes, are secreted, being activated after secretion. Also called pro-enzymes, or enzyme precursors

Further reading

Bender D A 2004 Oxford dictionary of food and nutrition. Oxford University Press, Oxford

Bender D A, Bender A E 1999 Benders' dictionary of nutrition and food technology, 7th edn. Soodhead Publishing, Cambridge

On-line Medical Dictionary: http://cancerweb.ncl.ac. uk/omd/index.html

Other nutrient groups have been considered prior to this as follows. Trace elements (1996), Carbohydrate, fat, non-starch polysaccharides (1990), energy and protein (1985).

Population requirement safe ranges (1996):

Basal   Lower limit of safe ranges of population mean intakes

Normative   Population mean intake sufficient to meet normative requirements. This

value is used in most of the tables in the Appendix

Maximum   Upper limit of safe ranges of population mean intakes

Recommended intakes (1974)   Average requirement augmented by a factor that takes into account interindividual variability. The amounts are considered sufficient for the maintenance of health in nearly all people.

UNITS

These vary for different nutrients.

Energy (kcal/day, kJ/day or MJ/day)

All energy values are based on the Schofield equations (FAO/WHO/UNU 1985) and so should be similar for each source. Any variation occurs because the equations are based on weight and activity within broad age bands.

Carbohydrate and fat

These are expressed as a percentage of total energy intake including 5% alcohol or as a percentage of food energy, excluding alcohol.

Protein (g/day or g/kg/day)

Protein requirements are all based on the FAO/WHO/UNU 1985 Report and, like energy values,

they should be similar from various sources, the only difference being the average weight chosen for each age group.

Most nutrients (g/day or mg/day or μg/day)

Some exceptions are:
niacin: mg/1000 kcal or mg/MJ
vitamin B_6: mg/g protein
vitamin E: mg/g polyunsaturated fatty acids.

Iron, zinc

Requirements depend on the bioavailability of the diet which may be low, moderate or high (see Ch. 12). In this Appendix levels were chosen for medium availability from WHO values. The UK and USA values assume Western diets of high availability.

AGE BANDS

The different national and international sources of data have used slightly different age bands in some instances. Where necessary these have been adjusted

to correspond as closely as possible with the most frequently used age bands.

References

Department of Health 1991 Report on health and social subjects 41. Dietary reference values for food energy and nutrients for the United Kingdom. Committee on Medical Aspects of Food Policy. HMSO, London

EC Scientific Committee for Food Report 1993 (31st series) Nutrient and energy intakes for the European Community. Directorate-General, Industry, Luxembourg

FAO/WHO 1988 Requirements for vitamin A, iron, folate and vitamin B_{12}. Report of a joint FAO/WHO

expert consultation. Food and Nutrition Series. Food and Agriculture Organization (FAO), Rome

FAO/WHO/UNU 1985 Energy and protein requirements. Report of a joint FAO/WHO/UNU expert consultation. Technical Report Series 724. World Health Organization (WHO), Geneva

Food and Nutrition Board, Institute of Medicine 1997 Dietary reference intakes for calcium, phosphorus, magnesium, vitamin D and fluoride. National Academy Press, Washington, DC

Food and Nutrition Board, Institute of Medicine 1998 Dietary reference intakes for thiamin, riboflavin, niacin, vitamin B6, folate, vitamin B12, pantothenic acid, biotin and choline. National Academy Press, Washington, DC

Food and Nutrition Board, Institute of Medicine 2000 Dietary reference intakes for vitamin C, vitamin E, selenium and carotenoids. National Academy Press, Washington, DC

Food and Nutrition Board, Institute of Medicine 2001 Dietary reference intakes for vitamin A, vitamin K, arsenic, boron, chromium, copper, iodine, iron manganese, molybdenum, nickel, silicon, vanadium and zinc. National Academy Press, Washington, DC

Food and Nutrition Board, Institute of Medicine, 2002 Dietary reference intakes for energy, carbohydrate, fibre, fat, fatty acids, cholesterol, protein and amino acids. National Academy Press, Washington, DC

James W P T 1988 Healthy nutrition. Preventing nutrition-related diseases in Europe. WHO Regional Publications, European Series No. 24, WHO, Copenhagen

WHO 1990 Diet, nutrition, and the prevention of chronic diseases. Technical Report Series 797, WHO, Geneva

WHO 1996 Trace elements in human nutrition and health. WHO, in collaboration with FAO, AEA, Geneva

WHO/FAO 1987 α-Tocopherol. In: Toxicological evaluation of certain food additives and contaminants. WHO Food Additives Series 21, Cambridge, p 55–69

TABLES OF DIETARY REFERENCE VALUES

Table A1a **Dietary reference values for energy for males**

Age	UK and WHO EAR[1]		USA AEA[2]		Europe	
	(MJ/day)	(kcal/day)	(MJ/day)	(kcal/day)	Lower[3,4] (MJ/day)	Higher[5] (MJ/day)
0–3 months	2.28	545	2.7	650	2.2	
4–6 months	2.89	690	2.7	650	3.0	
7–9 months	3.44	825	3.5	850	3.5	
10–12 months	3.85	920	3.5	850	3.9	
1–3 years	5.15	1230	5.4	1300	5.1	
4–6 years	7.16	1715	7.5	1800	7.1	
7–10 years	8.24	1970	8.3	2000	8.3	
11–14 years	9.27	2220	10.4	2500	9.8	
15–18 years	11.51	2755	12.5	3000	11.8	
19–50 years	10.60	2550	12.1	2900	11.3	12.0
51–59 years	10.60	2550	9.6	2300	11.3	12.0
60–64 years	9.93	2380	9.6	2300	8.5	9.2
65–74 years	9.71	2330	9.6	2300	8.5	9.2
75+	8.77	2100	9.6	2300	7.5	8.5

[1]EAR, estimated average requirement.
[2]AEA, average energy allowance.
[3]No physical activity + desirable body weight for adults.
[4]Children's values are estimated average requirement.
[5]Desirable physical activity + desirable body weight for adults.

Table A1b Dietary reference values for energy for females

| Age | UK and WHO EAR[1] | | USA AEA[2] | | Europe | |
	(MJ/day)	(kcal/day)	(MJ/day)	(kcal/day)	Lower[3,4] (MJ/day)	Higher[5] (MJ/day)
0–3 months	2.16	515	2.7	650	2.1	
4–6 months	2.69	645	2.7	650	2.8	
7–9 months	3.20	765	3.5	850	3.3	
10–12 months	3.61	865	3.5	850	3.7	
1–3 years	4.86	1165	5.4	1300	4.8	
4–6 years	6.46	1545	7.5	1800	6.7	
7–10 years	7.28	1740	8.3	2000	7.4	
11–14 years	7.92	1845	9.2	2200	8.4	
15–18 years	8.83	2110	9.2	2200	8.9	
19–50 years	8.10	1940	9.2	2200	8.4	9.0
51–59 years	8.00	1900	9.2	2200	8.4	9.0
60–64 years	7.99	1900	9.2	2200	7.2	7.8
65–74 years	7.96	1900	9.2	2200	7.2	7.8
75+	7.61	1810	9.2	2200	6.7	7.6
Pregnancy	+0.80[6]	+200[6]	+1.2	+300	+0.75	
Lactation	+1.9–2.0	+450–480	+2.1	+500	+1.5–1.9	

[1]EAR, estimated average requirement.
[2]AEA, average energy allowance.
[3]No physical activity + desirable body weight for adults.
[4]Children's values are estimated average requirement.
[5]Desirable physical activity + desirable body weight for adults.
[6]Last trimester.

Table A2 Dietary reference values for protein (g/day)

| Age | UK and WHO | | USA RDA/ AI | European PRI[3] |
	EAR[1]	RNI[1]		
0–3 months	[2]–	12.5[2]	9.1[4]	
4–6 months	10.6	12.7	9.1[4]	14.0
7–9 months	11.0	13.7	13.5[4]	14.5
10–12 months	11.2	14.9	13.5[4]	14.5
1–3 years	11.7	14.5	13	14.7
4–6 years	14.8	19.7	19	19.0
7–10 years	22.8	28.3	19	27.3
Males				
11–14 years	33.8	42.1	34	42.0
15–18 years	46.1	55.2	52	48.5
19–50 years	44.4	55.5	56	56.0
50+ years	42.6	53.3	56	55.0
Females				
11–14 years	33.1	41.2	34	39.7
15–18 years	37.1	45.0	46	51.4
19–50+ years	36.0	45.0	46	47.0
50+ years	37.2	46.5	46	47.0
Pregnancy		+6	71	+10
Lactation		+11	71	+16

RNI, reference nutrient intake; RDA, recommended dietary allowance;
AI, adequate intake; PRI, population reference intake.
[1]Based on egg and milk protein; assume complete digestibility.
[2]No WHO value.
[3]Children's values are safe levels.
[4]AI.

Table A3 **Dietary reference values for fat and carbohydrate for adults as a percentage of daily total energy intake (percentage food energy)**

	UK			USA RDA	WHO (1990)		
	Individual minimum	Population average[1]	Individual maximum		Lower[2]	Upper[2]	European PRI[3] or goal[4]
Saturated fatty acids		10 (11)		10	0	10	10[4]
Cis-polyunsaturated fatty acids		6 (6.5)	10	7	3	7	
n-3	0.2						0.5[3]
n-6	1.0						2.0[3]
Cis-monounsaturated fatty acids		12 (13)					
Trans fatty acids		2 (2)					
Total fatty acids		30 (32.5)					
Total fat		33 (35)		30	15	30	20–30[4]
Non-milk extrinsic sugars	0	10 (11)			0	10	10[4]
Intrinsic milk sugars and starch		37 (39)					
Total carbohydrate		47 (50)		60	55	75	55–65[4]
Non-starch polysaccharide (g/day)	12	18	24		16	24	30[4]

[1]Total energy intake assumes 5% alcohol; food energy (in parenthesis) excludes alcohol.
[2]Population nutrient goal.
[3]Population reference intake.
[4]Ultimate goal.

Table A4 **Dietary reference values for vitamin A (μg retinol equivalent/day)**

Age	UK			USA RDA/AI	FAO/WHO	European PRI
	LRNI[1]	EAR	RNI			
0–12 months	150	250	350	500	375	
1–3 years	200	300	400	300	400	400
4–6 years	200	300	400	400	450	400
7–10 years	250	350	500	400	500	500
Males						
11–15 years	250	400	600	600	600	600
15–50+ years	300	500	700	900	600	700
Females						
11–50+ years	250	400	600	700	600	600
Pregnancy			+100	770	800	+100
Lactation			+350	1300		+350

[1]LRNI, lower reference nutrient intake.

Table A5 Dietary reference values for vitamin D (μg/day)

Age	UK RNI	USA AI	FAO/WHO	European PRI
Males and females				
0–6 months	8.5	5	5	10–25
7 months–3 years	7.0	5	5	10
4–6 years	0[1]	5	5	0–10
7–10 years	0[1]	5	5	0–10
11–24 years	0[1]	5	5	0–15
25–50+ years	0[1]	5	5	0–10
65+	10	10	15	10
Pregnancy and lactation	10	5	5	10

[1]If exposed to the sun.

Table A6 Dietary reference values for vitamin E (mg/day, α-tocopherol)

Age	UK safe intake	USA RDA/AI	WHO/FAO	European PRI
0–6 months	0.4 mg/g PUFA	4[1]	2.7	0.4 mg/g PUFA
7–12 months	0.4 mg/g PUFA	5[1]	2.7	0.4 mg/g PUFA
1–3 years	0.4 mg/g PUFA	6	5	0.4 mg/g PUFA
4–10 years		7	7	
Males				
11–50+ years	>4	15	10	>4
Females				
11–50+ years	>3	15	7.5	>3
Pregnancy		15	7.5	
Lactation		19		

PUFA, polyunsaturated fatty acid.
[1]AI.

Table A7 Dietary reference values for vitamin K (μg/day)

Age	UK safe intake	USA AI	FAO/WHO	European[1]
0–6 months	10	2.0	5	
7–12 months	10	2.5	10	
1–3 years		30	15	
4–10 years		55	20	
7–10 years		30	25	
Males				
11–14 years	1 μg/kg body weight	60	35–55	1 μg/kg body weight
15–18 years	1 μg/kg body weight	75	35–55	1 μg/kg body weight
19–24 years	1 μg/kg body weight	120	65	1 μg/kg body weight
25+ years	1 μg/kg body weight	120	65	1 μg/kg body weight
Females				
11–14 years	1 μg/kg body weight	60	35–55	1 μg/kg body weight
15–18 years	1 μg/kg body weight	75	35–55	1 μg/kg body weight
19–24 years	1 μg/kg body weight	90	55	1 μg/kg body weight
25+ years	1 μg/kg body weight	90	55	1 μg/kg body weight
Pregnancy	1 μg/kg body weight	90	55	1 μg/kg body weight
Lactation	1 μg/kg body weight	90	55	1 μg/kg body weight

[1]No recommendation, but statement of what appears adequate.

Table A8 **Dietary reference values for vitamin C (mg/day)**

Age	UK			USA RDA/AI	FAO/WHO	European PRI
	LRNI	EAR	RNI			
0–6 months	6	15	25	40[1]	25	
7–12 months	6	15	25	50[1]	30	20
1–3 years	8	20	30	15	30	25
4–6 years	8	20	30	25	30	25
7–10 years	8	20	30	25	35	30
Males						
11–14 years	9	22	35	45	40	35
15–50+ years	10	25	40	90	45	45
Females						
11–14 years	9	22	35	45	40	35
15–50+ years	10	25	40	75	45	40
Pregnancy			+10	85	55	55
Lactation			+30	120	70	70.

[1]AI.

Table A9 **Dietary reference values for thiamin**

Age	UK				USA RDA/AI (mg/day)	FAO/WHO (mg/day)	European PRI (mg/day)
	LRNI (mg/1000 kcal)	EAR (mg/1000 kcal)	RNI (mg/1000 kcal)	RNI (mg/day)			
0–6 months	0.2	0.23	0.3	0.2	0.2[2]	0.2	
7–12 months	0.2	0.23	0.3	0.3	0.3[2]	0.3	0.3
1–3 years	0.23	0.3	0.4	0.5	0.5	0.5	0.5
4–6 years	0.23	0.3	0.4	0.7	0.6	0.7	0.7
7–10 years	0.23	0.3	0.4	0.7	0.6	0.9	0.8
Males							
11–14 years	0.23	0.3	0.4	0.9	0.9	1.2	1.0
15–50+ years	0.23	0.3	0.4	0.9	1.2	1.2	1.1
Females							
11–14 years	0.23	0.3	0.4	0.7	0.9	1.1	0.9
15–50+ years	0.23	0.3	0.4	0.8	1.1	1.1	0.9
Pregnancy	0.23	0.3	0.4	+0.1[1]	1.4	1.4	1.0
Lactation	0.23	0.3	0.4	+0.2	1.4	1.5	1.1

[1]For last trimester only.
[2]AI.

Table A10 **Dietary reference values for riboflavin (mg/day)**

Age	UK			USA RDA/AI	FAO/WHO	European PRI
	LRNI	EAR	RNI			
0–6 months	0.2	0.3	0.4	0.3[1]	0.3	
7–12 months	0.2	0.3	0.4	0.4[1]	0.4	0.4
1–3 years	0.3	0.5	0.6	0.5	0.5	0.8
4–6 years	0.4	0.6	0.8	0.6	0.6	1.0
7–10 years	0.5	0.8	1.0	0.6	0.9	1.2
Males						
11–14 years	0.8	1.0	1.2	0.9	1.3	1.4
15–18 years	0.8	1.0	1.3	1.3	1.3	1.6
19–50 years	0.8	1.0	1.3	1.3	1.3	1.6
50+ years	0.8	1.0	1.3	1.3	1.3	1.6
Females						
11–14 years	0.8	0.9	1.1	0.9	1.0	1.2
15–50+ years	0.8	0.9	1.1	1.1	1.1	1.3
Pregnancy			+0.3	1.4	1.4	1.6
Lactation			+0.5	1.6	1.6	1.7

[1] AI.

Table A11 **Dietary reference values for niacin (nicotinic acid equivalent)**

Age	UK				USA RDA/AI (mg/day)	FAO/WHO (mg/day)	European PRI[2] (mg/day)
	LRNI (mg/1000 kcal)	EAR (mg/1000 kcal)	RNI (mg/1000 kcal)	RNI (mg/day)			
0–6 months	4.4	5.5	6.6	3	2[1]	2	
7–12 months	4.4	5.5	6.6	5	4[1]	4	5
1–3 years	4.4	5.5	6.6	8	6	6	9
4–6 years	4.4	5.5	6.6	11	8	8	11
7–10 years	4.4	5.5	6.6	12	8	12	13
Males							
11–14 years	4.4	5.5	6.6	15	12	16	15
15–18 years	4.4	5.5	6.6	18	16	16	18
19–50 years	4.4	5.5	6.6	17	16	16	18
50+ years	4.4	5.5	6.6	16	16	16	18
Females							
11–14 years	4.4	5.5	6.6	12	12	16	14
15–18 years	4.4	5.5	6.6	14	14	16	14
19–50 years	4.4	5.5	6.6	13	14	14	14
50+ years	4.4	5.5	6.6	12	14	14	14
Pregnancy	*	*	*	*	18	18	*
Lactation	*	*	+2.3 mg/day	+2	17	17	+2

*No increment.
[1] AI.
[2] 1.6 mg/MJ.

Table A12 **Dietary reference values for vitamin B$_6$**

Age	UK				USA RDA/AI (mg/day)	FAO/WHO (mg/day)	European PRI[2] (mg/day)
	LRNI (μg/g protein)	EAR (μg/g protein)	RNI (μg/g protein)	RNI (mg/day)			
0–6 months	3.5	6	8	0.2	0.1[1]	0.1	
7–9 months	6	8	10	0.3	0.3[1]	0.3	0.4
10–12 months	8	10	13	0.4	0.3[1]	0.3	0.4
1–3 years	8	10	13	0.7	0.5	0.5	0.7
4–6 years	8	10	13	0.9	0.6	0.6	0.9
7–10 years	8	10	13	1.0	0.6	1.0	1.1
Males							
11–14 years	11	13	15	1.2	1.0	1.3	1.3
15–18 years	11	13	15	1.5	1.3	1.3	1.5
19–50+ years	11	13	15	1.4	1.7	1.7	1.5
Females							
11–14 years	11	13	15	1.0	1.0	1.2	1.1
15–18 years	11	13	15	1.2	1.2	1.3	1.1
19–50+ years	11	13	15	1.2	1.5	1.5	1.1
Pregnancy	*	*	*	*	1.9	1.9	1.3
Lactation	*	*	*	*	2.0	2.0	1.4

*No increment.
[1]AI.
[2]15 μg/g protein.

Table A13 **Dietary reference values for folate (μg/day)**

Age	UK			USA RDA/AI	FAO/WHO	European PRI[2]
	LRNI	EAR	RNI			
0–3 months	30	40	50	65[1]	80	50
4–6 months	30	40	50	65[1]	80	50
7–12 months	30	40	50	80[1]	80	50
1–3 years	35	50	70	150	160	100
4–6 years	50	75	100	200	200	130
7–10 years	75	110	150	200	300	150
Males						
11–14 years	100	150	200	300	400	180
15–50+ years	100	150	200	400	400	200
Females						
11–14 years	100	150	200	300	400	180
15–50+ years	100	150	200	400	400	200
Pregnancy			+100	600	600	400
Lactation			+60	500	500	350

[1]AI.
[2]Assuming bioavailability half that of pure folic acid and 20% coefficient of variation.

Table A14 Dietary reference values for vitamin B$_{12}$ (µg/day)

Age	UK LRNI	EAR	RNI	USA/AI	FAO/WHO	European PRI
0–6 months	0.1	0.25	0.3	0.4[1]	0.4	
7–12 months	0.25	0.35	0.4	0.5[1]	0.5	0.5
1–3 years	0.3	0.4	0.5	0.9	0.9	0.7
4–6 years	0.5	0.7	0.8	1.2	1.2	0.9
7–10 years	0.6	0.8	1.0	1.2	1.8	1.0
Males						
11–14 years	0.8	1.0	1.2	1.8	2.4	1.3
15–50+ years	1.0	1.25	1.5	2.4	2.4	1.4
Females						
11–14 years	0.8	1.0	1.2	1.8	2.4	1.2
15–50+ years	1.0	1.25	1.5	2.4	2.4	1.4
Pregnancy			*	2.6	2.6	1.6
Lactation			+0.5	2.8	2.8	1.9

*No increment.
[1]AI.

Table A15 Dietary reference values for biotin (µg/day)

Age	UK safe intake	USA/AI	European acceptable range
0–6 months		5	
7–12 months		6	
1–3 years		8	
4–10 years		12–20	
Males and females			
11–50+ years	10–20	30	15–100

Table A16 Dietary reference values for pantothenic acid (mg/day)

Age	UK safe intake	USA/AI	European acceptable range
0–6 months	1.7	1.7	
7–12 months	1.7	1.8	
1–3 years	1.7	2	
4–10 years	3–7	3–4	
Males and females			
11–50+ years	3–7	5	3–12

Table A17 Dietary reference values for calcium (mg/day)

Age	UK			USA/AI	FAO/WHO	European PRI
	LRNI	EAR	RNI			
0–6 months	240	400	525	210	300	
6–12 months	240	400	525	270	400	400
1–3 years	200	275	350	500	500	400
4–6 years	275	350	450	800	600	450
7–10 years	325	425	550	800	700	550
Males						
11–14 years	450	750	1000	1300	1300	1000
15–18 years	450	750	1000	1300	1300	1000
19–24 years	400	525	700	1000	1000	700
25–50 years	400	525	700	1000	1000	700
50+ years	400	525	700	1200	1000	700
Females						
11–14 years	480	625	800	1300	1300	800
15–18 years	480	625	800	1300	1300	800
19–24 years	400	525	700	1000	1000	700
25–50 years	400	525	700	1000	1000	700
50+ years	400	525	700	1200	1300	700
Pregnancy	*	*	*	1000	1000	*
Lactation			+550	1000	1000	+500

*No increment.

Table A18 Dietary reference values for phosphorus (mg/day) (No WHO values available)

Age	UK RNI[1]	USA RDA/AI	European PRI
0–6 months	400	100[2]	
7–12 months	400	275[2]	300
1–3 years	270	460	300
4–10 years	350	500	350–450
Males			
11–18 years	775	1250	775
19–24 years	550	700	550
25–50 years	550	700	550
50+ years	550	700	550
Females			
11–18 years	625	1250	625
19–24 years	550	700	550
25–50+ years	550	700	550
Pregnancy	*	700	550
Lactation	+440	700	+400

*No increment.
[1]Phosphorus RNI is set equal to calcium in molar terms.
[2]AI.

Table A19 **Dietary reference values for magnesium (mg/day)**

Age	UK			USA RDA/AI	FAO/WHO	European acceptable range
	LRNI	EAR	RNI			
0–3 months	30	40	55	30[1]	26–36	
4–6 months	40	50	60	30[1]	26–36	
7–9 months	45	60	75	75[1]	53	
10–12 months	45	60	80	75[1]	53	
1–3 years	50	65	85	80	60	
4–6 years	70	90	120	130	73	
7–10 years	115	150	200	130	100	
Males						
11–14 years	180	230	280	240	250	
15–18 years	190	250	280	410	250	
19–50 + years	190	250	300	420	260	150–500
Females						
11–14 years	180	230	280	240	230	
15–18 years	190	250	300	360	230	
19–50 years	190	250	300	320	220	150–500
50 + years	150	200	270	320	220	
Pregnancy	*	*	*	350	270	
Lactation			+550	310	270	

*No increment.
[1]AI.

Table A20 **Dietary reference values for sodium (mg/day[1])**

Age	UK		USA minimum requirement[2]	WHO population average[3]	European acceptable range
	LRNI	RNI			
0–3 months	140	210	120		
4–6 months	140	280	120		
7–9 months	200	320	200		
10–12 months	200	350	200		
1–3 years	200	500	225		
4–6 years	280	700	300		575–3500
7–10 years	350	1200	400		575–3500
Males and females					
11–14 years	460	1600	500		575–3500
15–50+ years	575	1600	500	3900	575–3500
Pregnancy	*	*			*
Lactation	*	*			*

*No increment.
[1]1 mmol sodium = 23 mg.
[2]No allowance for large losses from the skin through sweat.
[3]Upper limit.

Table A21 **Dietary reference values for potassium (mg/day[1]). (No WHO values available)**

Age	UK		USA minimum requirement[2]	European PRI
	LRNI	RNI		
0–3 months	400	800	500	
4–6 months	400	850	500	
7–9 months	400	700	700	800
10–12 months	450	700	700	800
1–3 years	450	800	1000	800
4–6 years	600	1100	1400	1100
7–10 years	950	2200	1600	2000
Males and females				
11–14 years	1600	3100	2000	3100
15–50+ years	2000	3500	2000	3100
Pregnancy	*	*	*	*
Lactation	*	*	*	*

*No increment.
[1]1 mmol potassium = 39 mg.
[2]Desirable intakes may exceed these values (3500 mg for adults).

Table A22 **Dietary reference values for chloride (mg/day). (No WHO values available)**

Age	UK RNI[1]	USA minimum requirement[2]	European acceptable range[1]
0–3 months	320	180	
4–6 months	400	300	
7–9 months	500	300	
10–12 months	500	300	
1–3 years	800	350	
4–6 years	1100	500	
7–10 years	1100	600	
Males and females			
11–50+ years	2500	750	Should match sodium intake
Pregnancy	*	*	*
Lactation	*	*	*

*No increment.
[1]Corresponds to sodium. 1 mmol = 35.5 mg.
[2]No allowance for large losses from the skin through sweat.

Table A23 **Dietary reference values for iron[1] (mg/day)**

Age	UK			USA RDA/AI	FAO/WHO[3]	European[4]
	LRNI	EAR	RNI			
0–3 months	0.9	1.3	1.7	0.27[2]	–	
4–6 months	2.3	3.3	4.3	0.27[2]	–	
7–12 months	4.2	6.0	7.8	11	6	6
1–3 years	3.7	5.3	6.9	7	4	4
4–6 years	3.3	4.7	6.1	10	4	4
7–10 years	4.7	6.7	8.7	10	6	6
Males						
11–14 years	6.1	8.7	11.3	8	10	10
15–18 years	6.1	8.7	11.3	11	12	13
19–50+ years	4.7	6.7	8.7	8	9	9
Females						
11–14 years	8.0	11.4	14.8[5]	8	9	18–22[6]
15–50 years	8.0	11.4	14.8[5]	15	22	17–21[6]
50+ years	4.7	6.7	8.7	8	8	8
Pregnancy	*	*	*	27	10	*
Lactation	*	*	*	9	10	10

*No increment.
[1] 1 μmol iron = 55.9 μg.
[2] AI.
[3] Median basal requirement on intermediate bioavailability diet.
[4] Bioavailability 15%.
[5] Insufficient for women with high menstrual losses who may need iron supplements.
[6] Lower value for 90% of population, upper value for 95% of population.

Table A24 **Dietary reference values for zinc (mg/day)**

Age	UK			USA RDA/AI	FAO/WHO	European PRI
	LRNI	EAR	RNI			
0–3 months	2.6	3.3	4.0	2.0[1]	2.8	
4–6 months	2.6	3.3	4.0	2.0[1]	2.8	
7–12 months	3.0	3.8	5.0	3	4.1	4.0
1–3 years	3.0	3.8	5.0	3	4.1	4.0
4–6 years	4.0	5.0	6.5	5	5.1	6.0
7–10 years	4.0	5.4	7.0	5	5.6	7.0
Males						
11–14 years	5.3	7.0	9.0	8	9.7	9.0
15–18 years	5.5	7.3	9.5	11	9.7	9.0
19–50+ years	5.5	7.3	9.5	11	7.0	9.5
Females						
11–14 years	5.3	7.0	9.0	8	7.8	9.0
15–18 years	4.0	5.5	7.0	9	7.8	7.0
19–50+ years	4.0	5.5	7.0	8	4.9	7.0
Pregnancy	*	*	*	11	5.5–10	*
Lactation						
0–4 months			+6.0	12.0	9.5	+5.0
4+ months			+2.5	12.0	8.8	+5.0

*No increment.
[1] AI.

Table A25 **Dietary reference values for copper[1] (mg/day)**

Age	UK RNI	USA	WHO[3] (1996)	European PRI
0–3 months	0.3	0.2	0.33–0.55[2]	
4–6 months	0.3	0.2	0.37–0.62[2]	
7–12 months	0.3	0.2	0.60	0.3
1–3 years	0.4	0.34	0.56	0.4
4–6 years	0.6	0.44	0.57	0.6
7–10 years	0.7	0.44	0.75	0.7
Males				
11–14 years	0.8	0.7	1.00	0.8
15–18 years	1.0	0.89	1.33	1.0
19–50+ years	1.2	0.90	1.15	1.1
Females				
11–14 years	0.8	0.7	1.00	0.8
15–18 years	1.0	0.89	1.15	1.0
19–50+ years	1.2	0.90	1.15	1.1
Pregnancy		1.0		
Lactation	+0.3	1.3	1.25	+0.3

[1]μmol = 63.5 μg.
[2]Upper levels should not be habitually exceeded because of toxicity.
[3]Normative requirement.

Table A26 **Dietary reference values for selenium[1] (μg/day)**

Age	UK		USA RDA/AI	WHO[2] (1996)	European PRI
	LRNI	RNI			
0–3 months	4	10	15[3]	6	
4–6 months	5	13	15[3]	9	
7–9 months	5	10	20[3]	12	8
10–12 months	6	10	20[3]	12	8
1–3 years	7	15	20	20	10
4–6 years	10	20	30	24	15
7–10 years	16	30	30	25	25
Males					
11–14 years	25	45	40	36	35
15–18 years	40	70	55	40	45
19–50+ years	40	75	55	40	55
Females					
11–14 years	25	45	40	30	35
15–18 years	40	60	55	30	45
19–50+ years	40	60	55	30	55
Pregnancy	*	*	60	35	*
Lactation	+15	+15	70	40	+15

*No increment.
[1]1 μmol selenium = 79 μg.
[2]Normative requirement.
[3]AI.

Table A27 **Dietary reference values for iodine (μg/day)**

Age	UK		USA RDA/AI	WHO (1996)[1]	European PRI
	LRNI	RNI			
0–3 months	40	50	110[2]	50	
4–6 months	40	60	110[2]	50	
7–12 months	40	60	130[2]	50	50
1–3 years	40	70	90	90	70
4–6 years	50	100	90	90	90
7–10 years	55	110	90	120	100
Males and females					
11–14 years	65	130	120	150	120
15–18 years	70	140	150	150	130
19–50+ years	70	140	150	150	130
Pregnancy	*	*	220	200	*
Lactation	*	*	290	200	160

*No increment.
[1]Normative requirement.
[2]AI.

Index

Please note that any page references to non-textual information such as Figures or Tables are in *italic* print and numbers are filed as if spelled out, e.g. 3-MCPD filed under 'three'

W

X

Y

ELSEVIER CD-ROM LICENSE AGREEMENT

PLEASE READ THE FOLLOWING AGREEMENT CAREFULLY BEFORE USING THIS PRODUCT. THIS PRODUCT IS LICENSED UNDER THE TERMS CONTAINED IN THIS LICENCE AGREEMENT ("Agreement"). BY USING THIS PRODUCT, YOU, AN INDIVIDUAL OR ENTITY INCLUDING EMPLOYEES, AGENTS AND REPRESENTATIVES ("You" or "Your"), ACKNOWLEDGE THAT YOU HAVE READ THIS AGREEMENT, THAT YOU UNDERSTAND IT, AND THAT YOU AGREE TO BE BOUND BY THE TERMS AND CONDITIONS OF THIS AGREEMENT. ELSEVIER LIMITED ("Elsevier") EXPRESSLY DOES NOT AGREE TO LICENSE THIS PRODUCT TO YOU UNLESS YOU ASSENT TO THIS AGREEMENT. IF YOU DO NOT AGREE WITH ANY OF THE FOLLOWING TERMS, YOU MAY, WITHIN THIRTY (30) DAYS AFTER YOUR RECEIPT OF THIS PRODUCT RETURN THE UNUSED PRODUCT AND ALL ACCOMPANYING DOCUMENTATION TO ELSEVIER FOR A FULL REFUND.

DEFINITIONS As used in this Agreement, these terms shall have the following meanings:

"Proprietary Material" means the valuable and proprietary information content of this Product including without limitation all indexes and graphic materials and software used to access, index, search and retrieve the information content from this Product developed or licensed by Elsevier and/or its affiliates, suppliers and licensors.

"Product" means the copy of the Proprietary Material and any other material delivered on CD-ROM and any other human readable or machine-readable materials enclosed with this Agreement, including without limitation documentation relating to the same.

OWNERSHIP This Product has been supplied by and is proprietary to Elsevier and/or its affiliates, suppliers and licensors. The copyright in the Product belongs to Elsevier and/or its affiliates, suppliers and licensors and is protected by the copyright, trademark, trade secret and other intellectual property laws of the United Kingdom and international treaty provisions, including without limitation the Universal Copyright Convention and the Berne Copyright Convention. You have no ownership rights in this Product. Except as expressly set forth herein, no part of this Product, including without limitation the Proprietary Material, may be modified, copied or distributed in hardcopy or machine-readable form without prior written consent from Elsevier. All rights not expressly granted to You herein are expressly reserved. Any other use of this Product by any person or entity is strictly prohibited and a violation of this Agreement.

SCOPE OF RIGHTS LICENSED (PERMITTED USES) Elsevier is granting to You a limited, non-exclusive, non-transferable licence to use this Product in accordance with the terms of this Agreement. You may use or provide access to this Product on a single computer or terminal physically located at Your premises and in a secure network or move this Product to and use it on another single computer or terminal at the same location for personal use only, but under no circumstances may You use or provide access to any part or parts of this Product on more than one computer or terminal simultaneously.

You shall not (a) copy, download, or otherwise reproduce the Product or any part(s) thereof in any medium, including, without limitation, online transmissions, local area networks, wide area networks, intranets, extranets and the Internet, or in any way, in whole or in part, except for printing out or downloading nonsubstantial portions of the text and images in the Product for Your own personal use; (b) alter, modify, or adapt the Product or any part(s) thereof, including but not limited to decompiling, disassembling, reverse engineering, or creating derivative works, without the prior written approval of Elsevier; (c) sell, license or otherwise distribute to third parties the Product or any part(s) thereof; or (d) alter, remove, obscure or obstruct the display of any copyright, trademark or other proprietary notice on or in the Product or on any printout or download of portions of the Proprietary Materials.

RESTRICTIONS ON TRANSFER This Licence is personal to You, and neither Your rights hereunder nor the tangible embodiments of this Product, including without limitation the Proprietary Material, may be sold, assigned, transferred or sublicensed to any other person, including without limitation by operation of law, without the prior written consent of Elsevier. Any purported sale, assignment, transfer or sublicense without the prior written consent of Elsevier will be void and will automatically terminate the Licence granted hereunder.

TERM This Agreement will remain in effect until terminated pursuant to the terms of this Agreement. You may terminate this Agreement at any time by removing from Your system and destroying the Product and any copies of the Proprietary Material.

Unauthorized copying of the Product, including without limitation, the Proprietary Material and documentation, or otherwise failing to comply with the terms and conditions of this Agreement shall result in automatic termination of this licence and will make available to Elsevier legal remedies. Upon termination of this Agreement, the licence granted herein will terminate and You must immediately destroy the Product and all copies of the Product and of the Proprietary Material, together with any and all accompanying documentation. All provisions relating to proprietary rights shall survive termination of this Agreement.

LIMITED WARRANTY AND LIMITATION OF LIABILITY Elsevier warrants that the software embodied in this Product will perform in substantial compliance with the documentation supplied in this Product, unless the performance problems are the result of hardware failure or improper use. If You report a significant defect in performance in writing to Elsevier within ninety (90) calendar days of your having purchased the Product, and Elsevier is not able to correct same within sixty (60) days after its receipt of Your notification, You may return this Product, including all copies and documentation, to Elsevier and Elsevier will refund Your money. In order to apply for a refund on your purchased Product, please contact the return address on the invoice to obtain the refund request form ("Refund Request Form"), and either fax or mail your signed request and your proof of purchase to the address indicated on the Refund Request Form. Incomplete forms will not be processed. Defined terms in the Refund Request Form shall have the same meaning as in this Agreement.

YOU UNDERSTAND THAT, EXCEPT FOR THE LIMITED WARRANTY RECITED ABOVE, ELSEVIER, ITS AFFILIATES, LICENSORS, THIRD PARTY SUPPLIERS AND AGENTS (TOGETHER "THE SUPPLIERS") MAKE NO REPRESENTATIONS OR WARRANTIES, WITH RESPECT TO THE PRODUCT, INCLUDING, WITHOUT LIMITATION THE PROPRIETARY MATERIAL. ALL OTHER REPRESENTATIONS, WARRANTIES, CONDITIONS OR OTHER TERMS, WHETHER EXPRESS OR IMPLIED BY STATUTE OR COMMON LAW, ARE HEREBY EXCLUDED TO THE FULLEST EXTENT PERMITTED BY LAW.

IN PARTICULAR BUT WITHOUT LIMITATION TO THE FOREGOING NONE OF THE SUPPLIERS MAKE ANY REPRESENTATIONS OR WARRANTIES (WHETHER EXPRESS OR IMPLIED) REGARDING THE PERFORMANCE OF YOUR PAD, NETWORK OR COMPUTER SYSTEM WHEN USED IN CONJUNCTION WITH THE PRODUCT, NOR THAT THE PRODUCT WILL MEET YOUR REQUIREMENTS OR THAT ITS OPERATION WILL BE UNINTERRUPTED OR ERROR-FREE.

EXCEPT IN RESPECT OF DEATH OR PERSONAL INJURY CAUSED BY THE SUPPLIERS' NEGLIGENCE AND TO THE FULLEST EXTENT PERMITTED BY LAW, IN NO EVENT (AND REGARDLESS OF WHETHER SUCH DAMAGES ARE FORESEEABLE AND OF WHETHER SUCH LIABILITY IS BASED IN TORT, CONTRACT OR OTHERWISE) WILL ANY OF THE SUPPLIERS BE LIABLE TO YOU FOR ANY DAMAGES (INCLUDING, WITHOUT LIMITATION, ANY LOST PROFITS, LOST SAVINGS OR OTHER SPECIAL, INDIRECT, INCIDENTAL OR CONSEQUENTIAL DAMAGES ARISING OUT OF OR RESULTING FROM: (I) YOUR USE OF, OR INABILITY TO USE, THE PRODUCT; (II) DATA LOSS OR CORRUPTION; AND/OR (III) ERRORS OR OMISSIONS IN THE PROPRIETARY MATERIAL.

IF THE FOREGOING LIMITATION IS HELD TO BE UNENFORCEABLE, OUR MAXIMUM LIABILITY TO YOU IN RESPECT THEREOF SHALL NOT EXCEED THE AMOUNT OF THE LICENCE FEE PAID BY YOU FOR THE PRODUCT. THE REMEDIES AVAILABLE TO YOU AGAINST ELSEVIER AND THE LICENSORS OF MATERIALS INCLUDED IN THE PRODUCT ARE EXCLUSIVE.

If the information provided In the Product contains medical or health sciences information, it is intended for professional use within the medical field. Information about medical treatment or drug dosages is intended strictly for professional use, and because of rapid advances in the medical sciences, independent verification of diagnosis and drug dosages should be made. The provisions of this Agreement shall be severable, and in the event that any provision of this Agreement is found to be legally unenforceable, such unenforceability shall not prevent the enforcement or any other provision of this Agreement.

GOVERNING LAW This Agreement shall be governed by the laws of England and Wales. In any dispute arising out of this Agreement, you and Elsevier each consent to the exclusive personal jurisdiction and venue in the courts of England and Wales.

Minimum system requirements

Windows®
Windows 98 or higher
Pentium® processor-based PC
16 MB RAM (32 MB recommended)

Macintosh®
Apple Power Macintosh
Mac OS version 9 or later
64 MB of available RAM

Using this product
This product is designed to run with Internet Explorer 5.0 or later and Netscape 4.7 or later (PC) and IE 5.1.5 or later and Netscape 4.7 or later (Mac). Please refer to the help files on those programs for problems specific to the browser.

Technical support

Technical support for this product is available between 7.30 a.m. and 7.00 p.m. CST,
8.00 a.m. and 1.00 a.m. UK, Monday through Friday.

Before calling, be sure that your computer meets the minimum system requirements to run this software.

Inside the United States and Canada, call 1-800-692-9010.
Inside the United Kingdom, call 0-0800-6929-0100.
Outside North America, call +1-314-872-8370.
You may also fax your questions to +1-314-997-5080,
or contact Technical Support through e-mail: technical.support@elsevier.com.